2011
YEAR BOOK OF
MEDICINE®

The 2011 Year Book Series

Year Book of Anesthesiology and Pain Management™: Drs Chestnut, Abram, Black, Gravlee, Lien, Mathru, and Roizen

Year Book of Cardiology®: Drs Gersh, Cheitlin, Elliott, Gold, Graham, and Thourani

Year Book of Critical Care Medicine®: Drs Dellinger, Parrillo, Balk, Dorman, Dries, and Zanotti-Cavazzoni

Year Book of Dermatology and Dermatologic Surgery™: Dr Del Rosso

Year Book of Diagnostic Radiology®: Drs Osborn, Abbara, Elster, Manaster, Oestreich, Offiah, Rosado de Christenson, Stephens, and Walker

Year Book of Emergency Medicine®: Drs Hamilton, Bruno, Handly, Mullin, Quintana, and Ramoska

Year Book of Endocrinology®: Drs Schott, Apovian, Clarke, Eugster, Ludlam, Meikle, Schinner, Schteingart, and Toth

Year Book of Gastroenterology™: Drs Talley, DeVault, Harnois, Murray, Pearson, Philcox, Picco, and Smith

Year Book of Hand and Upper Limb Surgery®: Drs Yao and Steinmann

Year Book of Medicine®: Drs Barker, Garrick, Gersh, Khardori, LeRoith, Panush, Talley, and Thigpen

Year Book of Neonatal and Perinatal Medicine®: Drs Fanaroff, Benitz, Donn, Neu, Papile, Polin, and Van Marter

Year Book of Neurology and Neurosurgery®: Drs Klimo and Rabinstein

Year Book of Obstetrics, Gynecology, and Women's Health®: Drs Dungan and Shulman

Year Book of Oncology®: Drs Arceci, Bauer, Chiorean, Gordon, Lawton, Murphy, Thigpen, and Tsao

Year Book of Ophthalmology®: Drs Rapuano, Cohen, Flanders, Fudemberg, Hammersmith, Milman, Myers, Nagra, Nelson, Penne, Pyfer, Sergott, Shields, Talekar, and Vander

Year Book of Orthopedics®: Drs Morrey, Beauchamp, Huddleston, Swiontkowski, and Trigg

Year Book of Otolaryngology-Head and Neck Surgery®: Drs Sindwani, Balough, Franco, Gapany, and Mitchell

Year Book of Pathology and Laboratory Medicine®: Drs Raab, Parwani, Bejarano, and Bissell

Year Book of Pediatrics®: Dr Stockman

Year Book of Plastic and Aesthetic Surgery™: Drs Miller, Gosain, Gurtner, Gutowski, Ruberg, Salisbury, and Smith

Year Book of Psychiatry and Applied Mental Health®: Drs Talbott, Ballenger, Buckley, Frances, Krupnick, and Mack

Year Book of Pulmonary Disease®: Drs Barker, Jones, Maurer, Raza, Tanoue, and Willsie

Year Book of Sports Medicine®: Drs Shephard, Cantu, Feldman, Jankowski, Khan, Lebrun, Nieman, Pierrynowski, and Rowland

Year Book of Surgery®: Drs Copeland, Behrns, Daly, Eberlein, Fahey, Huber, Klodell, Mozingo, and Pruett

Year Book of Urology®: Drs Andriole and Coplen

Year Book of Vascular Surgery®: Drs Moneta, Gillespie, Starnes, and Watkins

2011

The Year Book of MEDICINE®

Editors

James A. Barker
Renee Garrick
Bernard J. Gersh
Nancy M. Khardori
Derek LeRoith
Richard S. Panush
Nicholas J. Talley
James Tate Thigpen

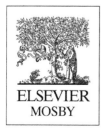

ELSEVIER
MOSBY

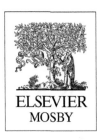

ELSEVIER
MOSBY

Vice President, Continuity: Kimberly Murphy
Developmental Editor: Rachel A. Glover
Production Supervisor, Electronic Year Books: Donna M. Skelton
Electronic Article Manager: Emily Ogle
Illustrations and Permissions Coordinator: Dawn Vohsen

2011 EDITION
Copyright 2011, Mosby, Inc. All rights reserved.

Composition by TNQ Books and Journals Pvt Ltd, India

Editorial Office:
Elsevier
Suite 1800
1600 John F. Kennedy Blvd
Philadelphia, PA 19103-2899

International Standard Serial Number: 0084-3873
International Standard Book Number: 978-0-323-08416-1

Printed and bound by CPI Group (UK) Ltd, Croydon, CR0 4YY
Transferred to Digital Print 2011

Editorial Board

Editors

James A. Barker, MD
Chief, Pulmonary, Critical Care Medicine, and Sleep Internal Medicine, Scott & White Health System; Professor of Medicine, Texas A&M Health Science Center, Temple, Texas

Renee Garrick, MD
Professor of Clinical Medicine and Vice Dean, New York Medical College; Nephrology Section Chief, Westchester Medical Center, Valhalla, New York

Bernard J. Gersh, MB, ChB, DPhil, FRCP
Professor of Medicine, Mayo Clinic College of Medicine; Consultant, Division of Cardiovascular Diseases, Mayo Clinic, Rochester, Minnesota

Nancy M. Khardori, MD, PhD
Professor of Internal Medicine, Division of Infectious Diseases; Professor of Microbiology and Molecular Cell Biology, Eastern Virginia Medical School, Norfolk, Virginia

Derek LeRoith, MD, PhD
Chief, Division of Endocrinology, Metabolism, and Bone Diseases, Department of Medicine, Mount Sinai School of Medicine, New York, New York

Richard S. Panush, MD
Professor of Medicine, Division of Rheumatology, Department of Medicine, Keck School of Medicine, University of Southern California, Los Angeles, California

Nicholas J. Talley, MD, PhD
Pro Vice-Chancellor, Dean of Health, and Professor of Medicine, University of Newcastle, Callaghan, New South Wales, Australia; Adjunct Professor, Mayo Clinic, Jacksonville, Florida; Adjunct Professor, University of North Carolina, Chapel Hill, North Carolina

James Tate Thigpen, MD
Professor of Medicine and Director, Division of Oncology, University of Mississippi Medical Center, Jackson, Mississippi

Contributors

Infectious Disease

Vidya Sundareshan, MD
Assistant Professor, Division of Infectious Diseases, Department of Internal Medicine, Southern Illinois University School of Medicine, Springfield, Illinois

Hematology and Oncology

E. Gabriela Chiorean, MD
Assistant Professor of Medicine, Medical Director, Gastrointestinal Oncology Program, Indiana University Melvin and Bren Simon Cancer Center, Indianapolis, Indiana

Table of Contents

Journals Represented

Journals represented in this YEAR BOOK are listed below.

Academic Emergency Medicine
AJR American Journal of Roentgenology
Alimentary Pharmacology & Therapeutics
American Heart Journal
American Journal of Cardiology
American Journal of Clinical Nutrition
American Journal of Emergency Medicine
American Journal of Gastroenterology
American Journal of Infection Control
American Journal of Kidney Diseases
American Journal of Medicine
American Journal of Respiratory and Critical Care Medicine
Anaesthesia and Intensive Care
Anesthesiology
Annals of Allergy, Asthma & Immunology
Annals of Internal Medicine
Annals of Surgery
Annals of the Rheumatic Diseases
Annals of Thoracic Surgery
Archives of Internal Medicine
Archives of Neurology
Arthritis Care & Research (Hoboken)
Arthritis Research & Therapy
Arthritis & Rheumatism
British Journal of Cancer
British Medical Journal
Canadian Medical Association Journal
Cancer
Chest
Circulation
Circulation Cardiovascular Quality and Outcomes
Clinical Gastroenterology and Hepatology
Clinical Infectious Diseases
Critical Care Medicine
Diabetes Care
Digestive Diseases and Sciences
European Heart Journal
European Respiratory Journal
Eye
Gastroenterology
Gut
Gynecologic Oncology
Heart
Heart Rhythm
Hepatology
Hypertension
International Journal of Colorectal Disease

International Journal of Gynaecology & Obstetrics
International Journal of Obesity
International Journal of Radiation Oncology Biology Physics
Journal of Allergy and Clinical Immunology
Journal of Bone Mineral Research
Journal of Clinical Endocrinology & Metabolism
Journal of Clinical Microbiology
Journal of Clinical Neuroscience
Journal of Clinical Oncology
Journal of Clinical Psychopharmacology
Journal of Experimental Medicine
Journal of Heart and Lung Transplantation
Journal of Hepatology
Journal of Hypertension
Journal of Immunology
Journal of Infectious Diseases
Journal of Neurosurgery
Journal of Pediatric Gastroenterology & Nutrition
Journal of Rheumatology
Journal of Surgical Research
Journal of the American Board of Family Medicine
Journal of the American College of Cardiology
Journal of the American College of Cardiology Interventions
Journal of the American Medical Association
Journal of the American Society of Nephrology
Journal of the National Cancer Institute
Journal of Thoracic and Cardiovascular Surgery
Journal of Trauma
Kidney International
Lancet
Mayo Clinic Proceedings
Medicine
Medicine (Baltimore)
Medicine and Science in Sports and Exercise
Nature Medicine
Neurology
New England Journal of Medicine
Obstetrics & Gynecology
Pediatric Infectious Disease Journal
Proceedings of the American Thoracic Society
Proceedings of the National Academy of Sciences of the United States of America
Rheumatology
Science
Sleep
Thorax
Thyroid
Transplantation
World Journal of Surgery

STANDARD ABBREVIATIONS

The following terms are abbreviated in this edition: acquired immunodeficiency syndrome (AIDS), cardiopulmonary resuscitation (CPR), central nervous system (CNS), cerebrospinal fluid (CSF), computed tomography (CT), deoxyribonucleic acid (DNA), electrocardiography (ECG), health maintenance organization (HMO), human immunodeficiency virus (HIV), intensive care unit (ICU), intramuscular (IM), intravenous (IV), magnetic resonance (MR) imaging (MRI), ribonucleic acid (RNA), and ultrasound (US).

NOTE

The YEAR BOOK OF MEDICINE is a literature survey service providing abstracts of articles published in the professional literature. Every effort is made to assure the accuracy of the information presented in these pages. Neither the editors nor the publisher of the YEAR BOOK OF MEDICINE can be responsible for errors in the original materials. The editors' comments are their own opinions. Mention of specific products within this publication does not constitute endorsement.

To facilitate the use of the YEAR BOOK OF MEDICINE as a reference tool, all illustrations and tables included in this publication are now identified as they appear in the original article. This change is meant to help the reader recognize that any illustration or table appearing in the YEAR BOOK OF MEDICINE may be only one of many in the original article. For this reason, figure and table numbers will often appear to be out of sequence within the YEAR BOOK OF MEDICINE.

PART ONE

RHEUMATOLOGY

RICHARD S. PANUSH, MD

Introduction

I am delighted to contribute the Rheumatology section* to this YEAR BOOK OF MEDICINE. It was a great pleasure and wonderful learning experience to serve as associate editor of the YEAR BOOK OF RHEUMATOLOGY since its inception and then as editor for 10 years. Most of the written literature never gets cited. Most, or certainly much, of the literature will not be important to the clinician or internist. Therefore, I try to select genuinely important or interesting articles for comment. These are articles that should change the way we think about, understand, or practice medicine. Or we may reflect on something that's just plain fun. During the past year, the key theme in my subspecialty is to recognize disease early, treat early and quickly, and treat aggressively. This offers the best opportunities to prevent progression of chronic inflammatory arthropathies, reduce disability, and indeed induce remission. This approach, along with the availability of potentially remittive therapies, has helped transform rheumatology from a specialty merely managing chronic disease to one in which we expect disease remissions.

Richard S. Panush, MD

---

*Portions of the commentaries in the Rheumatology section are adapted from *The Rheumatologist.*

1 Rheumatoid Arthritis

Different stages of rheumatoid arthritis: features of the synovium in the preclinical phase
van de Sande MG, de Hair MJ, van der Leij C, et al (Academic Med Ctr — Univ of Amsterdam, The Netherlands)
Ann Rheum Dis 70:772-777, 2011

Background.—The aetiology of rheumatoid arthritis (RA), a prototype immune-mediated inflammatory disorder, is poorly understood. It is currently unknown whether the disease process starts in the synovium, the primary target of RA, or at other sites in the body.

Objective.—To examine, in a prospective study, the presence of synovitis in people with an increased risk of developing RA.

Methods.—Thirteen people without evidence of arthritis, who were positive for IgM rheumatoid factor and/or anticitrullinated protein antibodies, were included in the study. To evaluate synovial inflammatory changes, all participants underwent dynamic contrast-enhanced MRI and arthroscopic synovial biopsy sampling of a knee joint at inclusion. Results were compared with knee MRI data and synovial biopsy data of 6 and 10 healthy controls, respectively.

Results.—MRI findings evaluated by measurement of maximal enhancement, rate of enhancement, synovial volume and enhancement shape curve distribution were similar between the autoantibody-positive subjects and the healthy controls. Consistent with these findings, all but one autoantibody-positive subject showed very low scores for phenotypic markers, adhesion molecules and vascularity, all in the same range as those in normal controls. The one person with higher scores had patellofemoral joint space narrowing.

Conclusion.—Subclinical inflammation of the synovium does not coincide with the appearance of serum autoantibodies during the pre-RA stage. Thus, systemic autoimmunity precedes the development of synovitis, suggesting that a 'second hit' is involved. This study supports the rationale for exploring preventive strategies aimed at interfering with the humoral immune response before synovial inflammation develops.

▶ When does the music stop? When does immunologic homeostasis' harmony, if you will, stop and disease begin? We now know that autoantibodies occur in individuals before development of (rheumatic) disease. When does disease, such as rheumatoid arthritis (RA), begin? And where? Why? When does the music become dissonant, why, and how can we fix it? I came across this study, which attempts to address this but left me somewhat unsatisfied. Fifty-five rheumatoid factor—positive or anticitrullinated protein antibody—positive otherwise-normal individuals underwent physical and dynamic contrast-enhanced-MRI examinations and arthroscopic synovial biopsy. All those studied had normal physical and MRI examination results (comparable with normal individuals who also underwent imaging and synovial biopsy). The one patient with some detectable cell/mediator abnormalities on biopsy had patellofemoral osteoarthritis. During 37 months of follow-up, 4 individuals developed clinical RA; their baseline findings could not be differentiated from others. While this was ambitious, I was disappointed that the results were not more helpful. No genetic information was provided. We know that more than just genetic predisposition is needed to express our diseases. So too it may be for just having autoantibodies. We really need to know what triggers disease and the transitions through the various stages of disease expression and evolution, how, when, under what circumstances, and where. Only when we have such information will we be able to try to truly prevent rheumatic disease. We'll doubtless see more and better studies elucidating this.

R. S. Panush, MD

Synovial fibroblasts spread rheumatoid arthritis to unaffected joints
Lefèvre S, Knedla A, Tennie C, et al (Justus-Liebig-Univ Giessen, Bad Nauheim, Germany)
Nat Med 15:1414-1420, 2009

Active rheumatoid arthritis originates from few joints but subsequently affects the majority of joints. Thus far, the pathways of the progression of the disease are largely unknown. As rheumatoid arthritis synovial fibroblasts (RASFs) which can be found in RA synovium are key players in joint destruction and are able to migrate in vitro, we evaluated the potential of RASFs to spread the disease in vivo. To simulate the primary joint of origin, we implanted healthy human cartilage together with RASFs subcutaneously into severe combined immunodeficient (SCID) mice. At the contralateral flank, we implanted healthy cartilage without cells. RASFs showed an active movement to the naive cartilage via the vasculature independent of the site of application of RASFs into the SCID mouse, leading to a marked destruction of the target cartilage. These findings support the hypothesis that the characteristic clinical phenomenon of destructive arthritis spreading between joints is mediated, at least in part, by the transmigration of activated RASFs.

▶ This elegant series of experiments attempted to address the question of how rheumatoid arthritis (RA) disseminates from a few to many joints. I must confess that I've usually encountered and perceived RA as a polyarthritis and presumed it was multicentric. I have certainly seen monoarticular or oligoarticular disease evolve to polyarthritis. So I accept that the problem is relevant and certainly of interest, while not necessarily the sole explanation for the propagation of RA. I congratulate the authors on their thinking, approach, experimental design, and controls. They implanted human tissues into immunodeficient (severe combined immunodeficiency disease) mice to show that RA synovial fibroblasts migrated to naive cartilage. These observations suggested that transmigration of these cells, at least in part, participates actively in the disease process. This is another obvious target for intervention. Expect to hear more about this.

R. S. Panush, MD

Disease activity score-driven therapy versus routine care in patients with recent-onset active rheumatoid arthritis: data from the GUEPARD trial and ESPOIR cohort

Soubrier M, Lukas C, Sibilia J, et al (Hôpital G Montpied, Clermont-Ferrand, France)
Ann Rheum Dis 70:611-615, 2011

Objectives.—To compare the efficacy of disease activity score in 28 joints (DAS28ESR)-driven therapy with anti-tumour necrosis factor (patients from the GUEPARD trial) and routine care in patients with recent-onset rheumatoid arthritis (patients of the ESPOIR cohort).

Results.—After matching GUEPARD and ESPOIR patients on the basis of a propensity score and a 1:2 ratio, at baseline all patients had comparable demographic characteristics, rheumatoid factor, anticyclic citrullinated peptide antibody positivity and clinical disease activity parameters: erythrocyte sedimentation rate, C-reactive protein, mean DAS (6.26 ± 0.87), Sharp/van der Heijde radiographic score (SHS), health assessment questionnaire (HAQ). Disease duration was longer in GUEPARD patients (5.6 ± 4.6 vs 3.5 ± 2.0 months, p<0.001). After 1 year, the percentage of patients in remission with an HAQ (<0.5) and an absence of radiological progression was higher in the tight control group (32.3% vs 10.2%, p=0.011) as well as the percentage of patients in low DAS with an HAQ (<0.5) and an absence of radiological progression (36.1% vs 18.9%, p=0.045). However, there was no difference in the decrease in DAS, nor in the percentage of EULAR (good and moderate), ACR20, ACR50 and ACR70 responses. More patients in the tight control group had an HAQ below 0.5 (70.2% vs 45.2%, p= 0.005). Overall, pain, patient and physician assessment and fatigue decreased more in the tight control group. The mean SHS progression was similar in the two groups as was the percentage of patients without progression.

Conclusions.—In patients with recent onset active rheumatoid arthritis, a tight control of disease activity allows more patients to achieve remission without disability and radiographic progression.

▶ "While we deliberate about beginning it is all ready too late to begin" (Quintilian, 35-96 BCE).

Early identification and treatment of rheumatoid arthritis (RA), with tight control, currently provide us our best opportunities to optimize outcomes for patients.[1-3] At present, we seek drug-induced suppression of symptoms for prevention of inflammatory damage and consequent disability. We hope for an occasional drug-free remission. We're disappointed, frustrated, and saddened when treatments fail and patients suffer, rather than benefit, from therapy, as is sometimes still inevitable. We struggle, not always successfully, to provide expensive state-of-the-art medications to all whom we think should receive them.

Early recognition and intervention for RA will be one of the epochal triumphs of this age of rheumatology. This is truly transformative in how we think about caring for patients. There is now urgency in finding patients with RA and getting them to rheumatologists or otherwise comparable therapeutic programs. We now have new classification criteria that facilitate early diagnosis (classification) of RA.[4] Too we have new tools available to quantifiably and reproducibly document outcomes of our care.[5] And finally we have a strict definition of remission.[6] These reflect the new paradigm of how we perceive RA and its optimal management. These changes are percolating into daily practice.

Why can't we implement this universally now? What yet must we know? Or do? The problems are procedural and perhaps also philosophical or even existential. When does disease begin? When exactly is the benefit of early aggressive treatment lost? What shall we do with individuals seropositive for rheumatoid factor or cyclic citrullinated peptides? With other phenotypic or genotypic markers or determinants? Is RA an oversimplification or group of heterogeneous syndromes? Are there multiple RAs? And, when we decide it's time to intervene, what is best? For how long? What will be the most effective yet safest regimen? What will we do when we have a vaccine? Or a genuinely curative therapy for established disease? Is RA (still) evolving, changing, before us independent of our interventions, as others have thought and predicted some years ago?[7,8]

There are potentially rather daunting procedural, logistical, practical, and societal problems too. How does a society or community screen a population to find these patients? Absent screening, how does referral information get effectively to primary care providers who would otherwise see these patients serendipitously? How do we assure adequate rheumatologists to promptly accommodate referrals? If we rheumatologists can't do this, are there others who could or could be trained? How do we ensure universal access to care? To costly contemporary therapies?

A colleague's preliminary experiences, establishing an early RA clinic for an underserved, indigent, and often transient population, emphasize the challenges in making the benefits of early appropriate care available to this patient population. Patients with RA, of varying duration, often wait as long as 12 months before their first rheumatologic evaluation, usually taking only nonsteroidal anti-inflammatory drugs. Once seen by our team, aggressive disease-modifying therapy is instituted (within budgetary and formulary limits of our county medical center) attempting to control disease as tightly as possible. We have not yet calculated the health cost(s) to patients stemming from our inability to initiate care for them sooner but presume it is not insignificant. Would such a situation be tolerated for patients with heart disease? Strokes? We suspect not. We must better educate those with leadership responsibilities to the moral, social, ethical, and economic imperative of providing no less to these patients.

Thus we near a threshold. We are able to control symptoms of RA and (probably) prevent long-term disability if only we can find patients with RA at onset of disease, start them on a therapeutic regimen, and reliably measure outcomes. Limitations to this are neither our current art nor science but rather our communal resources and will. It should be possible to do, or certainly do better. We owe it to our patients.[9]

"There are two mistakes one can make along the road to truth... not going all the way and not starting" (Gautama Siddhartha, 563-483 BCE).

R. S. Panush, MD

References

1. Verstappen SM, McCoy MJ, Roberts C, Dale NE, Hassell AB, Symmons DP, STIVEA Investigators. Beneficial effects of a 3-week course of intramuscular glucocorticoid injections in patients with very early inflammatory polyarthritis: results of the STIVEA trial. *Ann Rheum Dis.* 2010;69:503-509.
2. Smolen JS, Aletaha D, Bijlsma JW, et al. Treating rheumatoid arthritis to target: recommendations of an international task force. *Ann Rheum Dis.* 2010;69: 631-637.
3. Scirè CA, Verstappen SM, Mirjafari H, et al. Reduction of long-term disability in inflammatory polyarthritis by early and persistent suppression of joint inflammation: results from the Norfolk Arthritis Register. *Arthritis Care Res (Hoboken).* 2011;63:945-952.
4. Aletaha D, Neogi T, Silman AJ, et al. 2010 rheumatoid arthritis classification criteria: an American College of Rheumatology/European League Against Rheumatism collaborative initiative. *Arthritis Rheum.* 2010;62:2569-2581.
5. Aletaha D, Landewe R, Karonitsch T, et al. Reporting disease activity in clinical trials of patients with rheumatoid arthritis: EULAR/ACR collaborative recommendations. *Arthritis Rheum.* 2008;59:1371-1377.
6. Felson DT, Smolen JS, Wells G, et al. American College of Rheumatology/European League Against Rheumatism provisional definition of remission in rheumatoid arthritis for clinical trials. *Arthritis Rheum.* 2011;63:573-586.
7. Short CL. The antiquity of rheumatoid arthritis. *Arthritis Rheum.* 1974;17:193-205.
8. Buchanan WW, Murdoch RM. Hypothesis: that rheumatoid arthritis will disappear. *J Rheumatol.* 1979;6:324-329.
9. Ortiz EC, Torralba KD, O'Dell JR, Panush RS. Later comes earlier, nowadays [editorial]. *J Rheumatol.* 2011;38:2287-2289.

The growth factor progranulin binds to TNF receptors and is therapeutic against inflammatory arthritis in mice
Tang W, Lu Y, Tian QY, et al (New York Univ School of Medicine and NYU Hosp for Joint Diseases)
Science 332:478-484, 2011

The growth factor progranulin (PGRN) has been implicated in embryonic development, tissue repair, tumorigenesis, and inflammation, but its receptors remain unidentified. We report that PGRN bound directly to tumor necrosis factor receptors (TNFRs) and disturbed the TNFα-TNFR interaction. PGRN-deficient mice were susceptible to collagen-induced arthritis, and administration of PGRN reversed inflammatory arthritis. Atsttrin, an engineered protein composed of three PGRN fragments, exhibited selective TNFR binding. PGRN and Atsttrin prevented inflammation in multiple arthritis mouse models and inhibited TNFα-activated intracellular signaling. Collectively, these findings demonstrate that PGRN is a ligand of TNFR, an antagonist of TNFα signaling, and plays a critical role in the pathogenesis of inflammatory arthritis in mice. They also suggest new potential thera-peutic interventions for various TNFα-mediated pathologies and conditions, including rheumatoid arthritis.

▶ Progranulin (PGRN), an autocrine growth factor with cytokine-like proper-ties, binds to tumor necrosis factor (TNF) receptors and moderates the action of TNFα in experimental arthritis. It thus has promising therapeutic potential. May it be. This elegant study, as well as that by Wu and Siegel,[1] found that PGRN bound directly to TNFα receptors and antagonized TNFα actions, that PGRN-deficient mice had more severe collagen-induced arthritis than controls, that recombinant PGRN reversed disease, and that a protein containing 3 PGRN fragments, Atsttrin, was antiarthritic in mouse models and blocked TNFα-related intracellular signaling. The authors' cautious final statement was "the identification of PGRN and the PGRN-derived protein, ATSTTRIN, as antagonists of TNFR may lead to innovative therapeutics for various pathologies and conditions, such as rheumatoid arthritis." That would be nice indeed.

R. S. Panush, MD

Reference

1. Wu H, Siegel RM. Medicine. Progranulin resolves inflammation. *Science.* 2011; 332:427-428.

2 Osteoarthritis

Pomegranate extract inhibits the interleukin-1β-induced activation of MKK-3, p38α-MAPK and transcription factor RUNX-2 in human osteoarthritis chondrocytes
Rasheed Z, Akhtar N, Haqqi TM (MetroHealth Med Ctr/Case Western Reserve Univ, Cleveland, OH)
Arthritis Res Ther 12:R195, 2010

Introduction.—Pomegranate has been revered throughout history for its medicinal properties. p38-MAPK is a major signal-transducing pathway in osteoarthritis (OA) and its activation by interleukin-1β (IL-1β) plays a critical role in the expression and production of several mediators of cartilage catabolism in OA. In this study we determined the effect of a standardized pomegranate extract (PE) on the IL-1β-induced activation of MKK3/6, p38-MAPK isoforms and the activation of transcription factor RUNX-2 in primary human OA chondrocytes.

Methods.—Human chondrocytes were derived from OA cartilage by enzymatic digestion, treated with PE and then stimulated with IL-1β. Gene expression of p38-MAPK isoforms was measured by RT-PCR. Western immunoblotting was used to analyze the activation of MAPKs. Immunoprecipitation was used to determine the activation of p38-MAPK isoforms. DNA binding activity of RUNX-2 was determined using a highly sensitive and specific ELISA. Pharmacological studies to elucidate the involved pathways were executed using transfection with siRNAs.

Results.—Human OA chondrocytes expressed p38-MAPK isoforms p38α, -γ and -δ, but not p38β. IL-1β enhances the phosphorylation of the p38α-MAPK and p38γ-MAPK isoforms but not of p38δ-MAPK isoform in human OA chondrocytes. Activation of p38-MAPK in human OA chondrocytes was preferentially mediated via activation of MKK3. In addition, we also demonstrate that polyphenol rich PE inhibited the IL-1β-induced activation of MKK3, p38α-MAPK isoform and DNA binding activity of the transcription factor RUNX-2.

Conclusions.—Our results provide an important insight into the molecular basis of the reported cartilage protective and arthritis inhibitory effects of pomegranate extract. These novel pharmacological actions of PE on IL-1β stimulated human OA chondrocytes impart a new suggestion that PE or

PE-derived compounds may be developed as MKK and p38-MAPK inhibitors for the treatment of OA and other degenerative/inflammatory diseases.

▶ I came across this interesting report about potentially important biological effects of pomegranate extract. See also the study by Khalifé and Zafarullah.[1] The authors appreciated a long history attributing medicinal properties to pomegranate and noted its documented antioxidant effect. They therefore examined effects of pomegranate extract on pathways of cartilage catabolism and studied it in an animal model of osteoarthritis. They found that pomegranate extract affected intracellular signaling pathways that link receptor signals and nuclear gene transcription. Mitogen-activated protein kinases and transcription factors (RUNX-2) regulate several processes (apoptosis, nitric oxide synthase) and mediators (cytokines, monocytes/macrophages, neutrophils, T cells, matrix metalloproteinases) important in inflammation and cartilage damage. In animal models of arthritis, inhibition of the protein kinases was therapeutic. Thus these pathways are of considerable interest as potential targets for intervention in human disease. Should we be surprised that a food product has these biological effects?[2] From whence came aspirin? Colchicine? (Willow bark and meadow saffron, respectively, if you've forgotten.) Other potent agents in our armamentarium? It was probably more serendipity than science that brought gold, antimalarials, and sulfasalazine into our practice. There are other food products with potentially relevant biological effects: resveratrol, chocolate, teas, curcumin, perhaps ginger, and others. And let's not forget the occasional patient with food sensitivity.[3] We do not care about the source of an idea—only its experimental validity. There are no complementary and alternative medicines—only evidence-based medicine. We have seen and will see more therapies derived from food or food products. And it should not surprise us.

R. S. Panush, MD

References

1. Khalifé S, Zafarullah M. Molecular targets of natural health products in arthritis. *Arthritis Res Ther.* 2011;13:102.
2. Panush RS. Shift happens: complementary and alternative medicine for rheumatologists. *J Rheumatol.* 2002;29:656-658.
3. Panush RS, Stroud RM, Webster EM. Food-induced (allergic) arthritis. Inflammatory arthritis exacerbated by milk. *Arthritis Rheum.* 1986;29:220-226.

The effects of doxycycline on reducing symptoms in knee osteoarthritis: results from a triple-blinded randomised controlled trial

Snijders GF, NOAC study group (Sint Maartenskliniek, Nijmegen, The Netherlands)

Ann Rheum Dis 70:1191-1196, 2011

Objectives.—Evidence suggests that doxycycline might have disease-modifying properties in osteoarthritis. However, the clinically relevant question as to whether doxycycline also modifies symptoms in knee osteoarthritis is unanswered. The objective of this study was to investigate the effectiveness of doxycycline on pain and daily functioning in symptomatic knee osteoarthritis.

Methods.—A 24-week, randomised, triple-blind, placebo controlled trial on the symptomatic effectiveness of doxycycline twice a day 100 mg in knee osteoarthritis patients according to the clinical and radiological American College of Rheumatology classification criteria. The primary endpoint was the difference in the proportion of participants in both study groups achieving a clinical response defined by the OMERACT-OARSI set of responder criteria. Secondary endpoints included pain, stiffness, daily functioning, patient global assessment, quality of life, osteoarthritis-related medication and side effects.

Results.—232 patients were randomly assigned. At study end, 31% of participants met the primary endpoint in both groups. Except for more adverse events in the doxycycline group, no differences were also found on the secondary endpoints.

Conclusions.—Doxycycline is not effective in reducing symptoms in knee osteoarthritis patients over a 24-week study period, but is associated with an increased risk of adverse events. Although a possible structure-modifying effect of doxycycline was previously suggested, this is not accompanied by symptom relief in the short and medium term. Dutch Trial Register no NTR1111.

▶ I had grown sort of fond of doxycycline. I recall the studies of Bob Pinals and colleagues (on tetracycline), published when I was finishing fellowship,[1] showing its inefficacy in rheumatoid arthritis (RA). Then, Jim O'Dell and collaborators[2], and others, documented that tetracyclines (minocycline) were effective in and had a role in RA. Ken Brandt and associates noted that tetracyclines protected against experimental osteoarthritis (OA) in animals (poor dogs).[3] So I kind of hoped that tetracyclines, presumably as metalloproteinase inhibitors here, would turn out to have some value in treating patients with OA too. They don't. At least in this study, under these circumstances, for 24 weeks, twice-daily doxycycline was no better than placebo at relieving symptoms of OA. Adverse effects were considered to offer an unfavorable risk-benefit ratio. Disappointing. It's hard to contemplate trying higher doses or longer duration of treatment. Maybe earlier in disease. Maybe preventively or prophylactically, insofar as possible. Maybe another metalloproteinase inhibitor.

R. S. Panush, MD

References

1. Skinner M, Cathcart ES, Mills JA, Pinals RS. Tetracycline in the treatment of rheumatoid arthritis. A double blind controlled study. *Arthritis Rheum.* 1971;14:727-732.
2. O'Dell JR, Haire CE, Palmer W, et al. Treatment of early rheumatoid arthritis with minocycline or placebo: results of a randomized, double-blind, placebo-controlled trial. *Arthritis Rheum.* 1997;40:842-848.
3. Yu LP Jr, Smith GN Jr, Brandt KD, Myers SL, O'Connor BL, Brandt DA. Reduction of the severity of canine osteoarthritis by prophylactic treatment with oral doxycycline. *Arthritis Rheum.* 1992;35:1150-1159.

3 Gout and Other Crystal Diseases

Efficacy and tolerability of pegloticase for the treatment of chronic gout in patients refractory to conventional treatment: two randomized controlled trials
Sundy JS, Baraf HS, Yood RA, et al (Duke Univ Med Ctr, Durham, NC)
JAMA 306:711-720, 2011

Context.—Patients with chronic disabling gout refractory to conventional urate-lowering therapy need timely treatment to control disease manifestations related to tissue urate crystal deposition. Pegloticase, monomethoxypoly(ethylene glycol)-conjugated mammalian recombinant uricase, was developed to fulfill this need.

Objective.—To assess the efficacy and tolerability of pegloticase in managing refractory chronic gout.

Design, Setting, and Patients.—Two replicate, randomized, double-blind, placebo-controlled trials (C0405 and C0406) were conducted between June 2006 and October 2007 at 56 rheumatology practices in the United States, Canada, and Mexico in patients with severe gout, allopurinol intolerance or refractoriness, and serum uric acid concentration of 8.0 mg/dL or greater. A total of 225 patients participated: 109 in trial C0405 and 116 in trial C0406.

Intervention.—Twelve biweekly intravenous infusions containing either pegloticase 8 mg at each infusion (biweekly treatment group), pegloticase alternating with placebo at successive infusions (monthly treatment group), or placebo (placebo group).

Main Outcome Measure.—Primary end point was plasma uric acid levels of less than 6.0 mg/dL in months 3 and 6.

Results.—In trial C0405 the primary end point was reached in 20 of 43 patients in the biweekly group (47%; 95% CI, 31%-62%), 8 of 41 patients in the monthly group (20%; 95% CI, 9%-35%), and in 0 patients treated with placebo (0/20; 95% CI, 0%-17%; $P < .001$ and $<.04$ for comparisons between biweekly and monthly groups vs placebo, respectively). Among patients treated with pegloticase in trial C0406, 16 of 42 in the biweekly group (38%; 95% CI, 24%-54%) and 21 of 43 in the monthly group (49%; 95% CI, 33%-65%) achieved the primary end point; no placebo-treated patients reached the primary end point (0/23; 95% CI, 0%-15%; $P = .001$ and $< .001$, respectively). When data in the 2 trials were pooled, the primary end point was achieved in 36 of 85 patients in the biweekly group (42%; 95% CI, 32%-54%), 29 of 84 patients in the monthly group (35%; 95% CI, 24%-46%), and 0 of 43 patients in the placebo group (0%; 95% CI, 0%-8%; P < .001 for each comparison). Seven deaths (4 in patients receiving pegloticase and 3 in the placebo group) occurred between randomization and closure of the study database (February 15, 2008).

Conclusion.—Among patients with chronic gout, elevated serum uric acid level, and allopurinol intolerance or refractoriness, the use of pegloticase 8 mg either every 2 weeks or every 4 weeks for 6 months resulted in lower uric acid levels compared with placebo.

Trial Registration.—clinicaltrials.gov Identifier: NCT00325195.

▶ Do we need more or better treatments for gout? Sometimes. There are occasionally treatment-refractory or allopurinol-intolerant patients, and pegloticase (which degrades urate) may provide an alternative for some of these patients.

R. S. Panush, MD

4 Systemic Lupus Erythematosus

Cutting edge: IL-23 receptor deficiency prevents the development of lupus nephritis in C57BL/6-lpr/lpr mice
Kyttaris VC, Zhang Z, Kuchroo VK, et al (Beth Israel Deaconess Med Ctr, Boston, MA)
J Immunol 184:4605-4609, 2010

IL-17—producing T cells infiltrate kidneys of patients with lupus nephritis, and IL-23—treated lymph node cells from lupus-prone mice may transfer disease to *Rag1*-deficient mice. In this study, we show that IL-23R—deficient lupus-prone C57BL/6—*lpr/lpr* mice display decreased numbers of CD3(+) CD4(−)CD8(−) cells and IL-17A—producing cells in the lymph nodes and produce less anti-DNA Abs. In addition, clinical and pathology measures of lupus nephritis are abrogated. The presented experiments document the importance of IL-23R—mediated signaling in the development of lupus nephritis and urge the consideration of proper biologics for the treatment of the disease.

▶ Reports of associating selective perturbations of the immune system with specific clinical syndromes should not be surprising to rheumatologists. These observations are simply elegant and contemporary extension of principles familiar to us. They remind us of the intricacy and complexity of immune homeostasis and that there are doubtless many more such examples to be identified. This study shows that interleukin (IL)-23R-deficient lpr/lpr lupus-prone mice were protected from lupus nephritis; IL-23 is important for proinflammatory Th17 cells implicated in the pathogenesis of lupus. Nature here is trying to teach us something. This should suggest both clinical and therapeutic insights. What gene mutations will be associated with what symptoms? To what might heterozygotes be predisposed? Can we develop therapeutic interventions affecting IL-17/-22 without attenuating host defenses? We should look for such contributions in future literature.

R. S. Panush, MD

Efficacy and safety of belimumab in patients with active systemic lupus erythematosus: a randomised, placebo-controlled, phase 3 trial

Navarra SV, Guzmán RM, Gallacher AE, et al (Univ of Santo Tomas Hosp, Manila, Philippines)
Lancet 377:721-731, 2011

Background.—Systemic lupus erythematosus is a heterogeneous auto-immune disease that is associated with B-cell hyperactivity, autoantibodies, and increased concentrations of B-lymphocyte stimulator (BLyS). The efficacy and safety of the fully human monoclonal antibody belimumab (BLyS-specific inhibitor) was assessed in patients with active systemic lupus erythematosus.

Methods.—Patients (aged ≥18 years) who were seropositive with scores of at least 6 on the Safety of Estrogens in Lupus Erythematosus National Assessment-Systemic Lupus Erythematosus Disease Activity Index (SELENA-SLEDAI) were enrolled in a multicentre phase 3 study, which was done in Latin America, Asia-Pacific, and eastern Europe. Patients were randomly assigned by use of a central interactive voice response system in a 1:1:1 ratio to belimumab 1 mg/kg or 10 mg/kg, or placebo by intravenous infusion in 1 h on days 0, 14, and 28, and then every 28 days until 48 weeks, with standard of care. Patients, investigators, study coordinators, and sponsors were masked to treatment assignment. Primary efficacy endpoint was improvement in the Systemic Lupus Erythematosus Responder Index (SRI) at week 52 (reduction ≥4 points in SELENA-SLEDAI score; no new British Isles Lupus Assessment Group [BILAG] A organ domain score and no more than 1 new B organ domain score; and no worsening [<0·3 increase] in Physician's Global Assessment [PGA] score) versus baseline. Method of analysis was by modified intention to treat. This trial is registered with ClinicalTrials.gov, number NCT00424476.

Findings.—867 patients were randomly assigned to belimumab 1 mg/kg (n=289) or 10 mg/kg (n=290), or placebo (n=288). 865 were treated and analysed in the belimumab (1 mg/kg, n=288; 10 mg/kg, n=290) and placebo groups (n=287). Significantly higher SRI rates were noted with belimumab 1 mg/kg (148 [51%], odds ratio 1·55 [95% CI 1·10-2·19]; p=0·0129) and 10 mg/kg (167 [58%], 1·83 [1·30-2·59]; p=0·0006) than with placebo (125 [44%]) at week 52. More patients had their SELENA-SLEDAI score reduced by at least 4 points during 52 weeks with belimumab 1 mg/kg (153 [53%], 1·51 [1·07-2·14]; p=0·0189) and 10 mg/kg (169 [58%], 1·71 [1·21-2·41]; p=0·0024) than with placebo (132 [46%]). More patients given belimumab 1 mg/kg (226 [78%], 1·38 [0·93-2·04]; p=0·1064) and 10 mg/kg (236 [81%], 1·62 [1·09-2·42]; p=0·0181) had no new BILAG A or no more than 1 new B flare than did those in the placebo group (210 [73%]). No worsening in PGA score was noted in more patients with belimumab 1 mg/kg (227 [79%], 1·68 [1·15-2·47]; p=0·0078) and 10 mg/kg (231 [80%], 1·74 [1·18-2·55]; p=0·0048) than with placebo (199 [69%]). Rates of adverse events were similar in the groups given belimumab 1 mg/kg and 10 mg/kg, and placebo: serious infection was reported in 22 (8%), 13 (4%), and 17 (6%) patients, respectively, and severe or serious hypersensitivity reactions on an infusion day were reported in two (<1%), two (<1%), and no patients, respectively. No malignant diseases were reported.

Interpretation.—Belimumab has the potential to be the first targeted biological treatment that is approved specifically for systemic lupus erythematosus, providing a new option for the management of this important prototypic autoimmune disease.

▶ It took some rather arcane data manipulations and analyses to suggest even modest benefit for belimumab (a B lymphocyte stimulator inhibitor) in certain patients with lupus.[1] The Food and Drug Administration approved the treatment amidst considerable media fanfare. This therapy, the first new lupus therapy in 56 years, will probably be reasonably widely used, as we remain frustrated by the limited availability of safe and effective therapies for many patients with lupus. No doubt we will see further trials. I'd like to see better interventions.

R. S. Panush, MD

Reference

1. Stone JH. BLISS! Lupus learns its lessons. *Lancet.* 2011;377:693-694.

5 Vasculitis

Granulomatosis with polyangiitis (Wegener's): an alternative name for Wegener's granulomatosis
Falk RJ, Gross WL, Guillevin L, et al (Univ of North Carolina, Chapel Hill)
Arthritis Rheum 63:863-864, 2011

Background.—The American College of Rheumatology (ACR), American Society of Nephrology (ASN), and European League Against Rheumatism (EULAR) convened a panel of international experts in vasculitis to develop terminology for disease designations that do not use honorific eponyms. Instead the new terms use either disease-specific or etiology-based nomenclature. Wegener's granulomatosis is among the terms that have been retired.

Rationale.—Evidence indicates that Dr Friedrich Wegener was not the first to describe the disease in question. In addition, Dr Wegener was a member of the Nazi party both before and during World War II. Both of these facts support the decision to change.

Results.—The term adopted is granulomatosis with polyangiitis (wegener's) and can be abbreviated GPA. The parenthetical referral to Wegener's will be used for several years to ease people into the new name, avoid confusion in the medical literature, and facilitate electronic searches for the condition.

Conclusions.—The new terminology has been implemented by the journal Arthritis & Rheumatism already. It is anticipated that both the scientific and the medical communities will quickly adopt this new nomenclature.

▶ We all were notified electronically about the recommendations of the American College of Rheumatology (ACR), the American Society of Nephrology, and European League Against Rheumatism to begin shifting away from eponyms. This was prompted "by evidence that Dr. Friedrich Wegener was a member of Nazi party before and during World War II." He may also have been complicit with war crimes. Eric Matteson and I addressed these issues recently, reviewing the available information regarding Wegener and suggesting that the time had come to stop using eponyms.[1] Previously I, collaborating with Dan Wallace and assisted by Rabbi Elliot Dorff (a leading ethicist), had persuaded international rheumatology editors to abandon the term Reiter syndrome (Reiter was president of the Reich Health Office and responsible for all "experiments" in concentration camps) in exchange for "reactive arthritis." When Eph Engleman, who named Reiter syndrome in 1942, became aware of this, he agreed to retract his suggestion to use the term.[2] I was disappointed that the board or directors of the ACR then declined to consider this issue. I am, however, pleased that our organization and others, now confront challenging ethical issues. Kudos to them for their stand. They got this right.

R. S. Panush, MD

References

1. Matteson E, Panush RS. Eponyms should be abandoned. *Rheumatology News.* December 2007;6:12.
2. Panush RS, Wallace DJ, Dorff RE, Engleman EP. Retraction of the suggestion to use the term "Reiter's syndrome" sixty-five years later: the legacy of Reiter, a war criminal, should not be eponymic honor but rather condemnation. *Arthritis Rheum.* 2007;56:693-694.

Rituximab versus cyclophosphamide for ANCA-associated vasculitis
Stone JH, Merkel PA, Spiera R, et al (Massachusetts General Hosp, Boston)
N Engl J Med 363:221-232, 2010

Background.—Cyclophosphamide and glucocorticoids have been the cornerstone of remission-induction therapy for severe antineutrophil cytoplasmic antibody (ANCA)-associated vasculitis for 40 years. Uncontrolled studies suggest that rituximab is effective and may be safer than a cyclophosphamide-based regimen.

Methods.—We conducted a multicenter, randomized, double-blind, double-dummy, noninferiority trial of rituximab (375 mg per square meter of body-surface area per week for 4 weeks) as compared with cyclophosphamide (2 mg per kilogram of body weight per day) for remission induction. Glucocorticoids were tapered off; the primary end point was remission of disease without the use of prednisone at 6 months.

Results.—Nine centers enrolled 197 ANCA-positive patients with either Wegener's granulomatosis or microscopic polyangiitis. Baseline disease activity, organ involvement, and the proportion of patients with relapsing disease were similar in the two treatment groups. Sixty-three patients in the rituximab group (64%) reached the primary end point, as compared with 52 patients in the control group (53%), a result that met the criterion for noninferiority (P<0.001). The rituximab-based regimen was more efficacious than the cyclophosphamide-based regimen for inducing remission of relapsing disease; 34 of 51 patients in the rituximab group (67%) as compared with 21 of 50 patients in the control group (42%) reached the primary end point (P=0.01). Rituximab was also as effective as cyclophosphamide in the treatment of patients with major renal disease or alveolar hemorrhage. There were no significant differences between the treatment groups with respect to rates of adverse events.

Conclusions.—Rituximab therapy was not inferior to daily cyclophosphamide treatment for induction of remission in severe ANCA-associated vasculitis and may be superior in relapsing disease. (Funded by the National

Institutes of Allergy and Infectious Diseases, Genentech, and Biogen; ClinicalTrials.gov number, NCT00104299.)

▶ In the quest to identify therapies for systemic vasculitis that might be as effective as established immunosuppressive regimens but less toxic, rituximab was compared with cyclophosphamide. It wasn't demonstrably better as shown in this study as well as that by Jones et al.[1]

R. S. Panush, MD

Reference

1. Jones RB, Tervaert JW, Hauser T. Rituximab versus cyclophosphamide in ANCA-associated renal vasculitis. *N Engl J Med.* 2010;363:211-220.

6 Sjögren's Syndrome

Human tears contain a chemosignal
Gelstein S, Yeshurun Y, Rozenkrantz L, et al (Weizmann Inst of Science, Rehovot, Israel)
Science 331:226-230, 2011

Emotional tearing is a poorly understood behavior that is considered uniquely human. In mice, tears serve as a chemosignal. We therefore hypothesized that human tears may similarly serve a chemosignaling function. We found that merely sniffing negative-emotion-related odorless tears obtained from women donors induced reductions in sexual appeal attributed by men to pictures of women's faces. Moreover, after sniffing such tears, men experienced reduced self-rated sexual arousal, reduced physiological measures of arousal, and reduced levels of testosterone. Finally, functional magnetic resonance imaging revealed that sniffing women's tears selectively reduced activity in brain substrates of sexual arousal in men.

▶ Crying, emotional tearing, is uniquely human. These investigators, from the Weizmann Institute, carried out an imaginative, intricate, and compelling series of experiments that showed human tears contain a chemosignal with profound effects. Men who sniffed odorless tears, obtained from women in circumstances with no emotional content, experienced reduced sexual appeal for the women, less sexual arousal, reduced physiologic measures of arousal, lowered testosterone levels, and concomitant changes on brain MRI. Powerful stuff, these tears. "Not tonight, dear," would seem to be the simple message. An evolutionary signal. What else might be in tears? Where else might this or similar chemosignals be found? What are the active compounds? What is its mechanism of action? What else might it do? How might it be involved in the changes we see in our patients with eye disease?

R. S. Panush, MD

7 Other Topics in Rheumatology

A randomized, double-blind, controlled study of ultrasound-guided corticosteroid injection into the joint of patients with inflammatory arthritis
Cunnington J, Marshall N, Hide G, et al (Freeman Hosp and Newcastle Univ, Newcastle upon Tyne, UK)
Arthritis Rheum 62:1862-1869, 2010

Objective.—Most corticosteroid injections into the joint are guided by the clinical examination (CE), but up to 70% are inaccurately placed, which may contribute to an inadequate response. The aim of this study was to investigate whether ultrasound (US) guidance improves the accuracy and clinical outcome of joint injections as compared with CE guidance in patients with inflammatory arthritis.

Methods.—A total of 184 patients with inflammatory arthritis and an inflamed joint (shoulder, elbow, wrist, knee, or ankle) were randomized to receive either US-guided or CE-guided corticosteroid injections. Visual analog scales (VAS) for assessment of function, pain, and stiffness of the target joint, a modified Health Assessment Questionnaire, and the EuroQol 5-domain questionnaire were obtained at baseline and at 2 weeks and 6 weeks postinjection. The erythrocyte sedimentation rate and C-reactive protein level were measured at baseline and 2 weeks. Contrast injected with the steroid was used to assess the accuracy of the joint injection.

Results.—One-third of CE-guided injections were inaccurate. US-guided injections performed by a trainee rheumatologist were more accurate than the CE-guided injections performed by more senior rheumatologists (83% versus 66%; P = 0.010). There was no significant difference in clinical outcome between the group receiving US-guided injections and the group receiving CE-guided injections. Accurate injections led to greater improvement in joint function, as determined by VAS scores, at 6 weeks, as compared with inaccurate injections (30.6 mm versus 21.2 mm; P = 0.030). Clinicians who used US guidance reliably assessed the accuracy of joint injection (P < 0.001), whereas those who used CE guidance did not (P = 0.29).

Conclusion.—US guidance significantly improves the accuracy of joint injection, allowing a trainee to rapidly achieve higher accuracy than more experienced rheumatologists. US guidance did not improve the short-term outcome of joint injection.

▶ When they were younger, my children used to joke that it was okay for some things if you were just "close," that it wasn't necessary to be precise about everything; the analogy was that such things were like playing horseshoes or setting off hand grenades. I used to believe that was the case for joint injections. There is a literature that showed that only about 52% of injections, almost regardless of injectors' expertise and training, could be documented to be intra-articular—66% for knees, 83% for elbows, 10% for shoulders, 50% for wrists, and none in carpometacarpal, metacarpophalangeal, interphalangeal, or acromioclavicular joints. I was nonplussed by this; I thought we did better—certainly I thought I did (and I don't know that I don't!). This could be improved by imaging and by air arthrography.[1] So, would ultrasound (US)-guided injections be better and, perhaps more importantly, would it matter therapeutically? My colleague Karina Torralba, with expertise in musculoskeletal ultrasound, sees ultrasound as enhancing the physician examination (reminding us of or teaching us the relevant anatomy, which informs the examination), offering important diagnostic information (early rheumatoid arthritis, soft tissue disorders, and other situations), helping us follow outcomes for some clinical conditions, perhaps assisting us therapeutically (eg, grading synovitis), and providing educational value in simulations (for fellows and others); I expect to learn more from her.[2] This report (with its abstract) found that US indeed improved accuracy of injections but, interestingly, could not show that outcomes from therapeutic injections were better.

R. S. Panush, MD

References

1. Sergent JS, ed. *Year Book of Rheumatology.* St. Louis, MO: Mosby; 1995:317-318.
2. Panush RS, ed. *Year Book of Rheumatology.* St. Louis, MO: Mosby; 2002:58-59.

An autoinflammatory disease with deficiency of the interleukin-1-receptor antagonist

Aksentijevich I, Masters SL, Ferguson PJ, et al (Natl Inst of Arthritis and Musculoskeletal and Skin Diseases, Bethesda, MD)
N Engl J Med 360:2426-2437, 2009

Background.—Autoinflammatory diseases manifest inflammation without evidence of infection, high-titer autoantibodies, or autoreactive T cells. We report a disorder caused by mutations of IL1RN, which encodes the interleukin-1-receptor antagonist, with prominent involvement of skin and bone.

Methods.—We studied nine children from six families who had neonatal onset of sterile multifocal osteomyelitis, periostitis, and pustulosis. Response to empirical treatment with the recombinant interleukin-1-receptor antagonist anakinra in the first patient prompted us to test for the presence of mutations and changes in proteins and their function in interleukin-1-pathway genes including IL1RN.

Results.—We identified homozygous mutations of IL1RN in nine affected children, from one family from Newfoundland, Canada, three families from The Netherlands, and one consanguineous family from Lebanon. A nonconsanguineous patient from Puerto Rico was homozygous for a genomic deletion that includes IL1RN and five other interleukin-1-family members. At least three of the mutations are founder mutations; heterozygous carriers were asymptomatic, with no cytokine abnormalities in vitro. The IL1RN mutations resulted in a truncated protein that is not secreted, thereby rendering cells hyperresponsive to interleukin-1beta stimulation. Patients treated with anakinra responded rapidly.

Conclusions.—We propose the term deficiency of the interleukin-1-receptor antagonist, or DIRA, to denote this autosomal recessive autoinflammatory disease caused by mutations affecting IL1RN. The absence of interleukin-1-receptor antagonist allows unopposed action of interleukin-1, resulting in life-threatening systemic inflammation with skin and bone involvement. (ClinicalTrials.gov number, NCT00059748.)

▶ I probably won't look for patients with deficiency of the interleukin (IL)-1 receptor antagonist. These patients had neonatal sterile multifocal osteomyelitis, periostitis, pustulosis, osteopenia, lytic bone lesions, respiratory insufficiency, and thrombosis. Their absence of the IL-1 receptor antagonist (caused by autosomal recessive mutations) permitted unopposed action of IL-1 permitting elaboration and overproduction of proinflammatory chemokines and cytokines leading to these devastating clinical manifestations. Patients responded to treatment with anakinra.[1] Why though would this immunodeficiency be associated with these particular clinical symptoms?

R. S. Panush, MD

Reference

1. Reddy S, Jia S, Geoffrey R, et al. An autoinflammatory disease due to homozygous deletion of the IL1RN locus. *N Engl J Med.* 2009;360:2438-2444.

Are There Patients with Inflammatory Disease Who Do Not Respond to Prednisone?
Sen D, Rajbhandary R, Carlino A, et al (Saint Barnabas Med Ctr, Livingston, NJ; Univ of Dentistry and Medicine of New Jersey, Livingston, et al)
J Rheumatol 37:1559-1561, 2010

"Failure to observe the expected effects of prednisone therapy should bring to mind the fact that a very rare patient may lack the hepatic enzyme system that converts prednisone to prednisolone, its active metabolite; the keto group at position 11 must be converted to a hydroxyl group before any glucocorticoid activity is exhibited. Accelerated catabolism of the active metabolite may also result in clinical effects below those expected."

Might there be patients with inflammatory disorders who do not respond clinically as expected to prednisone but respond to prednisolone? Clinical medicine was transformed when corticosteroids were synthesized and made available for clinical use in the 1950s; this is considered one of the landmarks in medicine. [It seems appropriate that this work led to the awarding of the Nobel Prize to Philip S. Hench, MD, (the only rheumatologist to receive a Nobel Prize) and collaborators.] While we now know that corticosteroids are effective for certain patients with inflammatory diseases, there is no incontrovertible evidence to support uniform consensus for the selection of preparation, dosage, and duration for patients with differing conditions. Use of corticosteroids remains more art than science. Indeed, some of us learned and taught that there were some patients with inflammatory conditions who responded poorly to prednisone but did well on methylprednisolone. This was articulated by John Decker, MD, a distinguished and authoritative rheumatologist, director of the US National Institute of Arthritis and Metabolic Diseases, National Institutes of Health, and President of the American Rheumatology Association [now American College of Rheumatology (ACR)].

▶ Have you ever had a patient you expected to respond to steroids not do so? We have. I first learned this as a fellow at the old Robert Brigham Hospital, seeing a lupus nephritis patient. The patient, despite industrial-dose prednisone, did not improve. We were taught that when such patients did not manifest the anticipated physical and metabolic changes of corticosteroid administration (Cushingoid features, increase in appetite, weight gain, insomnia, leukocytosis, eosinopenia, and lymphopenia) to suspect unusual inability to convert prednisone to prednisolone, its active metabolite (the keto group at position 11 must be converted to a hydroxyl group before any glucocorticoid activity is exhibited). We offer such patients a trial of methylprednisolone therapy when we consider steroid therapy most appropriate for their condition before using other antirheumatic, antiinflammatory, or so-called immunomodulatory/immunosuppressive (second-line) agents.

This, we think, was first articulated by John Decker, MD, a distinguished and authoritative rheumatologist who was the director of the National Institute of Arthritis and Metabolic Diseases, National Institutes of Health, and a President of the American Rheumatology Association (now the ACR). Lack of 11 beta-hydroxysteroid dehydrogenase 1 (11β HSD1) enzyme activity leads to impaired conversion and poor availability of the active steroid molecule. In such instances, treatment with prednisolone or methylprednisolone, already in an active form, may be effective. Several studies have documented impaired conversion of prednisone to prednisolone in patients with liver disease and suggested that prednisolone be used preferentially in these conditions. Also, there are patients who have deficiency of the enzyme, 11β-HSD1, needed to convert prednisone to prednisolone. This condition, termed *acquired cortisone reductase deficiency*, was recognized as a partial deficiency of 11β-HSD1. 11β HSD 1 may modulate the levels of both endogenous and exogenous steroids at the tissue level; 11β HSD1 is ubiquitously present in the skin, central nervous system, adipose tissues, and other organs, including synovium, synovial fluid, and bone, that are responsive to endogenous cortisol.[1] Recently, polymorphisms within the 11β HSD1 gene and the gene coding for hexose 6 phosphate dehydrogenase (a coenzyme that supplies reducing equivalents to 11β HSD1) have been identified[2] with a population prevalence of 3% and 4%, respectively. This may have implications both for disease susceptibility and therapy. Physicians, perhaps especially of the younger generation(s), should be aware of this possible explanation for unexpected prednisone unresponsiveness. I think it is real, has a scientific basis, is not widely appreciated, and is important in optimally caring for our patients with chronic inflammatory diseases.

R. S. Panush, MD

References

1. Raza K, Hardy R, Cooper MS. The 11β-hydroxysteroid dehydrogenase enzymes—arbiters of the effects of glucocorticoids in synovium and bone. *Rheumatology (Oxford)*. 2010;49:2016-2023.
2. van Oosten MJ, Dolhain RJ, Koper JW, et al. Polymorphisms in the glucocorticoid receptor gene that modulate glucocorticoid sensitivity are associated with rheumatoid arthritis. *Arthritis Res Ther*. 2010;12:R159. http://arthritis-research.com/content/12/4/R159.

Autoantibodies against IL-17A, IL-17F, and IL-22 in patients with chronic mucocutaneous candidiasis and autoimmune polyendocrine syndrome type I

Puel A, Döffinger R, Natividad A, et al (Institut National de la Santé et de la Recherche Médicale (INSERM), Paris, France)
J Exp Med 207:291-297, 2010

Most patients with autoimmune polyendocrine syndrome type I (APS-I) display chronic mucocutaneous candidiasis (CMC). We hypothesized that this CMC might result from autoimmunity to interleukin (IL)-17 cytokines. We found high titers of autoantibodies (auto-Abs) against IL-17A, IL-17F, and/or IL-22 in the sera of all 33 patients tested, as detected by multiplex particle-based flow cytometry. The auto-Abs against IL-17A, IL-17F, and IL-22 were specific in the five patients tested, as shown by Western blotting. The auto-Abs against IL-17A were neutralizing in the only patient tested, as shown by bioassays of IL-17A activity. None of the 37 healthy controls and none of the 103 patients with other autoimmune disorders tested had such auto-Abs. None of the patients with APS-I had auto-Abs against cytokines previously shown to cause other well-defined clinical syndromes in other patients (IL-6, interferon [IFN]-gamma, or granulocyte/macrophage colony-stimulating factor) or against other cytokines (IL-1beta, IL-10, IL-12, IL-18, IL-21, IL-23, IL-26, IFN-beta, tumor necrosis factor [alpha], or transforming growth factor beta). These findings suggest that auto-Abs against IL-17A, IL-17F, and IL-22 may cause CMC in patients with APS-I.

▶ I may, however, consider the syndrome of autoimmune polyendocrinopathy type I with chronic mucocutaneous candidiasis. These patients have autoantibodies against IL-17A, IL-17F, and/or IL-22. (These cytokines have been shown important in host defense against *Candida* in the mouse, which formed the basis of the rationale for this study.)

R. S. Panush, MD

Chocolate consumption in relation to blood pressure and risk of cardiovascular disease in German adults
Buijsse B, Weikert C, Drogan D, et al (German Inst of Human Nutrition (DIfE) Potsdam-Rehbrücke, Arthur-Scheunert-Allee, Nuthetal, Germany)
Eur Heart J 31:1616-1623, 2010

Aims.—To investigate the association of chocolate consumption with measured blood pressure (BP) and the incidence of cardiovascular disease (CVD).

Methods and Results.—Dietary intake, including chocolate, and BP were assessed at baseline (1994-98) in 19 357 participants (aged 35-65 years) free of myocardial infarction (MI) and stroke and not using antihypertensive medication of the Potsdam arm of the European Prospective Investigation into Cancer and Nutrition. Incident cases of MI ($n = 66$) and stroke ($n = 136$) were identified after a mean follow-up of approximately 8 years. Mean systolic BP was 1.0 mmHg [95% confidence interval (CI) -1.6 to -0.4 mmHg] and mean diastolic BP 0.9 mmHg (95% CI -1.3 to -0.5 mmHg) lower in the top quartile compared with the bottom quartile of chocolate consumption. The relative risk of the combined outcome of MI and stroke for top vs. bottom quartiles was 0.61 (95% CI 0.44-0.87; P linear trend $= 0.014$). Baseline BP explained 12% of this lower risk (95% CI 3-36%). The inverse association was stronger for stroke than for MI.

Conclusion.—Chocolate consumption appears to lower CVD risk, in part through reducing BP. The inverse association may be stronger for stroke than for MI. Further research is needed, in particular randomized trials.

▶ Bloomberg News reported[1] on March 31, 2010, that "a daily nibble of dark chocolate may slash the risk of heart attacks and strokes by more than one-third." Intake of 6-gm chocolate daily was associated with statistically significantly slightly lowered blood pressure (about 1 mm Hg) and 39% less risk of stroke or myocardial infarction. How might this be? Flavonols in cocoa (chocolate) are quite biologically active. (Rheumatologists, with a rich tradition of using therapeutic agents such as colchicine, fish oils, plant oils, cyclosporine, and others shouldn't be surprised at these potential properties of plants/foodstuffs.) They lower blood pressure, decrease low-density lipoprotein oxidation, diminish C-reactive protein levels, increase endothelial-dependent dilation, reduce platelet reactivity, and modulate elaboration of cytokines and eicosanoids. Some years ago I wondered why we hadn't put statins in the drinking water already because of their array of salutary effects on health generally and perhaps rheumatic diseases too. Maybe we should be washing down our statins with some red wine (or probably white also) and a healthy bite of chocolate and advising our patients to do the same. I know I would except that wine and chocolate give me violent migraine-like headaches. Just as we've seen studies of statins for various rheumatic diseases, I expect to read about the experimental effects of chocolate on our disorders. But a note of warning: the April 26, 2010, issue of the *Archives of Internal Medicine*[2] reported an association of chocolate consumption with depression.

R. S. Panush, MD

References

1. Cortez MF. Dark chocolate aids heart in study. *Pittsburgh Post-Gazette*. March 31, 2010, http://www.post-gazette.com/pg/10090/1046788-114.stm. Accessed September 7, 2011.
2. Rose N, Koperski S, Golomb BA. Mood food: chocolate and depressive symptoms in a cross-sectional analysis. *Arch Intern Med*. 2010;170:699-703.

Correlation of rheumatology subspecialty choice and identifiable strong motivations, including intellectual interest
Rahbar L, Moxley G, Carleton D, et al (Virginia Commonwealth Univ, Richmond)
Arthritis Care Res (Hoboken) 62:1796-1804, 2010

Objective.—To describe motivations correlating with subspecialty choices, particularly rheumatology.

Methods.—A total of 179 respondents answered queries about various aspects affecting specialty and subspecialty choice with ordinal ratings of importance. Likert scale response data were analyzed to determine independent predictors of being a rheumatology fellow. Multivariate logistic regression analyses were used to develop models predicting rheumatology fellowship. Factor analysis methods to condense the individual responses into fewer underlying variables or factors were employed.

Results.—While every group ranked intellectual interest as more important than all other responses, its score in the rheumatology fellow group was significantly higher than that in the medical student group. A model using 4 composite variables based on prior literature did not fit well. Exploratory factor analysis identified 5 underlying motivations, which were designated as time, money, external constraints, practice content, and academics. All motivations except money were statistically significant, with the rheumatology fellow group attributing greater importance than medical students to time, practice content, and academics, and lesser importance than medical students to external constraints.

Conclusion.—Values and motivations leading toward rheumatology subspecialty choice can be traced to identifiable factors. Intellectual interest appears to be split between 2 distinct significant variables: practice content and academics. Time or controllable lifestyle, external constraints, practice content, and academic issues appear to be important influences on the choice of rheumatology fellowship. Such variables appear to reflect underlying values and motivations.

▶ Who are we? No, this isn't really intended to be an existential question. But this study at least touches on it. It seems appropriate to reflect on this as we begin again to advise students and residents about career choices and consider candidates for fellowship. We read applicants' personal statements, ask them "Why rheumatology?" and try to discern what kind of rheumatologists they will be. I've done that for decades, invested time reading the relevant literature, and concluded it just isn't possible to predict accurately. For the most part, "What's past is prologue" (The Tempest[1]); success, achievement, and accomplishment augur success, although occasionally I'm surprised. But the process is fun. Our colleagues at Virginia Commonwealth University surveyed fellows, medical residents, and medical students. They carried out a detailed analysis of a lot of data. Not surprising to us, they found rheumatology fellows tended to value intellectual activities; lifestyle and economic issues seemed less important.

My all-time favorite perspective on this goes back to something I saved and pass on to residents interested in fellowships before they write their personal statements.[2] Indeed, I just adapted this for part of my introductory remarks to our lectures on rheumatology for the first-year medical students. He wrote eloquently and timelessly, "Some years ago I spent many hours every year sitting on boards interviewing would-be medical students, and almost inevitably some member of the committee would round on the unfortunate boy or girl and ask what made them decide to take up medicine. The usual answer, thought up well beforehand as they knew this question was likely to be asked, was usually because they loved 'people' and wished to help them and so on. Members of the committee usually shifted uneasily in their chairs at this, as they had half-hoped for a rather more original (or possible truthful) answer. The best reply I ever had was from an Arab youth who answered 'Because it is not without interest and carries financial security.' I accepted him on that truthful answer, but alas, the political scene in his country changed and he never came back."

R. S. Panush, MD

References

1. Shakespeare W. *The Tempest.* Act 2, Scene 1, Line 279.
2. Hart FD. Why take up rheumatology? *Ann Rheum Dis.* 1980;39:97-98.

End-of-life care in rheumatology: Room for improvement
Crosby V, Wilcock A (Nottingham Univ Hosps NHS Trust, UK)
Rheumatology 50:1187-1188, 2011

Background.—Rheumatologists generally deal with supporting patients living with chronic conditions, but it may also be necessary to provide end-of-life care. Ways to ensure this care is of high quality were outlined.

Identifying End-of-Life.—Many deaths in developed countries result after a progressively deteriorating course and are expected. It can be hard to predict when the patient has reached end-of-life status. The rheumatologist should be aware of the natural history of the patient's disease and any markers of clinical deterioration. Sometimes patients refuse further disease-modifying treatments and choose "comfort care" only. The most pragmatic approach is to consider whether you would be surprised should the patient die within the next 12 months. If you would not be surprised, it is appropriate to offer advance care planning (ACP).

Communication.—The clinician's communication skills should enable him or her to sensitively explore what the patient wishes to be done concerning end-of-life care. This voluntary, patient-led discussion should identify the patient's concerns and desires, important values or personal goals for care, and preferences regarding care or treatment. A proactive ACP approach seeks to ensure the patient's wishes are clear and clearly communicated to the appropriate individuals or agencies so that they will be carried out. ACP can also include areas of special concern, such as the formal completion of an advance decision to refuse treatment (ADRT). Such a document should be communicated to emergency services so that unwanted resuscitation efforts are not carried out. If there is no ADRT and the patient lacks the capacity to make a decision about care, the responsible healthcare professional must ensure that the care provided is in the patient's best interests. Again, communication is a key element in achieving the patient's goals.

Place of Care.—Most people prefer to die at home, yet the majority of deaths take place in the hospital. Lack of proactive planning may contribute to this situation. A key element in ACP is understanding where the patient wants to receive care so that this can be accomplished. The preferred place of care can change over time and with varying circumstances. Clinicians must be prepared to seek confirmation in these cases. Should the patient prefer to die at home but be presently in the hospital, systems should be in place to permit rapid discharge to home with appropriate support.

End-of-Life Care Pathways.—Care in a patient's last days can be guided by end-of-life pathways, which embody the best practice for the provision of holistic palliative care for both the patient and his or her caregiver(s). Included is guidance on the management of common distressing symptoms (pain, nausea, agitation, and retained respiratory secretions, for example). Pathways help ensure the comfort and dignity of dying patients and include providing anticipatory prescriptions for drugs to achieve symptom relief.

Conclusions.—Rheumatologists have a duty to provide good end-of-life care. This is an important part of the patient's life and there is only one chance to get it right. Clinicians need to ensure that patients' wishes are understood and communicated to everyone involved in their care.

▶ Why have rheumatologists and internists not been more visible in leadership roles in palliative care? I thought about this after a recent rheumatology conference. The topic was new therapies for systemic sclerosis. One of our fellows presented a very nice distillation of some of the new studies. The therapeutic targets (endothelin, phosphodiesterase, platelets, combinations of these, platelet-derived growth factor, and vascular endothelial growth factor) reflected evolving thinking about the important events in the pathogenesis of disease and available interventions. Unfortunately, none worked consistently or impressively well. That seems to be the story of putative treatments for systemic sclerosis when ultimately investigated in rigorously controlled trials. The subsequent discussion at our conference focused on the role of these new therapies in managing systemic sclerosis patients. I mostly listened, because it's been a while since I actively cared for sick scleroderma patients. Afterward, I wondered about our discussion and the role of palliative care in scleroderma specifically and our diseases generally. Certainly it is our imperative to help our patients. Is it really evidence-based, compassionate practice to consider the standard to be recommending 1 or a combination of these essentially unproven treatments for primary Sjögren's syndrome despite the scant evidence for efficacy and the costs for some biologicals approaching $100 000 per year? Is that a rational and fair use of scarce resources? When our patients continue to progress to "end" stages and we have little of proven value to suggest, is that not when to consider instituting palliative care? Shouldn't this at least come up in some fashion in our conversation? Do we do this as well in rheumatology? In medicine? In my former life as a department chair and in my recent personal life experiencing the slow, painful demises of my parents, I came to learn how valuable palliative care is when done well. It is much underused and much underappreciated. It is certainly not a concession of failure. Death is always 100%. Palliative care reflects the realities of a situation and seeks to provide the most possible comfort and best quality of life possible under the circumstances as long as possible. We rheumatologists and internists should indeed be more familiar, active, proactive, and involved in this. It's good medicine, and it's good for our patients (at the appropriate time).

R. S. Panush, MD

IgG4-related systemic disease accounts for a significant proportion of thoracic lymphoplasmacytic aortitis cases
Stone JH, Khosroshahi A, Deshpande V, et al (Massachusetts General Hosp and Harvard Med School, Boston)
Arthritis Care Res (Hoboken) 62:316-322, 2010

Objective.—IgG4-related systemic disease, a disorder recognized only recently, can cause lymphoplasmacytic inflammation in the thoracic aorta. The percentage of cases caused by IgG4-related systemic disease is not known. We aimed to determine the percentage of noninfectious thoracic aortitis cases that are associated with IgG4-related systemic disease and to establish pathologic criteria for identifying involvement of the thoracic aorta by this disorder.

Methods.—We searched our Pathology Service database to identify patients with noninfectious thoracic aortitis who underwent resection over a 5-year time span. The histologic features of these cases were reviewed. All cases of lymphoplasmacytic aortitis and representative cases of giant cell aortitis and atherosclerosis were stained by immunohistochemistry for IgG4 and for the plasma cell marker CD138. We determined the fraction of plasma cells that stained for IgG4.

Results.—Of 638 resected thoracic aortas, 33 (5.2%) contained noninfectious aortitis. Four of these cases (12% of all patients with noninfectious aortitis) had histologic features of lymphoplasmacytic aortitis. Three of those 4 cases (9% of the noninfectious aortitis cases) demonstrated pathologic involvement by IgG4-related systemic disease, with an elevated proportion of plasma cells staining for IgG4 (mean ± SD 0.82 ± 0.08) compared with cases of giant cell aortitis (0.18 ± 0.13) and atherosclerosis (0.19 ± 0.08; P < 0.00001).

Conclusion.—IgG4-related systemic disease accounted for 75% of lymphoplasmacytic aortitis cases and 9% of all cases of noninfectious thoracic aortitis in our institution during a 5-year period. Immunohistochemical assessment of the percentage of plasma cells that stained for IgG4 in resected aortas was helpful in identifying patients with IgG4-related systemic disease.

▶ Until recently, most reports of IgG4-related systemic disease were single cases, focused on pathology or immunopathology, and were reported in obscure journals. We will probably encounter this as noninfectious aortitis or chronic periaortitis. These patients should have elevated serum IgG4 levels and may have systemic disease, such as Sjögren syndrome, or involvement of biliary tract, liver, lung, kidney, lymph nodes, pancreas, or retroperitoneum. The aortitis responds well to glucocorticoids as demonstrated in this study.

R. S. Panush, MD

Kawasaki disease in adults: report of 10 cases
Gomard-Mennesson E, Landron C, Dauphin C, et al (Université Claude Bernard Lyon 1, France)
Medicine (Baltimore) 89:149-158, 2010

Kawasaki disease (KD) is an acute multisystemic vasculitis occurring predominantly in children and rarely in adults. Diagnosis is made clinically using diagnostic guidelines; no specific test is available. "Incomplete" KD is a more recent concept, which refers to patients with fever lasting ≥5 days and 2 or 3 clinical criteria (rash, conjunctivitis, oral mucosal changes, changes of extremities, adenopathy), without reasonable explanation for the illness. To describe the clinical and laboratory features of classical (or "complete") KD, and incomplete KD in adults, we report 10 cases of adult KD, including 6 patients who fulfilled the criteria for incomplete KD, diagnosed either at presentation (n = 4) or retrospectively (n = 2). At the time of clinical presentation, complete KD was diagnosed in 4 patients, while 4 patients fulfilled the criteria for incomplete KD. For 3 of the 4 patients with incomplete KD, presence of severe inflammation, laboratory findings (hypoalbuminemia, anemia, elevation of alanine aminotransferase, thrombocytosis after 7 days, white blood cell count

≥15,000/mm, and urine ≥10 white blood cell/high power field), or echocardiogram findings were consistent with the diagnosis. In 2 patients, the diagnosis of KD was made retrospectively in the presence of myocardial infarction due to coronary aneurysms, after an undiagnosed medical history evocative of incomplete KD. Seven patients received intravenous immunoglobulins (IVIG), after a mean delay of 12.5 days, which appeared to shorten the course of the disease. This relatively large series of adult KD highlights the existence of incomplete KD in adults and suggests that the algorithm proposed by a multidisciplinary committee of experts to diagnose incomplete KD in children could be useful in adults. Further studies are needed to determinate whether prompt IVIG may avoid artery sequelae in adult patients with complete or incomplete KD.

▶ I was pleased to see a nice presentation of 10 cases and review of the world literature (84 cases) of Kawasaki disease (KD) in adults, which started to be recognized around 2005. I'm pretty sure I'd seen this before it was accepted; I recall commenting on rounds some years back that I would have offered this diagnosis if it occurred in adults, and now it does. Some patients fulfill diagnostic guidelines developed by the Centers for Disease Control and Prevention for children. Others are called "incomplete" KD (analogous to "incomplete" lupus) when they have typical coronary arterial involvement accompanied by fever and features of severe inflammation without other explanations for the illness.

R. S. Panush, MD

Peripherally applied Abeta-containing inoculates induce cerebral beta-amyloidosis
Eisele YS, Obermüller U, Heilbronner G, et al (Univ of Tübingen, Germany)
Science 330:980-982, 2010

The intracerebral injection of β-amyloid-containing brain extracts can induce cerebral β-amyloidosis and associated pathologies in susceptible hosts. We found that intraperitoneal inoculation with β-amyloid-rich extracts induced β-amyloidosis in the brains of β-amyloid precursor protein transgenic mice after prolonged incubation times.

▶ Is amyloid an infectious disease? It could be, according to this recent study. Despite the old precept of being wary of publications that have almost as many authors as data or subjects, this was a provocative study. Mouse brain lysates containing aggregates of amyloid beta peptide injected intraperitoneally into naive recipients caused plaque-associated pathological changes in brains. Why similar inoculations by intracerebral, intravenous, oral, intraocular, or intranasal routes failed to induce disease was unclear and certainly requires that the experiments be confirmed. The pathologic mechanism was reminiscent of prion transmission. This has implications for therapeutic strategies (attempts to block protein transmission) including a cautionary note for stem cell–based approaches.

R. S. Panush, MD

PART TWO

INFECTIOUS DISEASE

NANCY M. KHARDORI, MD, PHD

Introduction

The microbial ecology around us is conceptually a double-edged sword, and the role of nonpathogenic organisms in health maintenance is often ignored. This year's first selection discusses the inverse relationship between exposure to microbes in early life and health outcomes—in particular, asthma and atopy. Among the selections on bacterial infections are: (1) the role of concomitant organisms in creating passive resistance to antibiotics in otherwise susceptible bacteria by offering β-lactamases to the site of infection as well as promoting thicker biofilms; (2) a discussion of the worldwide concern caused by the newly described β-lactamase NDM-1. Knowing that the first enzyme able to destroy penicillin was described before the clinical use of penicillin in the mid 1940s, I must say again that the continued emergence of antibiotic resistance mechanisms pursuant to use and misuse of antibiotics is an expectation rather than "news"; (3) a wider view of the factors involved in continued high incidence of *Clostridium difficile* infection worldwide, both hospital-associated and community-associated; (4) an investigative view of the epidemiological and microbial studies needed to find a "point-source" for presumed food borne epidemics and the role of counseling in preventing these infections as exemplified by infection caused by *Mycobacterium bovis* in patients who use unpasteurized dairy products; (5) further emphasis on the loss of a boundary line between community-associated and hospital-acquired infections due to methicillin-resistant *Staphylococcus aureus*. The emphasis from a clinical point of view should be on antibiotic susceptibility patterns rather than acronyms.

Newer genome-based diagnostic tests for a number of bacteria, viruses, and fungi were described during the past year. In addition to decreasing the lag time compared with conventional culture-based methods, these tests offer the potential of group rather than single pathogen testing, resulting in more appropriate initial antimicrobial coverage. Among the newer antimicrobial agents brought to the clinical arena, fidaxomicin for *C difficile* infection and telavancin for pneumonia caused by methicillin-resistant *S aureus* are the most promising. In the area of viral infection, a much higher recurrence rate of herpes zoster in adults than previously believed was described, as was a much bigger role for norovirus in adult gastroenteritis. A novel deer-associated parapoxvirus in deer hunters in the United States was described, further expanding the repertoire of zoonotic diseases. One of the selections on HIV infection clearly shows that the HIV epidemic in the United States is alive and well despite extensive availability of resources for prevention and management. As in the previous volumes, there is a "healthy" emphasis on vaccine-related publications. For example, influenza vaccination of pregnant women was shown to reduce influenza-related hospitalizations in their less-than-6-month-old infants (for whom none of the currently available vaccines are effective). The addition of M2 protein on virus-like particles (VLPs) to inactivated influenza vaccine induced highly effective humoral and cellular immune responses. Unlike the current HA antigen—based influenza vaccination, this strategy has the potential of inducing broad and improved cross protection against multiple subtypes of influenza A virus. This brings us closer to season-independent universal influenza vaccine and lessens the threat of previously experienced devastation from pandemics. A capsid protein–based vaccine against human rhinovirus induced a polyclonal response in experimental animals with broad cross reactivity. This study paves the way for a recombinant rhinovirus vaccine for humans, offering protection against related and distantly related strains of human rhinovirus. While we are still working on a cure for the common cold, we seem to be much closer to preventing it. After all, vaccines to prevent infectious disease have had the greatest impact on the current level of human health and longevity.

Nancy M. Khardori, MD, PhD

8 Bacterial Infections

Exposure to Environmental Microorganisms and Childhood Asthma
Ege MJ, for the GABRIELA Transregio 22 Study Group (Univ Children's Hosp
Munich, Germany; et al)
N Engl J Med 364:701-709, 2011

Background.—Children who grow up in environments that afford them
a wide range of microbial exposures, such as traditional farms, are protected from childhood asthma and atopy. In previous studies, markers of
microbial exposure have been inversely related to these conditions.

Methods.—In two cross-sectional studies, we compared children living
on farms with those in a reference group with respect to the prevalence of
asthma and atopy and to the diversity of microbial exposure. In one
study — PARSIFAL (Prevention of Allergy — Risk Factors for Sensitization
in Children Related to Farming and Anthroposophic Lifestyle) — samples
of mattress dust were screened for bacterial DNA with the use of single-
strand conformation polymorphism (SSCP) analyses to detect environmental bacteria that cannot be measured by means of culture techniques.
In the other study — GABRIELA (Multidisciplinary Study to Identify the
Genetic and Environmental Causes of Asthma in the European Community
[GABRIEL] Advanced Study) — samples of settled dust from children's
rooms were evaluated for bacterial and fungal taxa with the use of culture
techniques.

Results.—In both studies, children who lived on farms had lower prevalences of asthma and atopy and were exposed to a greater variety of environmental microorganisms than the children in the reference group. In turn,
diversity of microbial exposure was inversely related to the risk of asthma
(odds ratio for PARSIFAL, 0.62; 95% confidence interval [CI], 0.44 to
0.89; odds ratio for GABRIELA, 0.86; 95% CI, 0.75 to 0.99). In addition,
the presence of certain more circumscribed exposures was also inversely
related to the risk of asthma; this included exposure to species in the fungal
taxon eurotium (adjusted odds ratio, 0.37; 95% CI, 0.18 to 0.76) and to
a variety of bacterial species, including *Listeria monocytogenes*, bacillus
species, corynebacterium species, and others (adjusted odds ratio, 0.57;
95% CI, 0.38 to 0.86).

Conclusions.—Children living on farms were exposed to a wider range
of microbes than were children in the reference group, and this exposure
explains a substantial fraction of the inverse relation between asthma

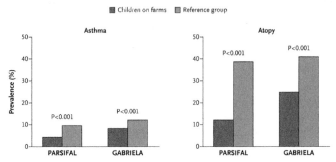

FIGURE 1.—Prevalence of Asthma and Atopy among Children Living on Farms as Compared with Reference Groups. The PARSIFAL study population included 6843 school-age children 6 to 13 years of age, and the GABRIELA study population included 9668 children between 6 and 12 years of age. Calculations of prevalence in GABRIELA were weighted on the basis of the total number of children who were eligible for inclusion in the study (34,491 children). (Reprinted from Ege MJ, for the GABRIELA Transregio 22 Study Group. Exposure to environmental microorganisms and childhood asthma. *N Engl J Med.* 2011;364:701-709. © 2011 of publication Massachusetts Medical Society.)

and growing up on a farm. (Funded by the Deutsche Forschungsgemeinschaft and the European Commission.) (Fig 1).

▶ The inverse relationship between exposure to microbes in the early years of life and health outcomes—in particular, asthma and atopy, has been reported.[1] This study describes two cross-sectional studies in which children living on farms were compared with reference groups attending the same schools in rural and suburban areas of Germany, Austria, and Switzerland. The focus was on the range of microbes to which the children in the 2 groups were exposed. In 1 study, samples of mattress dust were analyzed for bacterial DNA to detect environmental bacteria that conventional techniques cannot detect. In the second study, samples of settled dust from children's rooms were cultured to detect bacterial and fungal organisms. In both studies, the percentage of samples of mattress or settled mattress dust that were positive for bacteria or bacteria and fungi, respectively, were higher in the farm group compared with the reference group. They both point to the wider indoor range of microbial exposure for children living on farms compared with those that do not. This increased microbial exposure inversely related to the risk of asthma. The reduced risk of asthma was also seen with circumscribed exposure to a number of bacterial species including *Listeria monocytogenes, Bacillus* spp, and *Corynebacterium* spp (interestingly, all gram positive bacilli) and to the fungal species *Eurotium*. Gram negative bacilli were found to be protective against atopy. Previous studies have shown an inverse association between atopy and endotoxin exposure.[2,3] Children living on farms in both studies had lower prevalences of asthma and atopy than the children in the reference group (Fig 1). The authors explain these associations with 2 speculations: (1) summation of immunological stimuli by diverse microbes resulting in Type 1 helper T cell activation and counterbalancing of Type 2 helper T cells response that is characteristic of asthma and (2) prevention of colonization of the lower airways with harmful bacteria by the environmental exposure to a broad range of microbes. The bacterial colonization of airways has been associated with increased risk of asthma among children and adults.

N. M. Khardori, MD, PhD

References

1. von Mutius E, Radon K. Living on a farm: impact on asthma induction and clinical course. *Immunol Allergy Clin North Am.* 2008;28:631-647.
2. Braun-Fahrländer C, Riedler J, Herz U, et al. Environmental exposure to endotoxin and its relation to asthma in school-age children. *N Engl J Med.* 2002; 347:869-877.
3. Williams LK, Ownby DR, Maliarik MJ, Johnson CC. The role of endotoxin and its receptors in allergic disease. *Ann Allergy Asthma Immunol.* 2005;94:323-332.

Divergent Mechanisms for Passive Pneumococcal Resistance to β-Lactam Antibiotics in the Presence of *Haemophilus influenzae*
Weimer KED, Juneau RA, Murrah KA, et al (Wake Forest Univ School of Medicine, Winston-Salem, NC)
J Infect Dis 203:549-555, 2011

Background.—Otitis media, for which antibiotic treatment failure is increasingly common, is a leading pediatric public health problem.

Methods.—In vitro and in vivo studies using the chinchilla model of otitis media were performed using a β-lactamase-producing strain of nontypeable *Haemophilus influenzae* (NTHi 86-028NP) and an isogenic mutant deficient in β-lactamase production (NTHi 86-028NP *bla*) to define the roles of biofilm formation and β-lactamase production in antibiotic resistance. Coinfection studies were done with *Streptococcus pneumoniae* to determine if NTHi provides passive protection by means of β-lactamase production, biofilm formation, or both.

Results.—NTHi 86-028NP *bla* was resistant to amoxicillin killing in biofilm studies in vitro; however, it was cleared by amoxicillin treatment in vivo, whereas NTHi 86-028NP was unaffected in either system. NTHi 86-028NP protected pneumococcus in vivo in both the effusion fluid and bullar homogenate. NTHi 86-028NP *bla* and pneumococcus were both recovered from the surface-associated bacteria of amoxicillin-treated animals; only NTHi 86-028NP *bla* was recovered from effusion.

Conclusions.—Based on these studies, we conclude that NTHi provides passive protection for *S. pneumoniae* in vivo through 2 distinct mechanisms: production of β-lactamase and formation of biofilm communities.

▶ Epidemiologic studies have shown that coinfections with multiple bacterial species are common in both acute and chronic otitis media. The most common organisms are nontypeable *Haemophilus influenzae* (NTHi) and *Streptococcus pneumoniae*, accounting for more than 75% of infections.[1,2] This study addresses the important pediatric public health problem of increasing antibiotic treatment failure in otitis media. In vivo studies using a chinchilla model and in vitro studies were done using *S pneumoniae* plus a β-lactamase—producing strain of NTHi and/or a mutant of NT*Hi* deficient in β-lactamase production. In the in vitro biofilm studies, the β-lactamase—deficient NT*Hi* was not killed by amoxicillin, even though it was cleared in vivo, demonstrating the role of biofilm formation in antibiotic failures for susceptible bacteria.

β-lactamase—producing NTHi was unaffected by amoxicillin both in the in vitro biofilm model and in vivo. Furthermore, β-lactamase—producing *Haemophilus* was able to protect *S pneumoniae* from antibiotic action in vivo that was recovered from both the effusion fluid and bullar homogenate. Both *S pneumoniae* and β-lactamase—deficient *Haemophilus* were recovered from the surface (biofilm)-associated bacteria of amoxicillin-treated animals. Only β-lactamase—deficient *Haemophilus* was grown from effusion fluid (nonbiofilm). The findings show that β-lactamase produced by coexisting bacteria, ie, *Haemophilus,* was able to protect penicillin-susceptible *S pneumoniae* from amoxicillin leading to passive pneumococcal resistance. Even the β-lactamase nonproducing *Haemophilus* was able to protect *S pneumoniae* in the in vitro biofilm experiments as well as in the surface-associated (biofilm) bacteria in amoxicillin-treated animals. NT*Hi* and pneumococcus together form a much thicker biofilm than either organism alone.[3]

N. M. Khardori, MD, PhD

References

1. Benninger MS. Acute bacterial rhinosinusitis and otitis media: changes in pathogenicity following widespread use of pneumococcal conjugate vaccine. *Otolaryngol Head Neck Surg.* 2008;138:274-278.
2. Hendolin PH, Markkanen A, Ylikoski J, Wahlfors JJ. Use of multiplex PCR for simultaneous detection of four bacterial species in middle ear effusions. *J Clin Microbiol.* 1997;35:2854-2858.
3. Weimer KE, Armbruster CE, Juneau RA, Hong W, Pang B, Swordes WE. Coinfection with Haemophilus influenzae promotes pneumococcal biofilm formation during experimental otitis media and impedes the progression of pneumococcal disease. *J Infect Dis.* 2010;202:1068-1075.

A Case-Control Study of Community-associated *Clostridium difficile* Infection: No Role for Proton Pump Inhibitors

Naggie S, Miller BA, Zuzak KB, et al (Duke Univ Med Ctr, Durham, NC; et al)
Am J Med 124:276.e1-276.e7, 2011

Background.—The epidemiology of community-associated *Clostridium difficile* infection is not well known. We performed a multicenter, case-control study to further describe community-associated *C. difficile* infection and assess novel risk factors.

Methods.—We conducted this study at 5 sites from October 2006 through November 2007. Community-associated *C. difficile* infection included individuals with diarrhea, a positive *C. difficile* toxin, and no recent (12 weeks) discharge from a health care facility. We selected controls from the same clinics attended by cases. We collected clinical and exposure data at the time of illness and cultured residual stool samples and performed ribotyping.

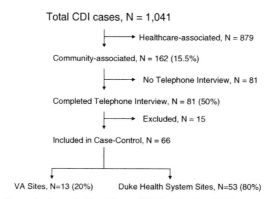

Total CDI cases, N = 1,041

→ Healthcare-associated, N = 879

Community-associated, N = 162 (15.5%)

→ No Telephone Interview, N = 81

Completed Telephone Interview, N = 81 (50%)

→ Excluded, N = 15

Included in Case-Control, N = 66

VA Sites, N=13 (20%)   Duke Health System Sites, N=53 (80%)

FIGURE 1.—Categorization of *Clostridium difficile* infection (CDI) cases from 5 hospitals. VA = Veterans Affairs. (Reprinted from The American Journal of Medicine, Naggie S, Miller BA, Zuzak KB, et al. A case-control study of community-associated clostridium difficile infection: no role for proton pump inhibitors. *Am J Med.* 2011;124:276.e1-276.e7. Copyright 2011, with permission from Elsevier.)

Results.—Of 1041 adult *C. difficile* infections, 162 (15.5%) met criteria for community-associated: 66 case and 114 control patients were enrolled. Case patients were relatively young (median 64 years), female (56%), and frequently required hospitalization (38%). Antimicrobials, malignancy, exposure to high-risk persons, and remote health care exposure were independently associated with community-associated *C. difficile* infection. In 40% of cases, we could not confirm recent antibiotic exposure. Stomach-acid suppressants were not associated with community-associated infection, and 3-hydroxy-3-methylglutaryl-coenzyme A reductase inhibitors appeared protective. Prevalence of the hypervirulent NAP-1/027 strain was infrequent (17%).

Conclusions.—Community-associated *C. difficile* infection resulted in a substantial health care burden. Antimicrobials are a significant risk factor for community-associated infection. However, other unique factors also may contribute, including person-to-person transmission, remote health care exposures, and 3-hydroxy-3-methylglutaryl-coenzyme A reductase inhibitors. A role for stomach-acid suppressants in community-associated *C. difficile* infection is not supported.

▶ Historically, the incidence of community-associated *Clostridium difficile* infection (CDI) has been low (range, 1 to 7.7 per 100 000 persons). As the incidence of hospital-acquired CDI has increased over the past decade, an increased proportion is identified as community associated.[1,2] Recent studies have reported the incidence of community-associated CDI to be as high as 22 per 100 000 persons.[3] The emergence of the hypervirulent strain ribotype 027 has been associated with risk factors, including the use of fluoroquinolones and gastric acid suppressants (proton pump inhibitors and histamine-2 blockers). The risk factors for community-associated CDI in the absence of antibiotic exposure are not clear. Two recent retrospective studies reported a significant change in the incidence and epidemiology of community-associated CDI.[3,4]

TABLE 1.—Characteristics of Community-Associated *Clostridium Difficile* Infection

Characteristic	Controls n = 114 (%)	Cases n = 66 (%)	P Value
Demographics			
Age, years (median/IQR)	63 (52-74)	64 (50-73)	.89
18-44, n (%)	14 (12)	12 (18)	
45-64	47 (41)	22 (33)	
≥65	53 (47)	32 (49)	
Female sex	63 (55)	37 (56)	.92
White race	77 (68)	54 (83)	.02
Charlson score (median/IQR)*	2 (1-2)	2 (0-3)	.767
Outpatient visit 3 mo (median/IQR)†	3 (2-5)	3 (2-6)	.58
Admit past >3 months-2 years‡	16 (14)	20 (30)	.01
Comorbidity			
Hypertension	76 (67)	36 (55)	.11
Cardiovascular disease	20 (18)	16 (24)	.28
Diabetes mellitus	31 (27)	14 (21)	.37
Gastroesophageal reflux	51 (45)	25 (38)	.37
Cancer (solid tumor)	7 (6)	11 (17)	.02
Bowel surgery (remote)	9 (8)	11 (17)	.07
Exposures (preceding 90 days)			
Antimicrobials	29 (25)	40 (61)	<.001
NSAID/aspirin	84 (74)	38 (58)	.03
Stomach acid-suppressants	44 (39)	22 (33)	.48
Steroid	15 (13)	13 (20)	.24
HMG-CoA reductase inhibitor	48 (42)	18 (27)	.05

HMG-CoA = 3-hydroxy-3-methylglutaryl-coenzyme A; IQR = interquartile range; NSAID = nonsteroidal anti-inflammatory drug.
*Charlson score = Modified Charlson Index.
†Any outpatient clinic visit to health care in the 3 months before community-associated *C. difficile* infection diagnosis.
‡Remote admission to acute care hospital more than 3 months and less than 2 years before community-associated *C. difficile* infection diagnosis.

This is a multicenter, case-control study to further characterize the epidemiology of community-associated CDI. From October 1, 2006, to November 30, 2007, a total of 1041 CDI patients were identified (Fig 1). Of these, 162 (15.5%) met the criteria for community-associated CDI. Of those, 66 patients were included in the case-control study and compared with 114 controls. The independent risk factors for community-associated CDI were antimicrobials, malignancy, exposure to high-risk persons, and remote exposure to health care. Recent antibiotic exposure could not be documented in 40% of cases, suggesting other risk factors. Proton pump inhibitor use did not appear to be associated with community-associated CDI, while the association between proton pump inhibitor/H2 blockers and health care—associated CDI has been consistently reported. Ribotyping identified 19 different strains. Interestingly, only 17% of community-associated *C difficile* belonged to the hypervirulent ribotype 027, the strain reported in health care—associated CDI. Risk factors not previously reported were person-to-person transmissions in the home and remote health care exposure. 3-Hydroxy-3-methylglutaryl-coenzyme A reductase inhibitors appeared protective (Table 1). Community-associated CDI, an important health care problem, seems to have a distinct epidemiology in comparison with health care—associated CDI.

N. M. Khardori, MD, PhD

References

1. Archibald LK, Bannerjee SN, Jarvis WR. Secular trends in hospital-acquired Clostridium difficile disease in the United States, 1987-2001. *J Infect Dis.* 2004;189: 1585-1589.
2. Norén T, Akerlund T, Bäck E, et al. Molecular epidemiology of hospital-associated and community-acquired Clostridium difficile infection in a Swedish county. *J Clin Microbiol.* 2004;42:3635-3643.
3. Kutty PK, Woods CW, Sena AC, et al. Risk factors for and estimated incidence of community-associated Clostridium difficile infection, North Carolina, USA. *Emerg Infect Dis.* 2010;16:197-204.
4. Naggie S, Frederick J, Pien BC, et al. Community-associated Clostridium difficile infection: experience of a veteran affairs medical center in the southeastern USA. *Infection.* 2010;38:297-300.

A Placebo-Controlled Trial of Antimicrobial Treatment for Acute Otitis Media

Tähtinen PA, Laine MK, Huovinen P, et al (Turku Univ Hosp, Finland; Univ of Turku, Finland)
N Engl J Med 364:116-126, 2011

Background.—The efficacy of antimicrobial treatment in children with acute otitis media remains controversial.

Methods.—In this randomized, double-blind trial, children 6 to 35 months of age with acute otitis media, diagnosed with the use of strict criteria, received amoxicillin–clavulanate (161 children) or placebo (158 children) for 7 days. The primary outcome was the time to treatment failure from the first dose until the end-of-treatment visit on day 8. The definition of treatment failure was based on the overall condition of the child (including adverse events) and otoscopic signs of acute otitis media.

Results.—Treatment failure occurred in 18.6% of the children who received amoxicillin–clavulanate, as compared with 44.9% of the children who received placebo (P<0.001). The difference between the groups was already apparent at the first scheduled visit (day 3), at which time 13.7% of the children who received amoxicillin–clavulanate, as compared with 25.3% of those who received placebo, had treatment failure. Overall, amoxicillin–clavulanate reduced the progression to treatment failure by 62% (hazard ratio, 0.38; 95% confidence interval [CI], 0.25 to 0.59; P<0.001) and the need for rescue treatment by 81% (6.8% vs. 33.5%; hazard ratio, 0.19; 95% CI, 0.10 to 0.36; P<0.001). Analgesic or antipyretic agents were given to 84.2% and 85.9% of the children in the amoxicillin–clavulanate and placebo groups, respectively. Adverse events were significantly more common in the amoxicillin–clavulanate group than in the placebo group. A total of 47.8% of the children in the amoxicillin–clavulanate group had diarrhea, as compared with 26.6% in the placebo group (P<0.001); 8.7% and 3.2% of the children in the respective groups had eczema (P = 0.04).

Conclusions.—Children with acute otitis media benefit from antimicrobial treatment as compared with placebo, although they have more side effects. Future studies should identify patients who may derive the greatest benefit, in order to minimize unnecessary antimicrobial treatment and the development of bacterial resistance. (Funded by the Foundation for Paediatric Research and others; ClinicalTrials.gov number, NCT00299455.)

▶ This is a randomized, double-blind trial in children 6 to 35 months of age who have acute otitis media diagnosed by strict criteria. Amoxicillin-clavulanate for 7 days was compared with placebo to determine the efficacy of antimicrobial treatment. There was a significant difference in primary treatment failure rates, 44.9% for the placebo group and 18.6% for the treatment group ($P < .0001$). Adverse events were significantly more common in the treatment group. The need for rescue treatment after initial failure (secondary outcomes) was reduced by 81% in the treatment group compared with the placebo group (Fig 3 in original article). Acute otitis media in the other ear developed in 8.2% of children in the treatment group compared with 18.6% in the placebo group. The use of antipyretic and analgesic did not differ between the 2 groups. Amoxicillin-clavulanate reduced day care attendee absenteeism by 9.4% compared with the placebo group. Fewer work days (12.1%) were missed by parents of children in the treatment arm compared with the parents of children in the placebo group (17.8), a reduction of 5.7%. At the end of the treatment visit, overall condition had not improved or had worsened in 6.8% of children receiving amoxicillin-clavulanate compared with 29.7% in the placebo group, a reduction of 22.9%. After treatment, fewer pathogenic bacteria were grown from nasopharynx of children receiving amoxicillin-clavulanate compared with the placebo group. One *Streptococcus pneumoniae* isolate changed from intermediate to full resistance during treatment. The study provides evidence that appropriate antibiotic therapy of acute otitis media in children 6 to 35 months of age is beneficial. What remains to be determined is which patients do not need antibiotic treatment based on prognostic markers and stringent diagnostic criteria.[1]

N. M. Khardori, MD, PhD

Reference

1. Vergison A, Dagan R, Arguedas A, et al. Otitis media and its consequences: beyond the earache. *Lancet Infect Dis.* 2010;10:195-203.

Clinical characteristics and therapeutic outcome of Gram-negative bacterial spinal epidural abscess in adults
Huang C-R, Lu C-H, Chuang Y-C, et al (Chang Gung Univ College of Medicine, Kaohsiung, Taiwan)
J Clin Neurosci 18:213-217, 2011

Gram-negative (G(−)) bacterial spinal epidural abscess (SEA) in adults is uncommon. Of the 42 adult patients with bacterial SEA admitted to the Chang Gung Memorial Hospital − Kaohsiung, between 2003 and 2007, 12 with G(−) SEA were included in this study. Of these 12 patients, seven were men and five were women; their ages ranged between 17 years and 81 years (median = 72.5 years, mean = 62.5 years). The patients were admitted at different stages of symptom onset (four were in the acute stage and four each in the subacute and chronic stages) and at different levels of neurologic deficit severity, ranging from back pain to paraplegia. Of these 12 patients, 11 had a medical and/or neurosurgical condition as the preceding event and four had a concomitant infection at other sites. Back pain (83%, 10/12) was the most common clinical presentation, followed by paraparesis (50%, 6/12), radiating pain (33%, 4/12), and urinary retention (25%, 3/12). The following causative G(−) pathogens were detected: *Klebsiella pneumoniae* (three patients), *Salmonella spp.* (three), *Escherichia coli* (two), *Enterobacter spp.* (two), *Aeromonas hydrophila* (one), and *Prevotella melaninogenica* (one). Both *Enterobacter* strains were resistant to multiple antibiotics. Of the 12 patients, eight (66.7%) had spontaneous SEA, whereas the remaining four had postneurosurgical SEA. Thoracic, lumbar, and thoracolumbar spine segments were the most commonly affected. After receiving medical and/or surgical treatment, 10 of the 12 patients (83%) survived, and all 10 recovered well. In conclusion, G(−) bacterial SEA accounted for 28.5% (12/42) of adult SEA. The causative G(−) pathogens found in this study were different from those reported in Western countries, and the strains noted in our study had multiple antibiotic resistance. Our findings suggest that the choice of initial empirical antibiotics for SEA should be carefully considered.

▶ Culture-proven cases of spinal epidural abscess (SEA) are caused mostly by gram-positive pathogens, especially *Staphylococcus aureus*.[1] The presumptive antibiotic therapy of SEA is based on this common microbiology. This study analyzes the clinical characteristics and therapeutic outcomes of 12 of 42 adult patients with SEA caused by gram-negative pathogens. The gram-negative organisms grown were *Klebsiella pneumoniae, Salmonella* spp, *Escherichia coli, Enterobacter* spp, *Aeromonas hydrophila*, and *Prevotella melaninogenica*. The other 29 patients grew *Staphylococcus aureus*. Four SEA were postneurosurgical, and 8 were spontaneous. Surgical intervention was used for 7 patients, 2 of whom died. Six patients were receiving appropriate antibiotics at the time culture and sensitivity became available. Therapy was adjusted for the other 6 patients. The 10 patients who survived recovered well and both patients who died had severe neurological deficits at presentation and multiple comorbidities. The spectrum of gram-negative bacteria from SEA in this study is similar to that reported in English literature (Table 2 in the original article). The major clinical implication of these data is in the choice of initial presumptive antibiotic therapy. Although 69% of SEA were caused by *S. aureus*, 29% incidence of gram-negative bacilli in SEA points to consideration of polymicrobial coverage initially.

N. M. Khardori, MD, PhD

Reference

1. Darouiche RO. Spinal epidural abscess. *N Engl J Med*. 2006;355:2012-2020.

Conceptual Model for Reducing Infections and Antimicrobial Resistance in Skilled Nursing Facilities: Focusing on Residents with Indwelling Devices

Mody L, Bradley SF, Galecki A, et al (Veterans Affairs/Univ of Michigan Patient Safety Enhancement Program, Ann Arbor; et al)

Clin Infect Dis 52:654-661, 2011

Infections in skilled nursing facilities (SNFs) are common and result in frequent hospital transfers, functional decline, and death. Colonization with multidrug-resistant organisms (MDROs) — including methicillinresistant *Staphylococcus aureus* (MRSA), vancomycin-resistant enterococci (VRE), and multidrug-resistant gram-negative bacilli (R-GNB) — is also increasingly prevalent in SNFs. Antimicrobial resistance among common bacteria can adversely affect clinical outcomes and increase health care costs. Recognizing a need for action, legislators, policy-makers, and consumer groups are advocating for surveillance cultures to identify asymptomatic patients with MDROs, particularly MRSA in hospitals and SNFs. Implementing this policy for all SNF residents may be costly, impractical, and ineffective. Such a policy may result in a large increase in the number of SNF residents placed in isolation precautions with the potential for reduced attention by health care workers, isolation, and functional decline. Detection of colonization and subsequent attempts to eradicate selected MDROs can also lead to more strains with drug resistance. We propose an alternative strategy that uses a focused multicomponent bundle approach that targets residents at a higher risk of colonization and infection with MDROs, specifically those who have an indwelling device. If this strategy is effective, similar strategies can be studied and implemented for other high-risk groups.

▶ Skilled nursing facilities in the United States carry more patients than the hospitals at any given time. Because of the host and the institutional factors involved, the risk for health care—associated infections, including those caused by multidrug resistant organisms (MDROs), the study proposed a strategy that uses a focused multicomponent bundle is high and constant.[1,2] The guidelines for infection prevention in these facilities have been adopted from those used in acute care settings and are often unaffordable and impractical. This approach targets residents at a higher risk of colonization and infection with MDROs. Patients with indwelling devices (eg, urinary catheters and feeding tubes) were specifically targeted. Indwelling devices in these patients are often colonized by MDROs, leading eventually to colonization of other sites and transfer of these organisms to the hands of health care workers. Horizontal transmission of MDROs from 1 resident to another through the hands of health care workers has been reported.[3]

The PRECEDE (Reinforcing and Enabling Factors in Educational and Health Diagnosis and Evaluation) model described in this study would intervene to break the chain of spread of microorganisms, especially MDROs, among health care workers and residents of skilled nursing facilities (Fig 2).

The facilities could promote the universal practice of hand hygiene as a part of the proposed bundle and use a multipronged approach to staff education,

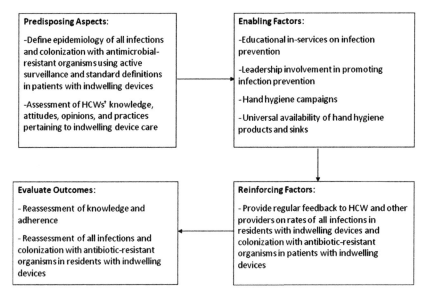

Predisposing Aspects:

-Define epidemiology of all infections and colonization with antimicrobial-resistant organisms using active surveillance and standard definitions in patients with indwelling devices

-Assessment of HCWs' knowledge, attitudes, opinions, and practices pertaining to indwelling device care

Enabling Factors:

-Educational in-services on infection prevention

-Leadership involvement in promoting infection prevention

-Hand hygiene campaigns

-Universal availability of hand hygiene products and sinks

Evaluate Outcomes:

- Reassessment of knowledge and adherence

- Reassessment of all infections and colonization with antibiotic-resistant organisms in residents with indwelling devices

Reinforcing Factors:

- Provide regular feedback to HCW and other providers on rates of all infections in residents with indwelling devices and colonization with antibiotic-resistant organisms in patients with indwelling devices

FIGURE 2.—PRECEDE (predisposing, reinforcing, and enabling factors in educational and health diagnosis and evaluation) model to implement interventions in high risk groups. HCW, health care worker. (Reprinted from Mody L, Bradley SF, Galecki A, et al. Conceptual model for reducing infections and anti-microbial resistance in skilled nursing facilities: focusing on residents with indwelling devices. *Clin Infect Dis.* 2011;52:654-661, by permission of the Infectious Diseases Society of America.)

including the role of indwelling devices as a reservoir of microorganisms. In my opinion, this strategy is highly likely to be effective, and similar strategies should be studied in other high-risk groups.

N. M. Khardori, MD, PhD

References

1. Rogers MA, Mody L, Chenoweth C, Kaufman SR, Saint S. Incidence of antibiotic-resistant infection in long-term residents of skilled nursing facilities. *Am J Infect Control.* 2008;36:472-475.
2. Smith PW, Bennett G, Bradley S, et al. SHEA/APIC guideline: infection prevention and control in the long-term care facility, July 2008. *Infect Control Hosp Epidemiol.* 2008;29:785-814.
3. Wingard E, Shlaes JH, Mortimer EA, Shlaes DM. Colonization and cross-colonization of nursing home patients with trimethoprim-resistant gram-negative bacilli. *Clin Infect Dis.* 1993;16:75-81.

Microbial profile and antibiotic susceptibility of culture-positive bacterial endophthalmitis
Melo GB, Bispo PJM, Yu MCZ, et al (Federal Univ of São Paulo, Brazil)
Eye 25:382-388, 2011

Purpose.—To assess the distribution of microorganisms isolated from patients with bacterial endophthalmitis and their antimicrobial susceptibility.

Methods.—Retrospective analysis of medical and microbiological records of patients with suspected diagnosis of endophthalmitis. The following information was assessed: number of presumed and culture-positive endophthalmitis cases, source of infection, microbiological result (aqueous and/or vitreous culture and Gram staining), microbial characterization and distribution, and antimicrobial susceptibility.

Results.—A total of 107 (46%) of 231 patients with bacterial endophthalmitis showed positive results by gram stain or culture. Of these, 97 (42%) patients were positive for culture only. Most of them (62%) were secondary to a surgical procedure (postoperative), 12% were posttraumatic and 26% were secondary to an unknown source or the data were unavailable. A total of 100 microorganisms were isolated (38 aqueous and 67 vitreous samples) from the 97 culture-positive cases (91% were gram-positive and 9% were gram-negative). Coagulase-negative *Staphylococcus* (CoNS) (48%) were the most frequently isolated, followed by *Streptococcus viridans* (18%), and *Staphylococcus aureus* (13%). The antimicrobial susceptibility for CoNS was as follows: amikacin—91.6%, cephalothin—97.9%, ceftriaxone—50%, ciprofloxacin—62.5%, chloramphenicol—91.8%, gatifloxacin—79.5%, gentamicin—72.9%, moxifloxacin—89.5%, ofloxacin—70.8%, oxacillin—58.3%, penicillin—33.3%, tobramycin—85.4%, and vancomycin—100%.

Conclusion.—Gram-positive bacteria were the major causes of infectious endophthalmitis in this large series, usually following surgery. CoNS was the most common isolate. Of interest, susceptibility to oxacillin and fourth-generation quinolones was lower than previously published.

▶ Bacterial endophthalmitis following surgery or trauma is a sight-threatening complication. The worldwide reported incidence varies from 0.05 to 0.4%.[1] The most common microbial source is the bacteria from the conjunctiva and the eyelid.

This retrospective study describes 231 patients with bacterial endophthalmitis between January 2006 and October 2009. The sources for microbiological studies included aqueous humor, vitreous tap, and vitrectomy samples. The microbiological spectrum from 107 gram-stain or culture-positive cases was similar to that reported in a previous study of patients from 2000 to 2005 by the same group (Table 2 in the original article).

In both studies, coagulase negative *Staphylococcus* (CNS), *Streptococcus viridans* and *Staphylococcus aureus*, in that order, were the 3 most common bacteria grown. This is consistent with the microbiology of conjunctival flora. In the data from 2000 to 2005, all CNS were susceptible to fourth-generation quinolones, moxifloxacin and gatifloxacin. However, in the current data (2006–2009) the in vitro sensitivity of CNS was 79.5% and 89.5% to moxifloxacin and gatifloxacin, respectively. The quinolone-resistant isolates were resistant to methicillin also, as has been reported in another recent study,[2] Other recently published studies report quinolone resistance in 65% to 96% of CNS from patients with endophthalmitis. Because the fourth-generation quinolones are routinely used in the prophylaxis in ophthalmic surgery and in the treatment of endophthalmitis, by both topical and systemic routes, the increasing resistance is of concern and needs further widespread evaluation.

N. M. Khardori, MD, PhD

References

1. Taban M, Behrens A, Newcomb RL, et al. Acute endophthalmitis following cataract surgery: a systematic review of the literature. *Arch Ophthalmol.* 2005;123: 613-620.
2. Hori Y, Nakazawa T, Maeda N, et al. Susceptibility comparisons of normal preoperative conjunctival bacteria to fluoroquinolones. *J Cataract Refract Surg.* 2009; 35:475-479.

Trimethoprim-Sulfamethoxazole or Clindamycin for Community-Associated MRSA (CA-MRSA) Skin Infections
Frei CR, Miller ML, Lewis JS II, et al (Univ of Texas at Austin; et al)
J Am Board Fam Med 23:714-719, 2010

Background.—In the United States, community-associated methicillin-resistant *Staphylococcus aureus* (CA-MRSA) has emerged as the predominant cause of skin infections. Trimethoprim-sulfamethoxazole (TMP-SMX) and clindamycin are often used as first-line treatment options, but clinical data are lacking.

Methods.—We conducted a retrospective cohort study of outpatients with skin and soft tissue infections managed from July 1 to December 31, 2006. Patients younger than 18 years of age were excluded, as were those who had no clinical admission or progress notes; were hospitalized within the 90 days before admission; were hospitalized with polymicrobial, surgical site, catheter-related, or diabetic foot infections; or were discharged to places other than home. Patient demographics, comorbidities, diagnoses, cultures, prescribed antibiotics, susceptibilities, surgical procedures, and health outcomes were extracted from electronic medical records. Patients were divided in 2 cohorts for further analysis: TMP-SMX and clindamycin. The primary study outcome was composite failure defined as an additional positive MRSA culture from any site 5 to 90 days after treatment initiation or an additional intervention during a subsequent outpatient or inpatient visit. Baseline characteristics and failure rates were compared using χ^2, Fisher's exact, and Wilcoxon rank sum tests.

Results.—A total of 149 patients were included in this study. These patients had a median age of 36 years, 55% were men, 71% were Hispanic, 42% were uninsured, and 60% received an incision and drainage procedure. Patients who did not receive incision and drainage were twice as likely to experience the composite failure endpoint (57% vs 29%; $P < .001$). Failure rates were 25% for patients who received incision and drainage plus antibiotics compared with 60% for patients who received incision and drainage minus antibiotics ($P = .03$). When patients who did not receive incision and drainage were excluded, there were no significant differences between the TMP-SMX (n = 54) and clindamycin (n = 20) cohorts with respect to composite failures (26% vs 25%), microbiologic failures (13% vs 15%), additional inpatient interventions (6% vs 5%), or additional outpatient interventions (20% vs 20%).

Conclusions.—Our findings reinforce the belief that incision and drainage and antibiotics are critical for the management of CA-MRSA skin infections. Patients who receive TMP-SMX or clindamycin for their CA-MRSA skin infections experience similar rates of treatment failure.

▶ More than half of *Staphylococcus aureus* skin and soft tissue infections documented in the outpatient setting in the United States are caused by community-associated methicillin-resistant strains.[1] Oral antibiotics, including clindamycin and trimethoprim-sulfamethoxazole (TMP/SMX), are used as first-line treatment options based on in vitro activity, high oral bioavailability, and excellent tissue penetration.

This retrospective cohort study describes 149 adult outpatients with skin and soft tissue infection caused by methicillin-resistant *S. aureus* (MRSA) over a 6-month period. The 2 cohorts consisted of those receiving TMP/SMX and those receiving clindamycin. All MRSA isolates were sensitive to vancomycin and TMP/SMX in vitro. The in vitro sensitivity to clindamycin was 94% in both groups. The in vivo sensitivity to doxycycline was 99% in the TMP/SMX-treated group and 97% in the clindamycin-treated group. Incision and drainage of the lesion was performed in 60% of patients. Composite treatment failure end point was twice as likely in patients not receiving incision and drainage (I & D) compared with those who did. Failure rate was 60% in patients receiving I & D without antibiotics compared with 25% for those who received a combination of I & D and antibiotics. Antibiotics prescribed included TMP/SMX (58%), clindamycin (23%), and cephalexin (6%). The most common TMP/SMX dose prescribed was 1 double-strength tablet twice daily rather than 2 double-strength tablets twice daily as supported by pharmacokinetic-pharmacodynamic literature.[2] In patients who received I & D plus TMP/SMX or clindamycin, composite treatment failure rates were similar (26% and 25%) between the 2 antibiotic groups. Overall, treatment failure rate was 39% in TIM/SMX group and 32% in clindamycin group (Table 5 in the original article). These data reinforce the role of combination of I & D and antibiotics as optimal management of skin and soft tissue infections caused by community associated MRSA.

N. M. Khardori, MD, PhD

References

1. Styers D, Sheehan DJ, Hogan P, Sahm DF. Laboratory-based surveillance of current antimicrobial resistance patterns and trends among *Staphylococcus aureus*: 2005 status in the United States. *Ann Clin Microbiol Antimicrob.* 2006;5:2.
2. Stevens DL, Bisno AL, Chambers HF, et al. Practice guidelines for the diagnosis and management of skin and soft-tissue infections. *Clin Infect Dis.* 2005;41: 1373-1406.

9 Nosocomial Infections

NDM-1 — A Cause for Worldwide Concern
Moellering RC Jr (Harvard Med School and Beth Israel Deaconess Med Ctr, Boston, MA)
N Engl J Med 363:2377-2379, 2010

Background.—Superbugs may not be more virulent or have greater pathogenicity, but they are resistant to multiple antimicrobial agents. Fifty years ago clinicians knew the major principles governing the nature, dissemination, and potential control of antibiotic resistance. This includes the inappropriate use of antibiotics, resistant organisms ability to spread in hospital settings, and the value of limiting antibiotic use in hospitals as a control measure. New Delhi metallo-beta-lactamase 1 (NDM-1) is a transmissible genetic element that encodes multiple resistance genes. It was initially isolated in 2008 from a strain of klebsiella from a patient who acquired the organism in New Delhi, India. By 2009 there were 24 carbapenem-resistant Enterobacteriaceae, 22 of which produce NDM-1. Isolates of Enterobacteriacea-containing NDM-1 are now widely found in India, Pakistan, Bangladesh, and Great Britain and turning up in many other countries.

Mechanisms of Resistance.—The first enzyme able to destroy penicillin was described before the clinical use of penicillin in the 1940s. Compounds resistant to beta-lactamases or able to inactivate them evolved, with more than 890 unique deactivating enzymes now identified. Most of these enzymes are found on transmissible genetic elements, so acquiring resistance genes is not difficult for organisms.

A new mechanism of resistance was found in staphylococci in German swine. It is attributable to genes that encoded a methylase able to change ribosomal binding sites for linezolid and caused cross-resistance to several other ribosomally active antimicrobials. Thus a single enzyme inactivated five classes of antibiotics. The gene encoding for this methylase is on a transmissible plasmid, and recent outbreaks of linezolid resistance suggest that soon *Staphylococcus aureus* may become resistant to linezolids.

The NDM-1 enzyme not only has the intrinsic ability to destroy most known beta-lactam antibiotics, but also contains a novel metallo-beta-lactamase that readily hydrolyzes penicillins, cephalosporins, and carbapenems (except aztreonam). This beta-lactamase was found on a large 180-kb resistance-conferring genetic element that readily transfers to other

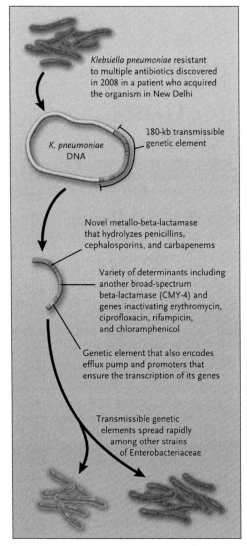

FIGURE 1.—The Origin and Spread of NDM-1. (Reprinted from Moellering RC Jr. NDM-1 — A cause for worldwide concern. *N Engl J Med.* 2010;363:2377-2379. © 2010 Massachusetts Medical Society.)

Enterobacteriaceae and contains various other resistance determinants, such as genes encoding CMY-4 and inactivating erythromycin, ciprofloxacin, rifampicin, and chloramphenicol. The genetic element encodes an efflux pump that can produce more antimicrobial resistance and growth promoters that ensure gene transcription. This, plus the ability of bacteria to overwhelm control efforts with superior numbers, the ability to reproduce with remarkable speed, and extremely efficient ways to exchange and promulgate resistance genes, makes widespread dissemination of NDM-1 a serious threat.

Conclusions.—Why NDM-1 emerged on the Indian subcontinent is unknown, but India has widespread nonprescription antibiotic use, poor sanitation, crowding, and a high prevalence of diarrheal disease. NDM-1 is just one threat. Major US outbreaks of infections caused by multidrug-resistant klebsiella containing KPC enzymes that can hydrolyze the carbapenems and other beta-lactam antibiotics have occurred. CTX beta-lactamases are increasing in Enterobacteriaceae isolates from outpatients worldwide and will compromise beta-lactamase usefulness. The Centers for Disease Control and Prevention believe NDM-1 can be contained with standard infection-control methods, but NDM-1 offers all the properties needed to turn organisms that contain it into superbugs (Fig 1).

▶ The development of antibiotic resistance in response to antibiotic exposure has been and remains an expected biological phenomenon. As demonstrated by the 3 *New England Journal of Medicine* archive articles from 1960 (Box from the original article), the fundamentals of nature, dissemination, and potential control of antibiotic resistance were discussed 50 years ago and were known before that. In the past few years, the emergence of methicillin-resistant *Staphylococcus aureus* (MRSA) in the community setting and other multiply resistant bacteria in the health care setting have made treatment options much more difficult based simply on the resistance to multiple antimicrobial agents. The acronym ESKAPE (*Enterococcus faecium, Staphylococcus aureus, Klebsiella pneumoniae, Acinetobacter baumannii, Pseudomonas aeruginosa* and *Enterobacter species*) summarizes the currently prevailing resistant bacteria well.[1] Last year, the professional and lay literature focused on the reports of a transmissible genetic element (NDM-1) encoding a multiply resistant gene that was initially isolated from a strain of *Klebsiella* obtained from a patient who acquired the organism in New Delhi, India,[2] as shown in Fig 1. Subsequently, members of the *Enterobacteriaceae* family containing this genetic element or its variants have been reported from around the world, including India, Pakistan, Bangladesh, and Britain. The resistance of this organism to all antimicrobial agents except polymyxins has become a worldwide concern.

Dr Moellering in this review puts in perspective the fact that NDM-1 is not the only worldwide threat posed by antibiotic resistance. Historically, penicillinase, capable of destroying penicillin, was described before the initial clinical use of penicillin in the early 1940s. Since then, bacteria have continued to undermine our best efforts to destroy them with antibiotics. The speed of multiplication and efficient ways to exchange resistance genes among bacteria lend them to currently known as well as unknown mechanisms of antibiotic resistance.

N. M. Khardori, MD, PhD

References

1. Rice LB. Federal funding for the study of antimicrobial resistance in nosocomial pathogens: no ESKAPE. *J Infect Dis*. 2008;197:1079-1081.

2. Kumarasamy KK, Toleman MA, Walsh TR, et al. Emergence of a new antibiotic resistance mechanism in India, Pakistan, and the UK: a molecular, biological, and epidemiological study. *Lancet Infect Dis.* 2010;10:597-602.

Clostridium difficile infection in Europe: a hospital-based survey

Bauer MP, for the ECDIS Study Group (Centre for Infectious Disease Control Netherlands, Bilthoven; et al)

Lancet 377:63-73, 2011

Background.—Little is known about the extent of *Clostridium difficile* infection in Europe. Our aim was to obtain a more complete overview of *C difficile* infection in Europe and build capacity for diagnosis and surveillance.

Methods.—We set up a network of 106 laboratories in 34 European countries. In November, 2008, one to six hospitals per country, relative to population size, tested stool samples of patients with suspected *C difficile* infection or diarrhoea that developed 3 or more days after hospital admission. A case was defined when, subsequently, toxins were identified in stool samples. Detailed clinical data and stool isolates were collected for the first ten cases per hospital. After 3 months, clinical data were followed up.

Findings.—The incidence of *C difficile* infection varied across hospitals (weighted mean 4·1 per 10 000 patient-days per hospital, range 0·0−36·3). Detailed information was obtained for 509 patients. For 389 of these patients, isolates were available for characterisation. 65 different PCR ribotypes were identified, of which 014/020 (61 patients [16%]), 001 (37 [9%]), and 078 (31 [8%]) were the most prevalent. The prevalence of PCR-ribotype 027 was 5%. Most patients had a previously identified risk profile of old age, comorbidity, and recent antibiotic use. At follow up, 101 (22%) of 455 patients had died, and *C difficile* infection played a part in 40 (40%) of deaths. After adjustment for potential confounders, an age of 65 years or older (adjusted odds ratio 3·26, 95% CI 1·08−9·78; p= 0·026), and infection by PCR-ribotypes 018 (6·19, 1·28−29·81; p= 0·023) and 056 (13·01; 1·14−148·26; p=0·039) were significantly associated with complicated disease outcome.

Interpretation.—PCR ribotypes other than 027 are prevalent in European hospitals. The data emphasise the importance of multicountry surveillance to detect and control *C difficile* infection in Europe.

▶ The past decade has seen increasing rates of *Clostridium difficile* infection (CDI) and a larger proportion of severe and recurrent cases in Canada and the United States. This higher incidence and increased virulence is partly explained by the spread of fluoroquinolone-resistant strains belonging to the Polymerase chain reaction-ribotype 027.[1-3] These strains produce a binary toxin of uncertain pathogenic significance in addition to the usual toxins A and B. The PCR-ribotype 027 has also been reported from Europe.

This study describes a network of 106 laboratories in 34 European countries that tested stool samples of patients with suspected CDIs or diarrhea that developed 3 or more days after hospital admission. A case was defined as CDI when toxins were identified in stool samples. Initial and 3-month follow-up clinical data and stool isolates were collected for the first 10 cases per hospital. The incidence of CDI varied among the participating hospitals with a weighted mean of 4.1 per 10 000 patient-days per hospital. A large number (65) of PCR-ribotypes were identified with PCR-ribotype 027 being responsible for only 5% of cases.

N. M. Khardori, MD, PhD

References

1. McDonald LC, Killgore GE, Thompson A, et al. An epidemic, toxin gene-variant strain of *Clostridium difficile*. N Engl J Med. 2005;353:2433-2441.
2. Loo VG, Poirier L, Miller MA, et al. A predominantly clonal multi-institutional outbreak of *Clostridium difficile*-associated diarrhea with high morbidity and mortality. N Engl J Med. 2005;353:2442-2449.
3. Kelly CP, LaMont JT. *Clostridium difficile*—more difficult than ever. N Engl J Med. 2008;359:1932-1940.

Incidence of and Risk Factors for Community-Associated Methicillin-Resistant *Staphylococcus aureus* Acquired Infection or Colonization in Intensive-Care-Unit Patients

Wang J-T, Liao C-H, Fang C-T, et al (Natl Taiwan Univ Hosp, Taipei; Far Eastern Memorial Hosp, Taipei County, Taiwan; et al)
J Clin Microbiol 48:4439-4444, 2010

The incidence of and risk factors for acquiring community-associated methicillin-resistant *Staphylococcus aureus* (CA-MRSA) among patients staying in intensive care units (ICUs) remain unclear. We enrolled patients staying in two ICUs at the Far Eastern Memorial Hospital during the period of 1 September 2008 to 30 September 2009 to clarify this issue. Surveillance cultures for MRSA were taken from nostril, sputum or throat, axillae, and the inguinal area in all enrolled patients upon admission to the ICU, every 3 days thereafter, and on the day of discharge from the ICU. For each MRSA isolate, we performed multilocus sequence typing, identified the type of staphylococcal cassette chromosome *mec*, detected the presence of the Panton-Valentine leukocidin gene, and conducted drug susceptibility tests. Among the 1,906 patients who were screened, 203 patients were carriers of MRSA before their admission to the ICU; 81 patients acquired MRSA during their stay in the ICU, including 31 who acquired CA-MRSA. The incidence rates of newly acquired MRSA and CA-MRSA during the ICU stay were 7.9 and 3.0 per 1,000 patient-days, respectively. Prior usage of antipseudomonal penicillins and antifungals and the presence of a nasogastric tube were found to be independent risk factors for acquiring CA-MRSA during the ICU stay when data for CA-MRSA carriers and patients without carriage of MRSA were compared ($P = 0.0035$, 0.0330, and 0.0262, respectively). Prior usage of carbapenems was found to be a protective factor against acquiring CA-MRSA when data for

TABLE 3.—Multivariate Analysis of Risk Factors for Acquiring CA-MRSA During ICU Stay

Parameter[a]	CA-MRSA vs no MRSA colonization Odds Ratio (95% CI)	P Value	CA-MRSA vs HA-MRSA Odds Ratio (95% CI)	P Value	P Value of Overall Model
Nasogastric tube	3.53 (1.16–10.75)	0.0262	0.50 (0.11–2.31)	0.3769	0.0001
Anti_2	3.09 (1.45–6.58)	0.0035	2.43 (0.93–6.38)	0.0704	0.0114
Anti_9	0.19 (0.02–1.45)	0.1085	0.08 (0.01–0.72)	0.0238	0.0240
Anti_14	3.45 (1.10–10.74)	0.033	1.74 (0.42–7.14)	0.4441	0.0411

[a]*Abbreviations*: Anti_2, antipseudomonal penicillins; Anti_9, carbapenems; Anti_14, antifungals.

patients with CA-MRSA and those with health care-associated MRSA acquired during ICU stay were compared ($P = 0.0240$).

▶ The past decade saw the emergence of *Staphylococcus aureus* USA 300 clone (CA-methicillin-resistant *Staphylococcus aureus* [MRSA]) as the predominant cause of skin and soft tissue infections in the community.[1,2] This clone was distinct from the strains involved in health care–associated (HA-MRSA) infections. Several studies have demonstrated that CA-MRSA strains are responsible for a significant proportion of health care–associated infections.[3]

This study reports an investigation of the incidence of and risk factors for acquisition of CA-MRSA strains in critically ill patients. Among 1906 patients screened, 203 were colonized by MRSA before admission to the intensive care unit (ICU) based on surveillance cultures taken from nostril, sputum or throat, axillae, and the inguinal area. Acquisition of MRSA during ICU stay was demonstrated in 81 patients. The incidence of acquiring MRSA was calculated to be 7.9 per 1000 patient days.

Of the 284 MRSA isolates (203 with colonization prior to the ICU study and 81 acquired during ICU stay), 52.8% were CA-MRSA strains. Among the patients who acquired MRSA during ICU stay, a significant proportion (31 of 81) were CA-MRSA strains. As shown in Table 3, presence of a nasogastric tube and use of antipseudomonal penicillins and antifungals were independent risk factors for acquiring CA-MRSA in the ICU. All patients with exposure to antifungals had exposure to broad-spectrum antibiotics including antipseudomonal penicillins. Prior use of a carbapenem was actually a protective factor against subsequent acquisition of CA-MRSA compared with acquisition of HA-MRSA. In vitro study showed that CA-MRSA (all susceptible) was 128 times more susceptible to imipenem than HA-MRSA. Interestingly, Talcano et al reported that in vitro activity of carbapenem against CA-MRSA but not HA-MRSA is superior to that of conventional anti-MRSA agents.[4] On the basis of this study, appropriate use of nasogastric tubes and broad-spectrum antibiotics might reduce the spread of CA-MRSA in the ICU setting.

N. M. Khardori, MD, PhD

References

1. King MD, Humphrey BJ, Wany YF, et al. Emergence of community-acquired methicillin-resistant Staphylococcus aureus USA 300 clone as the predominant cause of skin and soft tissue infections. *Ann Intern Med.* 2006;144:309-317.
2. Moran GJ, Krishnadasan A, Gorwitz RJ, et al. EMERGEncy ID Net Study Group. Methicillin-resistant S. aureus infections among patients in the emergency department. *N Engl J Med.* 2006;355:666-674.
3. Maree DL, Daum RS, Boyle-Vavra S. Community-associated methicillin-resistant Staphylococcus aureus isolated causing healthcare-associated infections. *Emerg Infect Dis.* 2007;13:236-242.
4. Takano T, Higuchi W, Yamanoto T. Superior in vitro activity of carbapenems over anti-methicillin-resistant Staphylococcus aureus (MRSA) and some related antimicrobial agents for community-acquired MRSA but not for hospital-acquired MRSA. *J Infect Chemother.* 2009;15:54-57.

Ventilator-Associated Tracheobronchitis in a Mixed Surgical and Medical ICU Population
Dallas J, Skrupky L, Abebe N, et al (Washington Univ School of Medicine, St Louis, MO; Barnes-Jewish Hosp, St Louis, MO; St Luke's Hosp, St Louis, MO)
Chest 139:513-518, 2011

Background.—Ventilator-associated tracheobronchitis (VAT) is considered an intermediate condition between bacterial airway colonization and ventilator-associated pneumonia (VAP). The purpose of this prospective cohort study was to further characterize VAT in terms of incidence, etiology, and impact on patient outcomes.

Methods.—Patients intubated for >48 h in the surgical and medical ICUs of Barnes-Jewish Hospital were screened daily for the development of VAT and VAP over 1 year. Patients were followed until hospital discharge or death, and patient demographics, causative pathogens, and clinical outcomes were recorded.

Results.—A total of 28 patients with VAT and 83 with VAP were identified corresponding to frequencies of 1.4% and 4.0%, respectively. VAP was more common in surgical than medical ICU patients (5.3% vs 2.3%; $P < .001$), but the occurrence of VAT was similar between surgical and medical patients (1.3% vs 1.5%; $P = .845$). VAT progressed to VAP in nine patients (32.1%) despite antibiotic therapy. There was no significant difference in hospital mortality between patients with VAP and VAT (19.3% vs 21.4%; $P = .789$). VAT was caused by a multidrug-resistant (MDR) pathogen in nine cases (32.1%).

Conclusion.—VAT occurs less commonly than VAP but at a similar incidence in medical and surgical ICU patients. VAT frequently progressed to VAP, and patients diagnosed with VAT had similar outcomes to those diagnosed with VAP, suggesting that antimicrobial therapy is appropriate for

VAT. VAT is also frequently caused by MDR organisms, and this should be taken into account when choosing antimicrobial therapy.

▶ Patients on mechanical ventilation are at high risk of airway colonization, including that by multiple drug-resistant (MDR) organisms. The colonization often precedes ventilator-associated pneumonia (VAP). For some patients, an intermediate condition of ventilator-associated tracheobronchitis (VAT) has been described.[1]

This prospective cohort study further characterizes the incidence, etiology, and patient outcomes in VAT compared with patients with VAP over a 365-day period starting January 19, 2009. A total of 2060 patients admitted to medical and surgical intensive care units required mechanical ventilation for more than 48 hours. Based on predefined criteria, 111 patients (5.4%) were identified as having either VAT (28) or VAP (83). These rates of 14% and 40%, respectively, were similar between surgical and medical patients. VAT was caused by MDR pathogens and progressed to VAP in one-third of patients. In-hospital mortality was similar between VAT (21.4%) and VAP (19.3%). The rate of VAT in this study was significantly lower than previously reported.[2] VAP occurred with and without preceding VAT. With mortality rates in VAT comparable to those of VAP, further studies are needed to identify patients needing antibiotics, the optimal duration of therapy, and the role of aerosolized antibiotics.

N. M. Khardori, MD, PhD

References

1. Craven DE, Chroneou A, Zias N, Hjalmarson KI. Ventilator-associated tracheobronchitis: the impact of targeted antibiotic therapy on patient outcomes. *Chest.* 2009;135:521-528.
2. Nseir S, Di Pompeo C, Pronnier P, et al. Nosocomial tracheobronchitis in mechanically ventilated patients: incidence, aetiology and outcome. *Eur Respir J.* 2002;20: 1483-1489.

10 Health Care Associated Infections

Antibiotic Prophylaxis for Dental Procedures to Prevent Indwelling Venous Catheter-related Infections
Hong CHL, Allred R, Napenas JJ, et al (Carolinas Med Ctr, Charlotte, NC; et al)
Am J Med 123:1128-1133, 2010

Background.—Chronic indwelling central venous catheters are used commonly for a variety of indications. A predominant limitation of their use is catheter-related infections. Some clinicians believe that bacteremia from an invasive dental procedure could cause catheter-related infections and that antibiotic prophylaxis may prevent this complication. The topic is controversial, in large part because of the lack of clinical trial data supporting this notion.

Methods.—We performed a systematic review to determine the level of evidence to support this practice. We retrieved studies, guidelines, recommendations, case reports, and editorials on prescribing prophylactic antibiotic therapy for indwelling central venous catheters before oral/dental procedures, using a search of PubMed, National Guideline Clearinghouse, and textbooks.

Results.—There were no clinical trials and no documented cases of a catheter-related infection associated with an invasive dental procedure. Despite the lack of evidence, there are numerous recommendations and guidelines available in the literature that support the administration of "dental" prophylaxis.

Conclusion.—There is no evidence to support the administration of prophylactic antibiotics to prevent catheter-related infections associated with an invasive oral procedure in patients with chronic indwelling central venous catheters.

▶ Infections continue to be a major complication of indwelling venous catheters.[1,2] About two-thirds of the infections originate from the skin, and 30% originate from the catheter hub. Only 5% of catheter-related infections arise from other mechanisms, including contamination of the infusate and hematogenous infection from a distant site.[3] Bacteremia from invasive dental procedures is considered a potential cause of venous-catheter-related infections, and systemic antibiotics are routinely recommended before dental procedures. This review is based on combined search of PubMed, the National Guidelines Clearinghouse, and standard textbooks to identify publications pertaining to prophylactic antibiotic therapy before oral/dental procedures in patients with central venous catheters. No clinical trials to support the use of prophylactic antibiotics prior to dental procedures were found. The common pathogens coagulase-negative *Staphylococci* (37.3%), *Enterococcus* spp (13.5%) and *Staphylococcus aureus* (12.6%) involved in venous-catheter-related infections are typically nonoral in origin, further indicating that antibiotic prophylaxis prior to dental procedures is unnecessary and potentially harmful. Oral bacterial flora contains more than 700 species, most common being gram-positive facultative anaerobic cocci and bacilli. Gram-positive cocci, especially viridian group streptococci and gram-negative bacilli are among the oral pathogens that are reported to cause distant site infections. Because those species are also found in upper respiratory tract and gastrointestinal tract flora, the oral source for these infections are difficult to determine. Based on extensive review of literature and microbiological differences between catheter-related infections pathogens and oral pathogens, there is no evidence to support the use of prophylactic systemic antibiotics for invasive oral procedures to prevent infections of indwelling venous catheters.

N. M. Khardori, MD, PhD

References

1. Mermel LA, Allon M, Bouza E, et al. Clinical practice guidelines for the diagnosis and management of intravascular catheter-related infection: 2009 Update by the Infectious Diseases Society of America. *Clin Infect Dis.* 2009;49:1-45.
2. Bouza E, Burillo A, Muñoz P. Catheter-related infections: diagnosis and intravascular treatment. *Clin Microbiol Infect.* 2002;8:265-274.
3. Yildizeli B, Laçin T, Batirel HF, Yüksel M. Complications and management of long-term central venous access catheters and ports. *J Vasc Access.* 2004;5: 174-178.

11 Clinical Diagnostics

Molecular Probes for Diagnosis of Clinically Relevant Bacterial Infections in Blood Cultures
Hansen WLJ, Beuving J, Bruggeman CA, et al (Maastricht Univ Med Ctr, Netherlands)
J Clin Microbiol 48:4432-4438, 2010

Broad-range real-time PCR and sequencing of the 16S rRNA gene region is a widely known method for the detection and identification of bacteria in clinical samples. However, because of the need for sequencing, such identification of bacteria is time-consuming. The aim of our study was to develop a more rapid 16S real-time PCR-based identification assay using species- or genus-specific probes. The Gram-negative bacteria were divided into *Pseudomonas* species, *Pseudomonas aeruginosa*, *Escherichia coli*, and other Gram-negative species. Within the Gram-positive species, probes were designed for *Staphylococcus* species, *Staphylococcus aureus*, *Enterococcus* species, *Streptococcus* species, and *Streptococcus pneumoniae*. The assay also included a universal probe within the 16S rRNA gene region for the detection of all bacterial DNA. The assay was evaluated with a collection of 248 blood cultures. In this study, the universal probe and the probes targeting *Pseudomonas* spp., *P. aeruginosa*, *E. coli*, *Streptococcus* spp., *S. pneumoniae*, *Enterococcus* spp., and *Staphylococcus* spp. all had a sensitivity and specificity of 100%. The probe specific for *S. aureus* showed eight discrepancies, resulting in a sensitivity of 100% and a specificity of 93%. These data showed high agreement between conventional testing and our novel real-time PCR assay. Furthermore, this assay significantly reduced the time needed for identification. In conclusion, using pathogen-specific probes offers a faster alternative for pathogen detection and could improve the diagnosis of bloodstream infections.

▶ Blood stream infections (BSIs) remain a major worldwide cause of morbidity and mortality. Conventional culture-based methods of diagnosis are time dependent and therefore not very helpful in choosing appropriate antimicrobial therapy during the initial 48 to 72 hours. Molecular techniques for the direct detection of bacteria and viral pathogens are already in use. However, most of these assays do not offer broad-range pathogen detection and are targeted toward single bacterial or viral agents. Several polymerase chain reaction (PCR) assays have been developed recently that target panels of most relevant bacterial and fungal pathogens in BSIs. Factors that hamper direct detection in whole blood include presence of PCR inhibitors and background DNA and low bacterial load.[1] In addition to

TABLE 1.—Probes Designed for Use in Multiplex PCR

Probe	Sequence (5′−3′)[a]
Pseudomonas species	NED-CCTTCCTCCCAACTTAAAGTGCTT-MGB
P. aeruginosa	JOE-CCAAAACTACTGAGCTAGAGTACG-BHQ1
E. coli	JOE-GGAGTAAAGTTAATACCTTTGCTCATT-BHQ1
Staphylococcus species	NED-AATCTTCCGCAATGGGCGAAAGC-MGB
S. aureus	FAM-AGATGTGCACAGTTACTTACACATAT-BHQ1
Enterococcus species	JOE-TCCTTGTTCTTCTCTAACAACAGAG-BHQ1
Streptococcus species	NED-CCAGAAAGGGACSGCTAACT-MGB
S. pneumoniae	JOE-CCAAAGCCTACTATGGTTAAGCCA-BHQ1

[a]NED, fluorescent label (Applied Biosystems); MGB, minor groove binder; JOE, 6-carboxy-4,5-dichloro-2,7-dimethyoxyfluorescein; BHQ1, black hole quencher 1; FAM, 6-carboxyfluorescein.

broad-range real-time RCR, sequencing of the 16s rRNA gene region has been widely used for detection and identification of bacteria in clinical samples.[2] These assays for identification of bacteria are time-consuming because of the need for sequencing.

This study aimed at developing a more rapid 16s real-time PCR-based identification assay using species or genus specific probes. The assay was particularly intended for gram stain positive blood samples. Table 1 lists the probes and their sequence used to detect common gram positive and gram negative BSI pathogens. A universal probe within the 16s RNA gene region for the detection of all bacterial DNA was included. The universal probe and the probe targeting *Pseudomonas* spp, *Pseudomonas aeruginosa*, *Escherichia coli*, *Streptococcus* spp, *Streptococcus pneumoniae*, *Enterococcus* spp, and *Staphylococcus* spp had a sensitivity and specificity of 100%. *Streptococcus aureus* probe showed a sensitivity of 100% and specificity of 93%. The correlation with conventional testing was high. The assay was completed in 2 hours and designed for blood culture material to do susceptibility testing. The turnaround time could be further shortened by using whole blood samples. A further use of such assays will be in quantitation of genomic bacterial load and virulence factors, both of which have major clinical implications.

N. M. Khardori, MD, PhD

References

1. Hansen WL, Bruggeman CA, Wolffs PF. Evaluation of new preanalysis sample treatment tools and DNA isolation protocols to improve bacterial pathogen detection in whole blood. *J Clin Microbiol.* 2009;47:2629-2631.
2. Wellinghausen N, Kochem AJ, Disqué C, et al. Diagnosis of bacteremia in whole-blood samples by use of a commercial universal 16s rRNA gene-based PCR and sequence analysis. *J Clin Microbiol.* 2009;47:2759-2765.

PCR Diagnosis of Invasive Candidiasis: Systematic Review and Meta-Analysis

Avni T, Leibovici L, Paul M (Tel-Aviv Univ, Israel)
J Clin Microbiol 49:665-670, 2011

Invasive candidiasis (IC) is a significant cause of morbidity and mortality. Diagnosis relies on culture-based methods, which lack sensitivity and delay diagnosis. We conducted a systematic review assessing the diagnostic accuracy of PCR-based methods to detect *Candida* spp. directly in blood samples. We searched electronic databases for prospective or retrospective cohort and case-control studies. Two reviewers abstracted data independently. Meta-analysis was performed using a hierarchical logistic regression model. Random-effects metaregression was performed to assess the effects of study methods and infection characteristics on sensitivity or specificity values. We included 54 studies with 4,694 patients, 963 of whom had proven/probable or possible IC. Perfect (100%) sensitivity and specificity for PCR in whole-blood samples was observed when patients with cases had candidemia and controls were healthy people. When PCR was performed to evaluate patients with suspected invasive candidiasis, the pooled sensitivity for the diagnosis of candidemia was 0.95 (confidence interval, 0.88 to 0.98) and the pooled specificity was 0.92 (0.88 to 0.95). A specificity of >90% was maintained in several analyses considering different control groups. The use of whole-blood samples, rRNA, or P450 gene targets and a PCR detection limit of ≤10 CFU/ml were associated with improved test performance. PCR positivity rates among patients with proven or probable IC were 85% (78 to 91%), while blood cultures were positive for 38% (29 to 46%). We conclude that direct PCR using blood samples had good sensitivity and specificity for the diagnosis of IC and offers an attractive method for early diagnosis of specific *Candida* spp. Its effects on clinical outcomes should be investigated.

▶ Invasive candidiasis (IC) has emerged as a serious cause of morbidity and mortality, with patients in intensive care units being at the highest risk.[1] Antemortem diagnosis of IC is missed in 50% of patients.[2] The laboratory diagnosis from blood cultures takes 24 to 48 hours to become positive and more time to identify species. This makes the use of empiric antifungal treatment for high-risk patients prevalent with inherent cost, adverse effects, and development of resistance to antifungal agents. DNA detection by polymerase chain reaction (PCR) and other nonculture–based methods has been developed for rapid diagnosis of IC.

This article analyzed data from prospective, retrospective cohort and case-control studies and performed a systematic review to assess the diagnostic accuracy of direct PCR on blood samples for IC. In comparison to whole-blood cultures (positive for 29%—46%), the sensitivity of PCR-based tests for proven or probable IC was 85% and specificity was greater than 90%.

In the studies that compared patients with candidemia with healthy control subjects, the sensitivity and specificity of PCR of whole-blood samples targeting panfungal genes was 100%. In addition to the advantage of earlier diagnosis, PCR assays offer the possibility of monitoring the persistence or resolution of infection. Persistent positive candida PCR results on blood have been associated with higher mortality. PCR assays have added to targeted therapy against candida species as early as 6 hours after the onset of sepsis. The authors recommend testing of patients with suspected IC by PCR accompanied by blood cultures and serial sampling for patients at high risk.

The use of panfungal PCR applied to whole-blood samples would allow the use of the same assay for early diagnosis of invasive aspergillus and invasive candidiasis in high-risk patients.

N. M. Khardori, MD, PhD

References

1. Wisplinghoff H, Bischoff T, Tallent SM, Seifert H, Wenzel RP, Edmond MB. Nosocomial bloodstream infections in US hospitals: analysis of 24,179 cases from a prospective nationwide surveillance study. *Clin Infect Dis.* 2004;39:309-317.
2. Ellepola AN, Morrison CJ. Laboratory diagnosis of invasive candidiasis. *J Microbiol.* 2005;43:65-84.

Rapid Stool-Based Diagnosis of *Clostridium difficile* Infection by Real-Time PCR in a Children's Hospital

Luna RA, Boyanton BL Jr, Mehta S, et al (Baylor College of Medicine, Houston, TX; Beaumont Hosps, Royal Oak, MI; et al)
J Clin Microbiol 49:851-857, 2011

Clostridium difficile is a major cause of nosocomial antibiotic-associated infectious diarrhea and pseudomembranous colitis. Detection of *C. difficile* by anaerobic bacterial culture and/or cytotoxicity assays has been largely replaced by rapid enzyme immunoassays (EIA). However, due to the lack of sensitivity of stool EIA, we developed a multiplex real-time PCR assay targeting the *C. difficile* toxin genes *tcdA* and *tcdB*. Stool samples from hospitalized pediatric patients suspected of having *C. difficile*-associated disease were prospectively cultured on cycloserine-cefoxitin-fructose agar following alcohol shock. Six testing modalities were evaluated, including stool EIA, culture EIA, and real-time PCR (*tcdA* and *tcdB*) of cultured isolates and stool samples. Real-time PCR detection was performed with *tcdA* and *tcdB* gene-specific primers and hydrolysis probes using the Light-Cycler platforms (Roche Diagnostics, Indianapolis, IN). A total of 157 samples from 96 pediatric patients were analyzed. The sensitivities of stool real-time PCR and stool EIA were 95% and 35%, respectively, with a specificity of 100% for both methods. The lower limit of detection of the stool real-time PCR was 30 CFU/ml of stool sample per reaction for *tcdA* and *tcdB*. This study highlights the poor performance of stool toxin EIAs in pediatric settings. Direct detection of *C. difficile* toxin genes in stool samples by real-time PCR showed sensitivity superior to that of stool and culture EIAs and performance comparable to that of real-time PCR assay of cultured isolates. Real-time PCR of DNA from stool samples

TABLE 1.—Performance Characteristics of Various Testing Modalities Compared to Those of Our Defined Reference Standard[a] for the Detection of Toxigenic *C. difficile* in Patients[b] Clinically Suspected of Having CDAD

| | EIA | | | Real-Time PCR | | | | |
| | Stool | | | Culture | | | Stool sample | |
Result or Parameter	Sample[e]	Culture	*tcdA*	*tcdB*	*tcdAB*[f]	*tcdA*	*tcdB*	*tcdAB*[f]
No. of samples:								
True positive	7	15	17	18	18	18	18	19
True negative	118	118	118	118	118	118	118	118
False positive	0	0	0	0	0	0	0	0
False negative	13	5	3	2	2	2	2	1
% Sensitivity	35	75	85	90	90	90	90	95
% Specificity	100	100	100	100	100	100	100	100
PPV (%)[c]	100	100	100	100	100	100	100	100
NPV (%)[d]	90	96	98	98	98	98	98	99
TAT[e]	<2 h	3—5 days	3—5 days	3—5 days	3—5 days	<4 h	<4 h	<4 h

[a]The reference standard was any stool specimen positive by at least four of the following six testing modalities: (i) stool EIA, (ii) culture EIA, (iii) culture real-time PCR (*tcdA*), (iv) culture real-time PCR (*tcdB*), (v) stool real-time PCR (*tcdA*), and (vi) stool real-time PCR (*tcdB*). The performance characteristics of each individual testing modality were subsequently compared to those of this reference standard.
[b]Total *n* = 138.
[c]PPV, positive predictive value.
[d]NPV, negative predictive value.
[e]TAT, turnaround time.
[f]Combination of singleplex assay results for *tcdA* and *tcdB*.

is a rapid and cost-effective diagnostic modality for children that should facilitate appropriate patient management and halt the practice of serial testing by EIA.

▶ *Clostridium difficile* was originally described as a member of the commensal microflora in neonates. Although neonatal colonization with toxin-producing *C difficile* is well documented, recent studies suggest an increase in the incidence of *C difficile*—associated diarrhea (CDAD) in children, including infants.[1,2] The prevalence of CDAD in children including infants increased by 53% between 2001 and 2006 with 26% of patients being less than 1 year old. Routine culture methods for *C difficile* (which lack the discrimination between toxigenic and nontoxigenic isolates) and cytotoxic assays have largely been replaced by rapid-detection testing (glutamate dehydrogenase) and toxin immunoassays. Both types of assays lack desired sensitivity and specificity to confirm or rule out the diagnosis of CDAD reliably. The lighter bacterial load in children may further decrease the sensitivity of these assays. These shortfalls in current assays has led to investigation of real-time polymerase chain reaction (PCR) for diagnosis of CDAD.

This prospective study describes a multiplex real-time PCR assay targeting the *C difficile* toxin genes *tcdA* and *tcdB*. Stool samples from hospitalized patients (15 days to 25 years, median 4 years) suspected of having CDAD were tested by stool culture, stool enzyme immunoassay (EIA), culture EIA, real-time PCR of stool sample, and cultured isolates. Table 1 compares the performance of various tests. All tests had a specificity of 100%. The sensitivity of PCR-based tests was 90% to 95% compared with 35% for EIA on stool samples. Turnaround time for stool sample EIA was less than 2 hours and for stool sample PCR was less than 4 hours. This real-time PCR assay using stool samples was highly sensitive with a short turnaround time for the diagnosis of CDAD in hospitalized children. This would make it a cost-effective means of diagnosis without the need for serial testing by EIA.

N. M. Khardori, MD, PhD

References

1. Baker SS, Faden H, Sayej W, et al. Increasing incidence of community associated atypical *Clostridium difficile* disease in children. *Clin Pediatr (Phila)*. 2010;49: 644-647.
2. Zilberberg MD, Tillotson GS, McDonald C. *Clostridium difficile* infections among hospitalized children, United States, 1997–2006. *Emerg Infect Dis*. 2010;16: 604-609.

12 Fungal Infections

Candida **bloodstream infections in intensive care units: Analysis of the extended prevalence of infection in intensive care unit study**
Kett DH, for the Extended Prevalence of Infection in the ICU Study (EPIC II) Group of Investigators (The Univ of Miami Miller School of Medicine and Jackson Memorial Hosp, FL; et al)
Crit Care Med 39:665-670, 2011

Objectives.—To provide a global, up-to-date picture of the prevalence, treatment, and outcomes of *Candida* bloodstream infections in intensive care unit patients and compare *Candida* with bacterial bloodstream infection.

Design.—A retrospective analysis of the Extended Prevalence of Infection in the ICU Study (EPIC II). Demographic, physiological, infection-related and therapeutic data were collected. Patients were grouped as having *Candida*, Gram-positive, Gram-negative, and combined *Candida/*bacterial bloodstream infection. Outcome data were assessed at intensive care unit and hospital discharge.

Setting.—EPIC II included 1265 intensive care units in 76 countries.

Patients.—Patients in participating intensive care units on study day.

Interventions.—None.

Measurement and Main Results.—Of the 14,414 patients in EPIC II, 99 patients had *Candida* bloodstream infections for a prevalence of 6.9 per 1000 patients. Sixty-one patients had candidemia alone and 38 patients had combined bloodstream infections. *Candida albicans* (n = 70) was the predominant species. Primary therapy included monotherapy with fluconazole (n = 39), caspofungin (n = 16), and a polyene-based product (n = 12). Combination therapy was infrequently used (n = 10). Compared with patients with Gram-positive (n = 420) and Gram-negative (n = 264) bloodstream infections, patients with candidemia were more likely to have solid tumors ($p < .05$) and appeared to have been in an intensive care unit longer (14 days [range, 5−25 days], 8 days [range, 3−20 days], and 10 days [range, 2−23 days], respectively), but this difference was not statistically significant. Severity of illness and organ dysfunction scores were similar between groups. Patients with *Candida* bloodstream infections, compared with patients with Gram-positive and Gram-negative bloodstream infections, had the greatest crude intensive care unit mortality rates (42.6%, 25.3%, and 29.1%, respectively) and longer intensive care unit lengths of stay (median [interquartile range]) (33 days [18−44], 20 days [9−43], and 21 days [8−46], respectively); however, these differences were not statistically significant.

Conclusion.—Candidemia remains a significant problem in intensive care units patients. In the EPIC II population, *Candida albicans* was the most common organism and fluconazole remained the predominant anti-fungal agent used. *Candida* bloodstream infections are associated with high intensive care unit and hospital mortality rates and resource use.

▶ Blood stream infections (BSI) due to *Candida* spp are the third and fourth leading cause of BSIs in intensive care unit (ICU) and non-ICU hospitalized patients in the United States.[1] Invasive candidiasis including *Candida* BSIs are the most common fungal infections among hospitalized patients. The crude mortality rate from these infections is 35% to 67%. In addition, the estimated economic burden associated with an episode of *Candida* BSI is 25,000 to 55 000 US dollars. Although fluconazole remains an effective agent for treatment of BSI, especially when used early, recent treatment guideline from the Infectious Diseases Society of America favor the use of echinocandins for primary therapy in moderately to severely ill patients.[2] The geographic and regional differences is the incidence of different *Candida* spp are well documented. In the United States, *Candida albicans* followed by *Candida glabrata* are the most common species involved in blood stream infections. Susceptibility of various classes of antifungal agents varies among species.

The Extended Prevalence of Infection in Intensive Care study provided a global picture (1256 intensive care units in 76 countries) of the extent and patterns of infections in ICUs.[3] This is a retrospective study of prevalence, epidemiology, treatment choices, and outcomes of *Candida* BSI in this world-wide sample of ICU patients. Of the 14 414 adult patients in this study, 99 had *Candida* BSI with a prevalence of 6.87 per 1000 ICU patients. Both candida and bacterial BSI was documented in 38 patients. *Candida albicans* was the predominant species (70% of isolates) in all regions (Table 1 in the original article). Fluconazole monotherapy (40% followed by monotherapy) with echinocandins (16.2%) and amphotericin B—based agents (12.4%) was similar among various regions. ICU mortality rates were 42.6 for candida, 25.3% for gram-positive BSI, 29.1% for gram-negative, and 31% for combination BSI, respectively. Because of high ICU and hospital mortality rates and difficulty in early diagnosis of *Candida* BSI, a high index of suspicion based on risk factor and early presumptive therapy should it be considered.

N. M. Khardori, MD, PhD

References

1. Wisplinghoff H, Bischoff T, Tallent SM. Nosocomial bloodstream infections in US hospitals: analysis of 24,179 cases from a prospective nationwide surveillance study. *Clin Infect Dis.* 2004;39:309-317.
2. Pappas PG, Kauffman CA, Andes D, et al. Clinical practice guidelines for the management of candidiasis: 2009 update by the Infectious Diseases society of America. *Clin Infect Dis.* 2009;48:503-535.
3. Vincent JL, Rello J, Marshall J, et al. International study of the prevalence and outcomes of infection in intensive care units. *JAMA.* 2009;302:2323-2329.

Efficacy and Safety of Posaconazole for Chronic Pulmonary Aspergillosis

Felton TW, Baxter C, Moore CB, et al (The Univ of Manchester, UK)

Clin Infect Dis 51:1383-1391, 2010

Background.—Chronic pulmonary aspergillosis (CPA) is a severe, progressive respiratory infection characterized by multiple pulmonary cavities and increased levels of antibodies to *Aspergillus* species. We report the first use of posaconazole in patients with CPA.

Methods.—A retrospective study was performed. A composite clinical and radiological evaluation was used to assess response to posaconazole therapy. The rates of clinical response and failure after 6 and 12 months of therapy were determined. Kaplan-Meier survival models were developed to describe the time to clinical response and failure. The underlying diagnosis, the type of therapy (primary or salvage), *Aspergillus* antibody titer, and posaconazole serum concentrations were assessed as covariates. *Aspergillus* species were identified and minimum inhibitory concentrations (MICs) of triazoles were determined using standard techniques.

Results.—There were 79 patients that initially received posaconazole 400 mg twice per day. The median age of patients was 61 years, and 57% were male. Response to posaconazole was observed in 61% of patients at 6 months and in 46% at 12 months. Kaplan-Meier plots showed that the first response to posaconazole was observed in some patients only after approximately 1 year of therapy. Covariates were not significant. Adverse reactions were observed in 12 patients (15%) (nausea in 5, rash in 5, headache in 1, and lethargy in 1), leading to withdrawal of treatment for 9 patients. *Aspergillus* species were recovered from 22 patients. A posaconazole MIC of >8 mg/L was found in 4 isolates; in 1 of these isolates, this emerged during therapy. Treatment failed in all 4 patients from whom these 4 isolates had been recovered.

Conclusion.—Posaconazole is a safe and partially effective treatment for CPA. Prospective comparative studies are now required.

▶ Chronic pulmonary aspergillosis (CPA) is a cavitary fungal infection of lung with a progressive course and 5-year mortality comparable to that for cancers.[1] It is typically seen in patients with underlying structural lung disease and adds significantly to respiratory and systemic symptoms.[2] The long-term administration of intravenous antifungal agents such as amphotericin B and echinocandins is impractical and expensive. Oral triazole antifungal agents have been the mainstay of treatment of CPA.[3] The long-term use of itraconazole and voriconazole is complicated by toxicity and emergence of resistance in the case of itraconazole. Posaconazole, a newer broad-spectrum triazole agent has proven effective and safe for prevention and treatment of a number of invasive fungal infections and has potent activity against *Aspergillus* species.

This is a retrospective study of patients with CPA treated with posaconazole at a single referral center in the United Kingdom. Posaconazole was used in 79 patients, in 21 for primary therapy and in 58 for salvage therapy. The median duration of therapy for the primary and salvage groups was 28 and 31 weeks, respectively. Sixty-seven patients received the drug for at least 6 months. At 6 months, treatment was successful for 61% (41 of 67 patients) and failed for 39%. At 12 months, posaconazole therapy was successful for 46% and failed for 54%. Posaconazole therapy was well tolerated, including by the patients with adverse events from other triazoles. Of the patients with *Aspergillus* sp infection resistant to itraconazole (minimum inhibitory concentrations [MIC] of > 8 mg/L) and susceptible to posaconazole (MIC < 1 mg/L), 50% responded to posaconazole therapy. All patients infected by isolates with posaconazole MIC greater than 8 mg/L failed to respond to therapy. Although this was not a comparative study, posaconazole seems to be at least as effective as other agents for CPA and is well tolerated.

N. M. Khardori, MD, PhD

References

1. Nam HS, Jeon K, Um SW, et al. Clinical characteristics and treatment outcomes of chronic necrotizing pulmonary aspergillosis: a review of 43 cases. *Int J Infect Dis.* 2010;14:e479-e482.
2. Denning DW, Riniotis K, Dobrashian R, Sambatakou H. Chronic cavitary and fibrosing pulmonary and pleural aspergillosis: case series, proposed nomenclature change, and review. *Clin Infect Dis.* 2003;37:S265-S280.
3. Walsh TJ, Anaissie EJ, Denning DW, et al. Treatment of aspergillosis: clinical practice guidelines of the Infectious Diseases Society of America. *Clin Infect Dis.* 2008; 46:327-360.

13 New Antibiotics

Fidaxomicin versus Vancomycin for *Clostridium difficile* Infection
Louie TJ, for the OPT-80-003 Clinical Study Group (Univ of Calgary, Alberta, Canada; et al)
N Engl J Med 364:422-431, 2011

Background.—*Clostridium difficile* infection is a serious diarrheal illness associated with substantial morbidity and mortality. Patients generally have a response to oral vancomycin or metronidazole; however, the rate of recurrence is high. This phase 3 clinical trial compared the efficacy and safety of fidaxomicin with those of vancomycin in treating C. *difficile* infection.

Methods.—Adults with acute symptoms of C. *difficile* infection and a positive result on a stool toxin test were eligible for study entry. We randomly assigned patients to receive fidaxomicin (200 mg twice daily) or vancomycin (125 mg four times daily) orally for 10 days. The primary end point was clinical cure (resolution of symptoms and no need for further therapy for C. *difficile* infection as of the second day after the end of the course of therapy). The secondary end points were recurrence of C. *difficile* infection (diarrhea and a positive result on a stool toxin test within 4 weeks after treatment) and global cure (i.e., cure with no recurrence).

Results.—A total of 629 patients were enrolled, of whom 548 (87.1%) could be evaluated for the per-protocol analysis. The rates of clinical cure with fidaxomicin were noninferior to those with vancomycin in both the modified intention-to-treat analysis (88.2% with fidaxomicin and 85.8% with vancomycin) and the per-protocol analysis (92.1% and 89.8%, respectively). Significantly fewer patients in the fidaxomicin group than in the vancomycin group had a recurrence of the infection, in both the modified intention-to-treat analysis (15.4% vs. 25.3%, P = 0.005) and the per-protocol analysis (13.3% vs. 24.0%, P = 0.004). The lower rate of recurrence was seen in patients with non–North American Pulsed Field type 1 strains. The adverse-event profile was similar for the two therapies.

Conclusions.—The rates of clinical cure after treatment with fidaxomicin were noninferior to those after treatment with vancomycin. Fidaxomicin was associated with a significantly lower rate of recurrence of C. *difficile* infection associated with non–North American Pulsed Field type 1 strains. (Funded by Optimer Pharmaceuticals; ClinicalTrials.gov number, NCT00314951.)

▶ *Clostridium difficile* infection (CDI) has been increasing in incidence, severity, and mortality. Much of this increase has been ascribed to the emergence of hypervirulent strain of *C difficile* referred to collectively as *NAP1/BI/027*.[1,2] CDI is now reported in populations previously considered to be at low risk, including young, healthy people in the community and peripartum women. The reduced rates of clinical response to metronidazole and vancomycin along with increased recurrence rates seen currently have led to the study of alternate therapies.

This study compares vancomycin with a new agent, fidaxomicin, in a prospective, multicenter, double-blind, randomized, parallel group phase 3 clinical trial conducted between May 9, 2000, and August 21, 2008. After diagnosis based on symptoms and a positive result on stool toxin test, patients were assigned randomly to receive fidaxomicin (200 mg twice daily) or vancomycin (125 mg 4 times daily) orally for 10 days. In the intention-to-treat analyses of a total of 596 patients, 287 received fidaxomicin, and 309 received vancomycin. A total of 548 patients were included in the per-protocol analysis (265 in the fidaxomicin subgroup and 283 in the vancomycin subgroup). In this group, clinical cure occurred in 92.1% of fidaxomicin and 89.8% of vancomycin recipients (Fig 2 in original article). The difference in recurrence rates was significant between the 2 groups (13.3% for fidaxomicin versus 24% for vancomycin) as was the difference in global cure, 77.7% for fidaxomicin versus 67.1% for vancomycin. Global cure was defined as cure with no recurrence. *C difficile* isolates belonging to the 027 strain were present in 35.5% and 36.4% of fidaxomicin and vancomycin groups, respectively, with no difference in recurrence rates between the groups. A lower rate of recurrence was seen in patients with non-027 strains. Significantly, fidaxomicin caused a 69% relative reduction in recurrence rate compared with vancomycin. No difference in adverse events or serious adverse events was noted between the 2 treatment groups. This trial has shown that fidaxomicin, a macrocyclic antibiotic, is safe and as effective as vancomycin in the treatment of CDI with significantly lower rates of recurrence in infections with non-027 strains.

N. M. Khardori, MD, PhD

References

1. McDonald LC, Killgore GE, Thompson A, et al. An epidemic, toxin gene-variant strain of *Clostridium difficile*. N Engl J Med. 2005;353:2433-2441.
2. Zilberberg MD, Shorr AF, Kollef MH. Increase in adult *Clostridium difficile*-related hospitalizations and case fatality rate, United States 2000–2005. *Emerg Infect Dis*. 2008;14:929-931.

Telavancin versus Vancomycin for Hospital-Acquired Pneumonia due to Gram-positive Pathogens
Rubinstein E, for the ATTAIN Study Group (Univ of Manitoba, Winnipeg, Canada; et al)
Clin Infect Dis 52:31-40, 2011

Background.—Telavancin is a lipoglycopeptide bactericidal against gram-positive pathogens.

Methods.—Two methodologically identical, double-blind studies (0015 and 0019) were conducted involving patients with hospital-acquired pneumonia (HAP) due to gram-positive pathogens, particularly methicillin-resistant *Staphylococcus aureus* (MRSA). Patients were randomized 1:1 to telavancin (10 mg/kg every 24 h) or vancomycin (1 g every 12 h) for 7–21 days. The primary end point was clinical response at follow-up/test-of-cure visit.

Results.—A total of 1503 patients were randomized and received study medication (the all-treated population). In the pooled alltreated population, cure rates with telavancin versus vancomycin were 58.9% versus 59.5% (95% confidence interval [CI] for the difference, −5.6% to 4.3%). In the pooled clinically evaluable population ($n = 654$), cure rates were 82.4% with telavancin and 80.7% with vancomycin (95% CI for the difference, −4.3% to 7.7%). Treatment with telavancin achieved higher cure rates in patients with monomicrobial *S. aureus* infection and comparable cure rates in patients with MRSA infection; in patients with mixed gram-positive/gram-negative infections, cure rates were higher in the vancomycin group. Incidence and types of adverse events were comparable between the treatment groups. Mortality rates for telavancin-treated versus vancomycin-treated patients were 21.5% versus 16.6% (95% CI for the difference, −0.7% to 10.6%) for study 0015 and 18.5% versus 20.6% (95% CI for the difference, −7.8% to 3.5%) for study 0019. Increases in serum creatinine level were more common in the telavancin group (16% vs 10%).

Conclusions.—The primary end point of the studies was met, indicating that telavancin is noninferior to vancomycin on the basis of clinical response in the treatment of HAP due to gram-positive pathogens.

▶ Hospital-acquired pneumonia (HAP) is the leading cause of mortality attributable to nosocomial infections.[1] Among the bacterial causes, *Staphylococcus aureus*, particularly methicillin-resistant *S aureus* (MRSA), is now a significant cause of HAP.[2] Currently vancomycin and linezolid are recommended for HAP caused by MRSA.[3] Vancomycin has the disadvantage of poor penetration into tissues including lung tissue. Linezolid has bacteriostatic activity against *S aureus*.

This article describes 2 identical randomized, double-blind, comparator-controlled, parallel-group Phase III trials for the Assessment of telavancin for Treatment of Hospital Acquired Pneumonia (ATTAIN). Adult patients older than 18 years were enrolled between January 2005 and June 2007. Telavancin is a lipoglycopeptide bactericidal agent against gram-positive pathogens. It acts by a dual mechanism of inhibition of cell wall synthesis and disruption of membrane barrier function. It penetrates well into the lung achieving 8-fold concentration in epithelial lining fluid and 85-fold concentration in alveolar macrophages of healthy subjects compared with minimum inhibitory concentration required for 90% of MRSA strains. In this study, telavancin was compared with vancomycin for the treatment of HAP. Microbiological characteristics of the patients are shown in Table 2 in the original article. *S aureus* was the most predominant organism The efficacy results of 2 telavancin groups (from 2 studies) were similar to that of vancomycin (ie, 58.9% for telavancin and 59.5% for vancomycin). The incidence of adverse events was comparable between the 2 groups.

N. M. Khardori, MD, PhD

References

1. Kollef MH. Prevention of hospital-associated pneumonia and ventilator-associated pneumonia. *Crit Care Med.* 2004;32:1396-1405.
2. Kollef MH, Shorr A, Tabak YP, Gupta V, Liu LZ, Johannes RS. Epidemiology and outcomes of health-care-associated pneumonia: results from a large US database of culture-positive pneumonia. *Chest.* 2005;128:3854-3862.
3. American Thoracic Society; Infectious Diseases Society of America. Guidelines for the management of adults with hospital-acquired, ventilator-associated, and healthcare-associated pneumonia. *Am J Respir Crit Care Med.* 2005;171: 388-416.

Anti-BK Virus Mechanisms of Sirolimus and Leflunomide Alone and in Combination: Toward a New Therapy for BK Virus Infection

Liacini A, Seamone ME, Muruve DA, et al (Univ of Calgary, Alberta, Canada)
Transplantation 90:1450-1457, 2010

Background.—Human BK polyomavirus is the causative agent of BK nephropathy which is now the leading cause of early renal graft loss. Although no randomized clinical trials have supported this therapy, reduction of immunosuppressive drugs is the current BK nephropathy treatment. We hypothesized that inhibition of the intracellular protein kinase pathways activated by BK virus may be a more effective therapeutic strategy than reduction of immunosuppression.

Methods and Results.—Four days after infection of renal epithelial cells lines CCD1103, CCD1105 and human primary tubular epithelial cells with BK virus, we found increased phosphorylation of 3'-phosphoinositide-dependent kinase-1 (PDK-1), the protein kinase Akt (Akt), mammalian target of rapamycin (mTOR), and 70 kDa ribosomal protein S6 kinase (p70S6K). To inhibit this pathway, we used sirolimus, which repressed p70S6K phosphorylation and reduced BK virus large T antigen expression in a dose-dependent manner. We then used the tyrosine kinase inhibitor leflunomide (using the active metabolite A77 1726), which decreased PDK1 and Akt phosphorylation and inhibited BK virus genome replication and early gene expression. The combination of sirolimus and leflunomide inhibited BK virus genome replication, large T antigen expression, PDK1, Akt, mammalian target of rapamycin, and p70S6K phosphorylation.

Conclusions.—On the basis of these results, we suggest that inhibition of protein kinase pathways with a combination of sirolimus and leflunomide may be an effective therapy for BK virus reactivation. Because both sirolimus and leflunomide possess immunosuppressive activity, combination therapy may reduce BK pathogenesis while maintaining appropriate transplant immunosuppression.

▶ Infections caused by BK virus, a polyomavirus, have emerged as a cause of renal transplant dysfunction and loss secondary to BK nephropathy.[1] The current approach to management is the reduction of immunosuppressive therapy with the rationale of allowing host immune mechanism to restrict viral replication.[2] This approach risks an increase in acute and subclinical rejection of the transplant. Simian virus 40 (SV40) and murine polyomavirus have been studied well. Polyomaviruses trigger host intracellular signaling, cause host DNA replication, and activate protein translational pathways.

This investigation studied the potential of impairing the host intracellular (protein kinase activation) signaling pathways activated by BK virus and its effect on viral proliferation in renal epithelial cell lines. They used sirolimus and leflunomide alone or in combination to inhibit protein kinase pathways in BK virus.

The combination of sirolimus and leflunomide inhibited multiple functions in the BK virus, including genome replication and large T tumor antigen. These data pave a way for further studies of therapeutic agents for the treatment of BK nephropathy.

N. M. Khardori, MD, PhD

References

1. Hirsch HH, Randhawa P; AST Infectious Diseases Community of Practice. BK virus in solid organ transplant recipients. *Am J Transplant.* 2009;9:S136-S146.
2. Hardinger KL, Koch MJ, Bohl DJ, Storch GA, Brennan DC. BK-virus and the impact of pre-emptive immunosuppression reduction: 5-year results. *Am J Transplant.* 2010;10:407-415.

14 Viral Infections

Herpes zoster and meningitis due to reactivation of varicella vaccine virus in an immunocompetent child
Han J-Y, Hanson DC, Way SS (Univ of Minnesota Med School, Minneapolis)
Pediatr Infect Dis J 30:266-268, 2011

Neurologic complications from varicella zoster virus (VZV) reactivation are rare. In this article, we describe a previously immunized child who developed herpes zoster with meningitis. Vaccine strain of VZV was recovered from a skin swab and the cerebrospinal fluid. Reactivation of the vaccine strain of VZV should be recognized as a potential cause of meningitis in children.

▶ Recent studies have demonstrated that the vaccine strain of varicella zoster virus (VZV) is a potential cause of reactivation herpes zoster in immunocompetent and immunocompromised children.[1] The clinical severity of VZV disease is milder in vaccinated children compared with those with wild-type VZV infection. In general, VZV reactivation disease involving the central nervous system is a rare complication.

This report describes a 7-year-old previously healthy boy with right arm pain and rash consistent with herpes zoster. The child was vaccinated at age 12 months. There was no evidence of meningitis or alteration in mental status. The cerebrospinal fluid (CSF) showed 16 white blood cell count with 71% lymphocytes, protein was 29 mg/dL, and glucose was 57 mg/dL. CSF and a swab from a skin lesion were positive for VZV by polymerase chain reaction, and both VZV isolates were identified as the vaccine strain. No clinical or laboratory evidence of immunodeficiency was detected. Patient recovered completely after a 21-day course of intravenous acyclovir (10 mg/kg every 8 hours). The authors speculate that the incidence of meningitis caused by the reactivation of vaccine VZV strain may be on the rise given the routine childhood immunization. The VZV isolated from patients presenting with meningitis should be tested to establish the incidence and risk of this rare vaccine complication. On a more general clinical note, the likelihood of VZV meningitis should not be excluded totally because of prior vaccination.

N. M. Khardori, MD, PhD

Reference

1. Galea SA, Sweet A, Beninger P, et al. The safety profile of varicella vaccine: a 10-year review. *J Infect Dis.* 2008;197:S165-S169.

Herpes Zoster Recurrences More Frequent Than Previously Reported

Yawn BP, Wollan PC, Kurland MJ, et al (Olmsted Med Ctr, Rochester, MN; et al)
Mayo Clin Proc 86:88-93, 2011

Objective.—To present population-based estimates of herpes zoster (HZ) recurrence rates among adults.

Patients and Methods.—To identify recurrent cases of HZ, we reviewed the medical records (through December 31, 2007) of all Olmsted County, Minnesota, residents aged 22 years or older who had an incident case of HZ between January 1, 1996, and December 31, 2001. Kaplan-Meier curves and Cox regression models were used to describe recurrences by age, immune status, and presence of prolonged pain at the time of the incident HZ episode.

Results.—Of the 1669 persons with a medically documented episode of HZ, 95 had 105 recurrences (8 persons with >1 recurrence) by December 31, 2007, an average follow-up of 7.3 years. The Kaplan-Meier estimate of the recurrence rate at 8 years was 6.2%. With a maximum follow-up of 12 years, the time between HZ episodes in the same person varied from 96 days to 10 years. Recurrences were significantly more likely in persons with zoster-associated pain of 30 days or longer at the initial episode (hazard ratio, 2.80; 95% confidence interval, 1.84-4.27; $P<.001$) and in immunocompromised individuals (hazard ratio, 2.35; 95% confidence interval, 1.35-4.08; $P=.006$). Women and anyone aged 50 years or older at the index episode also had a greater likelihood of recurrence.

Conclusion.—Rates of HZ recurrence appear to be comparable to rates of first HZ occurrence in immunocompetent individuals, suggesting that recurrence is sufficiently common to warrant investigation of vaccine prevention in this group.

▶ Published data on recurrences of herpes zoster (HZ), or shingles, are scant and appear as anecdotal reports of cases collected over varying durations of time using different methods.[1] The incidence of recurrence is likely to increase with time after the first episode of HZ.

This study (the largest to date) presents population-based estimates of the recurrence of HZ in adults over on average follow-up period of 7.3 years. As shown in Table 1 in the original article, the recurrence rates were 2% at 2 years after the initial HZ episode and increased to 3.6% at 1 year, 4.9% at 6 years, and 6.2% at 8 years. The age range was 22 to 100 years, with a median of 59.4 years. The time between HZ episodes in the same person varied from 90 days to 10 years, with a maximum follow-up of 12 years. The site of recurrence was in a different part of the body for 45% of the episodes than the site of the index episode. The recurrence rates were about 2.4 times higher among immunocompromised patients (at the time of initial episode). However, most episodes of recurrent HZ (85.7%) occurred in immunocompetent people—people who are eligible to receive currently available zoster vaccine.

In the immunocompetent adult population, the HZ recurrence rates are comparable with those of the first episode of HZ. Both initial episode and recurrent HZ diseases can be prevented by the currently available vaccine indicated at age > 50 years.

N. M. Khardori, MD, PhD

Reference

1. Chien AJ, Olerud JE. Why do so many clinicians believe that recurrent zoster is common? *Dermatol Online J.* 2007;13:2.

Human Herpesvirus 8 Infection in Children and Adults in a Population-based Study in Rural Uganda

Butler LM, Were WA, Balinandi S, et al (University of California, San Francisco; Ctrs for Disease Control and Prevention (CDC)—Uganda, Entebbe; et al)
J Infect Dis 203:625-634, 2011

Background.—Human herpesvirus 8 (HHV-8) infection is endemic in sub-Saharan Africa. We examined sociodemographic, behavioral, and biological factors associated with HHV-8 infection in children and adults to determine HHV-8 seroprevalence and potential routes of transmission.

Methods.—Participants were 1383 children and 1477 adults from a population-based sample in a rural community in Uganda. Serum samples were tested for HHV-8 antibodies with use of an enzyme immunoassay against K8.1.

Results.—HHV-8 seroprevalence increased from 16% among children aged 1.5–2 years to 32% among children aged 10–13 years (P <.001) and from 37% among participants aged 14–19 years to 49% among adults aged $\geq$50 years (P <.05). HHV-8 seropositivity in children was independently associated with residing with a seropositive parent (P <.001) and residing with $\geq$1 other seropositive child aged <14 years (P <.001). History of sharing food and/or sauce plates was marginally associated with HHV-8 infection in children (P =.05). Among 1404 participants aged $\geq$15 years, there was no association between correlates of sexual behavior (eg, number of lifetime sex partners and HIV infection) and HHV-8 seropositivity (P <.10).

Conclusions.—Our data suggest that HHV-8 is acquired primarily through horizontal transmission in childhood from intrafamilial contacts and that transmission continues into adulthood potentially through nonsexual routes.

▶ Human Herpes Virus 8 (HHV-8) endemic in sub-Saharan Africa is now known to be the etiologic agent for Kaposi sarcoma (KS) and is associated with body cavity-based lymphoma and multicentric Castelman disease.[1-3] Estimated HHV-8 seroprevalence in adults ranges from 14% to 83%. East and Central equatorial Africa ("the KS belt") has the highest seroprevalence rates.

The study was conducted on 1383 children and 1477 adults from a population-based sample in a rural community in Uganda. Seroprevalence rate was 15% in children < 2 years old, increased to 32% in children 10 to 13 years old, to 37% in the 14- to 19-year age group, and 49% in the > 50-year population (Fig 1 in original article). There was no association between HHV-8 seropositivity and sexual behavior among participants > 15 years. Among children, seropositivity was independently associated with residing with a seropositive parent and residing with > 1 other seropositive child aged < 14 years. Herpes simplex virus type 1 (HSV1), Epstein-Barr virus (EBV) or cytomegalovirus (CMV) co-infection was demonstrated in at least 90% of children. HHV-8 seropositivity in adults > 14 years was associated with residing in a household with > 2 HHV-8 seropositive persons and inversely associated with household density. No association between HHV-8 infection and sexual behavior was demonstrated in adults. Evidence of HSV-1, EBV, or CMV infection was seen in 90% of adults, the same as in children, demonstrating that these 3 viral infections were acquired early in childhood. The seroprevalence of HHV-8 increased with age (16% in 1.5- to 2-year-olds to 49% in adults aged > 50 years) suggesting that transmission is ongoing in adulthood, most likely by nonsexual routes. This study clearly shows the importance of horizontal transmission of HHV-8, although the specific routes remain unclear.

N. M. Khardori, MD, PhD

References

1. Chang Y, Cesarman E, Pessin MS, et al. Identification of herpesvirus-like DNA sequences in AIDS-associated Kaposi's sarcoma. *Science.* 1994;266:1865-1869.
2. Cesarman E, Chang Y, Moore PS, Said JW, Knowles DM. Kaposi's sarcoma-associated herpesvirus-like DNA sequences in AIDS-related body-cavity-based lymphomas. *N Engl J Med.* 1995;332:1186-1191.
3. Soulier J, Grollet L, Oksenhendler E, et al. Kaposi's sarcoma-associated herpesvirus-like DNA sequences in multicentric Castleman's disease. *Blood.* 1995;86: 1276-1280.

Increasing Rates of Gastroenteritis Hospital Discharges in US Adults and the Contribution of Norovirus, 1996–2007
Lopman BA, Hall AJ, Curns AT, et al (Natl Ctr for Immunization and Respiratory Diseases, Atlanta, GA)
Clin Infect Dis 52:466-474, 2011

Background.—Diarrhea remains an important cause of morbidity, but until the mid 1990s, hospital admissions for diarrhea in the US adult population were declining. We aimed to describe recent trends in gastroenteritis hospitalizations and to determine the contribution of norovirus.

Methods.—We analyzed all gastroenteritis-associated hospital discharges during 1996–2007 from a nationally representative data set of hospital inpatient stays. Annual rates of discharges by age were calculated. Time-series regression models were fitted using cause-specified discharges as explanatory variables; model residuals were analyzed to estimate norovirus- and rotavirus-associated discharges. We then calculated the annual hospital charges for norovirus-associated discharges.

Results.—Sixty-nine percent of all gastroenteritis discharges were cause-unspecified and rates increased by ≥50% in all adult and elderly age groups (≥18 years of age) from 1996 through 2007. We estimate an annual mean of 71,000 norovirus-associated hospitalizations, costing $493 million per year, with surges to nearly 110,000 hospitalizations per year in epidemic seasons. We also estimate 24,000 rotavirus hospitalizations annually among individuals aged ≥5 years.

Conclusions.—Gastroenteritis hospitalizations are increasing, and we estimate that norovirus is the cause of 10% of cause-unspecified and 7% of all-cause gastroenteritis discharges. Norovirus should be routinely considered as a cause of gastroenteritis hospitalization.

▶ This study describes recent trends in gastroenteritis in US adults based on hospital admission and defines the relative roles of common pathogens. As shown in Fig 1 in the original article, a cause-unspecified gastroenteritis ICD code made up the majority (69%) of all-cause gastroenteritis discharges. The rates increased by 41% from 1996–1997 to 2006–2007. The rates decreased in children (by 21%) in 0 to 4 year olds and 8% in 5 to 17 year olds), whereas an increase of 50% occurred in all adult and elderly age groups. Rates increased from 27 discharges per 10 000 persons in 1979 to 1995 (from another study) to 49.2 discharges per 10 000 persons in 2006 to 2007.[1] There was a marked increase in discharges coded as *Clostridium difficile* infection over the study period, but this did not account for all of the increase in cause-unspecified discharges. The peaks of December or January in all age groups most years was highly consistent with the norovirus seasonality. Because norovirus is rarely tested for (outside the public health laboratories for outbreak investigators), indirect methods used in this study to investigate the role of this etiology agent are highly acceptable. The study estimates norovirus to be the cause of 10% of cause-unspecified and 7% of all-cause gastroenteritis discharge among adults. With the rise in population of those living in long-term care institutions, the risk of being involved in outbreaks and transmission with the living environment is higher. Norovirus disproportionally affect the elderly requiring hospitalization.[2] The economic burden is at $493 million per year. Given the increasing number, morbidity, and economic burden of norovirus associated hospitalizations, rapid and reliable diagnostic tests need to be made available.

N. M. Khardori, MD, PhD

References

1. Mounts AW, Holman RC, Clarke MJ, Bresee JS, Glass RI. Trends in hospitalizations associated with gastroenteritis among adults in the United States, 1979-1995. *Epidemiol Infect.* 1999;123:1-8.
2. Lew JF, Glass RI, Gangarosa RE, Cohen IP, Bern C, Moe CL. Diarrheal deaths in the United States, 1979 through 1987. A special problem for the elderly. *JAMA.* 1991;265:3280-3284.

Novel Deer-Associated Parapoxvirus Infection in Deer Hunters

Roess AA, Galan A, Kitces E, et al (Ctrs for Disease Control and Prevention, Atlanta, GA; Yale Univ School of Medicine, New Haven, CT; Richmond Dermatology and Laser Specialists, VA)
N Engl J Med 363:2621-2627, 2010

Parapoxviruses are a genus of the double-stranded DNA family of poxviruses that infect ruminants, and zoonotic transmission to humans often results from occupational exposures. Parapoxvirus infection in humans begins with an incubation period of 3 to 7 days, followed by the development of one or more erythematous maculopapular lesions that evolve over the course of several weeks into nodules. In 2009, parapoxvirus infection was diagnosed in two deer hunters in the eastern United States after the hunters had field-dressed white-tailed deer. We describe the clinical and pathological features of these infections and the phylogenetic relationship of a unique strain of parapoxvirus to other parapoxviruses. Deer populations continue to increase, leading to the possibility that there will be more deer-associated parapoxvirus infections.

▶ Parapoxviruses, a genus of the family of poxviruses (including small pox and cow pox virus), are double-stranded DNA viruses that cause infection in ruminants (sheep, goats, and cattle) throughout the world. The disease in the animals presents as proliferation dermatitis in the mouth, teats, and skin and can be fatal in young animals. Orf virus infection occurs in sheep and goats, and bovine popular stomatitis and pseudocowpox virus infection occurs in cattle. As a zoonotic disease, human infection with parapoxviruses occur after direct contact with infected animals and possibly from fomites.[1] Parapoxviruses have been isolated from reindeer in northern Europe and red deer in New Zealand. In the United States, parapoxvirus has not been isolated or shown to cause illness in the free-ranging white-tailed deer. This increased population of deer in the United States provides opportunities for transmission of parapoxvirus to deer through contact with cattle.

This study reports parapoxvirus infection in 2009 in the eastern United States (eastern Virginia and Connecticut) in 2 deer hunters. The route of infection was trauma to the finger while dressing a white-tailed deer in both instances. The clinical lesions are shown in Fig 1 in the original article. The 2 cases were reported to the Centers for Disease Control within 1 week of each other, where the results of the "para-pox" universal polymerase chain reaction (PCR) assay and the parapoxvirus-specific real-time PCR assay confirmed the presence of parapoxvirus infection in both patients. The lesions in both patients healed after excision and biopsy. DNA analysis suggested that the causative agent is a unique parapoxvirus strain.

Parapoxvirus was compared with the ones involved in 3 previously reported cases of infection associated with deer contact. Nonhealing, complicated infections in humans caused by parapoxvirus can be confused with more serious diseases such as anthrax or other pox virus infections. It is important to ask about exposure and travel history as well as patient's hobbies and obtain a biopsy diagnosis.

N. M. Khardori, MD, PhD

Reference

1. Leavell UW Jr, McNamara MJ, Muelling R, Talbert WM, Rucker RC, Dalton AJ. ORF. Report of 19 human cases with clinical and pathological observations. *JAMA.* 1968;204:657-664.

Detection of prion infection in variant Creutzfeldt-Jakob disease: a blood-based assay
Edgeworth JA, Farmer M, Sicilia A, et al (UCL Inst of Neurology, UK; et al)
Lancet 377:487-493, 2011

Background.—Variant Creutzfeldt-Jakob disease (vCJD) is a fatal neurodegenerative disorder originating from exposure to bovine-spongiform-encephalopathy-like prions. Prion infections are associated with long and clinically silent incubations. The number of asymptomatic individuals with vCJD prion infection is unknown, posing risk to others via blood transfusion, blood products, organ or tissue grafts, and contaminated medical instruments. We aimed to establish the sensitivity and specificity of a blood-based assay for detection of vCJD prion infection.

Methods.—We developed a solid-state binding matrix to capture and concentrate disease-associated prion proteins and coupled this method to direct immunodetection of surface-bound material. Quantitative assay sensitivity was assessed with a serial dilution series of 10^{-7} to 10^{-10} of vCJD prion-infected brain homogenate into whole human blood, with a baseline control of normal human brain homogenate in whole blood (10^{-6}). To establish the sensitivity and specificity of the assay for detection of endogenous vCJD, we analysed a masked panel of 190 whole blood samples from 21 patients with vCJD, 27 with sporadic CJD, 42 with other neurological diseases, and 100 normal controls. Samples were masked and numbered by individuals independent of the assay and analysis. Each sample was tested twice in independent assay runs; only samples that were reactive in both runs were scored as positive overall.

Findings.—We were able to distinguish a 10^{-10} dilution of exogenous vCJD prion-infected brain from a 10^{-6} dilution of normal brain (mean chemiluminescent signal, $1 \cdot 3 \times 10^{5}$ [SD $1 \cdot 1 \times 10^{4}$] for vCJD vs $9 \cdot 9 \times 10^{4}$ [$4 \cdot 5 \times 10^{3}$] for normal brain; p<$0 \cdot 0001$)—an assay sensitivity that was orders of magnitude higher than any previously reported. 15 samples in the masked panel were scored as positive. All 15 samples were from patients with vCJD, showing an assay sensitivity for vCJD of 71·4% (95% CI 47·8-88·7) and a specificity of 100% (95% CIs between 97·8% and 100%).

Interpretation.—These initial studies provide a prototype blood test for diagnosis of vCJD in symptomatic individuals, which could allow development of large-scale screening tests for asymptomatic vCJD prion infection.

▶ Variant Creutzfeldt-Jakob (vCJD) disease is a uniformly fatal neurodegenerative disease caused by a prion. Other prion diseases with similar course and outcome include Creutzfeldt-Jakob disease (CJD), Gerstmann-Straussler-Scheinker disease, fatal familial insomnia and kuru in humans, bovine spongiform encephalopathy (BSE) in cattle, and chronic wasting disease of deer and elk and scrapie in sheep. It has been confirmed that vCJD originated from exposure to BSE in cattle.[1] The UK population has had widespread exposure to BSE. The disease is characterized by subclinical carrier state and a long incubation period.[2] There is a risk of iatrogenic transmission of vCJD prion infection by transfusion of blood and blood products and many forms of surgical and dental interventions. The National Health Team in the United Kingdom has implemented very costly risk-reducing strategies that are of uncertain efficacy and necessity.

Prions are infectious agents composed mostly of a misfolded form of host cellular prion protein (PrP^c). PrP^c, although expressed ubiquitously, is at its highest concentration in the central nervous system (CNS) and cells of the immune system. PrP^c is remodeled to aggregated, detergent insoluble isoform-designated PrP^{sc}, which is conformationally different from PrP^c during the pathogenesis of prion disease. PrP^{sc} levels in the CNS and lymphoreticular tissues correlate with prion infectivity.[3] The development of diagnostic tests has been hampered by the absence of agent-specific nucleic acid and lack of a host humoral response. Conventional immunoassays (ELISA and Western Blot) are able to detect sufficient quantities of PrP^{sc} in the neural tissues during the symptomatic phase of illness. However, the level of infectivity in the blood is very low, and the ratio of background PrP^c to PrP^{sc} in the blood is much higher than in other tissues contributing to nonspecific background signals.

This study makes use of the findings that prions can bind avidly to some surfaces, including metals, to detect the low concentrations of PrP^{sc} in the blood. Stainless steel (45/μm) particles were used as capture matrix to which blood samples were added and incubated overnight at 18°C with agitation. This was followed by direct immunodetection of surface bound PrP. The blood samples had been intentionally spiked with vCJD of normal brain homogenate. The sensitivity and specificity of the test for vCJD were 71.4% and 100%, respectively. This type of assay could be further enhanced to develop a large-scale screening test for vCJD prion infection.

N. M. Khardori, MD, PhD

References

1. Collinge J, Sidle KC, Meads J, Ironside J, Hill AF. Molecular analysis of prion strain variation and the aetiology of 'new variant' CJD. *Nature.* 1996;383: 685-690.

2. Collinge J, Whitfield J, McKintosh E, et al. Kuru in the 21st century—an acquired human prion disease with very long incubation periods. *Lancet.* 2006;367: 2068-2074.
3. Tattum MH, Jones S, Pal S, Collinge J, Jackson GS. Discrimination between prion-infected and normal blood samples by protein misfolding cyclic amplification. *Transfusion.* 2010;50:996-1002.

15 Human Immunodeficiency Virus

Epidemiology of HIV Infection in the United States: Implications for Linkage to Care

Moore RD (Johns Hopkins Univ, Baltimore, MD)

Clin Infect Dis 52:S208-S213, 2011

The epidemiology of human immunodeficiency virus (HIV) infection in the United States has changed significantly over the past 30 years. HIV/acquired immune deficiency syndrome (HIV/AIDS) is currently a disease of greater demographic diversity, affecting all ages, sexes, and races, and involving multiple transmission risk behaviors. At least 50,000 new HIV infections will continue to be added each year; however, one-fifth of persons with new infections may not know they are infected, and a substantial proportion of those who know they are infected are not engaged in HIV care. Barriers to early engagement in care may be specific to a demographic group. In this paper, the current epidemiology of HIV/AIDS in the United States is reviewed in order to understand the challenges, successes, and best practices for removing the barriers to effective diagnosis and receipt of HIV care within specific demographic groups.

▶ Since the early 1980s, the epidemiology of human immunodeficiency virus (HIV) infection in the United States has changed significantly. This has created more challenges and barriers to effective care.

This article provides a review of data on the current epidemiology of HIV/AIDS in the United States and its impact on infected patients. In 2006, the Centers for Disease Control (CDC) used a stratified extrapolation approach to estimate the HIV incidence among persons aged more than 13 years in 22 states. The total was extrapolated to all 50 states and the District of Columbia. The estimated incidence in 2006 was 56 300 new infections per year, 40% higher than the previous estimate of 40 000 based on a less precise method, not an actual increase in HIV incidence. Because an estimated 21% of infected persons have not been diagnosed, the overall HIV prevalence in the United States cannot be calculated directly. The extended back calculation method based on 80% of states reporting name-based HIV diagnosis, as of January 2006, estimates a prevalence rate of

447.8 per 100 000 population. HIV prevalence is 8 times higher among blacks than whites, even though blacks account for only 12% of the US population. The prevalence of HIV infection in the United States is higher than ever before because current highly active antiretroviral therapy prolongs life and improves quality of life for these patients. The significant demographic change has been a greater proportion of infections than ever before in the poor, minority racial/ethnic groups, and women. Heterosexual transmission is responsible for an increasing number of new infections. To increase early diagnosis and treatment of HIV infection, the CDC has recommended universal testing for HIV during routine medical care. Americans aged 13 to 64 years should be routinely tested, and persons over 65 years with risk factors for HIV infection should be counseled to get tested. Barriers specific to demographic groups may need to be addressed to engage patients who are aware of their infection status in HIV-related care and treatment. The HIV epidemic in the United States is alive and well despite availability of current management strategies.

V. Sundareshan, MD

Concordance of *CCR5* Genotypes that Influence Cell-Mediated Immunity and HIV-1 Disease Progression Rates
Catano G, Chykarenko ZA, Mangano A, et al (Univ of Texas Health Science Ctr, San Antonio; Dnepropetrovsk State Med Academy, Ukraine; Hospital de Pediatría "J. P. Garrahan," Buenos Aires, Argentina; et al)
J Infect Dis 203:263-272, 2011

We used cutaneous delayed-type hypersensitivity responses, a powerful in vivo measure of cell-mediated immunity, to evaluate the relationships among cell-mediated immunity, AIDS, and polymorphisms in *CCR5*, the HIV-1 co-receptor. There was high concordance between *CCR5* polymorphisms and haplotype pairs that influenced delayed-type hypersensitivity responses in healthy persons and HIV disease progression. In the cohorts examined, *CCR5* genotypes containing −2459G/G (HHA/HHA, HHA/HHC, HHC/HHC) or −2459A/A (HHE/HHE) associated with salutary or detrimental delayed-type hypersensitivity and AIDS phenotypes, respectively. Accordingly, the *CCR5*-Δ32 allele, when paired with non-Δ32-bearing haplotypes that correlate with low (HHA, HHC) versus high (HHE) *CCR5* transcriptional activity, associates with disease retardation or acceleration, respectively. Thus, the associations of *CCR5*-Δ32 heterozygosity partly reflect the effect of the non-Δ32 haplotype in a background of *CCR5* haploinsufficiency. The correlations of increased delayed-type hypersensitivity with −2459G/G-containing *CCR5* genotypes, reduced *CCR5* expression, decreased viral replication, and disease retardation suggest that *CCR5* may influence HIV infection and AIDS, at least in part, through effects on cell-mediated immunity.

▶ Cutaneous delayed-type hypersensitivity (DTH) responses can be a function of immune status (cell-mediated immunity [CMI]) in vivo and can be correlated with T cell responses in vitro. This innovative study looks at the associations of CCR5 (the major human immunodeficiency virus [HIV]-1 coreceptor) genotypes with cutaneous DTH in healthy persons and compared them with CCR5 variations in patients with acquired immunodeficiency disease (AIDS). The investigators explain that DTH status of patients with HIV predicts clinical outcome and immune responsiveness, both before and after initiation of antiretroviral therapy (ART). CCR5 polymorphisms are also known to influence HIV phenotype, infectivity, and susceptibility. The primary cohort for evaluation of the association of CCR5 genotypes with DTH responses to purified protein derivative (PPD) comprised a previously described cohort of 206 healthy HIV-uninfected adults from Australia in whom cutaneous DTH responses to the neoantigen keyhole limpet hemocyanin (KLH) were assessed. The analysis also included 2 separate cohorts of children infected with HIV.

Specific CCR5 single-nucleotide polymorphisms and genotypes that are associated with cutaneous DTH responses to 2 distinct antigens (KLH and PPD) in healthy adults as well as cohorts of HIV-infected children were identified. Concordance in the CCR5 genotypes was associated with DTH status in HIV-uninfected persons as well as those with disease progression rates. In the primary Ukrainian cohort, −2459G/G, HHE/HHF*2, and specific HHG*2 (Δ32)-containing genotypes were associated with disease retardation and increased DTH responses to KLH (except from the Δ32-containing genotypes). HHE/HHG*2 and HHE/HHE were associated with lower DTH responses and a faster rate of disease progression in Ukrainian children.

The strength of this study is in helping understand the genetic determinants of CMI, a less understood area in research. Moreover, 2 separate HIV-infected cohorts were included in the study for associations of CCR5 genotype with AIDS progression rates that revealed concordance in CCR5 genotype and association with AIDS and DTH status.

Reporter constructs bearing −2459G/−2135T (conflation of HHA to HHD) have lower transcriptional activity than those bearing −2459A/−2135C (conflation of HHE to HHG). Also noted is that CCR5 receptor density on CD4+ and CD14+ monocytes is lower in cells bearing CCR5 −2459G/G than in the G/A or A/A genotypes, with highest CCR5 expression in cells bearing −2459A/A. Finally, because CCR5 levels correlate with susceptibility to R5 virus infection, peripheral blood mononuclear cells from healthy whites bearing −2459G/G, A/G, and A/A genotypes, respectively, associate with low, medium, and high R5 viral propagation in vitro. The −2459G/G-containing genotypes are consistently noted with mitigated HIV and AIDS susceptibility.

Genotypes containing −2459G/G (noted with reduced CCR5 transcriptional activity/surface expression, viral replication, and HIV and AIDS susceptibility), caused HIV disease retardation and enhanced DTH responses in 2 HIV-uninfected cohorts. Genotypes containing −2459G/G may differ according to the ethnic/racial background of the cohorts studied.

CCR5 expression levels impact many different facets of HIV pathogenesis, namely HIV entry, HIV acquisition, AIDS progression rates, viral load, immune reconstitution during highly active antiretroviral therapy, efficacy of CCR5 blockers and entry inhibitors, and neutralizing activity of HIV-1—specific antibodies. Of note, low CCR5 surface expression and lower activity is associated with a protective phenotype. The authors suggest CCR5 may also influence HIV pathogenesis by immune-based mechanisms in addition to its function as a coreceptor. Other studies have noted that CCR5 expression is associated with Th1 and DTH responses. The CCR5-null state or antagonism of CCR5 is associated with reduced inflammation and transplant rejection. CCR5 expression is correlated with T-cell activation levels, and preseroconversion activation status is a predictor of disease progression. In summary, a high degree of concordance exists between the associations of CCR5 genotypes that influence DTH status and those that influence CCR5 transcriptional activity or surface expression, replication of HIV, and progression to AIDS.

V. Sundareshan, MD

Long-Term Survival of HIV-Infected Children Receiving Antiretroviral Therapy in Thailand: A 5-Year Observational Cohort Study

Collins IJ, for the Program for HIV Prevention and Treatment Study Team (Institut de Recherche pour le Développement IRD U174, Paris, France; et al)
Clin Infect Dis 51:1449-1457, 2010

Background.—There are scarce data on the long-term survival of human immunodeficiency virus (HIV)—infected children receiving antiretroviral therapy (ART) in lower-middle income countries beyond 2 years of follow-up.

Methods.—Previously untreated children who initiated ART on meeting immunological and/or clinical criteria were followed in a prospective cohort in Thailand. The probability of survival up to 5 years from initiation was estimated using Kaplan-Meier methods, and factors associated with mortality were assessed using Cox regression analyses.

Results.—Five hundred seventy-eight children received ART; of these, 111 (19.2%) were followed since birth. At start of ART (baseline), the median age was 6.7 years, 128 children (22%) were aged <2 years, and the median CD4 cell percentage was 7%. Median duration of follow-up was 53 months; 42 children (7%) died, and 38 (7%) were lost to follow-up. Age <12 months, low CD4 cell percentage, and low weight-for-height z score at ART initiation were independently associated with mortality ($P < .001$). The probability of survival among infants aged <12 months at baseline was 84.3% at 1 year and 76.7% at 5 years of ART, compared with 95.7% and 94.8%, respectively, among children aged ≥1 year. Low CD4 cell percentage and wasting at baseline had a strong association with mortality among older children but weak or no association among infants.

Conclusions.—Children who initiated ART as infants after meeting immunological and/or clinical criteria had a high risk of mortality which persisted beyond the first year of therapy. Among older children, those with severe wasting or low CD4 cell percentage at treatment initiation were at high risk of mortality during the first 6 months of therapy. These findings support the scale-up of early HIV diagnosis and immediate treatment in infants, before advanced disease progression in older children.

▶ There are plenty of data on the long-term success of highly active antiretroviral therapy (HAART) in adults, but there is a lack of similar data in the pediatric human immunodeficiency virus (HIV) population. This prospective cohort study from Thailand looks at long-term survival in children from lower to middle income families who have been initiated on HAART. This study comprised a generic fixed-dosed combination of stavudine, lamivudine, and nevirapine, produced in Thailand, with the tablets divided into halves or quarters according to the child's body weight. This treatment is provided free in Thailand, and there have been many pilot programs in place since 1999 for research purposes. When started on treatment earlier than 2002 (the year of introduction of protease inhibitor), many children were on dual nucleoside reverse-transcriptase inhibitor (NRTI) regimens, some of whom later switched to HAART. In Thailand, there are currently > 15 000 children living with HIV. This study was able to assess a 5-year survival with HAART in this group and identify risk factors for mortality. A total of 111 children in this study were followed from birth. The mean age for starting HAART was 6.7 years with 128 children being < 2 years old. Thirty-eight percent of the children were lost to follow-up, and median time for loss to follow-up was 53 months. Forty-two children (7%) died in this study (mostly from infection such as pneumonia, diarrhea, tuberculosis, or sepsis). Age < 12 months, low CD4 percentage (< 7%), and low birth-to-height ratio were independent risk factor for mortality. Survival at 5 years of therapy was > 94% in children that were 1 year old at the time of initiation of treatment. These findings were similar to those in many countries in Africa and Australia. Notable from this study is that children who initiated ART as infants based on clinical or immunologic criteria had higher risk of mortality throughout the time of follow-up. Further studies are necessary to assess the impact of early HIV diagnosis and treatment strategies on infant and child survival. Continued follow-up of this cohort into adolescence and newer HAART regimens will be useful for further decisions and policies. As in many other infections, preventive and therapeutic interventions for HIV disease in childhood seem to have maximum long-term benefits when initiated after the immune system has reached a certain level of maturity.

V. Sundareshan, MD

Tuberculosis due to *Mycobacterium bovis* in Patients Coinfected with Human Immunodeficiency Virus

Park D, Qin H, Jain S, et al (Univ of California, San Diego; et al)
Clin Infect Dis 51:1343-1346, 2010

We reviewed 86 cases of human immunodeficiency virus and tuberculosis coinfection; 34.9% were caused by *Mycobacterium bovis*. Patients with *M. bovis* infection were more likely to have advanced immunosuppression

(CD4 T cell counts ≤200 cells/µL). Hispanic ethnicity, male sex, and abdominal disease were strongly associated with *M. bovis* disease.

▶ *Mycobacterium bovis*, one of the species in the *Mycobacterium tuberculosis* complex is an important cause of tuberculosis (TB) in certain populations and some parts of the world.[1,2] This is a retrospective case-control analysis of TB among human immunodeficiency virus (HIV)-infected patient followed in the Owen Clinic in San Diego from 2000 to 2007. In this review of 86 cases of HIV and culture-positive coinfection, 30 (34.9%) were caused by *M bovis*. Of these 83.3% had abdominal TB. The most likely explanation is the hypothetical source of *M bovis* to be unpasteurized, contaminated dairy products. Abdominal disease from possible gastrointestinal portal of entry and clinical features are similar to HIV-associated disseminated *Mycobacterium avium* complex disease. The risk factors among HIV-infected patients for *M bovis* infection were CD4 count less than 200 uL/mL, Hispanic ethnicity and male sex. Mortality was 10% for *M bovis* case patient compared with 36% for *M tuberculosis* case patients. None of the *M bovis* isolates were multidrug resistant. This study is in agreement with others regarding the role of unpasteurized dairy products in *M bovis* infection and indicates the need for counseling of patient at risk, including HIV-infected patients.

V. Sundareshan, MD

References

1. Hlavsa MC, Moonan PK, Cowan LS, et al. Human tuberculosis due to *Mycobacterium bovis* in the United States, 1995-2005. *Clin Infect Dis.* 2008;47:168-175.
2. Ayele WY, Neill SD, Zinsstag J, Weiss MG, Pavlik I. Bovine tuberculosis: an old disease but a new threat to Africa. *Int J Tuberc Lung Dis.* 2004;8:924-937.

16 Vaccines

Administering influenza vaccine to egg allergic recipients: a focused practice parameter update
Greenhawt MJ, Li JT, Bernstein DI, et al (The Univ of Michigan Food Allergy Ctr, Ann Arbor; The Mayo Clinic, Rochester, MN; Univ of Cincinnati—College of Medicine, OH; et al)
Ann Allergy Asthma Immunol 106:11-16, 2011

- The well-proven benefits of influenza immunization can now be made available to persons with a history of egg allergy. Individuals with diagnosed or suspected egg allergy who need an influenza vaccination should be evaluated by an allergist/immunologist for evaluation of egg allergy and for administration of the 2010–2011 trivalent influenza vaccine (TIV) if clinically indicated.
- Studies have suggested that influenza vaccines can be administered to patients with a history of anaphylaxis to egg without adverse effects. However, such studies are limited in number, and reactions to influenza vaccines in egg allergic persons can occur. Caution is warranted in patients with a history of anaphylaxis or where the severity of their clinical reactivity is uncertain, particularly when the ovalbumin content of the vaccine is unknown. Therefore, consultation with an allergist experienced in food allergy and anaphylaxis is strongly recommended.
- For the 2010–2011 influenza season, the routine practice of skin testing to the TIV is no longer recommended.
- Both the 2-dose (10%, 90%) and single-dose methods are appropriate for administering influenza vaccine to egg allergic individuals.

Egg allergic individuals can receive TIV without prior skin testing to the vaccine, with the vaccine being administered via a 2-step graded challenge: first administer 10% of the age-appropriate dose, with a 30-minute observation after administration for symptom development. If no symptoms develop, the remaining 90% can be administered, with a 30-minute observation for symptom development. The same TIV product brand should be used for booster vaccinations if possible, but it is not necessary to use the same lot.

Egg allergic individuals can receive TIV without prior skin testing to the vaccine as a single, age-appropriate dose without use of graded challenge. Individuals should be observed for 30 minutes after injection for evidence of a systemic reaction. The same TIV product brand should be used for booster vaccinations, but the same lot is not necessary.

▶ During the global pandemic of H1N1 influenza A virus in 2009 to 2011, the interest in the safety of administering this egg-based vaccine to egg-allergic individuals was renewed. Several manufacturers now list the ovalbumin content of their products. Other potentially allergic moieties in the egg protein have not been identified. Previous experience suggests that people with suspected or diagnosed egg allergy can safely receive trivalent influenza vaccine if certain precautions are followed.[1,2] The recommended precautions include prevaccination skin testing, desensitization and a 2-step graded dose challenge (10% followed by 90% of the age-appropriate dose) separated by a brief observation period. Because of the urgency during the 2009—2010 season, investigators reexamined the safety of influenza vaccine in egg-allergic individuals with significant changes in recommendations.

This practice parameter update offers guidelines on evaluation and management of egg allergy in patients about to receive influenza vaccine and outlines the latest evidence-based approaches to influenza vaccine administration. The highlights of the executive summary are provided below.

1. Influenza immunization can be made available to persons with a history of egg allergy. These individuals should be evaluated by a specialist in allergy/immunology, if clinically indicated.

2. Consultation with an allergist with experience in food allergy and anaphylaxis is strongly recommended for patients with history of anaphylaxis or uncertain clinical reactivity, particularly when the ovalbumin content of the vaccine is unknown.

3. The routine practice of skin testing to trivalent influenza vaccine (TIV) is no longer recommended.

4. Both the 2-dose (10% followed by 90%) and single-dose methods are appropriate for egg-allergic patients. In both cases, individuals should be observed for 30 minutes after injection for evidence of a systemic reaction. The same TIV product brand but not necessarily the same lot should be used for booster vaccination.

N. M. Khardori, MD, PhD

References

1. James JM, Zeiger RS, Lester MR, et al. Safe administration of influenza vaccine to patients with egg allergy. *J Pediatr.* 1998;133:624-628.
2. Li JT. Administering the H1N1 influenza vaccine in patients with suspected egg allergy. http://aaaai.org/media/h1n1/egg_allergy_li.pdf. Accessed August 20, 2010.

Adverse events associated with the 2009 H1N1 influenza vaccination and the vaccination coverage rate in health care workers

Park S-W, Lee J-H, Kim ES, et al (Seoul Natl Univ College of Medicine and Boramae Med Ctr, Seoul, Republic of Korea; Chonbuk Natl Univ Med School, Jeonju, Republic of Korea; Dongguk Univ Ilsan Hosp, Goyang, Republic of Korea; et al)
Am J Infect Control 39:69-71, 2011

We prospectively examined the 2009 H1N1 influenza vaccination coverage rate and the adverse events related to the monovalent vaccine in Korean health care workers. The H1N1 vaccination coverage rate was 91.7%. There were no significant adverse events discouraging the vaccination.

▶ Vaccination of health care workers (HCWs) against influenza, in addition to preventing influenza in HCWs, confers protection to hospitalized patients who have not been or cannot be vaccinated.[1] The known barriers to high vaccination rates among HCWs are fear of needles, misbelief that they are not at risk for influenza, and, most importantly, fear of adverse events, like anaphylactic reactions and Guillain-Barre syndrome. Between 1989 and 2000, the influenza vaccination rates among HCWs in the United States were < 45%.[2]

This study, conducted in 7 university-affiliated hospitals between October and November 2009, used vaccine provided free of charge by the Korean government. As shown in Table 2 in the original article, 91.7% (10 547 of 11 294 HCWs registered in the 7 hospitals) received the vaccine. The lowest vaccination rate of 84.7% was among physicians. The questionnaire return rate was 44.4%, and these data were used to assess the frequency and nature of adverse events. Any local and systemic reactions up to 9 days after vaccination were reported on the questionnaire. Any adverse event was reported by 38.1%, the most common being fatigue in 21.1% of subjects, followed by injection site soreness, reported by 20.1% (Table 3 in original article). The adverse events occurred for a median duration of < 4 days. No severe adverse events were reported. This study of significant public health importance conducted in a large cohort of HCWs has value in alleviating adverse event apprehensions among HCWs and communities at large anywhere in the world.

N. M. Khardori, MD, PhD

References

1. Stewart AM. Mandatory vaccination of health care workers. *N Engl J Med.* 2009; 361:2015-2017.
2. Lugo NR. Will carrots or sticks raise influenza immunization rates of health care personnel? *Am J Infect Control.* 2007;35:1-6.

Antibody responses to hepatitis A virus vaccination in Thai HIV-infected children with immune recovery after antiretroviral therapy

Sudjaritruk T, Sirisanthana T, Sirisanthana V (Chiang Mai Univ, Thailand)
Pediatr Infect Dis J 30:256-259, 2011

The prevalence of hepatitis A virus (HAV) protective antibody in 98 Thai HIV-infected children who achieved immune recovery after antiretroviral therapy was 12.2%. After a 2-dose HAV vaccination, 98.8% (85 of 86 children) seroconverted. The geometric mean titer was 520.95 mIU/mL. In a multivariate analysis, female gender, age <12 years and higher CD4 lymphocyte count at enrollment were predicting factors for high ($\geq$250 mIU/mL) HAV antibody response.

▶ Immunization in immunocompromised hosts has far-reaching benefits. Hepatitis A vaccine is one of the recommended vaccines by the Advisory Committee on Immunization Practices for patients with human immunodeficiency virus (HIV) disease because of a higher incidence of severe liver disease with HIV co-infection. Conversely, hepatitis A virus (HAV) can also make HIV disease worse. Infection with hepatotropic viruses in patients with HIV disease can also worsen the adverse reaction profile seen with antiretroviral therapy (ART).

In this study, protective antibody response to HAV in 98 Thai children infected with HIV was studied to determine the prevalence of protective HAV antibody levels in patients on ART as well as to establish the immunogenicity and safety of HAV vaccine in this cohort of children.

The prevalence of HAV infection was similar in the HIV population (12.2%) compared with that of healthy Thai children between the ages of 8 and 15 years. After the first dose of the vaccine, seroconversion occurred in 68.6% of the children and after the second dose, almost 100% of the children had seroconversion. Other studies conducted in the United States and Brazil found variable rates (from 84.5% to 100%) of seroconversion. Studies with lower rates of seroconversion included children with detectable HIV viremia. Median HAV antibody titre following 2 doses of the vaccine after 8 weeks of vaccination was 320 mIU/mL. With HIV, the mean postvaccination antibody titre was noted to be lower than in controls. Healthy individuals may remain protected with the effects of vaccination for more than 20 years but may not last as long in patients with HIV disease. Further, univariate and multivariate analysis found female sex, younger age (<12 years), higher CD4 (>500), and undetectable viral load as favorable factors for good antibody repose with HAV vaccination. Most children in this study had been on ART for more than 1 year with good virologic suppression. Based on this study, it is recommended to give 2 doses of HAV vaccine to children after CD4 counts normalize with ART.

N. M. Khardori, MD, PhD

Effectiveness of 2 Doses of Varicella Vaccine in Children

Shapiro ED, Vazquez M, Esposito D, et al (Yale Univ School of Medicine Graduate School of Arts and Sciences New Haven, CT; et al)
J Infect Dis 203:312-315, 2011

Background.—Because of ongoing outbreaks of varicella, a second dose of varicella vaccine was added to the routine immunization schedule for children in June 2006 by the Centers for Disease Control and Prevention.

Methods.—We assessed the effectiveness of 2 doses of varicella vaccine in a case-control study by identifying children ≥4 years of age with varicella confirmed by polymerase chain reaction assay and up to 2 controls matched by age and pediatric practice. Effectiveness was calculated using exact conditional logistic regression.

Results.—From July 2006 to January 2010, of the 71 case subjects and 140 matched controls enrolled, no cases (0%) vs 22 controls (15.7%) had received 2 doses of varicella vaccine, 66 cases (93.0%) vs 117 controls (83.6%) had received 1 dose, and 5 cases (7.0%) vs 1 control (0.7%) did not receive varicella vaccine ($P < .001$). The effectiveness of 2 doses of the vaccine was 98.3% (95% confidence level [CI]: 83.5%–100%; $P < .001$). The matched odds ratio for 2 doses vs 1 dose of the vaccine was 0.053 (95% CI: 0.002–0.320; $P < .001$).

Conclusion.—The effectiveness of 2 doses of varicella vaccine in the first 2.5 years after recommendation of a routine second dose of the vaccine for children is excellent. Odds of developing varicella were 95% lower for children who received 2 doses compared with 1 dose of varicella vaccine.

▶ Varicella vaccine was added to the routine immunization for children in the United States in 1995. Initially a single dose was recommended for children 12 months to 13 years old, and 2 doses were recommended for older susceptible persons.[1] This live attenuated vaccine led to a 90% fall in the incidence of varicella, a 60% decline in its mortality, and an 80% decrease in the rates of hospitalization for varicella.[2] However, over time the effectiveness of the vaccine decreased; seroconversion after 1 dose was reported to be only 76%, breakthrough varicella among immunized children was documented, and outbreaks continued to occur in schools and day care centers. The routine administration of a second dose of varicella vaccine to young children was recommended by the Centers for Disease Control in 2006. In addition, a catch-up second dose was recommended for older children. These recommendations were based on higher antibody titers after 2 doses, but the association with better protection from varicella was presumed.

This case-controlled study presents data on the clinical efficacy of 2 doses of varicella vaccine in children aged 4 years and older. As shown in Table 2 in the original article, of the 71 subjects with polymerase chain reaction assay—positive for varicella, 7% had received no vaccine, 93% had received 1 dose, and none had received 2 doses of varicella vaccine. Among the 140 matched controls, 0.7% had received no vaccine, 83.8% had received 1 dose, and 15% had received 2 doses. The effectiveness of 2 doses of vaccine in preventing varicella was 98.3%. The matched odds ratio of 2 doses versus 1 dose of the vaccine indicate that in the first 2.5 years after introduction of the 2-dose regimen, the odds of developing varicella was 95% lower in 2-dose recipients than those who received a single dose. This strategy may have the added benefit of decreasing latent infection with wild-type varicella zoster vaccine and subsequent development of herpes zoster.

N. M. Khardori, MD, PhD

References

1. Prevention of varicella: Recommendations of the Advisory Committee on Immunization Practices (ACIP). Centers for Disease Control and Prevention. *MMWR Recomm Rep*. 1996;45:1-36.
2. Nguyen HQ, Jumaan AO, Seward JF. Decline in mortality due to varicella after implementation of varicella vaccination in the United States. *N Engl J Med*. 2005;352:450-458.

Phase II, Randomized, Double-Blind, Placebo-Controlled, Multicenter Study to Investigate the Immunogenicity and Safety of a West Nile Virus Vaccine in Healthy Adults

Biedenbender R, Bevilacqua J, Gregg AM, et al (Eastern Virginia Med School, Norfolk, VA; Sanofi Pasteur, Totonto, Ontario, Canada; Sanofi Pasteur, Cambridge, MA; et al)
J Infect Dis 203:75-84, 2011

Background.—ChimeriVax-WN02 is a live, attenuated chimeric vaccine for protection against West Nile virus. This Phase II, randomized, double-blind, placebo—controlled, multicenter study assessed the immunogenicity, viremia, and safety of the ChimeriVax-WN02 vaccine.

Methods.—The 2-part study included adults in general good health. In part 1, subjects aged 18—40 years were randomized to 1 of 4 treatment groups: ChimeriVax-WN02 3.7×10^5 plaque-forming units (PFU), 3.7×10^4 PFU, 3.7×10^3 PFU, or placebo. In part 2, subjects aged 41—64 and ≥ 65 years were randomized to receive ChimeriVax-WN02 3.7×10^5 PFU or placebo.

Results.—In both part 1 and part 2, seroconversion was achieved at day 28 by >96% of subjects in active treatment groups. In part 1, neutralizing antibody titers at day 28 were higher and viremia levels lower with the highest dose, whereas the adverse event profile was similar between the dose groups. In part 2, antibody titers and viremia levels were higher in subjects aged ≥ 65 years, and more subjects in the 41—64 years cohort experienced adverse events.

Conclusions.—The ChimeriVax-WN02 vaccine was highly immunogenic in younger adults and the elderly, and it was well tolerated at all dose levels and in all age groups investigated. ClinicalTrials.gov identifier: NCT00442169.

▶ West Nile Virus (WNV) was first detected in 1999 in the Western hemisphere during an outbreak of human encephalitis in New York City.[1] Subsequently, WNV spread within the United States, South America, and the Caribbean. The virus belongs to the genus *Flavivirus* and can infect humans, birds, mosquitoes, horses, and some other mammals. The typical human illness lasts for 3 to 6 days and is characterized by fever, headache, backache, myalgia, and anorexia.[2] It may also cause a severe illness, most commonly meningoencephalitis, with significant morbidity and mortality. Mosquito control and avoidance of mosquito bites are currently the only methods for prevention. A live attenuated chimeric vaccine (ChimeriVax-WN02) protected hamsters and mice against challenge with wild-type WNV.[3] The vaccine was produced by insertion of the genes encoding the premembrane and envelope proteins of WNV (Strain NY 99) into the yellow fever 17D vaccine clone. It was modified to reduce neurovirulence by mutations at multiple sites producing a highly attenuated phenotype.

This phase II, randomized, double-blind, placebo-controlled multicenter study is the first to assess the safety, tolerability, viremia, and immunogenicity of ChimeriVax-WN02 vaccine in healthy adults, including the elderly. High seroconversion rates of >96% were observed in all dose and age groups. Neutralizing antibodies have been the major mediator of protective immunity against WNV. A transient low-grade viremia was observed in most subjects. The subjects who received the higher doses of vaccine had lower viremia levels. This may be a clue to lower immune response to lower dose of vaccine as has been observed with the 17D yellow fever vaccine. Viremia did not correlate with systemic side effects. The vaccine was well tolerated with no major differences between the younger and older age groups. There are 4 licensed WNV veterinary vaccines in the United States, including one similar to ChimerVax-WN02, that are used in this study. Several other approaches to human WNV vaccine include live attenuated, recombinant subunit, vectorized, and DNA vaccines. ChimeriVax-WN02, a live recombinant vaccine used in this study, was highly immunogenic and well tolerated in all age groups.

N. M. Khardori, MD, PhD

References

1. Nash D, Mostashari F, Fine A, et al. The outbreak of West Nile virus infection in the New York City area in 1999. *N Engl J Med.* 2001;344:1807-1814.
2. Sampathkumar P. West Nile virus: epidemiology, clinical presentation, diagnosis, and prevention. *Mayo Clin Proc.* 2003;78:1137-1143.
3. Arroyo J, Miller C, Catalan J, et al. ChimeriVax-West Nile virus live-attenuated vaccine: preclinical evaluation of safety, immunogenicity, and efficacy. *J Virol.* 2004;78:12497-12507.

Vaccination inducing broad and improved cross protection against multiple subtypes of influenza A virus
Song J-M, Van Rooijen N, Bozja J, et al (Emory Univ School of Medicine, Atlanta, GA; Vrije Universiteit Medisch Centrum, Amsterdam, The Netherlands; Zetra Biologicals, Tucker, GA)
Proc Natl Acad Sci U S A 108:757-761, 2011

Development of an influenza vaccine that provides broadly cross-protective immunity has been a scientific challenge for more than half a century. This study presents an approach to overcome strain-specific protection by supplementing conventional vaccines with virus-like particles (VLPs) containing the conserved M2 protein (M2 VLPs) in the absence of adjuvants. We demonstrate that an inactivated influenza vaccine supplemented with M2 VLPs prevents disease symptoms without showing weight loss and confers complete cross protection against lethal challenge with heterologous influenza A viruses including the 2009 H1N1 pandemic virus as well as heterosubtypic H3N2 and H5N1 influenza viruses. Cross-protective immunity was long-lived, for more than 7 mo. Immune sera from mice immunized with M2 VLP supplemented vaccine transferred cross protection to naive mice. Dendritic and macrophage cells were found to be important for this cross protection mediated by immune sera. The results provide evidence that supplementation of seasonal influenza vaccines with M2 VLPs is a promising approach for overcoming the limitation of strain-specific protection by current vaccines and developing a universal influenza A vaccine.

▶ The potential of modern-day pandemic influenza at regular intervals became a reality in 2009 with the rapid worldwide spread of a swine origin H1N1 influenza A virus. The seasonal influenza vaccine for 2009 prepared based on the epidemiologically expected viral strains failed to control the emergence and spread of H1N1 strain. Current influenza vaccines provide protection by neutralizing antibody responses to the highly variable hemagglutinin (HA) antigen of the strains present in the vaccine but not antigenically distinct heterogonous viruses. The continuous evolution of influenza viruses based on mutations in the surface antigens HA and neuraminidase (NA) is the reason for lack of cross-protective activity against strains not present in the seasonal vaccines. Scientific work to develop an influenza vaccine able to provide broad cross-protection has been ongoing since the first introduction of the vaccine. In contrast to HA and NA, M2 Protein (M2e) exposed on the surface of human influenza A virion is a highly conserved domain.[1] The antibody response to M2e is not seen after natural infection or vaccination indicating poor immunogenicity of this protein. In experimental studies, antibodies to M2e provided limited to no protection against lethal infection even in the presence of potent adjuvants, cholera toxin, and bacterial protein conjugates.

This study describes further progress in the approach by presenting M2 on viruslike particles (VLPs) in a membrane-anchored form (M2 VLPs). Vaccination with M2 VLPs alone did not confer significant protective immunity against influenza in mice. However, addition of M2 VLPs to be an inactivated influenza vaccine induced effective M2-specific humoral and cellular immune responses. The M2VLP supplemented A/PR 8 vaccine induced an effective immune response including long-lived cross protection against the distantly related 2009 H1N1 pandemic virus as well as H3N2 and H5N1 subtypes. This approach can overcome the inefficient cross-protection by current inactivated vaccines and make a leap toward developing a universal influenza A vaccine.

N. M. Khardori, MD, PhD

Reference

1. Lamb RA, Zebedee SL, Richardson CD. Influenza virus M2 protein is an integral membrane protein expressed on the infected-cell surface. *Cell.* 1985;40:627-633.

Antibodies induced with recombinant VP1 from human rhinovirus exhibit cross-neutralisation

Edlmayr J, Niespodziana K, Popow-Kraupp T, et al (Med Univ of Vienna, Austria; et al)

Eur Respir J 37:44-52, 2011

Human rhinoviruses (HRVs) are the major cause of the common cold and account for 30-50% of all acute respiratory illnesses. Although HRV infections are usually harmless and invade only the upper respiratory tract, several studies demonstrate that HRV is involved in the exacerbation of asthma.

VP1 is one of the surface-exposed proteins of the viral capsid that is important for the binding of rhinoviruses to the corresponding receptors on human cells. Here we investigated its potential usefulness for vaccination against the common cold.

We expressed VP1 proteins from two distantly related HRV strains, HRV89 and HRV14, in *Escherichia coli.* Mice and rabbits were immunised with the purified recombinant proteins.

The induced antibodies reacted with natural VP1 and with whole virus particles as shown by immunoblotting and immunogold electron microscopy. They exhibited strong cross-neutralising activity for different HRV strains. Therefore, recombinant VP1 may be considered a candidate HRV vaccine to prevent HRV-induced asthma exacerbations.

▶ Human rhinoviruses (HRV) (family Picornaviridae) are single-stranded RNA viruses. There are >100 distinct serotypes belonging to 2 genetic species (clades), HRV-A and HRV-B.[1] Recently, a third clade, HRV-C, was included among HRVs. Until recently, HRVs have been known as a cause of acute upper respiratory disease. Recent data have implicated them as triggers for exacerbations of asthma, chronic obstructive pulmonary disease, and cystic fibrosis.[2] In addition, their pathogenic role in lower respiratory tract infection of infants, elderly, and immunocompromised patients has been reported.[3] Highly sensitive-specific polymerase chain reaction—based technology has provided the basis for these recent studies.

Four capsid proteins (60 copies of each), VP1, VP2, VP3, and VP4, form the viral capsid of HRVs. VP1, VP2, and VP3 are located on the surface of the capsid and are responsible for antigenic diversity of HRVs. Of these, VP1 is the most exposed and immunodominant surface protein in HRVs. In addition, VP1 is important for binding of rhinovirus to the human cells.

In this experimental study, VP1 from 2 distantly related strains of HRV was expressed in *Escherichia coli.* The expressed protein absorbed to alum was used to immunize mice and rabbits. The antibodies raised in the animals reacted strongly with VP1 and belonged to a polyclonal immune response against several segments of the protein, which increased the potential for cross-reactivity. The antibodies raised against the recombinant VP1 proteins for 2 HRV strains inhibited the infection of cultured HeLa cells by a variety of rhinovirus strains. These results show that a recombinant rhinovirus vaccine for humans that can be easily produced under controlled conditions and has a broad cross-protective activity is feasible.

N. M. Khardori, MD, PhD

References

1. Ledford RM, Patel NR, Demenczuk TM, et al. VP1 sequencing of all human rhinovirus serotypes: insights into genus phylogeny and susceptibility to antiviral capsid-binding compound. *J Virol.* 2004;78:3663-3674.
2. Holgate ST. Rhinoviruses in the pathogenesis of asthma: the bronchial epithelium as a major disease target. *J Allergy Clin Immunol.* 2006;118:587-590.
3. Gerna G, Piralla A, Rovida F, et al. Correlation of rhinovirus load in the respiratory tract and clinical symptoms in hospitalized immunocompetent and immunocompromised patients. *J Med Virol.* 2009;81:1498-1507.

Universal Vaccine Based on Ectodomain of Matrix Protein 2 of Influenza A: Fc Receptors and Alveolar Macrophages Mediate Protection
El Bakkouri K, Descamps F, De Filette M, et al (Flanders Inst of Biotechnology (VIB), Ghent, Belgium; et al)
J Immunol 186:1022-1031, 2011

The ectodomain of matrix protein 2 (M2e) of influenza A virus is an attractive target for a universal influenza A vaccine: the M2e sequence is highly conserved across influenza virus subtypes, and induced humoral anti-M2e immunity protects against a lethal influenza virus challenge in animal models. Clinical phase I studies with M2e vaccine candidates have been completed. However, the in vivo mechanism of immune protection induced by M2e-carrier vaccination is unclear. Using passive immunization experiments in wild-type, $FcR\gamma^{-/-}$, $Fc\gamma RI^{-/-}$, $Fc\gamma RIII^{-/-}$, and $(Fc\gamma RI, Fc\gamma RIII)^{-/-}$ mice, we report in this study that Fc receptors are essential for anti-M2e IgG-mediated immune protection. M2e-specific IgG1 isotype Abs are shown to require functional $Fc\gamma RIII$ for in vivo immune protection but other anti-M2e IgG isotypes can rescue $Fc\gamma RIII^{-/-}$ mice from a lethal challenge. Using a conditional cell depletion protocol, we also demonstrate that alveolar macrophages (AM) play a crucial role in humoral M2e-specific immune protection. Additionally, we show that adoptive transfer of wild-type AM into $(Fc\gamma RI, Fc\gamma RIII)^{-/-}$ mice restores protection by passively transferred anti-M2e IgG. We conclude that AM and Fc receptor-dependent elimination of influenza A virus-infected cells are essential for protection by anti-M2e IgG.

▶ The protective immune response conferred by current inactivated influenza vaccine is strain specific. Antibodies against the hemagglutinin (HA) antigen in serum are believed to correlate with protection provided that the HA present in the vaccine corresponds fairly closely to that of circulating influenza strain.[1] Even with the time and resources used for producing and administering yearly seasonal influenza vaccine, the infrequent but unpredictable pandemics cannot be controlled effectively. Influenza pandemics remain a worldwide threat to health and economy. In addition, a vaccine mismatch can occur for any given season.

The ectodomain of matrix protein 2 (M2e) of influenza A virus, a very highly conserved domain, is an attractive target for a universal influenza A vaccine. The M2e sequence is highly conserved across all known human influenza A viruses. Following animal studies, phase 1 clinical studies with M2e vaccine candidates have been completed. This study reports on the immunologic mechanism involved in protective immunity against influenza induced by M2e-containing vaccines. The investigators identified the crucial role of Fc receptor and alveolar macrophage in protection by anti-M2e antibody. The results indicate that antibody-dependent cellular cytotoxicity and antibody-dependent cell-mediated phagocytosis are the major mechanisms involved. Antibody against M2e probably provided protection by interacting with virus-infected cells rather than the viral particles. The infected cells express abundant M2 at their surface early after infection. The anti-M2e immunoglobulin G (IgG)-mediated cellular cytotoxicity or phagocytosis allows removal of infected cells before the budding, and spread of progeny virus, opsonization of virions, by anti-M2e IgG would be a less effective mechanism given less abundance of M2 particles compared with HA and neuraminidase influenza virus particles. This and many other recent studies are significant steps forward on the way to having a universal influenza vaccine for clinical use.

N. M. Khardori, MD, PhD

Reference

1. Hobson D, Currt RK, Beare AS, Ward-Gardner A. The role of serum haemagglutination-inhibiting antibody in protection against challenge infection with influenza A2 and B viruses. *J Hyg (Lond)*. 1972;70:767-777.

17 Tuberculosis

Evaluation of Clinical Prediction Rules for Respiratory Isolation of Inpatients with Suspected Pulmonary Tuberculosis

Solari L, Acuna-Villaorduna C, Soto A, et al (Inst of Tropical Medicine, Antwerp, Belgium; Universidad Peruana Cayetano Heredia, Lima, Peru; Hospital Nacional Hipolito Unanue, Lima, Peru)
Clin Infect Dis 52:595-603, 2011

Background.—In the framework of hospital infection control, various clinical prediction rules (CPRs) for respiratory isolation of patients with suspected pulmonary tuberculosis (PTB) have been developed. Our aim was to evaluate their performance in an emergency department setting with a high prevalence of PTB.

Methods.—We searched the MEDLINE and OVID databases to identify CPRs to predict PTB. We used a previously collected database containing clinical, radiographical, and microbiological information on patients attending an emergency department with respiratory complaints, and we applied each CPR to every patient and compared the result with culture for *Mycobacterium tuberculosis* as the reference standard. We also simulated the proportion of isolated suspects and missed cases for PTB prevalences of 5% and 30%.

Results.—We withheld 13 CPRs for evaluation. We had complete data on 345 patients. Most CPRs achieved a high sensitivity but very low specificity and very low positive predictive value. Mylotte's score, which includes results of sputum smear as a predictive finding, was the best-performing CPR. It attained a sensitivity of 88.9% and a specificity of 63.9%. However, at a 30% PTB prevalence, 498 of 1000 individuals with suspected PTB would have to be isolated; 267 of these cases would be true PTB cases, and 33 cases would be missed. Two consecutive sputum smears had a sensitivity of 75.6% and a specificity of 99.7%.

Conclusions.—In a setting with a high prevalence of PTB, only 1 of the 13 assessed CPRs demonstrated high sensitivity combined with satisfactory specificity. Our results highlight the need for local validation of CPRs before their application.

▶ The failure of early identification and prevention of transmission of pulmonary tuberculosis (PTB) in health care settings has led to nosocomial outbreaks of both drug-susceptible and drug-resistant tuberculosis.[1,2] In resource-poor settings with moderate to high prevalence of PTB, adherence to Centers for Disease Control (CDC) Guidelines is not possible. The CDC guidelines recommend that a patient presenting to a health care facility with clinical symptoms compatible with those of PTB should be kept under airborne precautions until 3 consecutive sputum smears show no acid fast bacilli.[3] However compatible clinical symptoms are not well defined and are therefore left to clinicians' interpretation.

The authors in this study evaluated the performance of various clinical prediction rules (CPRs) for airborne precautions in patients with suspected PTB in an emergency department setting with a high prevalence of PTB. Complete data on 345 patients (clinical, radiological, and microbiological) was used to evaluate 13 CPRs obtained from a search of MEDLINE and OVID databases.

The results from 2 consecutive sputum smears had sensitivity of 75.6% and a specificity of 99.7%.[4] Of the CPRs that did not include sputum smear, Tattevius was the best performer, which makes it more suitable for health care facilities where smear results are not readily available. The study illustrates the significance of external and local validation before implementation of published articles on clinical decision rules.

N. M. Khardori, MD, PhD

References

1. Frieden TR, Sherman LF, Maw KL, et al. A multi-institutional outbreak of highly drug-resistant tuberculosis: epidemiology and clinical outcomes. *JAMA.* 1996; 276:1229-1235.
2. Sepkowitz KA, Friedman CR, Hafner A, et al. Tuberculosis among urban health care workers: a study using restriction fragment length polymorphism typing. *Clin Infect Dis.* 1995;21:1098-1101.
3. Jensen PA, Lambert LA, Iademarco MF, Ridzon R, Centers for Disease Control and Prevention. Guidelines for preventing the transmission of *Mycobacterium tuberculosis* in health-care settings, 2005. *MMWR Recomm Rep.* 2005;54:1-141.
4. Mylotte JM, Rodgers J, Fassl M, Seibel K, Vacanti A. Derivation and validation of a pulmonary tuberculosis prediction model. *Infect Control Hosp Epidemiol.* 1997; 18:554-560.

Inhaled Corticosteroids and Risk of Tuberculosis in Patients with Respiratory Diseases

Brassard P, Suissa S, Kezouh A, et al (Jewish General Hosp, Montreal, Quebec, Canada)
Am J Respir Crit Care Med 183:675-678, 2011

Rationale.—Treatment with substantial doses of oral corticosteroids (OCS) for prolonged periods increases the risk of tuberculosis (TB). However, little is known about the effect of inhaled corticosteroids (ICS) in this respect.

Objectives.—We quantified the independent contribution of ICS to the risk of TB in a population of patients with airway diseases.

Methods.—A population-based cohort design with a nested case-control analysis was used. A cohort of patients with airways disease was formed using the Quebec databases. TB cases were identified and age-matched control subjects were selected from all subjects who entered the cohort in the same month as the cases. TB incidence among the cohort was compared with the general population of Quebec using the standardized incidence ratio.

Measurements and Main Results.—The cohort consisted of 427,648 subjects. There were 564 cases of TB identified between 1990 and 2005. The standardized incidence ratio was 3.9 (95% confidence interval [CI], 2.6—5.4). Any and current users of ICS are at an increased risk of TB (rate ratio [RR], 1.27; 95% CI, 1.05—1.53; and RR, 1.33; 95% CI, 1.04—1.71, respectively). Among users of OCS, no significant relationship could be demonstrated. Among subjects without OCS exposure, adjusted RRs were significant for any ICS use (RR, 1.26; 95%CI, 1.02—1.56) and current use (RR, 1.48; 95% CI, 1.11—1.97) and at the current high dose exposure level (RR, 1.97; 95% CI, 1.18—3.3).

Conclusions.—Exposure to ICS is not associated with risk of TB in the presence of OCS but is associated with increased TB risk in nonusers of OCS.

▶ The well-documented association between prolonged use of oral corticosteroid (OCS) and risk of tuberculosis (TB) infection has been recently quantified.[1] Although inhaled corticosteroids (ICS) have fewer adverse effects than OCS, they are partially absorbed and can cause systemic effects associated with corticosteroids use such as skin bruising, accelerated bone loss, and subcapsular cataracts.[2]

This is a population-based cohort study to quantify the independent contribution of ICS to the risk of TB among patients with airway disease. Between 1990 and 2005, 564 cases of TB were identified in a cohort of 427 648 subjects. They were compared with 5640 control subjects. The current and any use of ICS was associated with increased risk of TB (Table 2 in the original article). High-dose ICS was associated with the highest relative risk of 1.94. However, the exposure to ICS did not add to the risk of TB in the presence of OCS even at high doses. These data suggest that the use of ICS should be limited to patients with reactive airway disease (a subset of patient with COPD and patients with asthma) and the lowest possible dose should be used.

N. M. Khardori, MD, PhD

References

1. Brassard P, Kezouh A, Suissa S. Antirheumatic drugs and the risk of tuberculosis. *Clin Infect Dis.* 2006;43:717-722.
2. Uboweja A, Malhotra S, Pandhi P. Effect of inhaled corticosteroids on risk of development of cataract: a meta-analysis. *Fundam Clin Pharmacol.* 2006;20: 305-309.

PART THREE

HEMATOLOGY AND ONCOLOGY

JAMES TATE THIGPEN, MD

18 Breast Cancer

Eribulin monotherapy versus treatment of physician's choice in patients with metastatic breast cancer (EMBRACE): a phase 3 open-label randomised study

Cortes J, on behalf of the EMBRACE (Eisai Metastatic Breast Cancer Study Assessing Physician's Choice Versus E7389) investigators (Vall d'Hebron Univ Hosp and Vall d'Hebron Inst of Oncology, Barcelona, Spain; et al)

Lancet 377:914-923, 2011

Background.—Treatments with survival benefit are greatly needed for women with heavily pretreated metastatic breast cancer. Eribulin mesilate is a non-taxane microtubule dynamics inhibitor with a novel mode of action. We aimed to compare overall survival of heavily pretreated patients receiving eribulin versus currently available treatments.

Methods.—In this phase 3 open-label study, women with locally recurrent or metastatic breast cancer were randomly allocated (2:1) to eribulin mesilate ($1·4$ mg/m^2 administered intravenously during 2–5 min on days 1 and 8 of a 21-day cycle) or treatment of physician's choice (TPC). Patients had received between two and five previous chemotherapy regimens (two or more for advanced disease), including an anthracycline and a taxane, unless contraindicated. Randomisation was stratified by geographical region, previous capecitabine treatment, and human epidermal growth factor receptor 2 status. Patients and investigators were not masked to treatment allocation. The primary endpoint was overall survival in the intention-to-treat population. This study is registered at ClinicalTrials.gov, number NCT00388726.

Findings.—762 women were randomly allocated to treatment groups (508 eribulin, 254 TPC). Overall survival was significantly improved in women assigned to eribulin (median $13·1$ months, 95% CI $11·8–14·3$) compared with TPC ($10·6$ months, $9·3–12·5$; hazard ratio $0·81$, 95% CI $0·66–0·99$; p $= 0·041$). The most common adverse events in both groups were asthenia or fatigue (270 [54%] of 503 patients on eribulin and 98 [40%] of 247 patients on TPC at all grades) and neutropenia (260 [52%] patients receiving eribulin and 73 [30%] of those on TPC at all grades). Peripheral neuropathy was the most common adverse event leading to discontinuation from eribulin, occurring in 24 (5%) of 503 patients.

Interpretation.—Eribulin showed a significant and clinically meaningful improvement in overall survival compared with TPC in women with heavily pretreated metastatic breast cancer. This finding challenges the notion that improved overall survival is an unrealistic expectation during evaluation of new anticancer therapies in the refractory setting.

▶ Eribulin mesylate is a nontaxane antimicrotubule agent with activity in breast cancer. In this trial, the investigators randomly assigned patients with 2 to 5 prior treatment regimens to either eribulin mesylate or physician's choice. Analysis of the intention-to-treat population for overall survival was the primary goal of the trial. The study demonstrated a survival advantage for those patients assigned to eribulin; the investigators enthusiastically note that this proves that attaining a survival advantage in this heavily pretreated patient population is thus feasible, contrary to what some have claimed and what all previous trials looking at overall survival as a primary end point have suggested, since none were positive. There are several considerations, however, that suggest that one should draw this conclusion with caution. Firstly, the potential confounding effect of postprogression therapy, a concern cited in trials of breast cancer, cannot be assessed adequately in this trial. Secondly, to quote an old expression, "even a blind hog finds an acorn every now and then," this is 1 trial, and there will occasionally, by chance alone, be positive trials that do not reflect reality. The trial does demonstrate that eribulin is active in heavily pretreated metastatic breast cancer, but it does not prove that overall survival is the best end point for a study in a setting in which multiple additional treatments will be given following progression.

J. T. Thigpen, MD

Iniparib plus Chemotherapy in Metastatic Triple-Negative Breast Cancer
O'Shaughnessy J, Osborne C, Pippen JE, et al (Baylor Charles A. Sammons Cancer Ctr, Dallas, TX; et al)
N Engl J Med 364:205-214, 2011

Background.—Triple-negative breast cancers have inherent defects in DNA repair, making this cancer a rational target for therapy based on poly(adenosine diphosphate—ribose) polymerase (PARP) inhibition.

Methods.—We conducted an open-label, phase 2 study to compare the efficacy and safety of gemcitabine and carboplatin with or without iniparib, a small molecule with PARP-inhibitory activity, in patients with metastatic triple-negative breast cancer. A total of 123 patients were randomly assigned to receive gemcitabine (1000 mg per square meter of body-surface area) and carboplatin (at a dose equivalent to an area under the concentration—time curve of 2) on days 1 and 8 — with or without iniparib (at a dose of 5.6 mg per kilogram of body weight) on days 1, 4, 8, and 11 — every 21 days. Primary end points were the rate of clinical benefit (i.e., the rate of objective response [complete or partial response] plus the rate of stable disease for ≥6 months) and safety. Additional end points included the rate of objective response, progression-free survival, and overall survival.

Results.—The addition of iniparib to gemcitabine and carboplatin improved the rate of clinical benefit from 34% to 56% (P = 0.01) and the rate of overall response from 32% to 52% (P = 0.02). The addition of iniparib also prolonged the median progression-free survival from 3.6 months to 5.9 months (hazard ratio for progression, 0.59; P = 0.01) and the median overall survival from 7.7 months to 12.3 months (hazard ratio for death, 0.57; P = 0.01). The most frequent grade 3 or 4 adverse events in either treatment group included neutropenia, thrombocytopenia, anemia, fatigue or asthenia, leukopenia, and increased alanine amino-transferase level. No significant difference was seen between the two groups in the rate of adverse events.

Conclusions.—The addition of iniparib to chemotherapy improved the clinical benefit and survival of patients with metastatic triple-negative breast cancer without significantly increased toxic effects. On the basis of these results, a phase 3 trial adequately powered to evaluate overall survival and progression-free survival is being conducted.(Funded by BiPar Sciences [now owned by Sanofi-Aventis]; ClinicalTrials.gov number, NCT00540358.)

▶ Poly(adenosine diphosphate—ribose) polymerase (PARP) inhibitors have attracted major interest because of early trials that indicated significant activity for these agents in *BRCA* mutation—associated breast and ovarian cancers. Cancers associated with *BRCA* mutations exhibit deficiencies of usual DNA repair mechanisms. This brings into play pathways such as PARP inhibitors, which are not thought normally to play a major role. More recently, attention has been focused on other DNA repair deficiencies that might expand the patient population amenable to treatment with PARP inhibitors. This particular study focuses on triple-negative breast cancers (estrogen negative, progesterone negative, and human epidermal growth factor receptor type 2 negative), which have inherent defects in DNA repair. The PARP inhibitor is iniparib, which some now think may actually exert its effect through mechanisms other than PARP inhibition. The study randomized patients to gemcitabine/carboplatin ± iniparib. The study is a randomized phase II study that is not sufficiently powered to provide a definitive answer as to the proper role for iniparib, but the results do suggest that the addition of iniparib improved both progression-free and overall survival as well as the primary end point of clinical benefit (complete response + partial response + stable disease). As the investigators indicate in their conclusions, this should trigger a phase III trial to define whether the agent has a defined role in the management of triple-negative breast carcinoma. Similar studies of gemcitabine/carboplatin plus iniparib were reported at the American Society of Clinical Oncology 2011 meeting in June 2011 at Chicago, but the uncontrolled phase II design of these trials makes it impossible to comment on activity in recurrent ovarian carcinoma without further studies.

J. T. Thigpen, MD

Multicenter Phase III Randomized Trial Comparing Docetaxel and Trastuzumab With Docetaxel, Carboplatin, and Trastuzumab As First-Line Chemotherapy for Patients With HER2-Gene-Amplified Metastatic Breast Cancer (BCIRG 007 Study): Two Highly Active Therapeutic Regimens

Valero V, Forbes J, Pegram MD, et al (The Univ of Texas M D Anderson Cancer Ctr, Houston; Univ of Newcastle, New South Wales, Australia; Univ of California, Los Angeles; et al)

J Clin Oncol 29:149-156, 2011

Purpose.—Docetaxel-trastuzumab (TH) is effective therapy for *HER2*-amplified metastatic breast cancer (MBC). Preclinical findings of synergy between docetaxel, carboplatin, and trastuzumab (TCH) prompted a phase III randomized trial comparing TCH with TH in patients with *HER2*-amplified MBC.

Patients and Methods.—Two hundred sixty-three patients were randomly assigned to receive eight 3-week cycles of TH (trastuzumab plus docetaxel 100 mg/m^2) or TCH (trastuzumab plus carboplatin at area under the serum concentration-time curve 6 and docetaxel 75 mg/m^2). Trastuzumab was given at 4 mg/kg loading dose followed by a 2 mg/kg dose once per week during chemotherapy, and then 6 mg/kg once every 3 weeks until progression.

Results.—Patient characteristics were balanced between groups. There was no significant difference between TH and TCH in terms of the primary end point, time to progression (medians of 11.1 and 10.4 months, respectively; hazard ratio, 0.914; 95% CI, 0.694 to 1.203; $P = .57$), response rate (72% for both groups), or overall survival (medians of 37.1 and 37.4 months, respectively; $P = .99$). Rates of grades 3 or 4 adverse effects for TH and TCH, respectively, were neutropenic-related complications, 29% and 23%; thrombocytopenia, 2% and 15%; anemia, 5% and 11%; sensory neuropathy, 3% and 0.8%; fatigue, 5% and 12%; peripheral edema, 3.8% and 1.5%; and diarrhea, 2% and 10%. Two patients given TCH died of sepsis, and one patient given TH experienced sudden cardiac death. Absolute left ventricular ejection fraction decline > 15% was seen in 5.5% of patients on the TH arm and 6.7% of patients on the TCH arm.

Conclusion.—Adding carboplatin did not enhance TH antitumor activity. TH (docetaxel, 100 mg/m^2) and TCH (docetaxel, 75 mg/m^2) demonstrated efficacy with acceptable toxicity in women with *HER2*-amplified MBC.

▶ This trial addresses whether carboplatin should be given with docetaxel and trastuzumab (TH) for *HER2*-overexpressing metastatic breast cancer. The results suggest that the addition of carboplatin is unnecessary because docetaxel, carboplatin, and trastuzumab (TCH) and TH both yield the same response rate, progression-free survival, and overall survival. When one combines this information with the fact that most *HER2*-overexpressing cancers do not benefit from inclusion of an anthracycline (because only 35% have coamplification of *TOP2A* and thus are more sensitive to an anthracycline), it would appear that TH would be a reasonable regimen in most patients with *HER2*-overexpressing metastatic breast cancer. There is one caveat to keep in mind. The dose of the docetaxel in this trial in the arm without carboplatin was 100 mg/m^2, which is substantially more toxic than the more commonly used 75 mg/m^2. This, in fact, is probably the reason that TH was not less toxic than TCH. Whether TH with a docetaxel dose of 75 mg/m^2 would yield the same results is purely speculative; hence, one would need to use the higher dose if this study is to be used as a basis for omitting carboplatin.

J. T. Thigpen, MD

RIBBON-1: Randomized, Double-blind, Placebo-Controlled, Phase III Trial of Chemotherapy With or Without Bevacizumab for First-Line Treatment of Human Epidermal Growth Factor Receptor 2—Negative, Locally Recurrent or Metastatic Breast Cancer
Robert NJ, Diéras V, Glaspy J, et al (Virginia Cancer Specialists, Fairfax; Univ of California, Los Angeles; Genentech, South San Francisco, CA; et al)
J Clin Oncol 29:1252-1260, 2011

Purpose.—This phase III study compared the efficacy and safety of bevacizumab (BV) when combined with several standard chemotherapy regimens versus those regimens alone for first-line treatment of patients with human epidermal growth factor receptor 2—negative metastatic breast cancer.

Patients and Methods.—Patients were randomly assigned in 2:1 ratio to chemotherapy plus BV or chemotherapy plus placebo. Before random assignment, investigators chose capecitabine (Cape; 2,000 mg/m^2 for 14 days), taxane (Tax)-based (nab-paclitaxel 260 mg/m^2, docetaxel 75 or 100 mg/m^2), or anthracycline (Anthra)-based (doxorubicin or epirubicin combinations [doxorubicin/cyclophosphamide, epirubicin/cyclophosphamide, fluorouracil/epirubicin/cyclophosphamide, or fluorouracil/doxorubicin/cyclophosphamide]) chemotherapy administered every 3 weeks. BV or placebo was administered at 15 mg/kg every 3 weeks. The primary end point was progression-free survival (PFS). Secondary end points included overall survival (OS), 1-year survival rate, objective response rate, duration of objective response, and safety. Two independently powered cohorts defined by the choice of chemotherapy (Cape patients or pooled Tax/Anthra patients) were analyzed in parallel.

Results.—RIBBON-1 (Regimens in Bevacizumab for Breast Oncology) enrolled 1,237 patients (Cape cohort, n = 615; Tax/Anthra cohort, n = 622). Median PFS was longer for each BV combination (Cape cohort: increased from 5.7 months to 8.6 months; hazard ratio [HR], 0.69; 95% CI, 0.56 to 0.84; log-rank *P* < .001; and Tax/Anthra cohort: increased from 8.0 months to 9.2 months; HR, 0.64; 95% CI, 0.52 to 0.80; log-rank *P* < .001). No statistically significant differences in OS between the placebo- and BV-containing arms were observed. Safety was consistent with results of prior BV trials.

Conclusion.—The combination of BV with Cape, Tax, or Anthra improves clinical benefit in terms of increased PFS in first-line treatment of metastatic breast cancer, with a safety profile comparable to prior phase III studies.

▶ This study is 1 of 3 trials looking at the addition of bevacizumab to chemotherapy in the management of patients with HER2-negative metastatic breast cancer. This and the other 2 trials all show benefit for the addition of bevacizumab in terms of the primary end point of each trial, progression-free survival (PFS). The hazard ratios (HR) for each are as follows: E2100 HR, 0.60, $P < .001$; AVADO HR, 0.77, $P = .006$. This trial had 2 hazard ratios: capecitabine cohort HR, 0.69 and taxane/anthracycline cohort HR, 0.64, both $P < .001$. Of particular importance is the consistency of the results. In each instance, the improvement is about a 30% reduction in the hazard of progression. These trials led to accelerated approval of the agent. This approval was withdrawn this year because of the lack of a significant improvement in overall survival, but this lack was not surprising in light of the additional therapy that all of these patients receive after progression. The withdrawal was also inconsistent with other decisions of the US Food and Drug Administration (FDA) such as the approval of lapatinib based on improvement in time to progression without a survival improvement. Ostensibly, the decision was based on the toxicity of bevacizumab, but the only consistently increased toxicity with bevacizumab is hypertension, which is easily managed in most patients. Based on the data rather than the FDA decision, the use of bevacizumab should be considered in metastatic breast cancer because of the clear and consistent improvement in PFS with manageable toxicity.

J. T. Thigpen, MD

Axillary Dissection vs No Axillary Dissection in Women With Invasive Breast Cancer and Sentinel Node Metastasis: A Randomized Clinical Trial
Giuliano AE, Hunt KK, Ballman KV, et al (John Wayne Cancer Inst at Saint John's Health Ctr, Santa Monica, CA; M D Anderson Cancer Ctr, Houston, TX; Mayo Clinic Rochester, MN; et al)
JAMA 305:569-575, 2011

Context.—Sentinel lymph node dissection (SLND) accurately identifies nodal metastasis of early breast cancer, but it is not clear whether further nodal dissection affects survival.

Objective.—To determine the effects of complete axillary lymph node dissection (ALND) on survival of patients with sentinel lymph node (SLN) metastasis of breast cancer.

Design, Setting, and Patients.—The American College of Surgeons Oncology Group Z0011 trial, a phase 3 noninferiority trial conducted at 115 sites and enrolling patients from May 1999 to December 2004. Patients were women with clinical T1-T2 invasive breast cancer, no palpable adenopathy, and 1 to 2 SLNs containing metastases identified by frozen section, touch preparation, or hematoxylin-eosin staining on permanent section.

Targeted enrollment was 1900 women with final analysis after 500 deaths, but the trial closed early because mortality rate was lower than expected.

Interventions.—All patients underwent lumpectomy and tangential whole-breast irradiation. Those with SLN metastases identified by SLND were randomized to undergo ALND or no further axillary treatment. Those randomized to ALND underwent dissection of 10 or more nodes. Systemic therapy was at the discretion of the treating physician.

Main Outcome Measures.—Overall survival was the primary end point, with a non-inferiority margin of a 1-sided hazard ratio of less than 1.3 indicating that SLND alone is noninferior to ALND. Disease-free survival was a secondary end point.

Results.—Clinical and tumor characteristics were similar between 445 patients randomized to ALND and 446 randomized to SLND alone. However, the median number of nodes removed was 17 with ALND and 2 with SLND alone. At a median follow-up of 6.3 years (last follow-up, March 4, 2010), 5-year overall survival was 91.8% (95% confidence interval [CI], 89.1%-94.5%) with ALND and 92.5% (95% CI, 90.0%-95.1%) with SLND alone; 5-year disease-free survival was 82.2% (95% CI, 78.3%-86.3%) with ALND and 83.9% (95% CI, 80.2%-87.9%) with SLND alone. The hazard ratio for treatment-related overall survival was 0.79 (90% CI, 0.56-1.11) without adjustment and 0.87 (90% CI, 0.62-1.23) after adjusting for age and adjuvant therapy.

Conclusion.—Among patients with limited SLN metastatic breast cancer treated with breast conservation and systemic therapy, the use of SLND alone compared with ALND did not result in inferior survival.

Trial Registration.—clinicaltrials.gov Identifier: NCT00003855.

▶ Previous studies have shown that sentinel node biopsy can accurately identify the presence of nodal involvement without the need for an axillary node dissection. The question has remained, however, as to whether a completion node dissection was indicated in those patients with evidence of lymph node involvement to improve overall and disease-free survival. This article reports the results of a prospective randomized phase III trial addressing precisely this point. The American College of Surgeons Oncology Group randomized 891 patients with clinical T1-T2 breast cancer and positive sentinel nodes to either no further surgery or an axillary node dissection. At a median of 6.3 years of follow-up, 5-year overall and disease-free survivals were virtually identical. This finding of no advantage for a follow-up axillary node dissection should not be a surprise. Previous National Surgical Adjuvant Breast and Bowel Project studies have shown no therapeutic advantage for axillary node dissection, and it is difficult to find any advantage for use of node dissection in any solid tumor. The bottom line is that, in the absence of grossly involved residual lymph nodes, axillary node dissection cannot be supported as a useful approach.

J. T. Thigpen, MD

Alteration of Topoisomerase II–Alpha Gene in Human Breast Cancer: Association with Responsiveness to Anthracycline-Based Chemotherapy

Press MF, Sauter G, Buyse M, et al (Univ of Southern California, Los Angeles, CA; Univ of California Los Angeles; City of Hope Natl Med Ctr, Duarte, CA; et al)
J Clin Oncol 29:859-867, 2011

Purpose.—Approximately 35% of *HER2*-amplified breast cancers have coamplification of the topoisomerase II-alpha (*TOP2A*) gene encoding an enzyme that is a major target of anthracyclines. This study was designed to evaluate whether *TOP2A* gene alterations may predict incremental responsiveness to anthracyclines in some breast cancers.

Methods.—A total of 4,943 breast cancers were analyzed for alterations in *TOP2A* and *HER2*. Primary tumor tissues from patients with metastatic breast cancer treated in a trial of chemotherapy plus/minus trastuzumab were studied for amplification/deletion of *TOP2A* and *HER2* as a test set followed by evaluation of malignancies from two separate, large trials for changes in these same genes as a validation set. Association between these alterations and clinical outcomes was determined.

Results.—Test set cases containing *HER2* amplification treated with doxorubicin and cyclophosphamide (AC) plus trastuzumab, demonstrated longer progression-free survival compared to those treated with AC alone (*P* = .0002). However, patients treated with AC alone whose tumors contain *HER2/TOP2A* coamplification experienced a similar improvement in survival (*P* = .004). Conversely, for patients treated with paclitaxel, *HER2/TOP2A* coamplification was not associated with improved outcomes. These observations were confirmed in a larger validation set, where *HER2/TOP2A* coamplification was again associated with longer survival when only anthracycline-containing chemotherapy was used for treatment compared with outcome in *HER2*-positive cancers lacking *TOP2A* coamplification.

Conclusion.—In a study involving nearly 5,000 breast malignancies, both test set and validation set demonstrate that *TOP2A* coamplification, not *HER2* amplification, is the clinically useful predictive marker of an incremental response to anthracycline-based chemotherapy. Absence of *HER2/TOP2A* coamplification may indicate a more restricted efficacy advantage for breast cancers than previously thought.

▶ *HER2* amplification has, since 1998, marked a group of patients as having breast cancer that requires treatment that is different from the treatment for those that do not overexpress *HER2*. In particular, *HER2* amplification has been associated with better patient outcomes in those treated with an anthracycline and with trastuzumab. More recently, interest has focused on *TOP2A* gene alterations in association with *HER2* overexpression as a marker for anthracycline sensitivity. Studies have variously reported that only those patients with coamplification of both *HER2* and *TOP2A* benefit from an anthracycline more so than with regimens not containing an anthracycline. This study reports an attempt to clarify the issue by evaluating the coamplification as a marker of anthracycline sensitivity. When one puts these results together with results from previous literature on this topic, the following conclusions would seem reasonable. (1) There is little evidence for an advantage of using anthracyclines in patients who do not exhibit coamplification of *HER2* and *TOP2A*. (2) In patients with *HER2* amplification without *TOP2A* coamplification, the use of trastuzumab with chemotherapy yields improved progression-free survival and overall survival, but it is not necessary to use anthracycline-based chemotherapy to achieve this. (3) In patients with coamplification of both *HER2* and *TOP2A*, inclusion of an anthracycline confers improved progression-free survival and overall survival even in the absence of trastuzumab. (4) In patients who do not overexpress *HER2*, there is no advantage to an anthracycline-based regimen.

J. T. Thigpen, MD

Dose-Dense Chemotherapy in Nonmetastatic Breast Cancer: A Systematic Review and Meta-analysis of Randomized Controlled Trials
Bonilla L, Ben-Aharon I, Vidal L, et al (Rabin Med Ctr, Petah Tikva, Israel)
J Natl Cancer Inst 102:1845-1854, 2010

Background.—Dose-dense chemotherapy has become a mainstay regimen in the adjuvant setting for women with high-risk breast cancer. We performed a systematic review and meta-analysis of the existing data from randomized controlled trials regarding the efficacy and toxicity of the dose-dense chemotherapy approach in nonmetastatic breast cancer.

Methods.—Randomized controlled trials that compared a dose-dense chemotherapy protocol with a standard chemotherapy schedule in the neoadjuvant or adjuvant setting in adult women older than 18 years with breast cancer were identified by searching The Cochrane Cancer Network register of trials, The Cochrane Library, and LILACS and MEDLINE databases (from January 1966 to January 2010). Hazard ratios (HRs) of death and recurrence and relative risks of adverse events were estimated and pooled. All statistical tests were two-sided.

Results.—Ten trials met the inclusion criteria and were classified into two categories based on trial methodology. Three trials enrolling 3337 patients compared dose-dense chemotherapy with a conventional chemotherapy schedule (similar agents). Patients who received dose-dense chemotherapy had better overall survival (HR of death = 0.84, 95% confidence interval [CI] = 0.72 to 0.98, P =.03) and better disease-free survival (HR of recurrence or death = 0.83, 95% CI = 0.73 to 0.94, P =.005) than those on the conventional schedule. No benefit was observed in patients with hormone receptor–positive tumors. Seven trials enrolling 8652 patients compared dose-dense chemotherapy with regimens that use standard intervals but with different agents and/or dosages in the treatment arms. Similar results were obtained for these trials with respect to overall survival (HR of death = 0.85, 95% CI = 0.75 to 0.96, P =.01) and disease-free survival (HR of recurrence or death = 0.81, 95% CI = 0.73

to 0.88, $P < .001$). The rate of nonhematological adverse events was higher in the dose-dense chemotherapy arms than in the conventional chemotherapy arms.

Conclusion.—Dose-dense chemotherapy results in better overall and disease-free survival, particularly in women with hormone receptor-negative breast cancer. However, additional data from randomized controlled trials are needed before dose-dense chemotherapy can be considered as the standard of care.

▶ For the past 3 decades, oncologists have generally held that dose and schedule were important in determining the efficacy of chemotherapy. Results of a CALGB trial in breast cancer demonstrated that dose-dense therapy (single agents or combinations given in sequence at shorter intervals than conventional therapy supported by growth factors) compared with conventional therapy produces superior disease-free and overall survival. Over the past 15 years, 10 Phase III trials comparing dose-dense therapy to conventional therapy have been published. This article presents a meta-analysis of these 10 trials to determine the level of any advantage associated with dose-dense therapy. The data show that dose-dense therapy is associated with a better disease-free survival (hazard ratio [HR] $= 0.83$, $P = .005$) and overall survival (HR $= 0.84$, $P = .03$) than conventional therapy. This establishes dose-dense therapy as a valid approach. Before such an approach becomes the standard of care, however, 3 caveats must be addressed. First, 7 of the 10 trials did not use the same agents in the dose-dense and conventional arms. This introduces additional variables that must be accounted for before a definitive conclusion can be reached about the dose-dense approach. Second, the small number of trials included in this meta-analysis leaves open the possibility that conclusions are subject to publication bias (negative trials not published because they were negative). Finally, it is clear that not all patients benefit from a dose-dense approach. For example, essentially half the patient population, those with HR + disease, do not gain an advantage from this approach. Further studies are needed to characterize fully the patient population that is likely to benefit before this becomes the standard of care.

J. T. Thigpen, MD

HER2, *TOP2A*, and TIMP-1 and Responsiveness to Adjuvant Anthracycline-Containing Chemotherapy in High-Risk Breast Cancer Patients
Ejlertsen B, Jensen M-B, Nielsen KV, et al (Danish Breast Cancer Cooperative Group Statistical Ctr, Copenhagen, Denmark; Copenhagen Univ Hosp, Denmark; Dako A/S, Glostrup, Denmark; et al)
J Clin Oncol 28:984-990, 2010

Purpose.—To evaluate whether the combination of HER2 with TIMP-1 (HT) or *TOP2A* with TIMP-1 (2T) more accurately identifies patients who benefit from cyclophosphamide, epirubicin, and fluorouracil (CEF) compared with cyclophosphamide, methotrexate, and fluorouracil (CMF) than these markers do when analyzed individually.

Patients and Methods.—The Danish Breast Cancer Cooperative Group (DBCG) 89D trial randomly assigned 980 high-risk Danish breast cancer patients to CMF or CEF. Archival tumor tissue was analyzed TIMP-1, and HER2-negative and TIMP-1 immunoreactive tumors were classified as HT nonresponsive and otherwise HT responsive. Similarly, the 2T panel was constructed by combining *TOP2A* and TIMP-1; tumors with normal *TOP2A* status and TIMP-1 immunoreactivity were classified as 2T-nonresponsive and otherwise 2T-responsive.

Results.—In total, 623 tumors were available for analysis, of which 154 lacked TIMP-1 immunoreactivity, 188 were HER2 positive, and 139 had a *TOP2A* aberration. HT status was a statistically significant predictor of benefit from CEF compared with CMF ($P_{interaction} = .036$ for invasive disease–free survival [IDFS] and .047 for overall survival [OS]). The 269 (43%) patients with a 2T-responsive profile had a significant reduction in IDFS events (adjusted hazard ratio, 0.48; 95% CI, 0.34 to 0.69; $P < .001$) and OS events (adjusted hazard ratio, 0.54; 95% CI, 0.38 to 0.77; $P < .001$). 2T status was a highly significant predictor of benefit from CEF compared with CMF ($P_{interaction} < .0001$ for IDFS and .004 for OS).

Conclusion.—The 2T profile is a more accurate predictor of incremental benefit from anthracycline-containing chemotherapy than HER2, TIMP-1, or *TOP2A* individually, and compared with these, 2T classifies a larger proportion of patients as sensitive to anthracyclines.

▶ Continuing the theme of looking for biological markers that will identify those patients most likely to benefit from anthracyclines, this study looks at *TOP2A* and TIMP-1 in addition to HER2. The study uses a 980-patient phase III trial comparing cyclophosphamide, epirubicin, and fluorouracil (CEF) with cyclophosphamide, methotrexate, and fluorouracil (CMF) as a basis for the trial. The bottom line is that abnormalities of either or both of *TOP2A* and TIMP-1 represent better predictors of anthracycline sensitivity than the commonly HER2 status. The importance of this observation is that we can now avoid giving an anthracycline with all of the attendant risks of cardiotoxicity to a number of patients who otherwise would have received the anthracycline in the belief that anthracycline-based combinations are better than alternatives such as CMF. This is supported by another article reviewed herein that suggested that coamplification of HER2 and *TOP2A* represented a better marker of anthracycline sensitivity than HER2 status alone. Both this article and the one reviewed earlier point out indirectly that assessment of the meaning of specific biologic abnormalities is far more complex than simply assessing the status of a single marker and thus led to the conclusion that we have to accrue a great deal more information before we can accurately predict optimal treatment from the biologic profile. This does not mean that we shouldn't use the information we have at hand now to benefit (hopefully) patients now, but it does mean that we have to reassess constantly our treatment paradigms in light of expanding biologic data.

J. T. Thigpen, MD

Long-Term Benefits of 5 Years of Tamoxifen: 10-Year Follow-up of a Large Randomized Trial in Women at Least 50 Years of Age With Early Breast Cancer

Hackshaw A, Roughton M, Forsyth S, et al (Cancer Res UK and Univ College London Cancer Trials Centre)
J Clin Oncol 29:1657-1663, 2011

Purpose.—The Cancer Research UK "Over 50s" trial compared 5 and 2 years of tamoxifen in women with early breast cancer. Results are reported after median follow-up of 10 years.

Patients and Methods.—Between 1987 and 1997, 3,449 patients age 50 to 81 years with operable breast cancer who had been taking 20 mg of tamoxifen for 2 years were randomly assigned to either stop or continue for an additional 3 years, if they were alive and recurrence free. Data on recurrences, new tumors, deaths, and cardiovascular events were obtained (April 2010).

Results.—There were 1,103 recurrences, 755 deaths as a result of breast cancer, 621 cardiovascular (CV) events, and 236 deaths as a result of CV events. Fifteen years after starting treatment, for every 100 women who received tamoxifen for 5 years, 5.8 fewer experienced recurrence, compared with those who received tamoxifen for 2 years. The risk of contralateral breast cancer was significantly reduced (hazard ratio, 0.70; 95% CI, 0.48 to 1.00). Among women age 50 to 59 years, there was a 35% reduction in CV events ($P = .005$) and 59% reduction in death as a result of a CV event ($P = .02$); in older women, the effect was much smaller and not statistically significant.

Conclusion.—Taking tamoxifen for the recommended 5 years reduces the risk of recurrence or contralateral breast cancer 15 years after starting treatment. It also lowers the risk of CV disease and death as a result of a CV event, particularly among those age 50 to 59 years. Women should therefore be encouraged to complete the full course. Although aromatase inhibitors improve disease-free survival, tamoxifen remains a cheap and highly effective alternative, particularly in developing countries.

▶ For women older than 50 who have ER-positive breast cancer, the use of hormonal therapy for 5 years as adjuvant treatment is reasonably well established. The original agent used in this setting in large clinical trials was tamoxifen, although recent evidence of a superior effect with aromatase inhibitors has led to the replacement of tamoxifen with an aromatase inhibitor. This study provides long-term follow-up of patients randomly assigned to either 2 or 5 years of tamoxifen on 1 of the earlier trials. Among a total of 3449 women in the randomization, the use of 5 rather than 2 years of tamoxifen led to a 5.8% reduction in recurrences. The beneficial effects associated with prolonged use of tamoxifen were greatest in the younger women on the trial (ages 50 to 59). In addition, this study shows a marked reduction in risk of cardiovascular events (35%) and of death related to cardiovascular events (59%). One reasonably assumes that at least the beneficial effects seen with regard to the reduction in recurrence of the breast cancer will hold for the use of 5 years of aromatase inhibitors, the current standard of care in the United States.

J. T. Thigpen, MD

19 Cancer Therapies

Treatment-Related Mortality With Bevacizumab in Cancer Patients: A Meta-analysis
Ranpura V, Hapani S, Wu S (Stony Brook Univ Med Ctr, NY)
JAMA 305:487-494, 2011

Context.—Fatal adverse events (FAEs) have been reported in cancer patients treated with the widely used angiogenesis inhibitor bevacizumab in combination with chemotherapy. Currently, the role of bevacizumab in treatment-related mortality is not clear.

Objective.—To perform a systematic review and meta-analysis of published randomized controlled trials (RCTs) to determine the overall risk of FAEs associated with bevacizumab.

Data Sources.—PubMed, EMBASE, and Web of Science databases as well as abstracts presented at American Society of Clinical Oncology conferences from January 1966 to October 2010 were searched to identify relevant studies.

Study Selection and Data Extraction.—Eligible studies included prospective RCTs in which bevacizumab in combination with chemotherapy or biological therapy was compared with chemotherapy or biological therapy alone. Summary incidence rates, relative risks (RRs), and 95% confidence intervals (CIs) were calculated using fixed- or random-effects models.

Data Synthesis.—A total of 10 217 patients with a variety of advanced solid tumors from 16 RCTs were included in the analysis. The overall incidence of FAEs with bevacizumab was 2.5% (95% CI, 1.7%-3.9%). Compared with chemotherapy alone, the addition of bevacizumab was associated with an increased risk of FAEs, with an RR of 1.46 (95% CI, 1.09-1.94; $P = .01$; incidence, 2.5% vs 1.7%). This association varied significantly with chemotherapeutic agents ($P = .045$) but not with tumor types ($P = .13$) or bevacizumab doses ($P = .16$). Bevacizumab was associated with an increased risk of FAEs in patients receiving taxanes or platinum agents (RR, 3.49; 95% CI, 1.82-6.66; incidence, 3.3% vs 1.0%) but was not associated with increased risk of FAEs when used in conjunction with other agents (RR, 0.85; 95% CI, 0.25-2.88; incidence, 0.8% vs 0.9%). The most common causes of FAEs were hemorrhage (23.5%), neutropenia (12.2%), and gastrointestinal tract perforation (7.1%).

Conclusion.—In a meta-analysis of RCTs, bevacizumab in combination with chemotherapy or biological therapy, compared with chemotherapy alone, was associated with increased treatment-related mortality.

▶ The recent decision to remove Food and Drug Administration (FDA) approval for bevacizumab in breast cancer because, in its judgment, the benefits were outweighed by the risks has focused attention on the toxicity of bevacizumab and on the question of whether progression-free survival improvement provided clear evidence of clinical benefit. This article addresses the first of these concerns, the toxicity associated with the addition of bevacizumab to chemotherapy. The meta-analysis was based on 16 randomized clinical trials published or presented at an American Society of Clinical Oncology (ASCO) meeting between January 2000 and October 30, 2010, and randomizing between chemotherapy and chemotherapy plus bevacizumab. The authors claim to have included all randomized clinical trials meeting these criteria. The 2 critical conclusions drawn by the authors were that the addition of bevacizumab to chemotherapy significantly increased the risk of a fatal adverse event (2.5% versus 1.7%; relative risk [RR], 1.46; $P = .01$) and that the association between bevacizumab and fatal adverse events was especially true for those receiving taxanes or platinum agents (3.3% versus 1.0%; RR, 3.49).

The results of this study, however, need to be regarded with major caution. First, the study has a glaring omission from the included randomized clinical trials. The number one plenary session article at ASCO in June 2010 was the report of the Gynecologic Oncology Group 218, a prospective randomized clinical trial of 1873 patients assigned to paclitaxel/carboplatin/placebo followed by placebo maintenance, paclitaxel/carboplatin/bevacizumab followed by placebo maintenance, or paclitaxel/carboplatin/bevacizumab followed by bevacizumab maintenance. This study showed no difference in adverse effects except for a higher frequency of hypertension among those receiving bevacizumab. All these patients received the 2 alleged high-risk drugs (a taxane and a platinum). This clearly could have affected the conclusions of the meta-analysis. Second, regarding the FDA decision in breast cancer, the meta-analysis shows an RR of 0.69 in breast cancer studies and thus suggests a decrease in fatalities among those patients with breast cancer who received bevacizumab. At least in breast cancer, there seems to be little evidence to suggest that the toxicity of bevacizumab outweighs whatever beneficial effects one might want to attribute to the improvement in progression-free survival.

J. T. Thigpen, MD

20 Gastrointestinal Cancer

Addition of cetuximab to oxaliplatin-based first-line combination chemotherapy for treatment of advanced colorectal cancer: results of the randomised phase 3 MRC COIN trial

Maughan TS, on behalf of the MRC COIN Trial Investigators (Cardiff Univ, UK; et al)
Lancet 377:2103-2114, 2011

Background.—In the Medical Research Council (MRC) COIN trial, the epidermal growth factor receptor (EGFR)-targeted antibody cetuximab was added to standard chemotherapy in first-line treatment of advanced colorectal cancer with the aim of assessing effect on overall survival.

Methods.—In this randomised controlled trial, patients who were fit for but had not received previous chemotherapy for advanced colorectal cancer were randomly assigned to oxaliplatin and fluoropyrimidine chemotherapy (arm A), the same combination plus cetuximab (arm B), or intermittent chemotherapy (arm C). The choice of fluoropyrimidine therapy (capecitabine or infused fluorouracil plus leucovorin) was decided before randomisation. Randomisation was done centrally (via telephone) by the MRC Clinical Trials Unit using minimisation. Treatment allocation was not masked. The comparison of arms A and C is described in a companion paper. Here, we present the comparison of arm A and B, for which the primary outcome was overall survival in patients with KRAS wild-type tumours. Analysis was by intention to treat. Further analyses with respect to NRAS, BRAF, and EGFR status were done. The trial is registered, ISRCTN27286448.

Findings.—1630 patients were randomly assigned to treatment groups (815 to standard therapy and 815 to addition of cetuximab). Tumour samples from 1316 (81%) patients were used for somatic molecular analyses; 565 (43%) had KRAS mutations. In patients with KRAS wild-type tumours (arm A, n=367; arm B, n=362), overall survival did not differ between treatment groups (median survival 17·9 months [IQR 10·3–29·2] in the control group vs 17·0 months [9·4–30·1] in the cetuximab group; HR 1·04, 95% CI 0·87–1·23, p=0·67). Similarly, there was no effect on progression-free survival (8·6 months [IQR 5·0–12·5] in the control group vs 8·6 months [5·1–13·8] in the cetuximab group; HR 0·96, 0·82–1·12, p=0·60). Overall response rate increased from 57% (n=209) with chemotherapy alone to 64% (n=232) with addition of cetuximab (p=0·049). Grade 3 and higher skin and gastrointestinal toxic effects were increased with cetuximab (14 vs 114 and 67 vs 97 patients in the control group vs the cetuximab group with KRAS wild-type tumours, respectively). Overall survival differs by somatic mutation status irrespective of treatment received: BRAF mutant, 8·8 months (IQR 4·5−27·4); KRAS mutant, 14·4 months (8·5−24·0); all wild-type, 20·1 months (11·5−31·7).

Interpretation.—This trial has not confirmed a benefit of addition of cetuximab to oxaliplatin-based chemotherapy in first-line treatment of patients with advanced colorectal cancer. Cetuximab increases response rate, with no evidence of benefit in progression-free or overall survival in KRAS wild-type patients or even in patients selected by additional mutational analysis of their tumours. The use of cetuximab in combination with oxaliplatin and capecitabine in first-line chemotherapy in patients with widespread metastases cannot be recommended.

▶ Epidermal growth factor receptor (EGFR)-targeted therapies have a well-defined role in metastatic *KRAS* wild-type colorectal cancer. The monoclonal antibody cetuximab is US Food and Drug Administration approved in combination with irinotecan for metastatic colorectal cancer after progression on irinotecan, and as single agent after failure of any prior chemotherapy. Cetuximab has also demonstrated improved progression-free and overall survival when combined with FOLFIRI (infusional 5-fluorouracil and irinotecan) in the first-line treatment of *KRAS* wild-type metastatic colorectal cancer, with an added 3.5 months' benefit on overall survival (hazard ratio [HR], 0.8) and 1.5 months in progression-free survival (PFS) (HR, 0.7).[1]

The Medical Research Council (MRC) COIN trial investigators have addressed the role of adding cetuximab to an oxaliplatin-based regimen in first-line metastatic colorectal cancer and also analyzed the effect of treatment interruptions on outcomes. Overall, 2445 patients were randomly assigned to have FOLFOX (infusional 5-fluorouracil and oxaliplatin) or XELOX (capecitabine and oxaliplatin) until disease progression (arm A), FOLFOX or XELOX plus cetuximab until disease progression (arm B), or intermittent FOLFOX or XELOX (12 weeks of treatment, and restart at progression; arm C). The primary endpoint was overall survival in KRAS wild-type tumors, and the secondary endpoint included overall survival in KRAS mutant, KRAS/NRAS/BRAF wild type, "any" mutant, progression-free survival, response, and quality of life. This article reports on the primary outcome. Approximately 65% versus 35% of patients were treated at the physician's discretion with XELOX versus FOLFOX. Among 367 patients with *KRAS* wild-type disease randomly assigned to FOLFOX/XELOX and 361 patients with *KRAS* wild-type disease randomly assigned to FOLFOX/XELOX plus cetuximab, there was no benefit in overall survival (17.9 vs 17 months) or PFS (8.6 months in both groups) but a modest improvement in response from 57% to 64% (*P* = .049). Patients with wild-type tumors for all genes tested, *KRAS*, *NRAS*, and *BRAF*, similarly did not demonstrate any benefit from the addition of cetuximab. Exploratory analysis for predictive factors on PFS, found that 5-fluorouracil, but not capecitabine treatment, was associated with improved

PFS when combined with cetuximab (HR 0.72, 95% confidence interval [CI] 0.53–0.98; $P = .037$).

An additional study, NORDIC VII, previously reported at ESMO 2010, had shown similarly disappointing results when bolus 5-fluorouracil and oxaliplatin (FLOX) were combined with cetuximab, indicating no benefit in PFS (7.9 months for FLOX with cetuximab vs 8.7 months with FLOX, HR 1.07).[2]

The possibility of the lack of benefit with cetuximab added to the chemotherapy backbone being caused by capecitabine due to increased toxicity, as suggested by the authors, is unlikely to explain entirely the findings, as the duration on treatment was similar in both groups in the COIN study, especially when corroborated further with the NORDIC study, which used 5-fluorouracil. These results clearly suggest that cetuximab should not be used in combination with oxaliplatin-fluoropyrimidine chemotherapy in metastatic colorectal cancer, and raise the concern of a significant negative drug-drug interaction.

E. G. Chiorean, MD

References

1. Van Cutsem E, Köhne CH, Láng I, et al. Cetuximab plus irinotecan, fluorouracil, and leucovorin as first-line treatment for metastatic colorectal cancer: updated analysis of overall survival according to tumor KRAS and BRAF mutation status. *J Clin Oncol*. 2011;29:2011-2019.
2. Tveit K, Guren T, Glimelius B, et al. Randomized phase III study of 5-fluorouracil/folinate/oxaliplatin given continuously or intermittently with or without cetuximab, as first line treatment of metastatic colorectal cancer: the NORDIC VII study by the Nordic Colorectal Cancer Biomodulation Group. *J Clin Oncol*. 2011;29 [abstract 365].

Addition of cetuximab to oxaliplatin-based first-line combination chemotherapy for treatment of advanced colorectal cancer: results of the randomised phase 3 MRC COIN trial
Maughan TS, on behalf of the MRC COIN Trial Investigators (Cardiff Univ, UK; et al)
Lancet 377:2103-2114, 2011

Background.—In the Medical Research Council (MRC) COIN trial, the epidermal growth factor receptor (EGFR)-targeted antibody cetuximab was added to standard chemotherapy in first-line treatment of advanced colorectal cancer with the aim of assessing effect on overall survival.

Methods.—In this randomised controlled trial, patients who were fit for but had not received previous chemotherapy for advanced colorectal cancer were randomly assigned to oxaliplatin and fluoropyrimidine chemotherapy (arm A), the same combination plus cetuximab (arm B), or intermittent chemotherapy (arm C). The choice of fluoropyrimidine therapy (capecitabine or infused fluorouracil plus leucovorin) was decided before randomisation. Randomisation was done centrally (via telephone) by the MRC Clinical Trials Unit using minimisation. Treatment allocation was not masked. The comparison of arms A and C is described in a companion paper. Here, we present the comparison of arm A and B, for which the primary outcome was overall survival in patients with *KRAS* wild-type tumours. Analysis was by intention to treat. Further analyses with respect to *NRAS, BRAF,* and *EGFR* status were done. The trial is registered, ISRCTN27286448.

Findings.—1630 patients were randomly assigned to treatment groups (815 to standard therapy and 815 to addition of cetuximab). Tumour samples from 1316 (81%) patients were used for somatic molecular analyses; 565 (43%) had *KRAS* mutations. In patients with *KRAS* wild-type tumours (arm A, n=367; arm B, n=362), overall survival did not differ between treatment groups (median survival 17·9 months [IQR 10·3–29·2] in the control group *vs* 17·0 months [9·4–30·1] in the cetuximab group; HR 1·04, 95% CI 0·87–1·23, p=0·67). Similarly, there was no effect on progression-free survival (8·6 months [IQR 5·0–12·5] in the control group *vs* 8·6 months [5·1–13·8] in the cetuximab group; HR 0·96, 0·82–1·12, p=0·60). Overall response rate increased from 57% (n=209) with chemotherapy alone to 64% (n=232) with addition of cetuximab (p=0·049). Grade 3 and higher skin and gastrointestinal toxic effects were increased with cetuximab (14 *vs* 114 and 67 *vs* 97 patients in the control group *vs* the cetuximab group with *KRAS* wild-type tumours, respectively). Overall survival differs by somatic mutation status irrespective of treatment received: *BRAF* mutant, 8·8 months (IQR 4·5–27·4); *KRAS* mutant, 14·4 months (8·5–24·0); all wild-type, 20·1 months (11·5–31·7).

Interpretation.—This trial has not confirmed a benefit of addition of cetuximab to oxaliplatin-based chemotherapy in first-line treatment of patients with advanced colorectal cancer. Cetuximab increases response rate, with no evidence of benefit in progression-free or overall survival in *KRAS* wild-type patients or even in patients selected by additional mutational analysis of their tumours. The use of cetuximab in combination with oxaliplatin and capecitabine in first-line chemotherapy in patients with widespread metastases cannot be recommended.

▶ The most commonly used regimens in colorectal cancers use oxaliplatin with a fluoropyrimidine (either fluorouracil or capecitabine). The addition of bevacizumab to this combination has been suggested by some trials to enhance overall survival. The other biological alternative is cetuximab, which has been used primarily with irinotecan-based regimens. This trial seeks to determine whether the addition of cetuximab to an oxaliplatin and fluoropyrimidine regimen is advantageous in those patients with *KRAS* wild-type. The data show no advantage and substantial toxicity disadvantages for the addition of cetuximab to an oxaliplatin-based regimen. At least for now, it would appear that the standard of care for the first-line treatment of metastatic colon cancer remains an oxaliplatin and fluoropyrimidine regimen with or without bevacizumab. Cetuximab would appear to be better reserved for use with irinotecan-based regimens in patients with wild-type *KRAS*.

J. T. Thigpen, MD

Randomized Trial of Two Induction Chemotherapy Regimens in Metastatic Colorectal Cancer: An Updated Analysis

Masi G, Vasile E, Loupakis F, et al (Istituto Toscano Tumori, Pisa, Italy; et al)
J Natl Cancer Inst 103:21-30, 2011

Background.—In a randomized trial with a median follow-up of 18.4 months, 6 months of induction chemotherapy with a three-drug regimen comprising 5-fluorouracil (by continuous infusion)—leucovorin, irinotecan, and oxaliplatin (FOLFOXIRI) demonstrated statistically significant improvements in response rate, radical surgical resection of metastases, progression-free survival, and overall survival compared with 6 months of induction chemotherapy with fluorouracil—leucovorin and irinotecan (FOLFIRI).

Methods.—From November 14, 2001, to April 22, 2005, we enrolled 244 patients with metastatic colorectal cancer. To evaluate if the superiority of FOLFOXIRI is maintained in the long term, we updated the overall and progression-free survival data to include events that occurred up to February 12, 2009, with a median follow-up of 60.6 months. We performed a subgroup and a risk-stratified analysis to examine whether outcomes differed in specific patient subgroups, and we analyzed the results of treatment after progression. Survival curves were estimated by the Kaplan—Meier method. Multivariable Cox regression models were fit to estimate hazard ratios (HRs) and 95% confidence intervals (CIs). All statistical tests were two-sided.

Results.—FOLFOXIRI demonstrated statistically significant improvements in median progression-free survival (9.8 vs 6.8 months, HR for progression $= 0.59$, 95% CI $= 0.45$ to 0.76, $P < .001$) and median overall survival (23.4 vs 16.7 months, HR for death $= 0.74$, 95% CI $= 0.56$ to 0.96, $P = .026$) with a 5-year survival rate of 15% (95% CI $= 9\%$ to 23%) vs 8% (95% CI $= 4\%$ to 14%). The improvements in progression-free survival and, to a lesser extent, in overall survival were evident even when the analysis excluded patients who received radical resection of metastases. With regard to the risk-stratified analysis, FOLFOXIRI results in longer progression-free survival and over-all survival than FOLFIRI in all risk subgroups.

Conclusions.—Six months of induction chemotherapy with FOLFOXIRI is associated with a clinically significant improvement in the long-term outcome compared with FOLFIRI with an absolute benefit in survival at 5 years of 7%.

▶ The outlook for the patient with metastatic colon cancer has improved substantially in the past 15 years as new active agents have been added to 5-fluorouracil. The addition of first irinotecan, then oxaliplatin, and subsequently the monoclonal antibodies cetuximab and bevacizumab have increased the overall median survival from less than a year to more than 2 years. Two chemotherapy doublets have become the standard backbones for treatment: FOLFOX and FOLFIRI. This trial examines a regimen that includes all 3 chemotherapeutic agents as compared with one of the doublets, FOLFIRI. The results suggest an improvement in response rate, progression-free survival, and overall survival with the 3-drug regimen at the expense of a substantial increase in toxicity. In particular, patients receiving the 3-drug regimen had a higher response rate, which led to a greater likelihood that residual disease could be resected after chemotherapy. These data look convincing, but they are contradicted by another phase III trial by the Hellenic Group that found the increased toxicity seen in this trial but no advantage for the 3-drug regimen. These conflicting results have resulted in the continued use of doublets of chemotherapy in combination with bevacizumab as the basis for the therapy of most patients with metastatic disease.

J. T. Thigpen, MD

Association Between Time to Initiation of Adjuvant Chemotherapy and Survival in Colorectal Cancer: A Systematic Review and Meta-Analysis

Biagi JJ, Raphael MJ, Mackillop WJ, et al (Queen's Univ, Kingston, Ontario, Canada)
JAMA 305:2335-2342, 2011

Context.—Adjuvant chemotherapy (AC) improves survival among patients with resected colorectal cancer. However, the optimal timing from surgery to initiation of AC is unknown.

Objective.—To determine the relationship between time to AC and survival outcomes via a systematic review and meta-analysis.

Data Sources.—MEDLINE (1975 through January 2011), EMBASE, the Cochrane Database of Systematic Reviews, and the Cochrane Central Register of Controlled Trials were searched to identify studies that described the relationship between time to AC and survival.

Study Selection.—Studies were only included if the relevant prognostic factors were adequately described and either comparative groups were balanced or results adjusted for these prognostic factors.

Data Extraction.—Hazard ratios (HRs) for overall survival and disease-free survival from each study were converted to a regression coefficient (β) and standard error corresponding to a continuous representation per 4 weeks of time to AC. The adjusted β from individual studies were combined using a fixed-effects model. Inverse variance ($1/SE^2$) was used to weight individual studies. Publication bias was investigated using the trim and fill approach.

Results.—We identified 10 eligible studies involving 15 410 patients (7 published articles, 3 abstracts). Nine of the studies were cohort or population based and 1 was a secondary analysis from a randomized trial of chemotherapy. Six studies reported time to AC as a binary variable and 4 as 3 or more categories. Meta-analysis demonstrated that a 4-week increase in time to AC was associated with a significant decrease in both overall survival (HR, 1.14; 95% confidence interval [CI], 1.10-1.17) and disease-free survival (HR, 1.14; 95% CI, 1.10-1.18). There was no significant heterogeneity among included studies. Results remained significant after adjustment for potential publication bias and when the analysis was repeated to exclude studies of largest weight.

Conclusion.—In a meta-analysis of the available literature on time to AC, longer time to AC was associated with worse survival among patients with resected colorectal cancer.

▶ The interval of time between surgery and the initiation of adjuvant chemotherapy is theoretically crucial to the efficacy of the adjuvant treatment. Surgical removal of the bulk of disease can theoretically accelerate the growth and rate at which mutations leading to drug resistance can occur in the residual micrometastases. Delays in the initiation of adjuvant therapy can therefore lead to decreased efficacy by allowing for greater likelihood of the emergence of disease that is resistant for whatever reason. Previous studies have suggested that clinical evidence supports that adjuvant therapy started more than 12 weeks after surgery will have little effect. This meta-analysis evaluated 10 trials that had data on time to start of adjuvant therapy available for study and that included 15 410 patients and found positive evidence that delays in the start of adjuvant therapy to more than 4 weeks after surgery compromised the effectiveness of the therapy. The investigators concluded that a delay to 8 weeks increased the hazard of death by 14% and that a delay to 12 weeks increased the hazard of death by 30%. The one flaw in the study is that no data from the oxaliplatin era are included among the 10 studies evaluated. By the same token, no data from studies including bevacizumab are included either. The bottom line is that adjuvant therapy should be started as soon as possible after surgery and that the start should occur, if possible, no later than 4 weeks after surgery.

J. T. Thigpen, MD

DNA Mismatch Repair Status and Colon Cancer Recurrence and Survival in Clinical Trials of 5-Fluorouracil-Based Adjuvant Therapy
Sinicrope FA, Foster NR, Thibodeau SN, et al (Mayo Clinic, Rochester, MN; et al)
J Natl Cancer Inst 103:863-875, 2011

Background.—Approximately 15% of colorectal cancers develop because of defective function of the DNA mismatch repair (MMR) system. We determined the association of MMR status with colon cancer recurrence and examined the impact of 5-fluorouracil (FU)-based adjuvant therapy on recurrence variables.

Methods.—We included stage II and III colon carcinoma patients (n = 2141) who were treated in randomized trials of 5-FU-based adjuvant therapy. Tumors were analyzed for microsatellite instability by polymerase chain reaction and/or for MMR protein expression by immunohistochemistry to determine deficient MMR (dMMR) or proficient MMR (pMMR) status. Associations of MMR status and/or 5-FU-based treatment with clinicopathologic and recurrence covariates were determined using χ^2 or

Fisher Exact or Wilcoxon rank-sum tests. Time to recurrence (TTR), disease-free survival (DFS), and overall survival (OS) were analyzed using univariate and multivariable Cox models, with the latter adjusted for covariates. Tumors showing dMMR were categorized by presumed germline vs sporadic origin and were assessed for their prognostic and predictive impact. All statistical tests were two-sided.

Results.—In this study population, dMMR was detected in 344 of 2141 (16.1%) tumors. Compared with pMMR tumors, dMMR was associated with reduced 5-year recurrence rates (33% vs 22%; $P < .001$), delayed TTR ($P < .001$), and fewer distant recurrences (22% vs 12%; $P < .001$). In multivariable models, dMMR was independently associated with delayed TTR (hazard ratio = 0.72, 95% confidence interval = 0.56 to 0.91, $P = .005$) and improved DFS ($P = .035$) and OS ($P = .031$). In stage III cancers, 5-FU-based treatment vs surgery alone or no 5-FU was associated with reduced distant recurrence for dMMR tumors (11% vs 29%; $P = .011$) and reduced recurrence to all sites for pMMR tumors ($P < .001$). The dMMR tumors with suspected germline mutations were associated with improved DFS after 5-FU-based treatment compared with sporadic tumors where no benefit was observed ($P = .006$).

Conclusions.—Patients with dMMR colon cancers have reduced rates of tumor recurrence, delayed TTR, and improved survival rates, compared with pMMR colon cancers. Distant recurrences were reduced by 5-FU-based adjuvant treatment in dMMR stage III tumors, and a subset analysis suggested that any treatment benefit was restricted to suspected germline vs sporadic tumors.

▶ Approximately 15% of colorectal cancers (CRC) occur because of a defective DNA mismatch repair (MMR) genetic system, giving rise to deficient MMR (dMMR) colorectal cancers. dMMR tumors are mostly caused by epigenetic alterations in *MLH1* (in sporadic CRC), while few are secondary to germline mutations in *MLH1*, *MSH2*, *MSH6*, and *PMS2* (causing Lynch syndrome). Characteristically, dMMR CRC show high frequency of microsatellite instability (MSI-H), have clinical and pathologic characteristics, mainly located in the proximal colon, and have better clinical outcomes, based on retrospective data. In addition, several studies suggest no benefit from 5-fluorouracil (5-FU) for dMMR colorectal cancers.[1,2] It is unclear whether the lack of survival benefit using 5-FU for stages 2 and 3 CRC varies depending on the epigenetic or mutational inactivation of the DNA mismatch repair genes.

In one of the largest studies reported to date, with a median follow-up of 8 years, Sinicrope et al analyzed the effect of dMMR on patterns of cancer relapse and survival as well as on the effects of 5-FU adjuvant therapy (with no additional oxaliplatin or irinotecan) on clinical outcomes for 2141 patients with stages 2 (n = 778) and 3 (n = 1363) colorectal cancers; participation in international, randomized adjuvant clinical trials with 5-FU; and available tissue specimens for analysis of MSI (by reverse transcriptase polymerase chain reaction) and MMR protein expression by immunohistochemistry (IHC). Several tumors (n = 111) were also tested for the *BRAF* V600E mutation.

Approximately 16% of all patients had dMMR tumors, and the dMMR tumors were more likely to be stage 2, proximal in location, and poorly differentiated. dMMR CRC patients had superior disease-free survival (DFS) (hazard ratio [HR], 0.73; $P = .004$) as well as superior overall survival (HR, 0.73; $P = .004$) compared with proficient MMR tumors, but the significant benefit was limited to patients with stage 3 disease.

In a prior study, Sargent et al[1] reported on the lack of efficacy of 5-FU adjuvant therapy for dMMR colorectal cancer. In the current study, 5-FU therapy was associated with fewer distant recurrences for stage 3 dMMR CRC, but an overall predictive analysis for stage 2 or 3 dMMR CRC was not performed. Nevertheless, the authors intended to analyze the possible predictive effect from 5-FU by categorizing dMMR cancers into sporadic and germline based on dMMR (either loss of *MSH2* and MSI-H and/or loss of *MLH1*) and an age cutoff of 55 years at diagnosis: sporadic if age over 55, and germline (Lynch syndrome) if age 55 or less. All tumors with loss of *MSH2* were presumed germline, and all tumors with *BRAF* mutation were presumed sporadic. Prognosis was similar for germline and sporadic dMMR CRC. Of note, in patients with presumed germline tumors (n = 66), 5-FU versus no therapy was associated with improved DFS (HR 0.29, $P = .006$), while no benefit was observed for sporadic dMMR CRC (n = 120). This benefit was restricted to stage 3 germline dMMR CRC. No formal analysis in stage 2 dMMR CRC was provided.

These results suggest that the benefit of 5-FU in stage 3 dMMR colorectal cancer depends on the mechanism of epigenetic or mutational inactivation of the MMR genes, and while hypothesis generating, will need validation from larger randomized studies.

The study's limitations reside in its retrospective design, pooling of the patients from multiple randomized trials with incomplete tissue availability, and the categorization of germline versus sporadic on the presumption of MMR analysis in tumor in combination with the age at diagnosis rather than molecular germline DNA testing. Most importantly, the authors have not reported an updated analysis on the predictive value of MMR deficiency on DFS and overall survival based on treatment with 5-FU or observation.

Despite these shortcomings, the implications for clinical practice are important, and while this study did not address the role of 5-FU in stage 2 dMMR CRC, it validated the benefit from 5-FU for stage 3 CRC, including for MSI-H and other dMMR CRC. The predictive value of dMMR on treatment with 5-FU plus oxaliplatin, per standard practice for many stage 3 CRC patients, is currently unknown but will be addressed in future trials.

E. G. Chiorean, MD

References

1. Sargent DJ, Marsoni S, Monges G, et al. Defective mismatch repair as a predictive marker for lack of efficacy of fluorouracil-based adjuvant therapy in colon cancer. *J Clin Oncol.* 2010;28:3219-3226.
2. Jover R, Zapater P, Castells A, et al. The efficacy of adjuvant chemotherapy with 5-fluorouracil in colorectal cancer depends on the mismatch repair status. *Eur J Cancer.* 2009;45:365-373.

Comparison of Two Neoadjuvant Chemoradiotherapy Regimens for Locally Advanced Rectal Cancer: Results of the Phase III Trial ACCORD 12/0405-Prodige 2

Gérard J-P, Azria D, Gourgou-Bourgade S, et al (Centre Antoine-Lacassagne, Nice cedex, France; Université Nice Sofia Antipolis, France; Centre Val d'Aurelle, Montpellier, France; et al)

J Clin Oncol 28:1638-1644, 2010

Purpose.—Neoadjuvant chemoradiotherapy is considered a standard approach for T3-4 M0 rectal cancer. In this situation, we compared neoadjuvant radiotherapy plus capecitabine with dose-intensified radiotherapy plus capecitabine and oxaliplatin.

Patients and Methods.—We randomly assigned patients to receive 5 weeks of treatment with radiotherapy 45 Gy/25 fractions with concurrent capecitabine 800 mg/m^2 twice daily 5 days per week (Cap 45) or radiotherapy 50 Gy/25 fractions with capecitabine 800 mg/m^2 twice daily 5 days per week and oxaliplatin 50 mg/m^2 once weekly (Capox 50). The primary end point was complete sterilization of the operative specimen (ypCR).

Results.—Five hundred ninety-eight patients were randomly assigned to receive Cap 45 (n = 299) or Capox 50 (n = 299). More preoperative grade 3 to 4 toxicity occurred in the Capox 50 group (25 v 1%; $P < .001$). Surgery was performed in 98% of patients in both groups. There were no differences between groups in the rate of conservative surgery (75%) or postoperative deaths at 60 days (0.3%). The ypCR rate was 13.9% with Cap 45 and 19.2% with Capox 50 ($P = .09$). When ypCR was combined with yp few residual cells, the rate was respectively 28.9% with Cap 45 and 39.4% with Capox 50 ($P = .008$). The rate of positive circumferential rectal margins (between 0 and 2 mm) was 19.3% with Cap 45 and 9.9% with Capox 50 ($P = .02$).

Conclusion.—The benefit of oxaliplatin was not demonstrated and this drug should not be used with concurrent irradiation. Cap 50 merits investigation for T3-4 rectal cancers.

▶ T3 and T4 nonmetastatic rectal cancers are cured more often with the use of preoperative radiation therapy (RT). Furthermore, data from randomized trials support the addition of chemotherapy (5-fluorouracil) to the preoperative radiation regimen to increase pathologic complete response (CR) rates at the time of surgery. Thus, the question today regarding ways to improve the postchemotherapy pathologic CR rates (ypCR rates) center on RT dose and chemotherapy regimens. These authors have studied both questions in a phase III randomized trial, which has shown some complex results. The dose escalation arm of 50 Gy in 25 fractions was associated with more preoperative grade 3 and 4 toxicity than the 45 Gy arm. Yet the 50 Gy arm was given with both capecitabine and oxaliplatin not just capecitabine alone as in the 45 Gy arm. The 50 Gy arm did show a statistical improvement in the rate of positive circumferential radial margins, which is a surrogate for improved local control.

The challenge with these data lies in the treatment design where 2 variables were changed and the results are mixed. The authors do not support the addition of oxaliplatin in future trials but do encourage the use of dose escalation to 50 Gy. Clearly this recommendation warrants further investigation, but the data are encouraging.

C. A. Lawton, MD

Exposure to Oral Bisphosphonates and Risk of Esophageal Cancer
Cardwell CR, Abnet CC, Cantwell MM, et al (Queen's Univ Belfast, UK; Natl Insts of Health, Rockville, MD)
JAMA 304:657-663, 2010

Context.—Use of oral bisphosphonates has increased dramatically in the United States and elsewhere. Esophagitis is a known adverse effect of bisphosphonate use, and recent reports suggest a link between bisphosphonate use and esophageal cancer, but this has not been robustly investigated.

Objective.—To investigate the association between bisphosphonate use and esophageal cancer.

Design, Setting, and Participants.—Data were extracted from the UK General Practice Research Database to compare the incidence of esophageal and gastric cancer in a cohort of patients treated with oral bisphosphonates between January 1996 and December 2006 with incidence in a control cohort. Cancers were identified from relevant Read/Oxford Medical Information System codes in the patient's clinical files. Cox proportional hazards modeling was used to calculate hazard ratios and 95% confidence intervals for risk of esophageal and gastric cancer in bisphosphonate users compared with nonusers, with adjustment for potential confounders.

Main Outcome Measure.—Hazard ratio for the risk of esophageal and gastric cancer in the bisphosphonate users compared with the bisphosphonate nonusers.

Results.—Mean follow-up time was 4.5 and 4.4 years in the bisphosphonate and control cohorts, respectively. Excluding patients with less than 6 months' follow-up, there were 41 826 members in each cohort (81% women; mean age, 70.0 (SD, 11.4) years). One hundred sixteen esophageal or gastric cancers (79 esophageal) occurred in the bisphosphonate cohort and 115 (72 esophageal) in the control cohort. The incidence of esophageal and gastric cancer combined was 0.7 per 1000 person-years of risk in both the bisphosphonate and control cohorts; the incidence of esophageal cancer alone in the bisphosphonate and control cohorts was 0.48 and 0.44 per 1000 person-years of risk, respectively. There was no difference in risk of esophageal and gastric cancer combined between the cohorts for any bisphosphonate use (adjusted hazard ratio, 0.96 [95% confidence interval, 0.74-1.25]) or risk of esophageal cancer only (adjusted hazard ratio, 1.07 [95% confidence interval, 0.77-1.49]). There also was no difference in risk of esophageal or gastric cancer by duration of bisphosphonate intake.

Conclusion.—Among patients in the UK General Practice Research Database, the use of oral bisphosphonates was not significantly associated with incident esophageal or gastric cancer.

▶ Measuring bone density for both men and women in the United States has become commonplace. The result of this is that osteopenia and osteoporosis have been diagnosed at unprecedented numbers. Given the obesity in this country, these bone problems should not be a surprise to anyone, yet the results of this diagnosis is that thousands of Americans are being placed on bisphosphonate therapy.

Bisphosphonate therapy, like all medical interventions, has side effects. The effect on the jaw with regard to osteonecrosis with dental surgery is a well-documented potential toxicity of this therapy. Esophagitis and gastritis are other well-documented toxicities of bisphosphonate therapy. The concern of esophagitis and gastritis is related to the question of whether inflammation/irritation of a tissue could increase the risk of dysplasia and potentially lead to an increasing carcinoma risk.

These authors have looked at data from the United Kingdom general practice research database to try to assess this question in more than 82 000 patients with a mean follow-up of 4.5 years. They found no difference in the incidence of either esophageal or gastric carcinoma in patients on bisphosphonate therapy versus those not on the therapy, suggesting no association between these drugs and these cancers. Certainly one needs more data and longer follow-up to be certain of the lack of an association between bisphosphonates and esophageal and/or gastric malignancies. But these data are comforting in that if there were a significant risk of developing these cancers on these drugs, it likely would have been seen in this analysis. We await further work on this important topic.

C. A. Lawton, MD

21 Genitourinary Cancer

Active Surveillance Compared With Initial Treatment for Men With Low-Risk Prostate Cancer: A Decision Analysis

Hayes JH, Ollendorf DA, Pearson SD, et al (Harvard Med School, Boston, MA; et al)

JAMA 304:2373-2380, 2010

Context.—In the United States, 192 000 men were diagnosed as having prostate cancer in 2009, the majority with low-risk, clinically localized disease. Treatment of these cancers is associated with substantial morbidity. Active surveillance is an alternative to initial treatment, but long-term outcomes and effect on quality of life have not been well characterized.

Objective.—To examine the quality-of-life benefits and risks of active surveillance compared with initial treatment for men with low-risk, clinically localized prostate cancer.

Design and Setting.—Decision analysis using a simulation model was performed: men were treated at diagnosis with brachytherapy, intensity-modulated radiation therapy (IMRT), or radical prostatectomy or followed up by active surveillance (a strategy of close monitoring of newly diagnosed patients with serial prostate-specific antigen measurements, digital rectal examinations, and biopsies, with treatment at disease progression or patient choice). Probabilities and utilities were derived from previous studies and literature review. In the base case, the relative risk of prostate cancer–specific death for initial treatment vs active surveillance was assumed to be 0.83. Men incurred short- and long-term adverse effects of treatment.

Patients.—Hypothetical cohorts of 65-year-old men newly diagnosed as having clinically localized, low-risk prostate cancer (prostate-specific antigen level <10 ng/mL, stage ≤T2a disease, and Gleason score ≤6).

Main Outcome Measure.—Quality-adjusted life expectancy (QALE).

Results.—Active surveillance was associated with the greatest QALE (11.07 quality-adjusted life-years [QALYs]), followed by brachytherapy (10.57 QALYs), IMRT (10.51 QALYs), and radical prostatectomy (10.23 QALYs). Active surveillance remained associated with the highest QALE even if the relative risk of prostate cancer–specific death for initial treatment vs active surveillance was as low as 0.6. However, the QALE gains and the optimal strategy were highly dependent on individual preferences for living under active surveillance and for having been treated.

Conclusions.—Under a wide range of assumptions, for a 65-year-old man, active surveillance is a reasonable approach to low-risk prostate cancer based on QALE compared with initial treatment. However,

145

individual preferences play a central role in the decision whether to treat or to pursue active surveillance.

▶ Prostate cancer remains a challenge for the patients it afflicts as well as the physicians who guide the patient's decision after diagnosis. On one hand there are data that support the use of prostate-specific antigen (PSA) screening and treatment to reduce prostate cancer mortality. Yet the majority of patients diagnosed with prostate cancer fall into the "low-risk" category (PSA < 10, GS < 6, T-stage < T2a), where the risk of death related to the disease is very low.

Given the low risk of prostate cancer—related death in these patients, quality of life among the different forms of treatment and active surveillance is very important. These authors have looked at the quality-adjusted life expectancy (QALE) for patients treated for their prostate cancer with surgery, brachytherapy, intensity-modulated radiation therapy (IMRT), or active surveillance. QALE was superior for active surveillance patients as opposed to those who received upfront treatment. Yet this was highly dependent on the patient's preferences for the upfront treatment versus active surveillance. These data are important as they once again emphasize the need for all urologists and radiation oncologists to offer active surveillance as an excellent alternative and support patients who choose active surveillance as a way to address their localized prostate cancer.

C. A. Lawton, MD

Effect of Dutasteride on the Risk of Prostate Cancer

Andriole GL, for the REDUCE Study Group (Washington Univ School of Medicine in St Louis, MO; et al)
N Engl J Med 362:1192-1202, 2010

Background.—We conducted a study to determine whether dutasteride reduces the risk of incident prostate cancer, as detected on biopsy, among men who are at increased risk for the disease.

Methods.—In this 4-year, multicenter, randomized, double-blind, placebo-controlled, parallel-group study, we compared dutasteride, at a dose of 0.5 mg daily, with placebo. Men were eligible for inclusion in the study if they were 50 to 75 years of age, had a prostate-specific antigen (PSA) level of 2.5 to 10.0 ng per milliliter, and had one negative prostate biopsy (6 to 12 cores) within 6 months before enrollment. Subjects underwent a 10-core transrectal ultrasound-guided biopsy at 2 and 4 years.

Results.—Among 6729 men who underwent a biopsy or prostate surgery, cancer was detected in 659 of the 3305 men in the dutasteride group, as compared with 858 of the 3424 men in the placebo group, representing a relative risk reduction with dutasteride of 22.8% (95% confidence interval, 15.2 to 29.8) over the 4-year study period (P<0.001). Overall, in years 1 through 4, among the 6706 men who underwent a needle biopsy, there were 220 tumors with a Gleason score of 7 to 10 among 3299 men in the dutasteride group and 233 among 3407 men in the placebo group (P = 0.81). During years 3 and 4, there were 12 tumors with a Gleason score of 8 to 10 in the dutasteride group, as compared with only 1 in the placebo group (P = 0.003). Dutasteride therapy, as compared with placebo, resulted in a reduction in the rate of acute urinary retention (1.6% vs. 6.7%, a 77.3% relative reduction). The incidence of adverse events was similar to that in studies of dutasteride therapy for benign prostatic hyperplasia, except that in our study, as compared with previous studies, the relative incidence of the composite category of cardiac failure was higher in the dutasteride group than in the placebo group (0.7% [30 men] vs. 0.4% [16 men], P = 0.03).

Conclusions.—Over the course of the 4-year study period, dutasteride reduced the risk of incident prostate cancer detected on biopsy and improved the outcomes related to benign prostatic hyperplasia. (ClinicalTrials.gov number, NCT00056407.)

▶ Adenocarcinoma of the prostate is the second leading cause of cancer deaths in American men. It deserves our attention in terms of ways to decrease its incidence, especially in high-risk populations. One potential to decrease the incidence is the use of 5α-reductase inhibitors, which are used to treat benign prostate hypertrophy. These drugs block the conversion of testosterone to dihydrotestosterone, and this may decrease the risk of prostate cancer. The first study of these drugs used finasteride (the Prostate Cancer Prevention Trial). It did show a decrease in the incidence of prostate cancer, but of the tumors that were detected, there was an increase in the Gleason score of 7 to 10 tumors. So caution was the operative mode for consideration of finasteride to prevent prostate cancer.

This trial evaluated dutasteride, a drug that inhibits both forms of 5α-reductase in a double-blinded placebo-controlled parallel group study. Once again a decrease in prostate cancer incidence was found. In the first 4 years of the study, there was no difference in the detection of Gleason score of 7 to 10 tumors between the placebo versus the dutasteride groups. Yet during years 3 and 4, there was a large difference in the Gleason score of 8 to 10 tumors with 12 found in the dutasteride group and only 1 in the placebo group. The cause of these high-grade tumors in patients treated with these drugs is not known. Until it is better understood, caution should be used when considering 5α-reductase inhibitors to prevent prostate cancer.

C. A. Lawton, MD

Salvage radiotherapy for rising prostate-specific antigen levels after radical prostatectomy for prostate cancer: dose—response analysis
Bernard JR Jr, Buskirk SJ, Heckman MG, et al (Mayo Clinic, Jacksonville, FL; et al)
Int J Radiat Oncol Biol Phys 76:735-740, 2010

Purpose.—To investigate the association between external beam radiotherapy (EBRT) dose and biochemical failure (BcF) of prostate cancer in patients who received salvage prostate bed EBRT for a rising prostate-specific antigen (PSA) level after radical prostatectomy.

Methods and Materials.—We evaluated patients with a rising PSA level after prostatectomy who received salvage EBRT between July 1987 and October 2007. Patients receiving pre-EBRT androgen suppression were excluded. Cox proportional hazards models were used to investigate the association between EBRT dose and BcF. Dose was considered as a numeric variable and as a categoric variable (low, <64.8 Gy; moderate, 64.8–66.6 Gy; high, >66.6 Gy).

Results.—A total of 364 men met study selection criteria and were followed up for a median of 6.0 years (range, 0.1–19.3 years). Median pre-EBRT PSA level was 0.6 ng/mL. The estimated cumulative rate of BcF at 5 years after EBRT was 50% overall and 57%, 46%, and 39% for the low-, moderate-, and high-dose groups, respectively. In multivariable analysis adjusting for potentially confounding variables, there was evidence of a linear trend between dose and BcF, with risk of BcF decreasing as dose increased (relative risk [RR], 0.77 [5.0-Gy increase]; $p = 0.05$). Compared with the low-dose group, there was evidence of a decreased risk of BcF for the high-dose group (RR, 0.60; $p = 0.04$), but no difference for the moderate-dose group (RR, 0.85; $p = 0.41$).

Conclusions.—Our results suggest a dose response for salvage EBRT. Doses higher than 66.6 Gy result in decreased risk of BcF.

▶ Data from multiple randomized trials of adjuvant postoperative irradiation for patients with prostate cancer with pathologic T3 disease and/or positive margins show an obvious benefit to the postoperative radiation. Benefit has been measured in terms of clinical progression-free survival, biochemical progression-free survival, cause-specific survival, and overall survival. The doses of 60 to 64 Gy conventionally fractionated and the volumes treated are well accepted. Yet the majority of patients referred for postoperative radiation to date are not this group of patients, but those with rising prostate-specific antigen (PSA) after surgery. Many of these patients have pathologic T3 disease and/or positive surgical margins. The disease burden in these cases is likely greater and thus one would assume that the dose of radiation needed to eradicate the disease would also be greater.

These authors have looked at this question in terms of doses of a < 64.8 Gy, 64.8 to 66.6 Gy, and > 66.6 Gy (isocenter-defined doses). Their results show a trend toward an improvement in biochemical progression-free survival with the higher doses, although a direct comparison of 64.8 to 66.66 Gy versus > 66 Gy was not statistically different.

These data do not tell us the exact dose to use in these salvage cases. It certainly should make the treating radiation oncologist consider doses > 60 to 64 Gy as used in the adjuvant phase III trials when treating patients with rising PSA after surgery for adenocarcinoma of the prostate.

C. A. Lawton, MD

The rate of secondary malignancies after radical prostatectomy versus external beam radiation therapy for localized prostate cancer: a population-based study on 17,845 patients

Bhojani N, Capitanio U, Suardi N, et al (Univ of Montreal Health Ctr, Quebec, Canada; Vita-Salute San Raffaele, Milan, Italy; et al)

Int J Radiat Oncol Biol Phys 76:342-348, 2010

Purpose.—External-beam radiation therapy (EBRT) may predispose to secondary malignancies that include bladder cancer (BCa), rectal cancer (RCa), and lung cancer (LCa). We tested this hypothesis in a large French Canadian population-based cohort of prostate cancer patients.

Methods and Materials.—Overall, 8,455 radical prostatectomy (RP) and 9,390 EBRT patients treated between 1983 and 2003 were assessed with Kaplan-Meier and Cox regression analyses. Three endpoints were examined: (1) diagnosis of secondary BCa, (2) LCa, or (3) RCa. Covariates included age, Charlson comorbidity index, and year of treatment.

Results.—In multivariable analyses that relied on incident cases diagnosed 60 months or later after RP or EBRT, the rates of BCa (hazard ratio [HR], 1.4; $p = 0.02$), LCa (HR, 2.0; $p = 0.004$), and RCa (HR 2.1; $p < 0.001$) were significantly higher in the EBRT group. When incident cases diagnosed 120 months or later after RP or EBRT were considered, only the rates of RCa (hazard ratio 2.2; $p = 0.003$) were significantly higher in the EBRT group. In both analyses, the absolute differences in incident rates ranged from 0.7 to 5.2% and the number needed to harm (where harm equaled secondary malignancies) ranged from 111 to 19, if EBRT was used instead of RP.

Conclusions.—EBRT may predispose to clinically meaningfully higher rates of secondary BCa, LCa and RCa. These rates should be included in informed consent consideration.

▶ Secondary malignancies following radiation therapy for prostate cancer continue to be a concern for patients and radiation oncologists alike. While patients who develop 1 cancer such as prostate cancer certainly can develop other malignancies, concern for an increase in this problem via the addition of radiation therapy is important. Data exist that both support and refute the secondary malignancy concern. Thus, we as oncologists must continue to evaluate new research on the topic so as to best understand the risk, if present.

The data from this trial performed through the Quebec Health Plan represent a large population of prostate cancer patients treated with radiation therapy 9390 or surgery 8455 with reasonable follow-up. Interestingly, if one assumes that it takes at least 10 years for radiation therapy to cause a secondary malignancy than these data suggest, then lung cancer may be an important problem. If one uses the 5-year cutoff, then bladder, rectum, and lung cancers are concerns for secondary malignancies.

Certainly, 1 huge question for this data set is the question of smoking. Since smoking is so correlated with lung and bladder cancer, one would need to know whether patients were smokers or not to really understand the potential correlation or lack thereof with radiation therapy. Not knowing the smoking status and finding fewer secondary malignancy correlates at 10 years than 5 years are of concern for adopting these results. Yet we continue to need more studies to get a real handle on the potential for secondary malignancies after radiation therapy for prostate cancer.

C. A. Lawton, MD

Time of decline in sexual function after external beam radiotherapy for prostate cancer

Siglin J, Kubicek GJ, Leiby B, et al (Jefferson Med College of Thomas Jefferson Univ, Philadelphia, PA; Thomas Jefferson Univ Hosp, Philadelphia, PA; et al)

Int J Radiat Oncol Biol Phys 76:31-35, 2010

Purpose.—Erectile dysfunction is one of the most concerning toxicities for patients in the treatment of prostate cancer. The inconsistent evaluation of sexual function (SF) and limited follow-up data have necessitated additional study to clarify the rate and timing of erectile dysfunction after external beam radiotherapy (EBRT) for prostate cancer.

Methods and Materials.—A total of 143 men completed baseline data on SF before treatment and at the subsequent follow-up visits. A total of 1187 validated SF inventories were analyzed from the study participants. Multiple domains of SF (sex drive, erectile function, ejaculatory function, and overall satisfaction) were analyzed for ≤8 years of follow-up.

Results.—The median follow-up was 4.03 years. The strongest predictor of SF after EBRT was SF before treatment. For all domains of SF, the only statistically significant decrease in function occurred in the first 24 months after EBRT. SF stabilized 2 years after treatment completion, with no statistically significant change in any area of SF >2 years after the end of EBRT.

Conclusion.—These data suggest that SF does not have a continuous decline after EBRT. Instead, SF decreases maximally within the first 24 months after EBRT, with no significant changes thereafter.

▶ Discussion of side effects of radiation therapy for patients with prostate cancer usually centers on bowel and bladder issues. Yet sexual function remains a very important aspect of the patient's overall health and in some cases, patients place it as a number one concern for potential toxicity. In addition, it is well known that patient-reported toxicities versus physician-reported ones are different with patient-reported outcomes being much more reliable (ie, real). These authors have done an excellent job of assessing the effects of radiation therapy on sexual function by evaluating over 1000 patient-reported and validated sexual function inventories on 143 men treated with radiation therapy for localized prostate cancer.

With a median follow-up of just over 4 years, these authors have shown that contrary to the traditional belief that sexual function declines continuously after radiation therapy, their data show a maximal decrease in sexual function within the first 24 months after radiation and no significant changes after that. These data do confirm previous reports that the strongest predictor of sexual function after radiation therapy is sexual functioning prior to radiation therapy.

C. A. Lawton, MD

22 Gynecologic Cancer

Phase III, Open-Label, Randomized Study Comparing Concurrent Gemcitabine Plus Cisplatin and Radiation Followed by Adjuvant Gemcitabine and Cisplatin Versus Concurrent Cisplatin and Radiation in Patients With Stage IIB to IVA Carcinoma of the Cervix

Dueñas-González A, Zarbá JJ, Patel F, et al (Universidad Nacional Autónoma de México; Med Ctr, San Roque, Tucumán, Argentina; Eli Lilly Interamerica, Buenos Aires, Argentina; et al)

J Clin Oncol 29:1678-1685, 2011

Purpose.—To determine whether addition of gemcitabine to concurrent cisplatin chemoradiotherapy and as adjuvant chemotherapy with cisplatin improves progression-free survival (PFS) at 3 years compared with current standard of care in locally advanced cervical cancer.

Patients and Methods.—Eligible chemotherapy- and radiotherapy-naive patients with stage IIB to IVA disease and Karnofsky performance score ≥70 were randomly assigned to arm A (cisplatin 40 mg/m^2 and gemcitabine 125 mg/m^2 weekly for 6 weeks with concurrent external-beam radiotherapy [XRT] 50.4 Gy in 28 fractions, followed by brachytherapy [BCT] 30 to 35 Gy in 96 hours, and then two adjuvant 21-day cycles of cisplatin, 50 mg/m^2 on day 1, plus gemcitabine, 1,000 mg/m^2 on days 1 and 8) or to arm B (cisplatin and concurrent XRT followed by BCT only; dosing same as for arm A).

Results.—Between May 2002 and March 2004, 515 patients were enrolled (arm A, n = 259; arm B, n = 256). PFS at 3 years was significantly improved in arm A versus arm B (74.4% *v* 65.0%, respectively; *P* = .029), as were overall PFS (log-rank *P* = .0227; hazard ratio [HR], 0.68; 95% CI, 0.49 to 0.95), overall survival (log-rank *P* = .0224; HR, 0.68; 95% CI, 0.49 to 0.95), and time to progressive disease (log-rank *P* = .0012; HR, 0.54; 95% CI, 0.37 to 0.79). Grade 3 and 4 toxicities were more frequent in arm A than in arm B (86.5% *v* 46.3%, respectively; *P* < .001), including two deaths possibly related to treatment toxicity in arm A.

Conclusion.—Gemcitabine plus cisplatin chemoradiotherapy followed by BCT and adjuvant gemcitabine/cisplatin chemotherapy improved survival outcomes with increased but clinically manageable toxicity when compared with standard treatment.

▶ In February 1999, the National Cancer Institute of the United States released a clinical alert to notify all oncologists that 5 randomized trials including 6 comparisons showed that the concurrent use of cisplatin-based chemotherapy with radiation in the treatment of stages IB to IVA carcinoma of the cervix resulted in a significant reduction in mortality ranging from 24% to 51%. Since then, the standard of care for patients with stages IB to IVA carcinoma of the cervix has been the concurrent use of radiation plus weekly cisplatin, 40 mg/m². This trial reports the use of combination chemotherapy (gemcitabine plus cisplatin) concurrently with chemotherapy followed by 2 additional cycles of chemotherapy (gemcitabine plus cisplatin). This regimen was compared with weekly cisplatin plus radiation and showed a superior progression-free and overall survival at the expense of some increase in toxicity of tolerable magnitude. These results suggest that combination chemotherapy might yield superior results to the use of single-agent cisplatin. At least in the hands of the Gynecologic Oncology Group (GOG), the combination of paclitaxel/cisplatin is superior to gemcitabine/cisplatin, and these results have now become the basis for an international study using the paclitaxel/cisplatin combination in place of gemcitabine/cisplatin in a randomized trial similar to that reported here. For now, the standard remains weekly cisplatin plus radiation for stages IB to IVA carcinoma of the cervix.

J. T. Thigpen, MD

A phase II study of two topotecan regimens evaluated in recurrent platinum-sensitive ovarian, fallopian tube or primary peritoneal cancer: a Gynecologic Oncology Group Study (GOG 146Q)
Herzog TJ, Sill MW, Walker JL, et al (Columbia Univ, NY; Roswell Park Cancer Inst, Buffalo, NY; Univ of Oklahoma; et al)
Gynecol Oncol 120:454-458, 2011

Objective.—To evaluate the efficacy and safety of topotecan in patients with recurrent ovarian, primary peritoneal, and fallopian tube carcinomas.

Methods.—A randomized phase II analysis of platinum-sensitive patients with measurable disease was performed independently assessing intravenous topotecan 1.25 mg/m² daily × 5 every 21 days (regimen I) and topotecan 4.0 mg/m²/day on days 1, 8, and 15 of a 28-day cycle (regimen II). All patients were treated until disease progression, unmanageable toxicity, or patient refusal. Insufficient accrual related to regimen I resulted in a redesign of the study as a single arm phase II trial assessing only regimen II. More complete efficacy data is presented for regimen II as enrollment on regimen I was insufficient for some analyses.

Results.—A total of 81 patients were enrolled. One patient was ineligible. Fifteen patients received regimen I, while 65 patients were treated with regimen II. The response rate on regimen I (daily × 5) was 27% (90% CI: 10—51%) and 12% (90% CI: 6—21%) on regimen II (weekly). The median PFS and OS were 4.8 and 27.8 months, respectively, for regimen II. Grade 3/4 neutropenia rate was 93% with daily × 5 dosing and 28% for weekly treatment. Febrile neutropenia was very low in both groups.

Conclusion.—The weekly regimen of topotecan appeared less active but resulted in less toxicity than the daily regimen in platinum-sensitive recurrent ovarian cancer patients.

▶ This study is an attempt to determine whether the commonly used weekly schedule of topotecan yields efficacy similar to that of the Food and Drug Administration—approved 5-day schedule. As with most studies involving the 5-day schedule, the Gynecology Oncology Group (GOG) had trouble accruing to the study and finished the trial as a phase II study of the weekly schedule. The results, however, are sufficiently interesting to cause hesitation in opting for the weekly schedule. Only 27 patients were administered the 5-day schedule before closure of that arm, but the response rate of 27% is essentially identical to the 33% seen in an earlier GOG trial of the 5-day schedule in platinum-sensitive patients. The 12% response rate seen with the weekly schedule is consistent with reported phase II trials in the literature and is only half as effective in inducing objective responses as the 5-day schedule. These observations are consistent with preclinical data on the topoisomerase inhibitors, which show that duration of exposure to these agents is the predominant determinant of efficacy. While patient and physician convenience is certainly important, efficacy should be our primary consideration; hence the 5-day schedule should still be the preferred schedule unless toxicity considerations prevent its use.

J. T. Thigpen, MD

Addition of bevacizumab to weekly paclitaxel significantly improves progression-free survival in heavily pretreated recurrent epithelial ovarian cancer
O'Malley DM, Richardson DL, Rheaume PS, et al (The Ohio State Univ College of Medicine, Columbus)
Gynecol Oncol 121:269-272, 2011

Objective.—Weekly paclitaxel has been shown to be an effective cytotoxic regimen for recurrent epithelial ovarian cancer (EOC), and may act through inhibition of angiogenesis. Bevacizumab, a potent angiogenesis inhibitor, has also been shown to have activity in patients with EOC. Therefore, we sought to determine if the addition of bevacizumab to weekly paclitaxel led to an increased survival compared to weekly paclitaxel alone.

Methods.—A single institutional review was conducted for patients with recurrent EOC treated with weekly paclitaxel ($60-70$ mg/m^2) on days 1, 8, 15, and 22 of a 28 day cycle and those treated with weekly paclitaxel and bevacizumab ($10-15$ mg/kg on day 1 and 15). Response rates (RR) were calculated, and progression-free survival (PFS), and overall survival (OS) were compared using Kaplan—Meier survival analysis.

Results.—Twenty-nine patients treated with weekly paclitaxel and 41 patients treated with paclitaxel/bevacizumab were identified. The groups were similar in demographics, initial optimal cytoreduction, stage, histology, grade, platinum sensitivity, and median number of previous regimens (4 vs. 4, p=0.69).The overall response rate (ORR) was 63% (complete response (CR) 34% and partial response (PR) 29%) for paclitaxel/bevacizumab and 48% (CR 17% and PR 31%) for weekly paclitaxel (p=0.23). Improvement in PFS was seen in those treated with paclitaxel/bevacizumab in comparison to weekly paclitaxel alone (median PFS 13.2 vs. 6.2 months, p<.01). There was a trend towards improved OS for paclitaxel/bevacizumab (median OS 20.6 vs. 9.1 months; p=0.12). Toxicities were similar between the two regimens although more bowel perforations (2 vs. 0) were seen in the paclitaxel/ bevacizumab group.

Conclusion.—A significant increase in PFS with a trend towards improved OS was demonstrated in this heavily pretreated population treated with paclitaxel/bevacizumab as compared to weekly paclitaxel alone. This data should be helpful in guiding future trials to determine the optimal care for women with recurrent EOC.

▶ Bevacizumab had been evaluated extensively in ovarian carcinoma. Initial phase II data from the Gynecologic Oncology Group showed a 21% objective response rate and 40% of patients progression free at 6 months. These data led to the initiation of 2 large phase III trials in newly diagnosed disease, GOG 218 (Unites States) and ICON7 (United Kingdom). These studies were both reported in the summer of 2010 as showing a significant improvement in progression-free survival (PFS) and a trend toward improved overall survival (OS) in those patients who received bevacizumab with paclitaxel/carboplatin up front followed by bevacizumab maintenance (15 total months in GOG 218 and 12 total months in ICON 7). In June 2011, a phase III of gemcitabine/carboplatin bevacizumab showed the same thing: significantly improved PFS and a trend toward improved OS. These studies all support the conclusion that bevacizumab is a very active agent in ovarian carcinoma. This trial looks at bevacizumab in combination with weekly paclitaxel in patients with recurrent disease. The sample size is relatively small, so no definitive conclusions can be reached. However, the trends toward improvements in PFS and OS strongly support the use of the drug in this setting. The burning question that remains is whether a patient who received bevacizumab frontline would, when progression of disease occurs, still benefit from the drug in the recurrent disease setting. There is no definitive answer as of yet, but it would be reasonable to consider using bevacizumab in combination with chemotherapy in the recurrent disease setting.

J. T. Thigpen, MD

Clinical Activity of Gemcitabine Plus Pertuzumab in Platinum-Resistant Ovarian Cancer, Fallopian Tube Cancer, or Primary Peritoneal Cancer
Makhija S, Amler LC, Glenn D, et al (Emory Univ, Atlanta, GA; Genentech, South San Francisco, CA; Sharp Rees-Stealy Med Group, San Diego, CA; et al)
J Clin Oncol 28:1215-1223, 2010

Purpose.—Pertuzumab is a humanized monoclonal antibody that inhibits human epidermal growth factor receptor 2 (HER2) heterodimerization and has single-agent activity in recurrent epithelial ovarian cancer. The primary objective of this phase II study was to characterize the safety and estimate progression-free survival (PFS) of pertuzumab with gemcitabine in patients with platinum-resistant ovarian cancer.

Patients and Methods.—Patients with advanced, platinum-resistant epithelial ovarian, fallopian tube, or primary peritoneal cancer who had received a maximum of one prior treatment for recurrent cancer were randomly assigned to gemcitabine plus either pertuzumab or placebo. Collection of archival tissue was mandatory to permit exploration of biomarkers that would predict benefit from pertuzumab in this setting.

Results.—One hundred thirty patients (65 per arm) were treated. Baseline characteristics were similar between arms. The adjusted hazard ratio (HR) for PFS was 0.66 (95% CI, 0.43 to 1.03; $P = .07$) in favor of gemcitabine + pertuzumab. The objective response rate was 13.8% in patients who received gemcitabine + pertuzumab compared with 4.6% in patients who received gemcitabine + placebo. In patients whose tumors had low HER3 mRNA expression (< median, n = 61), an increased treatment benefit was observed in the gemcitabine + pertuzumab arm compared with the gemcitabine alone arm (PFS HR = 0.32; 95% CI, 0.17 to 0.59; $P = .0002$). Grade 3 to 4 neutropenia, diarrhea, and back pain were increased in patients treated with gemcitabine + pertuzumab. Symptomatic congestive heart failure was reported in one patient in the gemcitabine + pertuzumab arm.

Conclusion.—Pertuzumab may add activity to gemcitabine for the treatment of platinum-resistant ovarian cancer. Low HER3 mRNA expression may predict pertuzumab clinical benefit and be a valuable prognostic marker.

▶ Patients with ovarian cancer who either have failed to achieve a complete response with prior platinum-based therapy or who relapse within 6 months of achieving a complete response are categorized as clinically platinum resistant. These patients are treated with active agents other than a platinum compound. This patient population is the focus of this trial. Gemcitabine is an active agent in this setting with an objective response rate reportedly in the midteens. This study assigned all patients to treatment with gemcitabine and randomly assigned half of the patients to receive concurrent pertuzumab, a monoclonal antibody that inhibits human epidermal growth factor (HER) 2 dimerization. Patients receiving pertuzumab exhibited a superior response rate in this randomized phase II trial. The trial included an exploration of biomarkers, and this aspect of the study revealed that those whose tumors exhibited low levels of HER3 expression benefited most from the addition of pertuzumab (hazard ratio = 0.32). These data suggest that HER3 might be a valuable prognostic marker for response to pertuzumab. Phase III trials are planned.

J. T. Thigpen, MD

Clinical predictors of bevacizumab-associated gastrointestinal perforation

Tanyi JL, McCann G, Hagemann AR, et al (Univ of Pennsylvania Health System, Philadelphia)

Gynecol Oncol 120:464-469, 2011

Objectives.—Bevacizumab is a generally well-tolerated drug, but bevacizumab-associated gastrointestinal perforations (BAP) occur in 0 to 15% of patients with ovarian carcinoma. Our goal was to evaluate the clinical predictors of BAP in order to identify factors, which may preclude patients from receiving treatment.

Methods.—We conducted a review of patients with recurrent epithelial ovarian carcinoma treated with bevacizumab between 2006 and 2009. Demographic and treatment data were collected for statistical analysis.

Results.—Eighty-two patients were identified; perforation occurred in 8 (9.76%). Among patients with perforation, a significantly higher incidence of prior bowel surgeries ($p = 0.0008$) and prior bowel obstruction or ileus ($p < 0.0001$) were found compared to non-perforated patients. The median age at onset of bevacizumab in the perforated group was 3 years younger (60 vs. 63 years, $p = 0.61$). The incidence of thromboembolic events, GI comorbidities, number of prior chemotherapies, and body mass index were similar between the groups. None of the patients in the perforated group developed grade 3 or 4 hypertension, compared to a 32.4% incidence among the non-perforated patients ($p = 0.09$). Upon multivariate analysis, when controlled for age greater or less than 60, prior bowel surgery, obstruction/ileus, and grade 3 or 4 hypertension, only the presence of obstruction/ileus was noted to be a significant predictor of perforation ($p = 0.04$).

Conclusions.—Predicting BAP remains a challenge. Bowel obstruction or ileus appears to be associated with increased risk of BAP.

▶ Gastrointestinal perforation is one of the most substantial adverse effects associated with bevacizumab in patients with ovarian carcinoma. Although not definitive, early phase II data on bevacizumab in ovarian carcinoma suggested that patients with multiple prior treatments for recurrent disease were more likely to develop the problem. The highest reported frequency was in a study that permitted 3 or more prior lines of therapy. Whether this higher frequency reflected the number of prior lines of chemotherapy or other management approaches was not clear. This article reviews results in a series of 82 patients with 8 episodes of bowel perforation. Two factors were significantly related to the occurrence of bowel perforation: prior bowel surgeries and prior episodes of bowel obstruction or ileus. Particularly in patients with recurrent ovarian carcinoma who may have had multiple prior surgeries, use of bevacizumab should be considered earlier in the disease course (frontline or first recurrence) to avoid a clinical setting in which the likelihood of this complication is increased.

J. T. Thigpen, MD

Decreased hypersensitivity reactions with carboplatin-pegylated liposomal doxorubicin compared to carboplatin-paclitaxel combination: Analysis from the GCIG CALYPSO relapsing ovarian cancer trial
Joly F, Ray-Coquard I, Fabbro M, et al (Centre François Baclesse, Caen, France; Centre Leon Bérard, Lyon, France; CRLC Val d'Aurelle, Montpellier, France; et al)
Gynecol Oncol 122:226-232, 2011

Objective.—To describe and analyze observed hypersensitivity reactions (HSR) from the randomized, multicenter phase III CALYPSO trial that evaluated the efficacy and safety of the combination of carboplatin and pegylated liposomal doxorubicin (CD) compared with standard carboplatin-paclitaxel (CP) in patients with platinum—sensitive relapsed ovarian cancer (ROC).

Methods.—HSR documented within case report forms and SAE reports were specifically analyzed. Analyses were based on the population with allergy of any grade and for grade >2 allergy.

Results.—Overall 976 patients were recruited to this phase III trial, with toxicity data available for 466 and 502 on the CD and CP arms, respectively. There was a 15.5% HSR rate associated with CD (2.4% grade >2) versus 33.1% with CP (8.8% grade >2), $p<0.001$. HSRs occurred more often during first cycle in the CD (46%) arm than in the CP arm (16%). Multivariate predictors of allergy were chemotherapy regimen and age; patients randomized to CD and patients ≥70 years old on CP had less allergy. Few patients (<6%) stopped treatment due to allergy. Allergy rates were higher in patients who did not receive prior supportive treatment; however there was no relationship between allergy and the type of carboplatin product received, or response rate.

Conclusions.—Use of PLD with carboplatin instead of paclitaxel and older age were the only 2 factors predicting a low rate of HSRs in patients with ROC. CD has previously demonstrated superior progression-free survival and therapeutic index than CP. Taken together these data support the use of CD as a safe and effective therapeutic option for platinum-sensitive ROC.

▶ The paradigm in place for the management of recurrent ovarian cancer for the past 20 years has been to categorize patients as platinum sensitive or platinum resistant based on response to prior platinum-based therapy. Those who achieve a complete response that lasts at least 6 months are categorized as platinum sensitive, whereas the rest are considered platinum resistant. Patients categorized as platinum sensitive have generally been recommended to receive platinum-based therapy at relapse. Three large phase III trials in the past 8 years have shown platinum-based doublets to be superior to single-agent platinum: paclitaxel/carboplatin, gemcitabine/carboplatin, and now pegylated liposomal doxorubicin (PLD)/carboplatin. The last doublet was actually compared with another doublet, paclitaxel/carboplatin, and demonstrated a superior progression-free survival (PFS) (the CALYPSO trial). This particular ancillary study looks at the patients who experienced a carboplatin hypersensitivity reaction on the CALYPSO trial. The number of patients involved was not insignificant (15.5% on the PLD/carboplatin regimen versus 33.1% on the paclitaxel/carboplatin regimen). The data suggest that significantly fewer hypersensitivity reactions were observed among those patients receiving PLD/carboplatin, although the mechanism responsible for this decrease is not clear. This observation, combined with the PFS advantage with PLD/carboplatin, suggests that this doublet should be the regimen of choice in the patient with platinum-sensitive disease.

J. T. Thigpen, MD

Development of a Multimarker Assay for Early Detection of Ovarian Cancer

Yurkovetsky Z, Skates S, Lomakin A, et al (Univ of Pittsburgh Cancer Inst, PA; Univ of Pittsburgh, PA; Fox Chase Cancer Ctr, Philadelphia, PA; et al)
J Clin Oncol 28:2159-2166, 2010

Purpose.—Early detection of ovarian cancer has great promise to improve clinical outcome.

Patients and Methods.—Ninety-six serum biomarkers were analyzed in sera from healthy women and from patients with ovarian cancer, benign pelvic tumors, and breast, colorectal, and lung cancers, using multiplex xMAP bead-based immunoassays. A Metropolis algorithm with Monte Carlo simulation (MMC) was used for analysis of the data.

Results.—A training set, including sera from 139 patients with early-stage ovarian cancer, 149 patients with late-stage ovarian cancer, and 1,102 healthy women, was analyzed with MMC algorithm and cross validation to identify an optimal biomarker panel discriminating early-stage cancer from healthy controls. The four-biomarker panel providing the highest diagnostic power of 86% sensitivity (SN) for early-stage and 93% SN for late-stage ovarian cancer at 98% specificity (SP) was comprised of CA-125, HE4, CEA, and VCAM-1. This model was applied to an independent blinded validation set consisting of sera from 44 patients with early-stage ovarian cancer, 124 patients with late-stage ovarian cancer, and 929 healthy women, providing unbiased estimates of 86% SN for stage I and II and 95% SN for stage III and IV disease at 98% SP. This panel was selective for ovarian cancer showing SN of 33% for benign pelvic disease, SN of 6% for breast cancer, SN of 0% for colorectal cancer, and SN of 36% for lung cancer.

Conclusion.—A panel of CA-125, HE4, CEA, and VCAM-1, after additional validation, could serve as an initial stage in a screening strategy for epithelial ovarian cancer.

▶ Ovarian carcinoma is the second most common invasive cancer of the female genital tract, but it is by far the most common cause of death from gynecologic cancer. Some have assumed that this is because ovarian cancer is not responsive to current treatment modalities, but trials in advanced ovarian cancer report that essentially 75% of patients achieve a clinical complete response, far higher than any other solid tumor other than germ cell tumors. The problem rather lies in the fact that 75% to 80% of patients present with stage III to IV disease because of the lack of an effective early diagnostic test (compare this to 92% of breast cancers presenting as stage I to II and 88% of endometrial cancers presenting as stage I to II). Numerous studies have been reported to evaluate the use of serial CA-125 and transvaginal sonography as a screening approach. The most recent US trial, the Prostate, Lung, Colorectal, and Ovarian Cancer Screening Trial, involving more than 78 000 women screened for ovarian cancer in this fashion, produced a positive predictive value of 1.3% and no change in the mortality rate. The key to any screening test is its ability to reduce mortality related to the disease. This article presents the results of early studies of a panel of 4 markers and suggests that this panel is promising as a potential screening approach for ovarian cancer. The data presented, however, do not support the use of this approach as a screening test. The total number of women in the study is far too small for any conclusion that the approach is effective, and the results to date do not address the issue of mortality reduction. Other attempts at such an approach, including the use of proteomic profiling, have also failed. The authors are correct to conclude that further studies of a randomized design including much larger numbers of women will be required before any conclusions can be drawn. We remain without a confirmed screening approach for ovarian cancer.

J. T. Thigpen, MD

Docetaxel plus trabectedin appears active in recurrent or persistent ovarian and primary peritoneal cancer after up to three prior regimens: A phase II study of the Gynecologic Oncology Group

Monk BJ, Sill MW, Hanjani P, et al (Creighton Univ School of Medicine at St Joseph's Hosp and Med Ctr, Phoenix, AZ; Univ at Buffalo, NY; Abington Memorial Hosp, PA; et al)
Gynecol Oncol 120:459-463, 2011

Objective.—This study aims to estimate the activity of docetaxel 60 mg/m^2 IV over 1 h followed by trabectedin 1.1 mg/m^2 over 3 h with filgrastim, pegfilgrastim, or sargramostim every 3 weeks (one cycle).

Methods.—Patients with recurrent and measurable disease, acceptable organ function, PS≤2, and ≤3 prior regimens were eligible. A two-stage design was utilized with a target sample size of 35 subjects per stage. Another Gynecologic Oncology Group study within the same protocol queue involving a single agent taxane showed a response rate (RR) of (16%) (90% CI 8.6−28.5%) and served as a historical control for direct comparison. The present study was designed to determine if the current regimen had an RR of ≥36% with 90% power.

Results.—Seventy-one patients were eligible and evaluable (prior regimens: 1 = 28%, 2 = 52%, 3 = 20%). The median number of cycles was 6 (438 total cycles, range 1−22). The number of patients responding was 21 (30%; 90% CI 21−40%). The odds ratio for responding was 2.2 (90% 1-sided CI 1.07−Infinity). The median progression-free survival and overall survival were 4.5 months and 16.9 months, respectively. The median response duration was 6.2 months. Numbers of subjects with grade 3/4 toxicity included neutropenia 7/14; constitutional 8/0; GI (excluding nausea/vomiting) 11/0; metabolic 9/1; pain 6/0. There were no treatment-related deaths nor cases of liver failure.

Conclusions.—This combination was well tolerated and appears more active than the historical control of single agent taxane therapy in those with recurrent ovarian and peritoneal cancer after failing multiple lines of chemotherapy. Further study is warranted.

▶ Trabectedin is an agent derived from the sea squirt. In a prior phase III trial comparing pegylated liposomal doxorubicin trabectedin, the combination produced a significantly longer progression-free survival (PFS) and a trend toward improved overall survival. The Food and Drug Administration (FDA) refused to approve the drug in ovarian carcinoma because the FDA does not accept PFS as a valid end point in ovarian carcinoma contrary to what the proceedings of an FDA/ASCO/AACR conference on end points in ovarian carcinoma state on the FDA Web site (the conference concluded that PFS was a surrogate for survival unless extensive postprogression therapy blurred the correlation). This Gynecologic Oncology Group (GOG) study of trabectedin combined with another active agent in platinum-resistant ovarian carcinoma suggests, based on comparison with a historical GOG control of docetaxel alone in this setting, that the addition of trabectedin to this agent in a recurrent disease population improved response rate (30% vs 16%). Since this is not a randomized comparison, no definitive conclusions can be drawn, but the results do support the conclusions of the phase III trial with pegylated liposomal doxorubicin that adding trabectedin to other active drugs improves the efficacy of the regimen.

J. T. Thigpen, MD

Effect of Screening on Ovarian Cancer Mortality: The Prostate, Lung, Colorectal and Ovarian (PLCO) Cancer Screening Randomized Controlled Trial

Buys SS, for the PLCO Project Team (Univ of Utah Health Sciences Ctr, Salt Lake City; et al)
JAMA 305:2295-2303, 2011

Context.—Screening for ovarian cancer with cancer antigen 125 (CA-125) and transvaginal ultrasound has an unknown effect on mortality.

Objective.—To evaluate the effect of screening for ovarian cancer on mortality in the Prostate, Lung, Colorectal and Ovarian (PLCO) Cancer Screening Trial.

Design, Setting, and Participants.—Randomized controlled trial of 78 216 women aged 55 to 74 years assigned to undergo either annual screening (n = 39 105) or usual care (n = 39 111) at 10 screening centers across the United States between November 1993 and July 2001.

Intervention.—The intervention group was offered annual screening with CA-125 for 6 years and transvaginal ultrasound for 4 years. Participants and their health care practitioners received the screening test results and managed evaluation of abnormal results. The usual care group was not offered annual screening with CA-125 for 6 years or transvaginal ultrasound but received their usual medical care. Participants were followed up for a maximum of 13 years (median [range], 12.4 years [10.9-13.0 years]) for cancer diagnoses and death until February 28, 2010.

Main Outcome Measures.—Mortality from ovarian cancer, including primary peritoneal and fallopian tube cancers. Secondary outcomes included ovarian cancer incidence and complications associated with screening examinations and diagnostic procedures.

Results.—Ovarian cancer was diagnosed in 212 women (5.7 per 10 000 person-years) in the intervention group and 176 (4.7 per 10 000 person-years) in the usual care group (rate ratio [RR], 1.21; 95% confidence interval [CI], 0.99-1.48). There were 118 deaths caused by ovarian cancer (3.1 per 10 000 person-years) in the intervention group and 100 deaths (2.6 per 10 000 person-years) in the usual care group (mortality RR, 1.18; 95% CI, 0.82-1.71). Of 3285 women with false-positive results, 1080 underwent surgical follow-up; of whom, 163 women experienced at least 1 serious complication (15%). There were 2924 deaths due to other causes (excluding ovarian, colorectal, and lung cancer) (76.6 per 10 000 person-years) in the intervention group and 2914 deaths (76.2 per 10 000 person-years) in the usual care group (RR, 1.01; 95% CI, 0.96-1.06).

Conclusions.—Among women in the general US population, simultaneous screening with CA-125 and transvaginal ultrasound compared with usual care did not reduce ovarian cancer mortality. Diagnostic evaluation following a false-positive screening test result was associated with complications.

Trial Registration.—clinicaltrials.gov Identifier: NCT00002540.

▶ This article reports the results of a trial evaluating annual cancer antigen 125 (CA-125) and transvaginal sonography as a screening tool for the detection of early ovarian cancer in 78 216 women randomized to screening or no screening. The primary end point of the study was overall mortality. The trial showed no overall reduction in mortality as a result of screening, and there were numerous complications among the women who underwent surgery for a positive screen result. The results of this study must be taken in the context of a British trial reported in *The Lancet*, which showed a positive predictive value of 35% for a screening approach that analyzed the CA-125 data with a mathematical algorithm (ROCA). Mortality is awaited from this trial, but the positive predictive value is strikingly better than the 1.3% seen in the study reported here. The bottom line is that no approach as yet has demonstrated the ability to reduce mortality from ovarian cancer, and all approaches have resulted in surgeries for false-positive findings with associated morbidity.

J. T. Thigpen, MD

Effects of bevacizumab and pegylated liposomal doxorubicin for the patients with recurrent or refractory ovarian cancers

Kudoh K, Takano M, Kouta H, et al (Ohki Memorial Kikuchi Cancer Clinic for Women, Tokorozawa, Saitama, Japan; et al)
Gynecol Oncol 122:233-237, 2011

Objectives.—Currently, pegylated liposomal doxorubicin (PLD) is regarded as one of the standard treatment options in recurrent ovarian cancers (ROC). Bevacizumab has shown significant antitumor activity for ROC in single-agent or in combination with cytotoxic agents. We have conducted a preliminary study to investigate effects of combination of bevacizumab and PLD for heavily pretreated patients with ROC.

Methods.—Thirty patients with ROC were treated with combination therapy with weekly bevacizumab and PLD, 2 mg/kg of continuous weekly bevacizumab and 10 mg/m^2 of PLD (3 weeks on, 1 week off). The treatment was continued until development of disease progression, or unmanageable adverse effects. Response evaluation was based upon Response Evaluation Criteria in Solid Tumors (RECIST) version 1.0, and Gynecologic Cancer Intergroup (GCIG) CA125 response criteria. Adverse effects were analyzed according to Common Terminology Criteria for Adverse Events (CTCAE) version 3.0.

Results.—Overall response rate was 33%, and clinical benefit rate (CR+PD+SD) was 73%. Median progression-free survival was 6 months (range: 2—20 months), and a 6-months progression-free survival was 47%. Any hematological toxicities more than grade 3 were not observed. Two cases developed non-hematologic toxicities more than grade 2; a case with grade 3 hand-foot syndrome, another with grade 3 gastrointestinal perforation (GIP). The case with GIP was conservatively treated and recovered after 2 months, and there was no case with treatment-related death.

Conclusion.—The present investigation suggested that combination therapy with bevacizumab and PLD was active and well tolerated for patients with ROC. We recommend the regimen be evaluated in further clinical studies.

▶ Patients with platinum-resistant recurrent ovarian cancer are generally treated with single agents with demonstrated activity in this patient population. There are now some 21 different agents with reported activity in the platinum-resistant setting. To date, no study has demonstrated a superior outcome for patients treated with combinations of agents as opposed to single agent therapy. The demonstration of activity for bevacizumab and the success of front-line trials combining chemotherapy and bevacizumab for newly diagnosed ovarian cancer suggests that combinations of cytotoxic agents with bevacizumab might offer an advantage in the platinum-resistant population. This phase II study is noteworthy for evaluating the combination of pegylated liposomal doxorubicin (PLD) and bevacizumab in a heavily pretreated ovarian cancer population. What the study tells us is primarily that PLD can be combined safely with bevacizumab. What it does not tell us is whether the combination offers any advantage over either agent alone. Firstly, the study is not randomized and thus cannot give an accurate read on whether the combination is better than PLD or bevacizumab alone. Secondly, the patient population is not sufficiently well described to allow conclusions from such a small series. For example, one of the patients had platinum-sensitive disease. Of the other 29, all we know is that they were classi- fied as platinum-resistant. Were any of them actually refractory (no response and no treatment-free interval) or were they all responders with progression at 5-6 months (a much better population with a greater likelihood of response)? In all likelihood, combinations of a cytotoxic agent with bevacizumab will yield better results in platinum-resistant disease than a single agent, and other agents can be logically combined with bevacizumab (eg, weekly paclitaxel). We need further study in controlled settings to determine this definitively.

J. T. Thigpen, MD

The Use of Recombinant Erythropoietin for the Treatment of Chemotherapy-Induced Anemia in Patients With Ovarian Cancer Does Not Affect Progression-Free or Overall Survival

Cantrell LA, Westin SN, Van Le L (Univ of Virginia, Charlottesville; The Univ of Texas M D Anderson Cancer Ctr, Houston; University of North Carolina, Chapel Hill)
Cancer 117:1220-1226, 2011

Background.—Studies have suggested that erythropoietin-stimulating agents (ESAs) may affect progression-free survival (PFS) and overall survival (OS) in a variety of cancer types. Because this finding had not been explored previously in ovarian or primary peritoneal carcinoma, the authors of this report analyzed their ovarian cancer population to deter- mine whether ESA treatment for chemotherapy-induced anemia affected PFS or OS.

Methods.—A retrospective review was conducted of women who were treated for ovarian cancer at the corresponding author's institution over a 10-year period (from January 1994 to May 2004). Treatment groups were formed based on the use of an ESA. Two analyses of survival were conducted to determine the effect of ESA therapy on PFS and OS. Disease status was modeled as a function of treatment group using a logistic regression model. Kaplan-Meier curves were generated to compare the groups, and a Cox proportional hazards model was fit to the data.

Results.—In total, 343 women were identified. The median age was 57 (interquartile range, 48-68 years). The majority of women were Caucasian (n = 255; 74%) and were diagnosed with stage III (n = 210; 61%), epithe- lial (n = 268; 78%) ovarian cancer. Although the disease stage at diagnosis and surgical staging significantly affected the rates of disease recurrence and OS, the receipt of an ESA had no effect on PFS ($P = .9$) or OS ($P = .25$).

Conclusions.—The current results indicated that there was no difference in cancer-related PFS or OS with use of ESA in this cohort of women treated for ovarian cancer.

▶ The use of erythropoietic agents in the management of patients with cancer was based on 3 phase III trials showing a significant improvement in quality of life in those who responded to such treatment. In addition, several retrospective studies, particularly in carcinoma of the cervix, suggested an improvement in survival coincident with an increase in hemoglobin to 12 g/dL. Use of these was widespread until the reports of studies in head and neck cancer suggesting that use of erythropoietin-stimulating agents (ESAs) was associated with a decrease in survival, the opposite of what had been reported in retrospective studies. The Food and Drug Administration subsequently issued a black box warning, suggesting that such use was associated with a decrease in survival, although, at least in the case of cervix cancer, the cited study did not show a significant decrease in survival, although the trials showing decreased survival occurred in the setting in which ESAs were being used well beyond the increase in hemoglobin to 12 g/dL. As a result of the black box warning, the use of ESAs has been sharply curtailed. This study looks at ovarian carcinoma to determine whether there was any evidence of a decrease in survival associated with the use of ESAs. As is noted in the abstract, no such decrease can be detected. The issue of whether there is an associated improvement in quality of life with improvement in hemoglobin was not addressed in the trial, although prior studies as noted above are associated with a significant improvement in quality of life. Should we therefore be using ESAs to improve quality of life despite the black box warning? Under current circumstances, which require that the patient sign a detailed and onerous consent, it is very difficult to use the ESAs—a shame, given the improvement in quality of life associated with their use.

J. T. Thigpen, MD

23 Head and Neck Cancer

Human Papillomavirus and Survival of Patients with Oropharyngeal Cancer

Ang KK, Harris J, Wheeler R, et al (Univ of Texas M D Anderson Cancer Ctr, Houston; Radiation Therapy Oncology Group Statistical Ctr, Philadelphia, PA; Huntsman Cancer Inst, Salt Lake City, UT; et al)
N Engl J Med 363:24-35, 2010

Background.—Oropharyngeal squamous-cell carcinomas caused by human papillomavirus (HPV) are associated with favorable survival, but the independent prognostic significance of tumor HPV status remains unknown.

Methods.—We performed a retrospective analysis of the association between tumor HPV status and survival among patients with stage III or IV oropharyngeal squamous-cell carcinoma who were enrolled in a randomized trial comparing accelerated-fractionation radiotherapy (with acceleration by means of concomitant boost radiotherapy) with standard-fractionation radiotherapy, each combined with cisplatin therapy, in patients with squamous-cell carcinoma of the head and neck. Proportional-hazards models were used to compare the risk of death among patients with HPV-positive cancer and those with HPV-negative cancer.

Results.—The median follow-up period was 4.8 years. The 3-year rate of overall survival was similar in the group receiving accelerated-fractionation radiotherapy and the group receiving standard-fractionation radiotherapy (70.3% vs. 64.3%; P=0.18; hazard ratio for death with accelerated-fractionation radiotherapy, 0.90; 95% confidence interval [CI], 0.72 to 1.13), as were the rates of high-grade acute and late toxic events. A total of 63.8% of patients with oropharyngeal cancer (206 of 323) had HPV-positive tumors; these patients had better 3-year rates of overall survival (82.4%, vs. 57.1% among patients with HPV-negative tumors; P<0.001 by the log-rank test) and, after adjustment for age, race, tumor and nodal stage, tobacco exposure, and treatment assignment, had a 58% reduction in the risk of death (hazard ratio, 0.42; 95% CI, 0.27 to 0.66). The risk of death significantly increased with each additional pack-year of tobacco smoking. Using recursive-partitioning analysis, we classified our patients as having a low, intermediate, or high risk of death on the basis of four factors: HPV status, pack-years of tobacco smoking, tumor stage, and nodal stage.

Conclusions.—Tumor HPV status is a strong and independent prognostic factor for survival among patients with oropharyngeal cancer. (ClinicalTrials.gov number, NCT00047008.)

▶ The propensity of human papillomaviruses (HPVs) to stimulate development of squamous cell carcinoma has been well understood in the context of cervical cancer. Unfortunately, there are a growing number of HPV-positive patients who have developed squamous cell carcinoma of the head and neck region, especially the oropharynx. One plus of these HPV-associated oropharyngeal cancers is that the prognosis in terms of survival is better than non-HPV—associated oropharyngeal squamous cell carcinomas. Yet until these data, the exact relationship of HPV versus other risk factors such as smoking, tumor, and nodal stage was not well understood.

One of the many benefits of data sets of large cooperative groups is the ability to do meta-analyses such as was performed here. The data and therefore the results are strengthened by the fact that single-institution biases are lessened dramatically and thus the results carry more statistical power.

These authors are to be commended for this work, which clearly demonstrates tumor HPV status as a strong independent prognostic factor for improved survival in patients with oropharyngeal squamous cell carcinoma. The next question will be, can these patients be treated differently, perhaps less intensively and still see excellent survival outcomes?

C. A. Lawton, MD

24 Neuro-Oncology

Randomized comparison of whole brain radiotherapy, 20 Gy in four daily fractions versus 40 Gy in 20 twice-daily fractions, for brain metastases
Graham PH, Bucci J, Browne L (St George Hosp, Kogarah, Australia)
Int J Radiat Oncol Biol Phys 77:648-654, 2010

Purpose.—The present study compared the intracranial control rate and quality of life for two radiation fractionation schemes for cerebral metastases.

Methods and Materials.—A total of 113 patients with a Eastern Cooperative Oncology Group performance status <3; and stable (>2 months), absent, or concurrent presentation of extracranial disease were randomized to 40 Gy in 20 twice-daily fractions (Arm A) or 20 Gy in four daily fractions (Arm B), stratified by resection status. The European Organization for Research and Treatment of Cancer Quality of Life 30-item questionnaire was administered monthly during Year 1, bimonthly during Year 2, and then every 6 months to Year 5.

Results.—The patient age range was 28–83 years (mean 62). Of the 113 patients, 41 had undergone surgical resection, and 74 patients had extracranial disease (31 concurrent and 43 stable). The median survival time was 6.1 months in Arm A and 6.6 months in Arm B, and the overall 5-year survival rate was 3.5%. Intracranial progression occurred in 44% of Arm A and 64% of Arm B patients ($p = .03$). Salvage surgery or radiotherapy was used in 4% of Arm A patients and 21% of Arm B patients ($p = .004$). Death was attributed to central nervous system progression in 32% of patients in Arm A and 52% of patients in Arm B ($p = .03$). The toxicity was minimal, with a minor increase in short-term cutaneous reactions in Arm A. The patients' quality of life was not impaired by the more intense treatment in Arm A.

Conclusion.—Intracranial disease control was improved and the quality of life was maintained with 40 Gy in 20 twice-daily fractions. This schema should be considered for better prognosis subgroups of patients with cerebral metastases.

▶ The use of whole brain radiotherapy in patients with cerebral metastasis has become a standard of care. Yet the overall survival for these patients remains in the range of approximately 6 months given that the short overall survival, quality of life, and time spent receiving treatment (which often affects quality of life) are important end points to study. These authors have evaluated 2 radiation fractionation schemes 20 Gy in 4 fractions versus 40 Gy in 20 fractions (twice a day) to assess the effects on quality of life and intracranial control rates. While their data certainly support a statistical increase in intracranial control and decrease in death attributed to central nervous system progression with the use of the 40 Gy arm, overall survival was not different (6.1 vs 6.6 months).

Going forward with these results, the obvious next question is to address centers on patients with limited extracranial disease. Perhaps a randomized trial of 40 Gy in 20 fractions (twice a day) versus more standard fractionation schemes of 30 in 10 fractions or 37.5 in 15 fractions. Yet for patients with extensive extracranial disease and intracranial metastasis, 20 Gy in 4 fractions remains a reasonable option, given the overall survival rate seen in this study.

C. A. Lawton, MD

25 Supportive Care

Randomized, Double-Blind Study of Denosumab Versus Zoledronic Acid in the Treatment of Bone Metastases in Patients With Advanced Cancer (Excluding Breast and Prostate Cancer) or Multiple Myeloma

Henry DH, Costa L, Goldwasser F, et al (Joan Karnell Cancer Ctr, Philadelphia, PA; Hosp de Santa Maria and Instituto de Medicina Molecular, Lisboa, Portugal; Teaching Hosp Cochin, Paris, France; et al)
J Clin Oncol 29:1125-1132, 2011

Purpose.—This study compared denosumab, a fully human monoclonal anti-receptor activator of nuclear factor kappa-B ligand antibody, with zoledronic acid (ZA) for delaying or preventing skeletal-related events (SRE) in patients with advanced cancer and bone metastases (excluding breast and prostate) or myeloma.

Patients and Methods.—Eligible patients were randomly assigned in a double-blind, double-dummy design to receive monthly subcutaneous denosumab 120 mg (n = 886) or intravenous ZA 4 mg (dose adjusted for renal impairment; n = 890). Daily supplemental calcium and vitamin D were strongly recommended. The primary end point was time to first on-study SRE (pathologic fracture, radiation or surgery to bone, or spinal cord compression).

Results.—Denosumab was noninferior to ZA in delaying time to first on-study SRE (hazard ratio, 0.84; 95% CI, 0.71 to 0.98; $P = .0007$). Although directionally favorable, denosumab was not statistically superior to ZA in delaying time to first on-study SRE ($P = .03$ unadjusted; $P = .06$ adjusted for multiplicity) or time to first-and-subsequent (multiple) SRE (rate ratio, 0.90; 95% CI, 0.77 to 1.04; $P = .14$). Overall survival and disease progression were similar between groups. Hypocalcemia occurred more frequently with denosumab. Osteonecrosis of the jaw occurred at similarly low rates in both groups. Acute-phase reactions after the first dose occurred more frequently with ZA, as did renal adverse events and elevations in serum creatinine based on National Cancer Institute Common Toxicity Criteria for Adverse Events grading.

Conclusion.—Denosumab was noninferior (trending to superiority) to ZA in preventing or delaying first on-study SRE in patients with advanced cancer metastatic to bone or myeloma. Denosumab represents a potential novel treatment option with the convenience of subcutaneous administration and no requirement for renal monitoring or dose adjustment.

▶ Denosumab is a fully humanized monoclonal antibody directed against receptor activator of nuclear factor κβ ligand to disrupt the cycle of bone resorption associated with bone metastases. This is one of 3 reports of phase III trials comparing denosumab with zoledronic acid. This particular one is in patients with either myeloma or solid tumors other than breast or prostate cancer and at reduced risk of skeletal-related events including pathologic fracture, surgery for cancer-related bone events, radiation to bone, or spinal cord compression. This study showed noninferiority of denosumab compared with zoledronic acid and a strong trend for superiority. In a further analysis, superiority of denosumab was shown in patients with solid tumors after removal of the patients with myeloma. The trials in breast and prostate cancer each showed superiority for denosumab. All 3 studies called for a pooled analysis, which also showed superiority for denosumab. These 3 trials led to the approval of denosumab by the Food and Drug Administration for use in all patients with solid tumor with bone metastases. Because the drug is superior to zoledronic acid in reducing the risk of skeletal-related events, it should be the treatment of choice. In the case of multiple myeloma, an ongoing phase III trial with an accrual target of 1500 patients with multiple myeloma should eventually determine whether the drug should be used in patients with this disease.

J. T. Thigpen, MD

26 Thoracic Cancer

Phase III Trial of Vandetanib Compared With Erlotinib in Patients With Previously Treated Advanced Non–Small-Cell Lung Cancer

Natale RB, Thongprasert S, Greco FA, et al (Cedars-Sinai Outpatient Cancer Ctr, Los Angeles, CA; Sarah Cannon Res Inst, Nashville, TN; Florida Cancer Specialists, Bradenton; et al)

J Clin Oncol 29:1059-1066, 2011

Purpose.—Vandetanib is a once-daily oral inhibitor of vascular endothelial growth factor receptor and epidermal growth factor receptor signaling. This phase III study assessed the efficacy of vandetanib versus erlotinib in unselected patients with advanced non–small-cell lung cancer (NSCLC) after treatment failure with one to two prior cytotoxic chemotherapy regimens.

Patients and Methods.—One thousand two hundred forty patients were randomly assigned to receive vandetanib 300 mg/d (n = 623) or erlotinib 150 mg/d (n = 617). The primary objective was to show superiority in progression-free survival (PFS) for vandetanib versus erlotinib. If the difference did not reach statistical significance for superiority, a noninferiority analysis was conducted.

Results.—There was no significant improvement in PFS for patients treated with vandetanib versus erlotinib (hazard ratio [HR], 0.98; 95.22% CI, 0.87 to 1.10; $P = .721$); median PFS was 2.6 months for vandetanib and 2.0 months for erlotinib. There was also no significant difference for the secondary end points of overall survival (HR, 1.01; $P = .830$), objective response rate (both 12%), and time to deterioration of symptoms for pain (HR, 0.92; $P = .289$), dyspnea (HR, 1.07; $P = .407$), and cough (HR, 0.94; $P = .455$). Both agents showed equivalent PFS and overall survival in a preplanned noninferiority analysis. Adverse events (AEs; any grade) more frequent with vandetanib than erlotinib included diarrhea (50% v 38%, respectively) and hypertension (16% v 2%, respectively); rash was more frequent with erlotinib than vandetanib (38% v 28%, respectively). The overall incidence of grade $\geq$ 3 AEs was also higher with vandetanib than erlotinib (50% v 40%, respectively).

Conclusion.—In patients with previously treated advanced NSCLC, vandetanib showed antitumor activity but did not demonstrate an efficacy advantage compared with erlotinib. There was a higher incidence of some AEs with vandetanib.

▶ The choice of systemic therapy for the first-line treatment of recurrent or advanced non—small cell lung cancer has been studied extensively in phase III trials. Second- and subsequent-line therapy, on the other hand, has generally been studied in phase II trials. Three approaches for second-line therapy, however, have been evaluated in phase III trials and have been shown to be of benefit: docetaxel, pemetrexed, and erlotinib. This study seeks to evaluate a fourth single agent compared with erlotinib. That approach is single-agent vandetanib, an inhibitor of vascular endothelial growth factor and endothelial growth factor receptor. The study was designed as a superiority study with a preplanned non-inferiority analysis if superiority was not demonstrated. The trial shows no supe-riority, but the noninferiority analysis shows no difference between the 2 approaches. One can therefore assume that vandetanib does in fact confer benefit as second-line therapy, but there is no reason to consider its use when there is no advantage and, in fact, greater toxicity, in this trial. The bottom line? Effective second-line therapy for non—small cell lung cancer is available.

J. T. Thigpen, MD

KIDNEY, WATER, AND ELECTROLYTES

RENEE GARRICK, MD

Introduction

METABOLIC FACTORS AND PROGRESSION OF CHRONIC KIDNEY DISEASE

Mitigation of the progression of chronic kidney injury continues to be an area of intense investigation and predicting patient outcomes in chronic kidney disease (CKD) continues to be an important clinical goal. It is known that cystatin C better predicts clinical outcomes in patients with chronic kidney disease than does serum creatinine. Using patients from the Multi-ethnic Study of Atherosclerosis (MESA), and the Cardiovascular Health Study (CHS), Peralta and colleagues demonstrated that the combination of cystatin C with creatinine-based equations is better able to identify patients at highest risk for complications than creatinine or creatinine-based equations alone.

Methven and colleagues demonstrated that a random urinary albumin to creatinine ratio and a urinary total protein to creatinine ratio were as effective (and much more convenient) as 24-hour urine samples for predicting all-cause mortality, the start of renal replacement therapy, and doubling of the serum creatinine level.

Laouari and colleagues used breeding experiments and genome-scan analysis to evaluate the genetic risk factors for progression of CKD. Their findings suggest that TGF-α, which they have previously shown to be a pivotal intermediate in renal lesions induced by angiotensin II, may be a key mediator in the genetic predisposition of CKD progression. TGF-α is a ligand for the epidermal growth factor receptor and, taken together, their data suggest that inhibition of EGFR may mitigate genetic susceptibility to progressive kidney disease.

Studies by Hu and colleagues demonstrated that Klotho, also known as a suppressor of aging (or the fountain of youth), is reduced in CKD. Widespread soft tissue vascular calcification is an almost universal complication of CKD. Their studies demonstrated that deficiency of Klotho is linked to vascular calcification and they suggest that Klotho replacement may have therapeutic potential. Other studies focusing on end organ damage in CKD by Kao and colleagues demonstrated allopurinol may improve left ventricular mass and endothelial dysfunction in chronic kidney disease. The SHARP and FAVORIT trials are the final selections of this section. The SHARP trial, which was the first randomized double-blind trial of patients with chronic kidney disease (either not yet on dialysis or on dialysis) to demonstrate that a reduction in LDL cholesterol with simvastatin (20 mg) and ezetimibe (10 mg) can safely reduce the occurrence of major atherosclerotic events in patients with advanced kidney disease.

On a more cautious note, The FAVORIT trial utilized B_6, B_{12}, and folic acid to control homocysteine levels in stable kidney transplant patients (GFR greater than 30 mL/min at time of enrollment). Even though treatment reduced homocysteine levels, there was no improvement in cardiovascular disease outcome, all-cause mortality, or in dialysis-dependent kidney failure.

GLOMERULAR DISEASE AND ACUTE KIDNEY INJURY

Several interesting studies involving acute kidney injury and glomerular disease are included in this year's reviews. Chronic kidney disease is approximately 4-fold more common in African Americans than in individuals of European descent. Last year, a great deal of interest was generated by the finding that Myosin Heavy Chain 9 (MYH9) mutations were linked to nondiabetic renal disease in African Americans. Fascinating studies by Genovese et al utilized the human genome project to demonstrate that the linkage is actually not with MYH9 but with a neighboring gene APOL. An additional twist to the story is that although genetic variation in APOL1 increases susceptibility to kidney disease, it confers protection against infection with the endemic parasite *Trypanosoma brucei*. The pathogenesis of the increased susceptibility to kidney disease remains to be definitively determined; in the meantime, we are reminded that medical science is rarely as straightforward as it might first appear. Other studies focused on anti-glomerular basement membrane disease and postinfectious glomerulonephritis in the elderly. Clinicians should be aware that the fairly common glomerular diseases often have different risk factors and clinical presentations in the elderly.

Studies by James and colleagues suggest that patients who are hospitalized with acute kidney injury during the weekend have a higher risk of death than do patients admitted on a weekday. The risk of death was more pronounced in smaller hospitals as compared with larger hospitals. These data should certainly increase our clinical vigilance as we strive to identify and correct the factors that contributed to this observation. Additional studies by James and studies by Grams and colleagues demonstrated that the presence and severity of underlying proteinuria and albuminuria are linked to the risk of incident acute kidney injury. Finally, the work of Chawla and colleagues emphasized that despite apparent recovery, there are potential long-term consequences of an episode of acute kidney injury, and that the severity of acute kidney injury can be useful to predict which patients are at greatest risk for progression to CKD.

DIABETES

The ACCORD trial investigated the effects of intensive pressure control in type 2 diabetes and determined that targeting systolic blood pressure to less than 120 mm Hg as compared to 140 mm Hg did not reduce the composite risk of major cardiovascular events. From the kidney perspective, these data are in keeping with the current guidelines, and using 120 mm Hg as the low-end systolic target remains reasonable, pending additional studies. The significance of micro and macroalbuminuria is well established in diabetic renal disease. The ROADMAP trial evaluated whether treatment with an angiotensin receptor blocker could delay or prevent the onset of microalbuminuria. Olmesartan therapy did just that; however, patients with high-grade pre-existing vascular and coronary disease demonstrated a higher rate of fatal cardiovascular events. The findings reinforce the need to carefully individualize and monitor therapy.

New diabetic therapies may be gaining ground. The BEAM trial in patients with advanced CKD and type 2 diabetes, demonstrated that 24 weeks of treatment with the oral antioxidant inflammatory modulator bardoxolone methyl was associated with an improvement in eGFR. Longer-term trials with this agent should be forthcoming. The data by Welsh and Uzu reinforce that cardiovascular and microvascular diseases are extremely common in diabetics. This must be appreciated when assessing surgical and postsurgical risk and, as suggested by Uzu, the presence of cerebral microvascular disease may be a harbinger of clinical renal disease. Finally, data from the On Target/Transcend Study, which included patients with diabetes or vascular disease, demonstrated that patients with albuminuria (a manifestation of microvascular disease) were more likely to have evidence of cognitive decline as compared with individuals without albuminuria. Moreover, the rate of cognitive decline was slowed by therapy with angiotensin receptor blockers and/or converting enzyme inhibitors.

CLINICAL NEPHROLOGY

Selections this year encompass a wide range of topics. Studies in polycystic kidney disease have demonstrated that sirolimus therapy can halt renal cyst growth, and octreotide may slow the progressive increase in both kidney and liver cyst volume. Studies focusing on diet and disease have demonstrated that low socioeconomic status is associated with higher serum phosphorus levels, which in turn have been associated with adverse outcomes in CKD. The data of Jalal and co-workers showed that diets high in fructose (typically derived from high fructose corn syrup) are associated with elevated blood pressure in patients without a history of hypertension. Studies also have demonstrated that low health care literacy alone is associated with increased mortality in CKD.

Regarding CKD awareness, interesting data from Europe stress that when caring for patients with hypertension, primary care providers must be more aware of CKD risk and treatment guidelines. These findings are echoed in studies by Greer and colleagues, which found that when caring for patients at high risk for CKD, primary care providers often did not discuss the presence of, or risk factors for, CKD progression.

Clinical nephrology research continues to translate basic science findings to the bedside. The last several selections focus on important clinical topics, including diuretic use in patients with decompensated heart failure, the risk of aggressive calcium supplementation as a precipitating factor for the modern version of the milk alkali syndrome, severe proteinuria as a complication of bevacizumab therapy, and the use of plasma resistin levels as a marker for hypertensive risk among nondiabetic women.

CHRONIC KIDNEY DISEASE AND DIALYSIS

In many ways, this section might be called "the more we know, the less we really know," as there have been several publications this year that call into question some of the prior guidelines and practice patterns regarding the treatment of patients with progressive CKD. O'Hare and colleagues discovered significant regional differences and treatment practices for older patients with end-stage renal disease. The data were not explained by differences in patient characteristics. Interestingly, the highest quintile of end-of-life intensity of care was less likely to be under the care of a nephrologist prior to the onset of dialysis and less likely to have a fistula at the time of dialysis initiation. Patients in those same regions were more likely to continue dialysis near the time of death rather than seeking hospice care.

During the last 10 years, dialysis has been initiated at increasingly higher levels of glomerular filtration rate. This was in part fueled by widely accepted treatment standards and practices. The results of the IDEAL trial from Australia and the studies of Clark and colleagues from Canada evaluated the association between the timing of the initiation of dialysis and patient mortality. The data from these 2 trials did not demonstrate that early initiation of therapy was associated with an improvement in survival. Winkelmayer and colleagues evaluated patients over the age of 67 with multiple comorbidities and were unable to demonstrate that early referral to a nephrologist (at least 3 months prior to the initiation of dialysis) improved 1-year dialysis survival. In view of the age, comorbidities, and dialysis survival rates in the elderly, it does seem possible that early referral may improve morbidity without significantly improving mortality rates. Taken as a group, these articles highlight the fact that care of the dialysis patient clearly must be individualized. This is an important role for the subspecialist nephrologist who has the additional expertise required to evaluate each patient's specific issues and, together with the patient, develop an appropriate plan of care.

Renee Garrick, MD

27 Metabolic Factors and Renal Disease Progression

Cystatin C Identifies Chronic Kidney Disease Patients at Higher Risk for Complications
Peralta CA, Katz R, Sarnak MJ, et al (San Francisco Veterans Affairs Med Ctr, CA; Univ of Washington, Seattle; Tufts-New England Med Ctr, Boston, MA; et al)
J Am Soc Nephrol 22:147-155, 2011

Although cystatin C is a stronger predictor of clinical outcomes associated with CKD than creatinine, the clinical role for cystatin C is unclear. We included 11,909 participants from the Multi-Ethnic Study of Atherosclerosis (MESA) and the Cardiovascular Health Study (CHS) and assessed risks for death, cardiovascular events, heart failure, and ESRD among persons categorized into mutually exclusive groups on the basis of the biomarkers that supported a diagnosis of CKD (eGFR <60 ml/min per 1.73 m^2): creatinine only, cystatin C only, both, or neither. We used CKD-EPI equations to estimate GFR from these biomarkers. In MESA, 9% had CKD by the creatinine-based equation only, 2% had CKD by the cystatin C-based equation only, and 4% had CKD by both equations; in CHS, these percentages were 12, 4, and 13%, respectively. Compared with those without CKD, the adjusted hazard ratios (HR) for mortality in MESA were: 0.80 (95% CI 0.50 to 1.26) for CKD by creatinine only; 3.23 (95% CI 1.84 to 5.67) for CKD by cystatin C only; and 1.93 (95% CI 1.27 to 2.92) for CKD by both; in CHS, the adjusted HR were 1.09 (95% CI 0.98 to 1.21), 1.78 (95% CI 1.53 to 2.08), and 1.74 (95% CI 1.58 to 1.93), respectively. The pattern was similar for cardiovascular disease (CVD), heart failure, and kidney failure outcomes. In conclusion, among adults diagnosed with CKD using the creatinine-based CKD-EPI equation, the adverse prognosis is limited to the subset who also have CKD according to the cystatin C-based equation. Cystatin C may have a role in identifying persons with CKD who have the highest risk for complications.

▶ Cystatin C is less influenced by muscle mass than is creatinine and has emerged as an interesting alternate marker of kidney function. Prior studies in both the elderly and the general population have demonstrated that cystatin C is a superior predictor of mortality and adverse cardiovascular outcomes than is serum creatinine.[1,2] In addition, a cystatin C level of greater than 1 mg/L in patients with an estimated glomerular filtration rate (GFR) (by Modification of Diet in Renal Disease calculation) of greater than 60 mL/min/1.73 m^2 has been used to classify patients as having preclinical renal disease, a finding that placed them at increased risk for cardiovascular disease and death.[3]

This study was designed to evaluate whether clinical outcomes are better predicted by cystatin C, or creatinine-based estimations of GFR. The study included 11 900 participants from the Multi-Ethnic Study of Atherosclerosis (MESA) and the Cardiovascular Health Study (CHS). Ambulatory adult classification of chronic kidney disease (CKD) based on the cystatin C estimation of GFR (eGFRcys) was compared with the estimated GFR based on serum creatinine (eGFR creatinine). The authors looked at the proportion of patients with an eGFR of less than 60 mL/min/1.73 m^2 on the basis of creatinine, cystatin C, both, or neither and compared the risk for mortality, cardiovascular events, heart failure, and kidney failure among these groups. In addition, the authors evaluated whether eGFR cystatin detected additional cases of decreased GFR among persons with an eGFR creatinine of greater than 60 mL/min. In MESA, 9% had CKD by the creatinine-based equation only, 2% had CKD by the cystatin C—based equation only, and 4% had CKD by both equations; in the CHS, these percentages were 12%, 4%, and 13%, respectively. These data suggest that there is a fair amount of variability among these GFR classifications. More interesting, however, was the finding that the adjusted hazard ratio for mortality for CKD by creatinine only was 0.80 (95% CI 0.50 to 1.26) and was 3.23 (95% CI 1.84 to 5.67) for CKD by cystatin C only. A similar pattern was detected for cardiovascular disease, heart failure, and kidney failure outcomes. The study does have limitations. For example, the MESA trial did not include information on the incidence of renal failure, and cystatin C itself has been shown to be associated with factors other than kidney function.[4] Strengths of the study included the large, ethnically diverse sample size.

In sum, the study is the first to demonstrate that cystatin C—based equations for the estimation of GFR can be used to define a subset of patients who are at the greatest risk for mortality and cardiovascular complications. If verified, this information may allow for risk stratification and would permit practitioners to give heightened attention to the subpopulation of patients at greatest risk for adverse outcomes.

R. Garrick, MD

References

1. Shlipak MG, Sarnak MJ, Katz R, et al. Cystatin C and the risk of death and cardiovascular events among elderly persons. *N Engl J Med.* 2005;352:2049-2060.
2. Astor BC, Levey AS, Stevens LA, Van Lente F, Selvin E, Coresh J. Method of glomerular filtration rate estimation affects prediction of mortality risk. *J Am Soc Nephrol.* 2009;20:2214-2222.
3. Shlipak MG, Katz R, Sarnak MJ, et al. Cystatin C and prognosis for cardiovascular and kidney outcomes in elderly persons without chronic kidney disease. *Ann Intern Med.* 2006;145:237-246.
4. Stevens LA, Schmid CH, Greene T, et al. Factors other than glomerular filtration rate affect serum cystatin C levels. *Kidney Int.* 2009;75:652-660.

Comparison of Urinary Albumin and Urinary Total Protein as Predictors of Patient Outcomes in CKD
Methven S, MacGregor MS, Traynor JP, et al (Crosshouse Hosp, Kilmarnock, UK; Monklands Hosp, Airdrie, UK; et al)
Am J Kidney Dis 57:21-28, 2010

Background.—Proteinuria is common and is associated with adverse patient outcomes. The optimal test of proteinuria to identify those at risk is uncertain. This study assessed albuminuria and total proteinuria as predictors of 3 patient outcomes: all-cause mortality, start of renal replacement therapy (RRT), and doubling of serum creatinine level.

Study Design.—Retrospective longitudinal cohort study.

Setting & Participants.—Nephrology clinic of a city hospital in Scotland; 5,586 patients with chronic kidney disease (CKD) and proteinuria measured in random urine samples (n = 3,378) or timed urine collections (n = 1,808).

Predictors.—Baseline measurements of albumin-creatinine ratio (ACR), total protein—creatinine ratio (PCR), 24-hour albuminuria, and total proteinuria.

Outcomes.—All-cause mortality, start of RRT, and doubling of serum creatinine level were assessed using receiver operating characteristic curves and Cox proportional hazards models.

Measurements.—Blood pressure, serum creatinine level, ACR, PCR, date of death, date of starting RRT.

Results.—Patients were followed up for a median of 3.5 (25th-75th percentile, 2.1-6.0) years. For all outcomes, adjusted HRs were similar for PCR and ACR (derived from random urine samples and timed collections): death, 1.41 (95% CI, 1.31-1.53) vs 1.38 (95% CI, 1.28-1.50); RRT, 1.96 (95% CI, 1.76-2.18) vs 2.33 (95% CI, 2.06-3.01); and doubling of serum creatinine level, 2.03 (95% CI, 1.87-2.19) vs 1.92 (95% CI, 1.78-2.08). Receiver operating characteristic curves showed almost identical performance for ACR and PCR for the 3 outcome measures. Adjusted HRs for ACR and PCR were similar when derived from random urine samples or timed collections and compared with 24-hour total protein and albumin excretion for each outcome measure.

Limitations.—This is a retrospective study.

Conclusions.—Total proteinuria and albuminuria perform equally as predictors of renal outcomes and mortality in patients with CKD. ACR and PCR were as effective as 24-hour urine samples at predicting outcomes and are more convenient for patients, clinicians, and laboratories. Both ACR and PCR stratify risk in patients with CKD.

▶ Microalbuminuria has been shown to be a predictor of renal events and mortality,[1-3] as well as serving as a predictor of cardiovascular events in both diabetic and nondiabetic patients.[4,5] In this study, Methven and colleagues sought to identify whether the urinary protein or urinary albumin has greater predictive value as a marker for patient outcomes in individuals with chronic kidney disease. Although retrospective, the study is important, because, with regard to mortality,

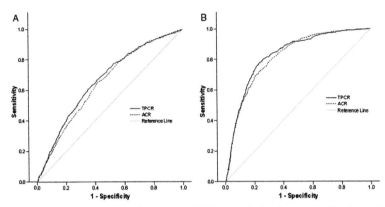

FIGURE 2.—Receiver operating characteristic (ROC) curves for baseline urinary albumin-creatinine ratio (ACR) and total protein—creatinine ratio (TPCR) to predict (A) all-cause mortality and (B) renal replacement therapy. ROC curves include ACR and TPCR derived from timed (24-hour) urine collections and spot urine samples. (Reprinted from *American Journal of Kidney Diseases*, Methven S, MacGregor MS, Traynor JP, et al. Comparison of urinary albumin and urinary total protein as predictors of patient outcomes in CKD. *Am J Kidney Dis.* 2010;57:21-28. Copyright 2010 with permission from the National Kidney Foundation.)

it remains uncertain whether proteinuria, the albumin-to-creatinine ratio (ACR), the albumin excretion rate (AER), or the protein creatinine ratio (PCR) is best used. The Glasgow Royal Infirmary electronic database was mined from 1999 onward. The database contains an extensive array of baseline clinical information (including the use of angiotensin-converting enzyme inhibitor and angiotensin receptor blocker therapy), as well as patient demographic and outcome data. Using a hierarchical Cox regression survival analysis and multiple covariance analysis, the hazard ratios for albumin and protein excretion were analyzed. As shown in Table 2, there were no significant differences between the results for ACR and PCR derived from the spot urine sample compared with those derived from timed urine collection. Because the timed samples and random samples showed similar predictive ability, these were combined and used to compare the ACR versus the PCR as predictors of mortality and progressive renal disease. As shown in Fig 2, both measurements were similarly powered to predict mortality. Because of the retrospective nature of the study, the authors were not able to study whether a combination of proteinuria and albuminuria excretion would improve the sensitivity of the predictive power of the observations.

Despite a retrospective nature, the results are very interesting. The authors demonstrated that in a large chronic kidney disease clinic comprised of both diabetic and nondiabetic patients (the majority were nondiabetic), both timed and untimed albumin creatinine ratios and protein creatinine ratios are equally powerful predictors of all-cause mortality and renal outcomes. Interestingly, even low levels of proteinuria (PCR 150 to 500 mg/g equivalent to protein excretion of 0.15 to 0.5 g/d) defined by the PCR was a strong marker of risk. These retrospectives will need to be verified with a prospective study before guideline recommendations can be made. However, with regard to daily clinical care, these data clearly suggest that either of these markers (as distinct from

TABLE 2.—Associations of Baseline Urine ACR and PCR With Subsequent Patient Outcomes

	No.	Death		RRT		Doubled SCr	
		HR	aHR	HR	aHR	HR	aHR
Spot ACR	3,264	1.42 (1.30-1.55)	1.49 (1.34-1.66)	3.28 (2.87-3.76)	2.41 (2.06-2.83)	1.90 (1.75-2.06)	1.95 (1.78-2.08)
Spot PCR	3,264	1.53 (1.40-1.66)	1.54 (1.38-1.71)	2.99 (2.69-3.33)	2.03 (1.77-2.32)	1.92 (1.78-2.07)	2.01 (1.82-2.21)
24-h ACR	1,676	1.48 (1.31-1.66)	1.26 (1.11-1.42)	2.82 (2.37-3.35)	2.24 (1.83-2.74)	2.06 (1.85-2.30)	1.91 (1.69-2.16)
24-h PCR	1,676	1.51 (1.37-1.66)	1.28 (1.14-1.44)	2.68 (2.32-3.09)	1.88 (1.59-2.23)	2.03 (1.85-2.23)	2.12 (1.84-2.45)
Spot and 24-h ACR (combined)	4,940	1.41 (1.31-1.51)	1.38 (1.28-1.50)	3.00 (2.69-3.36)	2.33 (2.06-3.01)	1.94 (1.81-2.08)	1.92 (1.78-2.08)
Spot and 24-h PCR (combined)	4,940	1.53 (1.43-1.63)	1.41 (1.31-1.53)	2.84 (2.59-3.11)	1.96 (1.76-2.18)	1.96 (1.84-2.08)	2.03 (1.87-2.19)

Note: N = 5,586 patients with CKD attending an outpatient clinic. HRs and aHRs (with 95% confidence intervals) from multivariate Cox regression analyses are presented, per 1−standard deviation difference in the variable. Age, sex, blood pressure, and SCr level are covariates in all models. SCr level is a time-dependent covariate for RRT. Age is a time-dependent covariate for doubling of SCr level. Spot ACR and PCR are derived from random urine samples; and 24-hour ACR and PCR are derived from timed urine collections.

Abbreviations: ACR, albumin-creatinine ratio; aHR, adjusted hazard ratio; PCR, total protein−creatinine ratio; HR, hazard ratio; RRT, renal replacement therapy; SCr, serum creatinine.

a full 24-hour collection) are useful and powerful predictors for all-cause mortality and renal outcomes in patients with chronic kidney disease.

R. Garrick, MD

References

1. van der Velde M, Halbesma N, de Charro F, et al. Screening for albuminuria identifies individuals at increased renal risk. *J Am Soc Nephrol.* 2009;20:852-862.
2. Heerspink HJL, Gansevoort RT, Brenner B, et al. Comparison of different measures of urinary protein excretion for prediction of renal events. *J Am Soc Nephrol.* 2010;21:1355-1360.
3. Rifkin DE, Katz R, Chonchol M, et al. Albuminuria, impaired kidney function and cardiovascular outcomes or mortality in the elderly. *Nephrol Dial Transplant.* 2010;25:1560-1567.
4. Hillege HL, Fidler V, Diercks GF, et al. Urinary albumin excretion predicts cardiovascular and noncardiovascular mortality in general population. *Circulation.* 2002;106:1777-1782.
5. Klausen K, Borch-Johnsen K, Feldt-Rasmussen B, et al. Very low levels of microalbuminuria are associated with increased risk of coronary heart disease and death independently of renal function, hypertension, and diabetes. *Circulation.* 2004; 110:32-35.

TGF-α Mediates Genetic Susceptibility to Chronic Kidney Disease

Laouari D, Burtin M, Phelep A, et al (Université Paris Descartes, France; et al)
J Am Soc Nephrol 22:327-335, 2011

The mechanisms of progression of chronic kidney disease (CKD) are poorly understood. Epidemiologic studies suggest a strong genetic component, but the genes that contribute to the onset and progression of CKD are largely unknown. Here, we applied an experimental model of CKD (75% excision of total renal mass) to six different strains of mice and found that only the FVB/N strain developed renal lesions. We performed a genome-scan analysis in mice generated by back-crossing resistant and sensitive strains; we identified a major susceptibility locus (Ckdp1) on chromosome 6, which corresponds to regions on human chromosome 2 and 3 that link with CKD progression. *In silico* analysis revealed that the locus includes the gene encoding the EGF receptor (EGFR) ligand TGF-α. TGF-α protein levels markedly increased after nephron reduction exclusively in FVB/N mice, and this increase preceded the development of renal lesions. Furthermore, pharmacologic inhibition of EGFR prevented the development of renal lesions in the sensitive FVB/N strain. These data suggest that variable TGF-α expression may explain, in part, the genetic susceptibility to CKD progression. EGFR inhibition may be a therapeutic strategy to counteract the genetic predisposition to CKD.

▶ It is well known that chronic kidney disease (CKD) inexorably progresses regardless of the inciting renal injury. The fact that some ethnicities are more susceptible to progressive injury than others[1] and that many forms of progressive renal disease demonstrate familial clustering[2] suggest that there are genetic factors that affect these susceptibilities. Most of the data on the mechanisms of renal disease progression were derived from animal models of renal mass reduction via subtotal nephrectomy.

Using a 75% nephrectomy model in 6 different strains of mice, Laouari et al identified a strain of mouse (FVB/N) that is most susceptible to the development of renal lesions after subtotal nephrectomy. These mice rapidly develop proteinuria, glomerulosclerosis, and interstitial fibrosis mimicking human focal segmental glomerulosclerosis. Other strains were identified that did not develop these lesions. Using experimental crosses, whole genome scan, and linkage analysis, they further identified a putative locus on chromosome 6 that includes the gene coding for transforming growth factor alpha (TGF-α). Because TGF-α is a known intermediate in angiotensin II—induced renal lesions,[3] it was not surprising that the expression of this cytokine was elevated in the susceptible mice compared with their nonsusceptible counterparts and was temporally associated with the development of renal failure.

Even more exciting is that pharmacologic blockade of epidermal growth factor receptor (EGFR), the target receptor for TGF-α, effectively minimized the progression of renal lesions in the affected mice. This fits very nicely both with the well-documented role of EGFR in activation of CKD and with the known stimulatory effects of angiotensin II on TGF-α expression.

This study brings us a step closer to understanding the genetic influences and ethnic differences that modify the progression of CKD. It also suggests useful avenues for clinical intervention should similar genetic linkages be found in humans.

M. Klein, MD, JD

References

1. Hsu CY, Lin F, Vittinghoff E, Shlipak MG. Racial differences in the progression from chronic renal insufficiency to end-stage renal disease in the United States. *J Am Soc Nephrol.* 2003;14:2902-2907.
2. Satko SG, Sedor JR, Iyengar SK, Freedman BI. Familial clustering of chronic kidney disease. *Semin Dial.* 2007;20:229-236.
3. Lautrette A, Li S, Alili R, et al. Angiotensin II and EGF receptor cross-talk in chronic kidney diseases: a new therapeutic approach. *Nat Med.* 2005;11:867-874.

Klotho Deficiency Causes Vascular Calcification in Chronic Kidney Disease
Hu MC, Shi M, Zhang J, et al (Univ of Texas Southwestern Med Ctr, Dallas)
J Am Soc Nephrol 22:124-136, 2011

Soft-tissue calcification is a prominent feature in both chronic kidney disease (CKD) and experimental Klotho deficiency, but whether Klotho deficiency is responsible for the calcification in CKD is unknown. Here, wild-type mice with CKD had very low renal, plasma, and urinary levels of Klotho. In humans, we observed a graded reduction in urinary Klotho starting at an early stage of CKD and progressing with loss of renal function. Despite induction of CKD, transgenic mice that overexpressed Klotho had preserved levels of Klotho, enhanced phosphaturia, better renal function, and much less calcification compared with wild-type mice with CKD. Conversely, Klotho-haploinsufficient mice with CKD had undetectable levels of Klotho, worse renal function, and severe calcification. The beneficial effect of Klotho on vascular calcification was a result of more than its effect on renal function and phosphatemia, suggesting a direct effect of Klotho on the vasculature. *In vitro*, Klotho suppressed Na^+-dependent uptake of phosphate and mineralization induced by high phosphate and preserved differentiation in vascular smooth muscle cells. In summary, Klotho is an early biomarker for CKD, and Klotho deficiency contributes to soft-tissue calcification in CKD. Klotho ameliorates vascular calcification by enhancing phosphaturia, preserving glomerular filtration, and directly inhibiting phosphate uptake by vascular smooth muscle. Replacement of Klotho may have therapeutic potential for CKD.

▶ Premature vascular and soft tissue calcifications are closely associated with high cardiovascular mortality in patients with chronic kidney disease (CKD). The etiology of this calcification has been intensely investigated. Alterations in several risk factors and biomarkers have been identified, including fibroblast growth factor 23 (FGF-23) and Klotho, a protein that acts as a cofactor for FGF-23 receptor activation. FGF-23 and Klotho increase urinary phosphate excretion. High serum phosphate levels are associated with increased mortality in patients with CKD and treatment with phosphate binders has been shown to improve survival in patients with CKD.[1,2]

Klotho-deficient rodents developed ectopic soft tissue calcification and premature aging, and because of the similarities between Klotho deficiency in rodents and CKD in humans, the authors postulated that Klotho deficiency may be causally related to the vascular calcification of CKD. To study this, the authors performed a series of elegant whole-animal and tissue-culture experiments to evaluate the role of Klotho in phosphate transport and vascular calcification. In addition, they measured urinary Klotho in patients with CKD with various stages of kidney disease.

Their findings demonstrated a graded reduction in human urinary Klotho levels beginning in the early stages of kidney disease. Klotho-deficient mice with CKD had worse renal outcomes and severe vascular calcification, whereas transgenic mice that overexpressed Klotho had enhanced phosphate excretion and preserved renal function, and developed less severe calcification. The studies of vascular smooth muscle cells in tissue culture suggested that in addition to its effects on cellular phosphate transport, Klotho may control the balance between differentiations in dedifferentiation of vascular smooth muscle cells. Together, the tissue culture data and the transgenic data demonstrate that Klotho overexpression slows the progression of CKD, improves phosphate metabolism, and protects against vascular calcification.

This very exciting translational research study demonstrates for the first time that human CKD is a state of Klotho deficiency and this deficiency has a causal role in the vascular calcification that is a hallmark of CKD. Moreover, the findings demonstrate that replacement of Klotho can ameliorate vascular calcification and preserve glomerular filtration rate. The finding that Klotho replacement slows the progression of kidney disease and reduces vascular calcification, which is one of the most important cardiovascular risk factors of CKD, should prompt many additional studies to evaluate the feasibility of Klotho supplementation in humans.

R. Garrick, MD

References

1. Kestenbaum B, Sampson JN, Rudser KD, et al. Serum phosphate levels and mortality risk among people with chronic kidney disease. *J Am Soc Nephrol.* 2005;16:520-528.
2. Isakova T, Gutiérrez OM, Chang Y, et al. Phosphorus binders and survival on hemodialysis. *J Am Soc Nephrol.* 2009;20:388-396.

Allopurinol Benefits Left Ventricular Mass and Endothelial Dysfunction in Chronic Kidney Disease

Kao MP, Ang DS, Gandy SJ, et al (Univ of Dundee, UK)
J Am Soc Nephrol 22:1382-1389, 2011

Allopurinol ameliorates endothelial dysfunction and arterial stiffness among patients without chronic kidney disease (CKD), but it is unknown if it has similar effects among patients with CKD. Furthermore, because arterial stiffness increases left ventricular afterload, any allopurinol-induced improvement in arterial compliance might also regress left ventricular hypertrophy (LVH). We conducted a randomized, double-blind, placebo-controlled, parallel-group study in patients with stage 3 CKD and LVH. We randomly assigned 67 subjects to allopurinol at 300 mg/d or placebo for 9 months; 53 patients completed the study. We measured left ventricular mass index (LVMI) with cardiac magnetic resonance imaging (MRI), assessed endothelial function by flow-mediated dilation (FMD) of the brachial artery, and evaluated central arterial stiffness by pulse-wave analysis. Allopurinol significantly reduced LVH $(P = 0.036)$, improved endothelial function $(P = 0.009)$, and improved the central augmentation index $(P = 0.015)$. This study demonstrates that allopurinol can regress left ventricular mass and improve endothelial function among patients with CKD. Because LVH and endothelial dysfunction associate with prognosis, these results call for further trials to examine whether allopurinol reduces cardiovascular events in patients with CKD and LVH.

▶ This study is important, as left ventricular hypertrophy (LVH) affects up to 75% of end-stage renal disease (ESRD) patients and up to 50% of patients with milder chronic kidney disease (CKD). The presence of LVH confers almost a 3-fold increased risk for total and cardiovascular mortality in ESRD patients.[1] The Losartan Intervention for Endpoint reduction (LIFE) study demonstrated that, independent of blood pressure changes, a regression in LVH reduces the risk of sudden death, atrial fibrillation, and heart failure.[2,3] Finding novel therapies to effectively reduce LVH in the CKD population is obviously quite appealing. In animal models, uric acid reduction has been shown to improve LVH,[4] and in non-CKD patients, allopurinol has consistently been found to improve endothelial/vascular function and arterial wave reflection, which, by lowering afterload, may improve LVH. However, no data exist as to the effects of allopurinol on LVH in patients with CKD. In the current 9-month, randomized, double-blind, placebo-controlled study in patients with stage 3 CKD and LVH, 67 patients were assigned to allopurinol at 300 mg/d or placebo. Fifty-three patients completed the study. Left ventricular mass index (LVMI) was measured with cardiac MRI, endothelial function was assessed by flow-mediated dilation of the brachial artery, and central arterial stiffness was evaluated by pulse-wave analysis. Allopurinol significantly reduced LVH ($P = .036$), improved endothelial function ($P = .009$), and improved the central augmentation index ($P = .015$).

This is the first study to show that allopurinol can improve left ventricular mass and endothelial function among patients with CKD. This effect was seen despite no significant improvement in blood pressure control or in urate levels. The data are quite intriguing and will likely spur larger clinical trials. However, on a cautionary note, 7 patients discontinued treatment because of rash, and the dosage studied resulted in only a modest reduction in LVMI. Whether larger dosages could safely result in a greater clinical effect will require carefully monitored dose-response trials.

A. Kapoor, MD

References

1. Silberberg JS, Barre PE, Prichard SS, Sniderman AD. Impact of left ventricular hypertrophy on survival in end-stage renal disease. *Kidney Int.* 1989;36:286-290.
2. Wachtell K, Okin PM, Olsen MH, et al. Regression of electrocardiographic left ventricular hypertrophy during antihypertensive therapy and reduction in sudden cardiac death: the LIFE Study. *Circulation.* 2007;116:700-705.
3. Okin PM, Wachtell K, Devereux RB, et al. Regression of electrocardiographic left ventricular hypertrophy and decreased incidence of new-onset atrial fibrillation in patients with hypertension. *JAMA.* 2006;296:1242-1248.
4. Xu X, Hu X, Lu Z, et al. Xanthine oxidase inhibition with febuxostat attenuates systolic overload-induced left ventricular hypertrophy and dysfunction in mice. *J Card Fail.* 2008;14:746-753.

The effects of lowering LDL cholesterol with simvastatin plus ezetimibe in patients with chronic kidney disease (Study of Heart and Renal Protection): a randomised placebo-controlled trial
Baigent C, on behalf of the SHARP Investigators (Univ of Oxford, UK; et al)
Lancet 377:2181-2192, 2011

Background.—Lowering LDL cholesterol with statin regimens reduces the risk of myocardial infarction, ischaemic stroke, and the need for coronary revascularisation in people without kidney disease, but its effects in people with moderate-to-severe kidney disease are uncertain. The SHARP trial aimed to assess the efficacy and safety of the combination of simvastatin plus ezetimibe in such patients.

Methods.—This randomised double-blind trial included 9270 patients with chronic kidney disease (3023 on dialysis and 6247 not) with no known history of myocardial infarction or coronary revascularisation. Patients were randomly assigned to simvastatin 20 mg plus ezetimibe 10 mg daily versus matching placebo. The key prespecified outcome was first major atherosclerotic event (non-fatal myocardial infarction or coronary death, non-haemorrhagic stroke, or any arterial revascularisation procedure). All analyses were by intention to treat. This trial is registered at ClinicalTrials.gov, NCT00125593, and ISRCTN54137607.

Findings.—4650 patients were assigned to receive simvastatin plus ezetimibe and 4620 to placebo. Allocation to simvastatin plus ezetimibe yielded an average LDL cholesterol difference of 0·85 mmol/L (SE 0·02; with about two-thirds compliance) during a median follow-up of 4·9 years and produced a 17% proportional reduction in major atherosclerotic events (526 [11·3%] simvastatin plus ezetimibe *vs* 619 [13·4%] placebo; rate ratio [RR] 0·83, 95% CI 0·74–0·94; log-rank p=0·0021). Non-significantly fewer patients allocated to simvastatin plus ezetimibe had a non-fatal myocardial infarction or died from coronary heart disease (213 [4·6%] vs 230 [5·0%]; RR 0·92, 95% CI 0·76–1·11; p=0·37) and there were significant reductions in non-haemorrhagic stroke (131 [2·8%] *vs* 174 [3·8%]; RR 0·75, 95% CI 0·60–0·94; p=0·01) and arterial revascularisation procedures (284 [6·1%] *vs* 352 [7·6%]; RR 0·79, 95% CI 0·68–0·93; p=0·0036). After weighting for subgroup-specific reductions in LDL cholesterol, there was no good evidence that the proportional effects on major atherosclerotic events differed from the summary rate ratio in any subgroup examined, and, in particular, they were similar in patients on dialysis and those who were not. The excess risk of myopathy was only two per 10 000 patients per year of treatment with this combination (9 [0·2%] *vs* 5 [0·1%]). There was no evidence of excess risks of hepatitis (21 [0·5%] *vs* 18 [0·4%]), gallstones (106 [2·3%] *vs* 106 [2·3%]), or cancer (438 [9·4%] *vs* 439 [9·5%], p=0·89) and there was no significant excess of death from any non-vascular cause (668 [14·4%] *vs* 612 [13·2%], p=0·13).

Interpretation.—Reduction of LDL cholesterol with simvastatin 20 mg plus ezetimibe 10 mg daily safely reduced the incidence of major atherosclerotic events in a wide range of patients with advanced chronic kidney disease.

▶ The SHARP (Study of Heart and Renal Protection) trial was a large multinational, randomized, controlled trial designed to assess the efficacy and safety of the combination of simvastatin plus ezetimibe in more than 9000 patients with moderate-to-severe kidney disease. The trial used this combination of agents to maximize cholesterol lowering while minimizing the risk of myopathy that has been associated with statin therapy in patients with chronic kidney disease. Patients were initially randomized 3 ways between simvastatin plus ezetimibe daily and simvastatin daily plus placebo. Those allocated to simvastatin alone were rerandomized after 1 year to simvastatin plus ezetimibe versus simvastatin plus placebo. Patients older than 40 years with serum creatinine level of > 1.5 mg/dL in women and 1.7 mg/dL in men were eligible to participate.

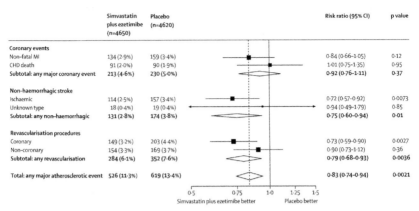

	Simvastatin plus ezetimibe (n=4650)	Placebo (n=4620)		Risk ratio (95% CI)	p value
Coronary events					
Non-fatal MI	134 (2.9%)	159 (3.4%)		0.84 (0.66–1.05)	0.12
CHD death	91 (2.0%)	90 (1.9%)		1.01 (0.75–1.35)	0.95
Subtotal: any major coronary event	213 (4.6%)	230 (5.0%)		0.92 (0.76–1.11)	0.37
Non-haemorrhagic stroke					
Ischaemic	114 (2.5%)	157 (3.4%)		0.72 (0.57–0.92)	0.0073
Unknown type	18 (0.4%)	19 (0.4%)		0.94 (0.49–1.79)	0.85
Subtotal: any non-haemorrhagic	131 (2.8%)	174 (3.8%)		0.75 (0.60–0.94)	0.01
Revascularisation procedures					
Coronary	149 (3.2%)	203 (4.4%)		0.73 (0.59–0.90)	0.0027
Non-coronary	154 (3.3%)	169 (3.7%)		0.90 (0.73–1.12)	0.36
Subtotal: any revascularisation	284 (6.1%)	352 (7.6%)		0.79 (0.68–0.93)	0.0036
Total: any major atherosclerotic event	526 (11.3%)	619 (13.4%)		0.83 (0.74–0.94)	0.0021

0.5   0.75   1.0   1.25   1.5
Simvastatin plus ezetimibe better   Placebo better

FIGURE 3.—Major atherosclerotic events subdivided by type. MI=myocardial infarction. CHD=coronary heart disease. (Reprinted from Baigent C, on behalf of the SHARP Investigators. The effects of lowering LDL cholesterol with simvastatin plus ezetimibe in patients with chronic kidney disease (Study of Heart and Renal Protection): a randomised placebo-controlled trial. *Lancet.* 2011;377:2181-2192.)

The trial is important because other large meta-analyses of randomized trials in patients without chronic kidney disease have found that statin therapy reduces the risk of major coronary events and ischemic stroke without substantially altering the risk of hemorrhagic stroke or other noncardiac vascular causes of death.[1,2] The prior trials included in these analyses did not definitively demonstrate whether reduction of low-density lipoprotein (LDL) cholesterol levels was associated with an improvement in cardiovascular outcome in patients with renal disease. The SHARP trial was specifically designed to value the effect of lowering LDL cholesterol with simvastatin plus ezetimibe on major atherosclerotic events across a wide range of chronic kidney diseases. The Prior Cholesterol Treatment Trialists Collaboration (CTT) showed that statin therapy reduced the risk of myocardial infarction or coronary death or stroke by about one-fifth per 1 mmol/L LDL cholesterol reduction.[2] In the SHARP trial an average reduction of 0.85 mmol/L of LDL produced a 17% reduction in major atherosclerotic events (Fig 3), a finding that was similar to the effects seen in the CTT trial.

It should be noted that on average, only two-thirds of the patients allocated to the simvastatin plus ezetimibe group were taking an LDL-lowering regimen. This raises the possibility that if patients with chronic kidney disease had taken the full regimen as prescribed, the results would be even more marked. Although the trial did not have sufficient power to independently assess atherosclerotic events in dialysis patients and nondialysis patients separately, about a third of the patients began dialysis after the initiation of the trial, and subgroup analysis suggested that the proportional effects on major atherosclerotic events were similar in dialysis and nondialysis patients.

No excess risk of cancer was noted, and the excess risk of myopathy was only 2 per 10 000 patients per year of treatment with this dosage regimen and medication combination. This latter finding is of particular importance in view of the most recent US Food and Drug Administration alert regarding the use of high-dose simvastatin (80 mg) in combination with other medications that can raise simvastatin levels and increase the risk of myopathy.[3] Cardiovascular disease is the most common cause of morbidity and mortality in patients with chronic kidney disease and those on dialysis. The results suggest that for every 1000 patients treated for 5 years, 30 to 40 major atherosclerotic deaths can be prevented. Although these benefits may not seem large in number, the SHARP trial is important because it is the first to demonstrate that statin therapy can be used safely and can reduce atherosclerotic events in patients with chronic kidney disease.

R. Garrick, MD

References

1. Baigent C, Keech A, Kearney PM, et al; Cholesterol Treatment Trialists' (CTT) Collaborators. Efficacy and safety of cholesterol-lowering treatment: prospective meta-analysis of data from 90,056 participants in 14 randomised trials of statins. *Lancet.* 2005;366:1267-1278.
2. Cholesterol Treatment Trialists' (CTT) Collaboration, Baigent C, Blackwell L, Emberson J, et al. Efficacy and safety of more intensive lowering of LDL cholesterol: a meta-analysis of data from 170,000 participants in 26 randomised trials. *Lancet.* 2010;376:1670-1681.
3. FDA drug safety communication: new restrictions, contraindications, and those limitations for Zocor (simvastatin) to reduce the risk of muscle injury. US Department of Health and Human Services Food and Drug Administration; June 8, 2011.

Homocysteine-Lowering and Cardiovascular Disease Outcomes in Kidney Transplant Recipients: Primary Results From the Folic Acid for Vascular Outcome Reduction in Transplantation Trial

Bostom AG, Carpenter MA, Kusek JW, et al (Rhode Island Hosp, Providence; Univ of North Carolina, Chapel Hill; Natl Inst of Diabetes and Digestive and Kidney Diseases, Bethesda, MD; et al)

Circulation 123:1763-1770, 2011

Background.—Kidney transplant recipients, like other patients with chronic kidney disease, experience excess risk of cardiovascular disease and elevated total homocysteine concentrations. Observational studies of patients with chronic kidney disease suggest increased homocysteine is a risk factor for cardiovascular disease. The impact of lowering total homocysteine levels in kidney transplant recipients is unknown.

Methods and Results.—In a double-blind controlled trial, we randomized 4110 stable kidney transplant recipients to a multivitamin that included either a high dose (n = 2056) or low dose (n = 2054) of folic acid, vitamin B6, and vitamin B12 to determine whether decreasing total homocysteine concentrations reduced the rate of the primary composite arteriosclerotic cardiovascular disease outcome (myocardial infarction, stroke, cardiovascular disease death, resuscitated sudden death, coronary artery or renal artery revascularization, lower-extremity arterial disease, carotid endarterectomy or angioplasty, or abdominal aortic aneurysm repair). Mean follow-up was 4.0 years. Treatment with the high-dose multivitamin reduced homocysteine but did not reduce the rates of the primary outcome (n = 547 total events; hazards ratio [95%

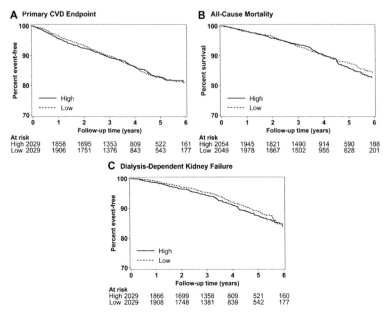

FIGURE 2.—Kaplan–Meier analyses for (**A**) primary CVD, (**B**) all-cause mortality, and (**C**) dialysis-dependent kidney failure outcomes. CVD indicates cardiovascular disease. (Reprinted from Bostom AG, Carpenter MA, Kusek JW, et al. Homocysteine-lowering and cardiovascular disease outcomes in kidney transplant recipients: primary results from the Folic Acid for Vascular Outcome Reduction in Transplantation trial. *Circulation.* 2011;123:1763-1770.)

confidence interval]=0.99 [0.84 to 1.17]), secondary outcomes of all-cause mortality (n = 431 deaths; 1.04 [0.86 to 1.26]), or dialysis-dependent kidney failure (n = 343 events; 1.15 [0.93 to 1.43]) compared to the low-dose multivitamin.

Conclusions.—Treatment with a high-dose folic acid, B6, and B12 multivitamin in kidney transplant recipients did not reduce a composite cardiovascular disease outcome, all-cause mortality, or dialysis-dependent kidney failure despite significant reduction in homocysteine level.

▶ Elevated levels of homocysteine are a marker for cardiovascular disease. It has been suggested that therapies aimed at lowering homocysteine levels may reduce cardiovascular risk. However, interestingly enough, prior studies in patients with diabetic renal disease have actually demonstrated that therapy with vitamin B complex (including B6, B12, and folic acid) can actually hasten the progression of renal disease.[1] The results of that study again demonstrated that observational data alone should not be used to guide clinical interventions across wide populations of patients.

The current double-blind randomized trial (FAVORIT) was designed to study the influence of folic acid on vascular outcome in clinically stable kidney transplant recipients. The study evaluated the influence of both high (5 mg folic acid, 50 mg B6, and 1.0 mg B12) and low (1.4 mg B6, 2 μg B12, and no folic acid) dose regimens in more than 4000 transplant patients with high homocysteine levels. The authors systematically evaluated whether therapy aimed at reducing homocysteine levels would reduce the rate of the cardiac, aortic, cerebral vascular, and/or peripheral vascular arteriosclerotic disease. The mean follow-up was 4 years. The findings demonstrated that although treatment with high-dose B-complex supplementation significantly reduced homocysteine levels, this reduction was not associated with a reduction in the composite cardiovascular disease outcomes, all-cause mortality, or dialysis-dependent renal disease (Fig 2). Unlike the findings in diabetic patients with renal disease, there were no deleterious effects of B-vitamin supplementation. However, similar to prior trials in patients with chronic kidney disease,[2] treatment did not improve cardiovascular outcomes in the transplant population. Thus, these data do not support the generalized use of these widely advertised, costly, and readily available nutraceuticals in the post renal—transplant population.

R. Garrick, MD

References

1. House AA, Eliasziw M, Cattran DC, et al. Effect of B-vitamin therapy on progression of diabetic nephropathy: a randomized controlled trial. *JAMA*. 2010;303: 1603-1609.
2. Heinz J, Kropf S, Domröse U. B vitamins and the risk of total mortality and cardiovascular disease in end-stage renal disease: results of a randomized, controlled trial. *Circulation*. 2010;121:1432-1438.

28 Glomerular Diseases and Renal Injury

A risk allele for focal segmental glomerulosclerosis in African Americans is located within a region containing APOL1 and MYH9
Genovese G, Tonna SJ, Knob AU, et al (Brigham and Women's Hosp and Harvard Med School, Boston, MA; et al)
Kidney Int 78:698-704, 2010

Genetic variation at the MYH9 locus is linked to the high incidence of focal segmental glomerulosclerosis (FSGS) and non-diabetic end-stage renal disease among African Americans. To further define risk alleles with FSGS we performed a genome-wide association analysis using more than one million single-nucleotide polymorphisms in 56 African-American and 61 European-American patients with biopsy-confirmed FSGS. Results were compared to 1641 European Americans and 1800 African Americans as unselected controls. While no association was observed in the cohort of European Americans, the case—control comparison of African Americans found variants within a 60 kb region of chromosome 22 containing part of the *APOL1* and *MYH9* genes associated with increased risk of FSGS. This region spans different linkage disequilibrium blocks, and variants associating with disease within this region are in linkage disequilibrium with variants which have shown signals of natural selection. *APOL1* is a strong candidate for a gene that has undergone recent natural selection and is known to be involved in the infection by *Trypanosoma brucei*, a parasite common in Africa that has recently adapted to infect human hosts. Further studies will be required to establish which variants are causally related to kidney disease, what mutations caused the selective sweep, and to ultimately determine if these are the same.

▶ As if drawn from the pages of a suspenseful crime novel, the recent rush to judgment on the presumed guilt of myosin heavy chain 9 (*MYH9*) mutations in causing nondiabetic renal disease in African Americans (AA),[1] has been seriously called into doubt. Using gene sequences from the "1000 genomes project," Genovese et al have convincingly demonstrated that, although the association of *MYH9* mutations with focal segmental glomerular sclerosis (FSGS) in AA remains robust and reproducible, the *MYH9* mutations were likely not responsible for the observed incidence of disease progression.

In actuality, 2 distinct genetic variants within the apolipoprotein 1 (*APOL1*) gene locus on chromosome 22 are independently associated with both FSGS and end-stage renal disease due to hypertensive nephropathy in AA. These variants were not found in patients with exclusively European ancestry. Furthermore, the *APOL1* locus is in linkage disequilibrium with the *MYH9* locus, thereby framing the latter as the polymorphism responsible for the excess progression of renal disease in nondiabetic AA.

Interestingly, the *APOL1* mutation and its gene product confer the ability to lyse trypanosoma brucei rhodesiense, thereby preventing "sleeping sickness" in affected individuals.[2] This polymorphism was found almost exclusively in subjects with African lineage.

Just as hemoglobin S has evolved to block malarial infection caused by *Plasmodium* species, this is another fascinating example of selective genetic pressure resulting in a genetic variant, which leads to a maladaptive clinical condition. The cause of the renal disease has yet to be elucidated but might include the initiation of cellular autophagy or apoptosis.

M. Klein, MD, JD

References

1. Kao W, Klag MJ, Meoni LA, et al. MYH9 is associated with nondiabetic end-stage renal disease in African Americans. *Nat Genet.* 2008;40:1185-1192.
2. Vanhamme L, Paturiaux-Hanocq F, Poelvoorde P, et al. Apolipoprotein L-I is the trypanosome lytic factor of human serum. *Nature.* 2003;422:83-87.

Postinfectious Glomerulonephritis in the Elderly
Nasr SH, Fidler ME, Valeri AM, et al (Mayo Clinic, Rochester, MI; Columbia Univ, NY)
J Am Soc Nephrol 22:187-195, 2011

Postinfectious glomerulonephritis (PIGN) is primarily a childhood disease that occurs after an upper respiratory tract infection or impetigo; its occurrence in older patients is not well characterized. Here, we report 109 cases of PIGN in patients ≥65 years old diagnosed by renal biopsy. The male to female ratio was 2.8:1. An immunocompromised background was present in 61%, most commonly diabetes or malignancy. The most common site of infection was skin, followed by pneumonia and urinary tract infection. The most common causative agent was staphylococcus (46%) followed by streptococcus (16%) and unusual gram-negative organisms. Hypocomplementemia was present in 72%. The mean peak serum creatinine was 5.1 mg/dl, and 46% of patients required acute dialysis. The most common light microscopic patterns were diffuse (53%), focal (28%), and mesangial (13%) proliferative glomerulonephritis. IgA-dominant PIGN occurred in 17%. Of the 72 patients with ≥3 months of follow-up (mean, 29 months), 22% achieved complete recovery, 44% had persistent renal dysfunction, and 33% progressed to ESRD. The presence of diabetes, higher creatinine at biopsy, dialysis at presentation, the presence of diabetic glomerulosclerosis, and greater tubular atrophy and interstitial fibrosis predicted ESRD. In summary, the epidemiology of PIGN is shifting as the population ages. Older men and patients with diabetes or malignancy are particularly at risk, and the sites of infection and causative organisms differ from the typical childhood disease. Prognosis for these older patients is poor, with fewer than 25% recovering full renal function.

▶ Among elderly patients with acute renal insufficiency coming to renal biopsy, the most common finding is pauci-immune crescentic glomerulonephritis (31% to 71%), followed by acute interstitial nephritis (7% to 19%). Postinfectious glomerulonephritis (PIGN) is less frequent, encountered in 3% to 6% of biopsy results, and is frequently unexpected clinically. This study is important because it effectively highlights some very distinct differences in the clinical presentation of adult and childhood PIGN.

PIGN is primarily a childhood disease and occurs after an upper respiratory tract infection or impetigo. *Streptococcus* is the most common responsible bacterium for PIGN in children. In patients older than 65 years, skin infection, pneumonia, and urinary tract infection are more common than upper respiratory tract infection, and staphylococcal infection is almost 3 times more common than streptococcal infection, followed by many unusual gram-negative organisms in adults. In adults, men are more commonly affected than women. PIGN is more common in immunocompromised patients (61% vs 32%) and diabetics (present in about 50% of patients), and alcoholism and aging have emerged as important risk factors. Malignancy, particularly carcinoma, was the second most common predisposing condition (14%).

The latent period between infection and onset of renal disease in children with PIGN is typically 1 to 6 weeks. In contrast, in nearly half of elderly patients in this report, the infection was first discovered at the onset of renal disease, suggesting that an infection may go unrecognized for some time. Signs of infection in the elderly population are often nonspecific. Fever is absent in 20% to 30% of patients, and complement levels are normal about 30% of the time. Elderly patients have a higher rate of more severe acute renal insufficiency at presentation. The mean peak serum creatinine level was 5.1 mg/dL, and unlike children in whom complete recovery is the rule, in adults the prognosis is less favorable with a complete recovery in only about 22% of patients.

PIGN should be considered in the differential diagnosis for elderly patients with severe acute renal failure and active urine sediment.

A. Kapoor, MD

Clinical Features and Outcomes of Anti–Glomerular Basement Membrane Disease in Older Patients

Cui Z, Zhao J, Jia X-Y, et al (Peking Univ First Hosp, Beijing, China)
Am J Kidney Dis 57:575-582, 2011

Background.—Anti–glomerular basement membrane (GBM) disease is being recognized increasingly in older patients. Disease presentation and outcomes of these patients are unclear.

Study Design.—Case series.

Setting & Participants.—221 consecutive Chinese patients with anti-GBM disease diagnosed in 1998-2008 in our tertiary referral center. Anti-GBM disease was defined as positive anti-GBM antibodies in circulation and/or linear immunoglobulin G deposition along the GBM on kidney biopsy.

Predictor.—Older age, defined as 65 years or older, and antineutrophil cytoplasmic antibody, detected using immunofluorescence and enzyme-linked immunosorbent assay, at presentation.

Outcomes.—Clinical features, kidney pathologic characteristics, end-stage renal disease (ESRD), and mortality. Multivariate Cox proportional hazard models were used to assess the contribution of age, sex, clinical measures, and treatments to ESRD and mortality.

Results.—50 of 221 (22.6%) patients were 65 years or older. Older patients had a male predominance (male/female ratio, 1.9:1). They had a higher proportion of positive antineutrophil cytoplasmic antibody results (46.0% vs 14.6%; $P < 0.001$), lower prevalence of hemoptysis (26.0% vs 46.2%; $P = 0.01$), lower urine protein excretion (1.4 ± 1.0 vs 3.9 ± 3.3 g/d; $P = 0.001$), and higher estimated glomerular filtration rate (eGFR) at presentation (8.4 vs 5.1 mL/min/1.73 m^2; $P = 0.007$) compared with younger patients. During follow-up, 30 of 37 (81.1%) and 21 of 37 (56.8%) patients developed ESRD and died in the older group compared with 115 of 139 (82.7%) and 35 of 139 (25.2%) in the younger group ($P = 0.1$ and $P = 0.001$, respectively). For older patients, multivariate Cox regression analysis showed that higher initial eGFR was an independent predictor for both ESRD (HR, 0.86; 95% CI, 0.78-0.96; $P = 0.005$) and death (HR, 0.79; 95% CI, 0.66-0.94; $P = 0.008$).

Limitations.—Not all patients underwent kidney biopsy, especially those with very old age or ESRD at presentation.

Conclusions.—Older patients with anti-GBM disease had milder kidney damage and less pulmonary involvement. Outcomes were predicted by initial eGFR. Thus, early diagnosis was crucial to improve outcomes (Fig 2).

▶ Anti–glomerular basement membrane (GBM) disease affects 2 distinct age groups: the first peak is in the second and third decade of life and the second is the sixth and seventh decade. This is an important study because it highlights the differences in the presentation of anti-GBM between the affected age groups. In the younger population, anti-GBM is typically a disease of male preponderance, and pulmonary hemorrhage is frequent. In the older population,

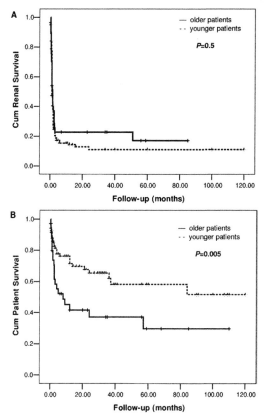

FIGURE 2.—Kaplan-Meier analysis for (A) kidney and (B) patient survival compared between older patients and younger patients with anti—glomerular basement membrane disease (logrank test). (Reprinted from American Journal of Kidney Diseases, Cui Z, Zhao J, Jia X-Y, et al. Clinical features and outcomes of anti—glomerular basement membrane disease in older patients. *Am J Kidney Dis.* 2011;57:575-582. Copyright 2011 with permission from the National Kidney Foundation, Inc.)

the incidence and biomarkers are less well studied. The current study identifies 221 consecutive patients between 1990 and 2008 in 1 center. One potential limitation to the study is that it was performed in an Asian population, and therefore, the results may not be fully applicable to all other genetic populations. Interestingly, of the entire population, approximately 20% were over the age of 65, and although renal disease was severe in both groups, the glomerular filtration rate (GFR) was slightly better preserved in the older population. However, as shown in Fig 2, this preservation of GFR did not correspond with an improved mortality or improved renal outcomes. Pulmonary complications were less frequent, the hemoglobin was better preserved, and proteinuria was less severe in the elderly. An additional finding was that the presence of both anti antineutrophil cytoplasmic—myeloperoxidase antibodies and anti-GBM antibodies was associated with a more aggressive presentation and a worse outcome in the elderly group. Overall, the presentation of anti-GBM disease is more subtle in the elderly, and this fact may lead to a delay in the diagnosis in this age range. Thus, because a satisfactory clinical response demands early aggressive intervention, it is extremely important for clinicians to consider anti-GBM disease in the differential diagnosis of progressive renal injury in the elderly.

R. Garrick, MD

Weekend Hospital Admission, Acute Kidney Injury, and Mortality
James MT, Wald R, Bell CM, et al (Univ of Calgary, Alberta, Canada; Univ of Toronto, Ontario, Canada; et al)
J Am Soc Nephrol 21:845-851, 2010

Admission to the hospital on weekends is associated with increased mortality for several acute illnesses. We investigated whether patients admitted on a weekend with acute kidney injury (AKI) were more likely to die than those admitted on a weekday. Using the Nationwide Inpatient Sample, a large database of admissions to acute care, nonfederal hospitals in the United States, we identified 963,730 admissions with a diagnosis of AKI between 2003 and 2006. Of these, 214,962 admissions (22%) designated AKI as the primary reason for admission (45,203 on a weekend and 169,759 on a weekday). We used logistic regression models to examine the adjusted odds of in-hospital mortality associated with weekend *versus* weekday admission. Compared with admission on a weekday, patients admitted with a primary diagnosis of AKI on a weekend had a higher odds of death [adjusted odds ratio (OR) 1.07, 95% confidence interval (CI) 1.02 to 1.12]. The risk for death with admission on a weekend for AKI was more pronounced in smaller hospitals (adjusted OR 1.17, 95% CI 1.03 to 1.33) compared with larger hospitals (adjusted OR 1.07, 95% CI 1.01 to 1.13). Increased mortality was also associated with weekend admission among patients with AKI as a secondary diagnosis across a spectrum of co-existing medical diagnoses. In conclusion, among patients hospitalized with AKI, weekend admission is associated with a higher risk for death compared with admission on a weekday.

▶ Over the last 10 years, multiple lines of investigation have demonstrated that clinical outcomes can be improved by standardizing care. Most of our attention has focused on the steps that clinicians should take to best standardize our approach to care. The current study focuses on whether standardization of hospital staffing and resources can truly alter clinical outcomes. Prior studies from Canada suggested that patients with renal failure who were admitted to the hospital on weekends had a 34% higher risk of in-hospital mortality.[1] The current study used admission and mortality data from nonfederal US acute care hospitals to determine if patients admitted with acute kidney injury (AKI) over the weekend would experience higher in-hospital mortality, independent of demographic and clinical characteristics, including severity of illness. The authors hypothesized that patients admitted with acute kidney injury over a weekend would experience a greater in-hospital mortality and that this variation would be greater in small hospitals compared with larger facilities. The authors evaluated 963 730 admissions with a diagnosis of AKI between the years 2003 and 2006. Data were adjusted for age, sex, race, comorbidities (using the Charlson comorbidity index), and the requirement for mechanical ventilation.

After adjustment, weekend admission with AKI was associated with a 22% increased odds of death by day 3 of admission. Larger facilities had a 24% increase in the adjusted risk of death by day 3, and smaller hospitals yielded a 35% increase in the adjusted odds of death over the same time. The authors noted that patients admitted over the weekend were less likely to receive dialysis (odds ratio, 0.94, 95% confidence interval, 0.90 to 0.97), regardless of hospital size (*P* interaction, 0.45), and suggested that this may have contributed to an increase in weekend morbidity. However, the need for dialysis was relatively small for both weekend (8.4%) and weekday (8.9%) AKI admissions, so other factors, such as the availability of subspecialists who are aware of and adhere to standardized AKI treatment guidelines, may have also contributed to the findings.

This study cannot definitively determine the reasons for excess mortality observed among patients admitted with AKI over a weekend. However, the findings are worrisome, and clinicians should be aware of these results. While the explanation for these findings is unraveled, clinicians should take extra steps to be especially attentive to this high-risk group during this period of excess risk.

R. Garrick, MD

Reference

1. Bell CM, Redelmeier DA. Mortality among patients admitted to hospital on weekends as compared with weekdays. *N Engl J Med*. 2001;345:633-638.

Glomerular filtration rate, proteinuria, and the incidence and consequences of acute kidney injury: a cohort study

James MT, for the Alberta Kidney Disease Network (Univ of Calgary, Alberta, Canada; et al)
Lancet 376:2096-2103, 2010

Background.—Low values of estimated glomerular filtration rate (eGFR) predispose to acute kidney injury, and proteinuria is a marker of kidney disease. We aimed to investigate how eGFR and proteinuria jointly modified the risks of acute kidney injury and subsequent adverse clinical outcomes.

Methods.—We did a cohort study of 920 985 adults residing in Alberta, Canada, between 2002 and 2007. Participants not needing chronic dialysis at baseline and with at least one outpatient measurement of both serum creatinine concentration and proteinuria (urine dipstick or albumin-creatinine ratio) were included. We assessed hospital admission with acute kidney injury with validated administrative codes; other outcomes were all-cause mortality and a composite renal outcome of end-stage renal disease or doubling of serum creatinine concentration.

Findings.—During median follow-up of 35 months (range 0–59 months), 6520 (0·7%) participants were admitted with acute kidney injury. In those with eGFR 60 mL/min per 1·73 m^2 or greater, the adjusted risk of admission with this disorder was about 4 times higher in those with heavy proteinuria measured by dipstick (rate ratio 4·4 *vs* no proteinuria, 95% CI 3·7–5·2). The adjusted rates of admission with acute kidney injury and kidney injury needing dialysis remained high in participants with heavy dipstick proteinuria for all values of eGFR. The adjusted rates of death and the composite renal outcome were also high in participants admitted with acute kidney injury, although the rise associated with this injury was attenuated in those with low baseline eGFR and heavy proteinuria.

Interpretation.—These findings suggest that information on proteinuria and eGFR should be used together when identifying people at risk of acute kidney injury, and that an episode of acute kidney injury provides further long-term prognostic information in addition to eGFR and proteinuria.

▶ It has previously been recognized that reduced baseline glomerular filtration rate (GFR) is a risk factor for acute kidney injury (AKI). This study, together with the findings of Grams and colleagues,[1] also reviewed, now demonstrate that proteinuria has a graded effect on the risk of AKI development. The studies are important because AKI is one of the leading causes of mortality in hospitalized patients.

This study used a province-wide sample of 920 985 adults in Alberta, Canada, to examine the associations of estimated GFR (eGFR) and proteinuria with risk of AKI. This cohort study included adults with at least 1 outpatient measurement of serum creatinine and 1 measurement of proteinuria between 2002 and 2007, and excluded those with end-stage renal disease at study entry (eGFR < 15 mL/min/1.73 m^2, chronic dialysis, or previous kidney transplant). The baseline eGFR was calculated using the Modification of Diet in Renal Disease equation after averaging all outpatient serum creatinine measurements taken within 6 months of the first creatinine measurement within the cohort study period, and proteinuria was measured by urine dipstick or albumin-to-creatinine ratio for the primary analysis. Proteinuria characterized as normal (dipstick negative), mild (dipstick trace to 1+), and heavy (dipstick ≥2+) OR urine albumin:creatine ratio measurements of normal (< 3.4 mg/mmol), mild (3.4–33.9 mg/mmol), or heavy (> 33.9 mg/mmol).

During median follow-up of 35 months, 6520 (0.7%) participants in the cohort were admitted with AKI and 516 (<0.01%) with AKI requiring dialysis. The incidence rates of AKI were stratified by level of eGFR and following adjustments for patient demographics and a number of comorbidities, including hypertension and diabetes, the rate ratios for both AKI and AKI requiring dialysis increased with higher levels of proteinuria.

Although the large sample size adds strength to the study, it does have limitations. The study used routine creatinine and proteinuria measurements that were obtained as part of clinical care, and this may have created a selection bias toward patients who were older or had more comorbidities. The reliance on administrative codes to identify hospitalizations with AKI may have also affected the results, as the coding may have not adequately represented the true event rate. Even given these limitations, the study does establish proteinuria as an independent risk factor for AKI, and shows that the effect of proteinuria is influenced by the severity of the underlying renal disease. Given the cumulative risks of AKI on mortality and long-term renal outcomes, these findings and those of Grams and colleagues[1] (from the ARIC database) are important and can help clinicians identify those patients at greater risk for an episode of AKI and, where possible, implement mitigation strategies.

A. Kapoor, MD

Reference

1. Grams ME, Astor BC, Bash LD, Matsushita K, Wang Y, Coresh J. Albuminuria and estimated glomerular filtration rate independently associate with acute kidney injury. *J Am Soc Nephrol.* 2010;21:1757-1764.

Albuminuria and Estimated Glomerular Filtration Rate Independently Associate with Acute Kidney Injury
Grams ME, Astor BC, Bash LD, et al (The Johns Hopkins Univ School of Medicine, Baltimore, MD; The Johns Hopkins Bloomberg School of Public Health, Baltimore, MD)
J Am Soc Nephrol 21:1757-1764, 2010

Acute kidney injury (AKI) is increasingly common and a significant contributor to excess death in hospitalized patients. CKD is an established risk factor for AKI; however, the independent graded association of urine albumin excretion with AKI is unknown. We analyzed a prospective cohort of 11,200 participants in the Atherosclerosis Risk in Communities (ARIC) study for the association between baseline urine albumin-to-creatinine ratio and estimated GFR (eGFR) with hospitalizations or death with AKI. The incidence of AKI events was 4.0 per 1000 person-years of follow-up. Using participants with urine albumin-to-creatinine ratios <10 mg/g as a reference, the relative hazards of AKI, adjusted for age, gender, race, cardiovascular risk factors, and categories of eGFR were 1.9 (95% CI, 1.4 to 2.6), 2.2 (95% CI, 1.6 to 3.0), and 4.8 (95% CI, 3.2 to 7.2) for urine albumin-to-creatinine ratio groups of 11 to 29 mg/g, 30 to 299 mg/g, and ≥300 mg/g, respectively. Similarly, the overall adjusted relative hazard of AKI increased with decreasing eGFR. Patterns persisted within subgroups of age, race, and gender. In summary, albuminuria and eGFR have strong, independent associations with incident AKI.

▶ Acute kidney injury (AKI) is known to increase hospital morbidity and can lead to chronic kidney disease (CKD), end-stage renal disease, and death. Risk factors for AKI include older age, CKD, black race, obesity, diabetes, and male gender.[1] Additionally, the presence of albuminuria has been positively correlated with the risk of dialysis dependent AKI.[2] Albuminuria is also a known marker for cardio-vascular risk.[3] It portends poorly for progression of CKD[3] and seems to be related to elevated risk for severe AKI. How much the degree of albuminuria affects the level of risk remains poorly defined. This study examined the association of various levels of albuminuria with the risk of AKI and looked for any relationship to the estimated glomerular filtration rate (eGFR).

The data for this study were drawn from the Atherosclerosis Risk in Communities Study (ARIC) database. Selected for this study were more than 11 000 individuals with complete data sets available, including the requisite urine albumin/creatinine ratios (UACR) and eGFR. Hospital discharges with the ICD code for AKI were collected during the follow-up period. The AKI incidence was stratified for the degree of albuminuria such that UACR less than 10 mg/g, 10 to 29 mg/g, 30 to 299 mg/g, and greater than 300 mg/g showed a stepwise increase in the incidence of AKI. This ranged from 2.6 events per 1000 person years in the lowest albumin group to 41.2 events per 1000 person years in the macroalbuminuric patients. The hazard ratio ranged from 1.9 to 8.0 using UACR <10 mg/g as a reference in the same groups, respectively. This correlation of albuminuria with occurrence of AKI was maintained at all levels of initial eGFR, as well as with all subgroups of age, gender, race, and CKD.

This interesting population-based study demonstrated a positive correlation between the degree of albuminuria and the risk of AKI. The magnitude of risk appeared to be independent of the initial eGFR and was worse at higher degrees of albuminuria. Elevated risk was noted even at levels of microalbuminuria previously felt to be insignificant.

So now we have good evidence that albuminuria is a risk not only for cardiovascular endpoints and CKD progression, but also for AKI at all levels of eGFR. This study should raise awareness as to the critical importance of urine albumin testing in assessing both cardiovascular and renal risk, acute and chronic.

M. Klein, MD, JD

References

1. Peterson JC, Adler S, Burkart JM, et al. Blood pressure control, proteinuria, and the progression of renal disease. The modification of diet in renal disease study. *Ann Intern Med.* 1995;123:754-762.
2. Hsu CY, Ordoñez JD, Chertow GM, Fan D, McCulloch CE, Go AS. The risk of acute renal failure in patients with chronic kidney disease. *Kidney Int.* 2008;74: 101-107.
3. Gerstein HC, Mann JF, Yi Q, et al. Albuminuria and risk of cardiovascular events, death, and heart failure in diabetic and nondiabetic individuals. *JAMA.* 2001;286: 421-426.

The severity of acute kidney injury predicts progression to chronic kidney disease

Chawla LS, Amdur RL, Amodeo S, et al (George Washington Univ Med Ctr, DC; Veterans Affairs Med Ctr, Washington, DC)
Kidney Int 79:1361-1369, 2011

Acute kidney injury (AKI) is associated with progression to advanced chronic kidney disease (CKD). We tested whether patients who survive

AKI and are at higher risk for CKD progression can be identified during their hospital admission, thus providing opportunities to intervene. This was assessed in patients in the Department of Veterans Affairs Healthcare System hospitalized with a primary diagnosis indicating AKI (ICD9 codes 584.xx). In the exploratory phase, three multivariate prediction models for progression to stage 4 CKD were developed. In the confirmatory phase, the models were validated in 11,589 patients admitted for myocardial infarction or pneumonia during the same time frame that had RIFLE codes R, I, or F and complete data for all predictor variables. Of the 5351 patients in the AKI group, 728 entered stage 4 CKD after hospitalization. Models 1, 2, and 3 were all significant with 'c' statistics of 0.82, 0.81, and 0.77, respectively. In model validation, all three were highly significant when tested in the confirmatory patients, with moderate to large effect sizes and good predictive accuracy ('c' 0.81–0.82). Patients with AKI who required dialysis and then recovered were at especially high risk for progression to CKD. Hence, the severity of AKI is a robust predictor of progression to CKD.

▶ Previous studies have found that patient outcome is worsened by even relatively small acute changes in the serum creatinine level.[1,2] And after multivariate risk adjustment, acute kidney injury has been shown to be an independent risk factor for death.[3] The incidence of acute kidney injury is increasing, and in view of the long-term sequelae, the authors sought to determine whether specific patient characteristics could be used to predict which patients were most at risk for progression to chronic kidney disease (CKD) following an episode of acute kidney injury. The study is important because the ability to predict which patients are at highest risk for progressive CKD following an episode of acute kidney injury would allow physicians to focus their follow-up and tailor their interventions toward the patient group most at risk.

The authors used the Department of Veterans Affairs health care system database to generate 3 different models to predict the risk of disease progression and then tested and validated the model in 11 589 patients admitted with myocardial infarction or pneumonia who had detailed concurrent acute kidney injury (AKI) data available. Multiple factors were included in each model, including age, sex, race, diagnosis of acute tubular necrosis, time at risk of acute renal failure, presence of diabetes, the estimated glomerular filtration rate (GFR), the need for renal replacement therapy, and several baseline laboratory values, including albumin and hemoglobin levels. Patients were then followed to determine the progress of the risk of progression to CKD stage IV (GFR of <30 mL/min/1.7 m^2). The authors identified advanced age, low serum albumin levels, the presence of diabetes, and the severity of the acute kidney injury as strong risk factors for progression to advanced CKD stage IV and for poor renal outcomes. The need for renal replacement therapy (even with recovery and cessation of dialysis) increased the likelihood of progression to CKD by more than 500 fold.

Because the study was largely based on coding data from the Department of Veterans Affairs, it will need to be validated in other groups. However, even with that limitation in mind, the clinical importance of this study is highlighted by their finding that slightly less than a third of the patients who had an episode of AKI that required dialysis were seen by a nephrologist within 1 month of discharge. Certainly our ability to predict which patients are at risk for CKD progression after an episode of AKI should help us better focus our discharge planning and follow-up care.

R. Garrick, MD

References

1. Chertow GM, Burdick E, Honour M, Bonventre JV, Bates DW. Acute kidney injury, mortality, length of stay, and costs in hospitalized patients. *J Am Soc Nephrol.* 2005;16:3365-3370.
2. Lassnigg A, Schmidlin D, Mouhieddine M, et al. Minimal changes of serum creatinine predict prognosis in patients after cardiothoracic surgery: a prospective cohort study. *J Am Soc Nephrol.* 2004;15:1597-1605.
3. Chertow GM, Levy EM, Hammermeister KE, Grover F, Daley J. Independent association between acute renal failure and mortality following cardiac surgery. *Am J Med.* 1998;104:343-348.

29 Diabetes

Effects of Intensive Blood-Pressure Control in Type 2 Diabetes Mellitus
The ACCORD Study Group (Memphis Veterans Affairs (VA) Med Ctr,
Memphis; Wake Forest Univ School of Medicine, Winston-Salem, NC; et al)
N Engl J Med 362:1575-1585, 2010

Background.—There is no evidence from randomized trials to support a strategy of lowering systolic blood pressure below 135 to 140 mm Hg in persons with type 2 diabetes mellitus. We investigated whether therapy targeting normal systolic pressure (i.e., <120 mm Hg) reduces major cardiovascular events in participants with type 2 diabetes at high risk for cardiovascular events.

Methods.—A total of 4733 participants with type 2 diabetes were randomly assigned to intensive therapy, targeting a systolic pressure of less than 120 mm Hg, or standard therapy, targeting a systolic pressure of less than 140 mm Hg. The primary composite outcome was nonfatal myocardial infarction, nonfatal stroke, or death from cardiovascular causes. The mean follow-up was 4.7 years.

Results.—After 1 year, the mean systolic blood pressure was 119.3 mm Hg in the intensive-therapy group and 133.5 mm Hg in the standard-therapy group. The annual rate of the primary outcome was 1.87% in the intensive-therapy group and 2.09% in the standard-therapy group (hazard ratio with intensive therapy, 0.88; 95% confidence interval [CI], 0.73 to 1.06; P = 0.20). The annual rates of death from any cause were 1.28% and 1.19% in the two groups, respectively (hazard ratio, 1.07; 95% CI, 0.85 to 1.35; P = 0.55). The annual rates of stroke, a prespecified secondary outcome, were 0.32% and 0.53% in the two groups, respectively (hazard ratio, 0.59; 95% CI, 0.39 to 0.89; P = 0.01). Serious adverse events attributed to antihypertensive treatment occurred in 77 of the 2362 participants in the intensive-therapy group (3.3%) and 30 of the 2371 participants in the standard-therapy group (1.3%) (P<0.001).

Conclusions.—In patients with type 2 diabetes at high risk for cardiovascular events, targeting a systolic blood pressure of less than 120 mm Hg, as compared with less than 140 mm Hg, did not reduce the rate of a composite outcome of fatal and nonfatal major cardiovascular events. (ClinicalTrials.gov number, NCT00000620.)

▶ The increased cardiovascular risk associated with hypertension in the setting of diabetic disease has been well established.[1,2] Blood pressure control has been one of the mainstay therapies of diabetic patients. Despite multiple prior investigations, the optimal target for blood pressure in diabetics remains elusive. The Action to Control Cardiovascular Risk and Diabetes (ACCORD) trial included 4733 participants with type II diabetes with hemoglobin A1c levels of 7.5% or higher with evidence of cardiovascular disease (40 years of age or older) or 55 years of age with anatomic evidence of atherosclerosis, albuminuria, left ventricular hypertrophy, and 2 additional risk factors for cardiovascular disease. The trial used a 2x2 design of either intensive or standard glycemic control followed by intensive (systolic blood pressure ≤120 mm Hg) or standard (systolic blood pressure ≤140 mm Hg) blood pressure control and included a parallel lipid control study. The primary composite outcome was nonfatal myocardial infarction, nonfatal stroke, or death from cardiovascular causes, and the mean follow-up was 4.7 years. A primary finding was that in patients with type 2 diabetes at high risk for cardiovascular events, targeting a systolic blood pressure of < 120 mm Hg compared with < 140 mm Hg did not reduce the rate of composite cardiovascular outcomes. However, patients in the intensive control group did have a greater number of syncopal and hypotensive episodes and a greater reduction in renal function as measured by an increase in the serum creatinine concentration.

The findings of the ACCORD trial, however, are not perfectly clear cut. First, perhaps because of the selection bias generated by the lipid-lowering arm of the study, the number of events in the standard therapy group was lower than would have been expected, and this may have skewed the results. In addition, in the setting of other aggressive therapy, such as glycemic control and lipid control, the follow-up time may not have been long enough to see a difference in cardiovascular endpoints from blood pressure control. Finally, patients with significant renal disease (serum creatinine > 1.5 mg/dL) were excluded, and therefore the results may not be safely generalized to patients with more advanced renal disease.

However, the findings do raise a risk-benefit flag of caution, and in the population studied, the data from ACCORD do not provide evidence to support lowering the systolic blood pressure to < 120 mm Hg.

R. Garrick, MD

References

1. Stamler J, Vaccaro O, Neaton JD, Wentworth D. Diabetes, other risk factors, and 12-yr cardiovascular mortality for men screened in the Multiple Risk Factor Intervention Trial. *Diabetes Care.* 1993;16:434-444.
2. Adler AI, Stratton IM, Neil HA, et al. Association of systolic blood pressure with macrovascular and microvascular complications of type 2 diabetes (UKPDS 36): prospective observational study. *BMJ.* 2000;321:412-419.

Olmesartan for the Delay or Prevention of Microalbuminuria in Type 2 Diabetes

Haller H, for the ROADMAP Trial Investigators (Hannover Med School, Germany; et al)

N Engl J Med 364:907-917, 2011

Background.—Microalbuminuria is an early predictor of diabetic nephropathy and premature cardiovascular disease. We investigated whether treatment with an angiotensin-receptor blocker (ARB) would delay or prevent the occurrence of microalbuminuria in patients with type 2 diabetes and normoalbuminuria.

Methods.—In a randomized, double-blind, multicenter, controlled trial, we assigned 4447 patients with type 2 diabetes to receive olmesartan (at a dose of 40 mg once daily) or placebo for a median of 3.2 years. Additional antihypertensive drugs (except angiotensin-converting—enzyme inhibitors or ARBs) were used as needed to lower blood pressure to less than 130/80 mm Hg. The primary outcome was the time to the first onset of microalbuminuria. The times to the onset of renal and cardiovascular events were analyzed as secondary end points.

Results.—The target blood pressure (<130/80 mm Hg) was achieved in nearly 80% of the patients taking olmesartan and 71% taking placebo; blood pressure measured in the clinic was lower by 3.1/1.9 mm Hg in the olmesartan group than in the placebo group. Microalbuminuria developed in 8.2% of the patients in the olmesartan group (178 of 2160 patients who could be evaluated) and 9.8% in the placebo group (210 of 2139); the time to the onset of microalbuminuria was increased by 23% with olmesartan (hazard ratio for onset of microalbuminuria, 0.77; 95% confidence interval, 0.63 to 0.94; P = 0.01). The serum creatinine level doubled in 1% of the patients in each group. Slightly fewer patients in the olmesartan group than in the placebo group had nonfatal cardiovascular events — 81 of 2232 patients (3.6%) as compared with 91 of 2215 patients (4.1%) (P = 0.37) — but a greater number had fatal cardiovascular events — 15 patients (0.7%) as compared with 3 patients (0.1%) (P = 0.01), a difference that was attributable in part to a higher rate of death from cardiovascular causes in the olmesartan group than in the placebo group among patients with preexisting coronary heart disease (11 of 564 patients [2.0%] vs. 1 of 540 [0.2%], P = 0.02).

Conclusions.—Olmesartan was associated with a delayed onset of microalbuminuria, even though blood-pressure control in both groups was excellent according to current standards. The higher rate of fatal cardiovascular events with olmesartan among patients with preexisting coronary heart disease is of concern. (Funded by Daiichi Sankyo; ClinicalTrials.gov number, NCT00185159.)

▶ The role of angiotensin-converting enzyme inhibitors and angiotensin receptor blockade (ARB) for the treatment of type 1 and type 2 diabetes has been well established. The current trial evaluated whether prophylactic therapy with the ARB olmesartan can prevent or delay the occurrence of microalbuminuria in patients with type 2 diabetes. The study is important because in type 2 diabetics, the development of microalbuminuria portends the earlier development of renal and cardiovascular events, as compared with diabetics without microalbuminuria. The investigators studied 4447 patients with type 2 diabetes. The median follow-up period was 3.2 years. Patients were randomly assigned to receive either olmesartan (40 mg daily) or placebo. The target blood pressure was 130/80 mm Hg and was achieved in 80% of the olmesartan group compared with 71% of the placebo group. In the olmesartan group, microalbuminuria developed in fewer patients, and the time to onset of micro albuminuria was delayed. The baseline characteristics of patients most likely to benefit from therapy included a higher systolic blood pressure (> 135 mm Hg) prior to treatment, better glycemic control, a glomerular filtration rate of < 84 mL/min/1.73 m^2 and a urinary albumin to creatinine ratio of > 4. These findings suggest that this constellation may help identify those patients with type 2 diabetes, without microalbuminuria, who would achieve the greatest benefit from ARB therapy. The rate of renal events (defined as doubling the serum creatinine level or a need for dialysis) was low and identical in the olmesartan and placebo groups.

The overall rate of cardiovascular and cerebrovascular events was low at about 2.9 cases per 1000 person-years. This may reflect the fact that patients had less severe renal disease than those in other diabetic/ARB trials, such as those with Losartan and Irbesartan.[1,2] Despite these positive findings, it is noteworthy that there was a higher rate of fatal cardiovascular events among patients treated with olmesartan compared with placebo. Several possible explanations have been put forward to explain this observation. First was the finding that most of the patients enrolled had between 2 and 4 comorbid conditions, and the majority of cardiovascular deaths occurred in patients who had preexisting coronary heart disease. Additionally, cardiac fatalities occurred most frequently in patients with underlying cardiovascular disease who were either in the lowest quartile of systolic blood pressure or had greatest change in systolic blood pressure during the treatment. This observation raised the possibility of development of cardiac underperfusion and a "J curve effect." The findings suggest that it would be premature to recommend the generalized use of olmesartan to prevent the development of microalbuminuria in type 2 diabetics with normal albumin excretion. Rather, an individualized risk-benefit analysis that includes cardiovascular risk factors and comorbid conditions should be done, and in the setting of underlying cardiovascular disease, target blood pressures of < 120/70 mm Hg should be avoided,[3] and perhaps the rate of change in pressure should be monitored.

R. Garrick, MD

References

1. Brenner BM, Cooper ME, de Zeeuw D, et al. Effects of losartan on renal and cardiovascular outcomes in patients with type 2 diabetes and nephropathy. *N Engl J Med.* 2001;345:861-869.
2. Lewis EJ, Hunsicker LG, Clarke WR, et al. Renoprotective effect of the angiotensin-receptor antagonist irbesartan in patients with nephropathy due to type 2 diabetes. *N Engl J Med.* 2001;345:851-860.
3. Mancia G, Laurent S, Agabiti-Rosei E, et al. Reappraisal of European guidelines on hypertension management: a European Society of Hypertension Task Force document. *J Hypertens.* 2009;27:2121-2158.

Bardoxolone Methyl and Kidney Function in CKD with Type 2 Diabetes

Pergola PE, for the BEAM Study Investigators (Renal Associates, San Antonio, TX; et al)
N Engl J Med 365:327-336, 2011

Background.—Chronic kidney disease (CKD) associated with type 2 diabetes is the leading cause of kidney failure, with both inflammation and oxidative stress contributing to disease progression. Bardoxolone methyl, an oral antioxidant inflammation modulator, has shown efficacy in patients with CKD and type 2 diabetes in short-term studies, but longer-term effects and dose response have not been determined.

Methods.—In this phase 2, double-blind, randomized, placebo-controlled trial, we assigned 227 adults with CKD (defined as an estimated glomerular filtration rate [GFR] of 20 to 45 ml per minute per 1.73 m^2 of body-surface area) in a 1:1:1:1 ratio to receive placebo or bardoxolone methyl at a target dose of 25, 75, or 150 mg once daily. The primary outcome was the change from baseline in the estimated GFR with bardoxolone methyl, as compared with placebo, at 24 weeks; a secondary outcome was the change at 52 weeks.

Results.—Patients receiving bardoxolone methyl had significant increases in the mean ($\pm$ SD) estimated GFR, as compared with placebo, at 24 weeks (with between-group differences per minute per 1.73 m^2 of 8.2 $\pm$ 1.5 ml in the 25-mg group, 11.4 $\pm$ 1.5 ml in the 75-mg group, and 10.4 $\pm$ 1.5 ml in the 150-mg group; P<0.001). The increases were maintained through week 52, with significant differences per minute per 1.73 m^2 of 5.8 $\pm$ 1.8 ml, 10.5 $\pm$ 1.8 ml, and 9.3 $\pm$ 1.9 ml, respectively. Muscle spasms, the most frequent adverse event in the bardoxolone methyl groups, were generally mild and dose-related. Hypomagnesemia, mild increases in alanine aminotransferase levels, and gastrointestinal effects were more common among patients receiving bardoxolone methyl.

Conclusions.—Bardoxolone methyl was associated with improvement in the estimated GFR in patients with advanced CKD and type 2 diabetes at 24 weeks. The improvement persisted at 52 weeks, suggesting that bardoxolone methyl may have promise for the treatment of CKD. (Funded by Reata Pharmaceuticals; BEAM ClinicalTrials.gov number, NCT00811889.)

▶ The demonstration that angiotensin receptor blockade (ARB) and enzyme inhibition slow the progression of diabetic renal disease was one of the most important advances in the care of patients with diabetic renal disease during the last several decades. Following that critical observation, the mainstays of therapy for diabetic renal disease have centered around blood pressure and antiproteinuria therapy using angiotensin-converting enzyme (ACE) inhibitors and ARB agents. However, despite such treatment, diabetic renal disease is often progressive, and this is believed to be related to chronic inflammation and attendant endothelial dysfunction and glomerular fibrosis. Bardoxolone methyl is an antioxidant-inflammatory modulator that activates Keap1-Nrf2, which has a key role in maintaining kidney structure. Bardoxolone methyl interacts with cysteine residues on

Keap1, which allows Nrf2 to translocate to the nucleus, which results in upregulation of several cytoprotective genes and inhibition of the proinflammatory nuclear factor κB pathway. The current study from the BEAM study investigators is extremely interesting, as it represents the first long-term (52-week) randomized, placebo-controlled assessment of the effect of bardoxolone methyl on renal function in 573 type 2 diabetics. Patients with type 1 diabetes and nondiabetic renal disease were excluded. Participants were stratified according to estimated glomerular infiltration rate (GFR) (< 30 mL or > 30 mL/min/1.73 m^2), and were randomly assigned to receive placebo or escalating doses (25, 75, or 150 mg) of bardoxolone methyl, which was then maintained for 52 weeks. Patients remained on stable doses of ACE inhibitors, ARB, or both. Eighty-one percent of the 25-mg group reached their target dose compared with 25% of the 150-mg group. Blood glucose levels were generally well controlled throughout all groups. Following 24 weeks of bardoxolone methyl therapy, the estimated GFR was better preserved in all treatment groups compared with the placebo arm. This trend persisted after 52 weeks of therapy.

The main side effects noted were muscle cramps, a slight increase in liver enzyme levels, and a decrease in the serum magnesium level of uncertain etiology. The study does have limitations, including the fact that a large percentage of patients failed to meet the target dose, which may have influenced the assessment of side effects. In addition, the surrogate estimated GFR was the only marker used to assess renal function. Whether the changes in GFR reflect hemodynamic effects (as suggested by the slight increase in albumin excretion) rather than an anti-inflammatory effect remains to be determined. Nonetheless, this initial 52-week trial is encouraging and suggests that further studies with bardoxolone methyl are warranted, as this novel agent may represent the newest member of the armamentarium against progressive diabetic-induced renal injury.

R. Garrick, MD

Cardiovascular Assessment of Diabetic End-Stage Renal Disease Patients Before Renal Transplantation
Welsh RC, Cockfield SM, Campbell P, et al (Univ of Alberta, Edmonton, Canada; et al)
Transplantation 91:213-218, 2011

Background.—Although consensus guidelines for preoperative cardiovascular (CV) assessment exist, diabetic patients with renal insufficiency (DM/RI) undergoing assessment for renal transplantation are a unique high-risk group that remains poorly investigated.

Methods.—A consecutive cohort of DM/RI patients being assessed for renal transplantation was studied. We analyzed the ability of clinical characteristics and noninvasive investigation to predict significant coronary artery disease (CAD) and incidence of major adverse CV events.

Results.—Baseline characteristics (n = 280) are as follows: mean age 48.6 years (± 11.5 standard deviation), 66% men, diabetes duration

22.6 years (mean ± 8.9 standard deviation), 92% hypertension, 46% hypercholesterolemia, 24% family history CAD, and 21% known CAD. Abnormal myocardial perfusion imaging was found in 27.8%, and 56.5% had CAD more than or equal to 50%. Although positive myocardial perfusion imaging was the only independent predictor of CAD (odds ratio 7.18, 95% confidence interval 2.98—17.3), a poor negative predicted value was observed with normal imaging in 50.3% of patients having CAD more than or equal to 50%, 35.4% CAD more than 70%, and 41.8% Duke angiographic score more than or equal to 4. At mean follow up of 4 years (median 3.9), 76 of 280 patients suffered major adverse cardiovascular events including 17% mortality. Angiographic evidence of CAD (≥70% odds ratio 1.81, 95% confidence interval 1.02—3.23) was the only independent predictor of major adverse cardiac events.

Conclusion.—DM/RI patients being assessed for renal transplantation have frequent CV risk factors, high likelihood of CAD, and a 28% incidence of major adverse cardiac events after 4 years. Myocardial perfusion imaging is of little clinical utility as a screening tool for CAD in this population. Only angiographic CAD was predictive of subsequent major adverse cardiac events. Further studies of risk stratification and revascularization in this high-risk population are warranted.

▶ Cardiovascular disease is ubiquitous in patients with chronic renal failure on maintenance dialysis and remains the leading cause of mortality in both the dialysis and renal transplant populations.[1] This study represents a prospective approach to cardiovascular screening in diabetic dialysis patients who are candidates for renal transplantation. The study is included because although transplant evaluation was once mainly the domain of nephrologists, cardiologists, and surgeons, many additional caregivers now participate in the pretransplant evaluation process. A key objective of the study was to determine what preoperative predictors of major adverse cardiac events could be used to develop a pretransplant cardiac risk stratification tool to predict posttransplant cardiac risk in diabetic dialysis patients.

The results of this 289-consecutive-patient cohort are quite interesting. First was the finding of a 29% incidence of major adverse cardiac events after 4 years of follow-up, including an 8.3% perioperative event rate. Second was the finding that noninvasive risk assessment with myocardial perfusion imaging carries a very high false-negative rate and therefore is of limited clinical use as a screening tool for coronary artery disease in this population. In addition, as the authors note, most patients denied symptomatic limitations (suggestive of asymptomatic ischemia in this diabetic dialysis population), and this further limits the sensitivity of some of the noninvasive screening tools. The results of this prospective study suggest that the risk of adverse cardiac events in this population can only be determined by cardiac angiography. The results of this study indicate that additional follow-up prospective data are needed, and those studies should also be designed to help assess the best treatment for these lesions once they have been detected.

R. Garrick, MD

Reference

1. Fleisher LA, Beckman JA, Brown KA, et al. ACC/AHA 2007 Guidelines on Peri-operative Cardiovascular Evaluation and Care for Noncardiac Surgery: Executive Summary: A Report of the American Heart Association Task Force on Practice Guidelines (Writing Committee to Revise the 2002 Guidelines on Perioperative Cardiovascular Evaluation for Noncardiac Surgery) Developed in Collaboration With the American Society of Echocardiography, American Society of Nuclear Cardiology, Heart Rhythm Society, Society of Cardiovascular Anesthesiologists, Society for Cardiovascular Angiography and Interventions, Society for Vascular Medicine and Biology, and Society for Vascular Surgery. *J Am Coll Cardiol.* 2007;50:1707-1732.

Cerebral Microvascular Disease Predicts Renal Failure in Type 2 Diabetes

Uzu T, Kida Y, Shirahashi N, et al (Shiga Univ of Med Science, Otsu, Japan; The Second Okamoto Hosp, Uji, Kyoto, Japan; Osaka City Univ, Japan; et al)
J Am Soc Nephrol 21:520-526, 2010

Abnormalities in small renal vessels may increase the risk of developing impaired renal function, but methods to assess these vessels are extremely limited. We hypothesized that the presence of small vessel disease in the brain, which manifests as silent cerebral infarction (SCI), may predict the progression of kidney disease in patients with type 2 diabetes. We recruited 608 patients with type 2 diabetes without apparent cerebrovascular or cardiovascular disease or overt nephropathy and followed them for a mean of 7.5 years. At baseline, 177 of 608 patients had SCI, diagnosed by cerebral magnetic resonance imaging. The risk for the primary outcome of ESRD or death was significantly higher for patients with SCI than for patients without SCI [hazard ratio, 2.44; 95% confidence interval (CI) 1.36 to 4.38]. The risk for the secondary renal end point of any dialysis or doubling of the serum creatinine concentration was also significantly higher for patients with SCI (hazard ratio, 4.79; 95% CI 2.72 to 8.46). The estimated GFR declined more in patients with SCI than in those without SCI; however, the presence of SCI did not increase the risk for progression of albuminuria. In conclusion, independent of microalbuminuria, cerebral microvascular disease predicted renal morbidity among patients with type 2 diabetes.

▶ It is well known that type 2 diabetes mellitus is a risk factor for both cardio-vascular[1] and renal[2] diseases. Most diabetics who have renal failure develop proteinuria during the early phases of the disease, suggesting that proteinuria contributes to the decline in estimated glomerular filtration rate (eGFR). Never-theless, many patients with progressive renal dysfunction in the setting of dia-betes do not have significant proteinuria. This implies that there is likely some nonglomerular pathology contributing to the excess prevalence of renal disease in diabetics. This pathology is presumed to be caused by the presence of renal microvascular disease.

There are several noninvasive indirect methods for assessing renal microvas-cular function. Indirectly, the renal arterial resistive index can be used to detect vascular compromise. Endothelial dysfunction and resultant vascular changes in the periphery may also be detected using laser flow Doppler spectroscopy and have been correlated with renal disease.[3] There are many similarities between the cerebral and renal microcirculations. Since silent cerebral ischemia (SCI) is a manifestation of cerebral vascular dysfunction, it is hypothesized to similarly predict the presence of microvascular disease in the kidneys.

Uzu et al prospectively followed up with 659 Japanese patients with type 2 diabetes admitted to the hospital for glucose control or other diabetic complications while monitoring for primary and secondary end points. Patients with a history of cerebrovascular, malignant, or overt renal diseases, specifically, proteinuria and decreased eGFR, were excluded. All subjects were screened with MRI for SCI. The patients were followed up for an average of 7.5 years. The primary end points of end-stage renal disease (ESRD) or death and the secondary end point of doubling of creatinine level were reached in a statistically higher percentage of patients with SCI compared with those without. Interestingly, the renal functional decline was independent of the degree of albuminuria and was unrelated in multivariate analysis to the higher blood pressure, which was noted in the SCI group. This suggests that SCI, as a reflection of renal microvascular dysfunction, predicts the progression to declining eGFR, ESRD, or death.

This study suggests another possible means of indirectly detecting renal microvascular function by correlating the presence of silent cerebral ischemia with the development of renal failure in this population of type 2 diabetics. It might be helpful if renal microvascular dysfunction could be estimated routinely; however, routine MRI scanning may be prohibitively expensive.

M. Klein, MD, JD

References

1. Haffner SM, Lehto S, Rönnemaa T, Pyörälä K, Laakso M. Mortality from coronary heart disease in subjects with type 2 diabetes and in nondiabetic subjects with and without prior myocardial infarction. *N Engl J Med.* 1998;339:229-234.
2. Brancati FL, Whelton PK, Randall BL, Neaton JD, Stamler J, Klag MJ. Risk of end-stage renal disease in diabetes mellitus: a prospective cohort study of men screened for MRFIT. Multiple risk factor intervention trial. *JAMA.* 1997;278: 2069-2074.
3. Stewart J, Kohen A, Brouder D, et al. Noninvasive interrogation of microvasculature for signs of endothelial dysfunction in patients with chronic renal failure. *Am J Physiol Heart Circ Physiol.* 2004;287:H2687-H2696.

Albuminuria and Decline in Cognitive Function: The ONTARGET/ TRANSCEND Studies

Barzilay JI, for the ONTARGET and TRANSCEND Investigators (Emory Univ School of Medicine, Atlanta, GA; et al)
Arch Intern Med 171:142-150, 2011

Background.—Microvascular disease of the kidney (manifesting as albuminuria) and of the brain (manifesting as cognitive decline) may share a common pathogenesis. Gaining an understanding of the concomitant history of these 2 conditions may inform clinical practice and lead to novel prevention and treatment approaches.

Methods.—A total of 28 384 participants with vascular disease or diabetes mellitus were examined. At baseline and year 5, participants underwent a Mini-Mental State Examination (MMSE) and urine testing for albumin excretion. Multivariable logistic regression was used to determine the association between albumin excretion and MMSE score, cross-sectionally and prospectively, and whether angiotensin-converting enzyme inhibitor and/or angiotensin receptor blocker use modified the association.

Results.—Compared with participants with normoalbuminuria, those with microalbuminuria (odds ratio [OR], 1.26; 95% confidence interval [CI], 1.11-1.44]) and macroalbuminuria (1.49; 1.20-1.85) were more likely to have a reduced MMSE score (<24). On follow-up, participants with baseline albuminuria had increased odds of cognitive decline (decrease in MMSE score ≥3 points) compared with those with normoalbuminuria (microalbuminuria: OR, 1.22; 95% CI, 1.07-1.38; macroalbuminuria: 1.21; 0.94-1.55). Participants who developed new albuminuria had increased odds of cognitive decline during follow-up compared with those who remained normoalbuminuric (new microalbuminuria: OR, 1.30; 95% CI, 1.12-1.52; new macroalbuminuria: 1.77; 1.24-2.54). Participants with baseline macroalbuminuria treated with an angiotensin-converting enzyme inhibitor and/or angiotensin receptor blocker had lower odds of MMSE decline than participants treated with placebo.

Conclusion.—Factors that contribute to albuminuria may contribute to cognitive decline, supporting the notion that both conditions share a common microvascular pathogenesis.

Trial Registration.—clinicaltrials.gov Identifier: NCT00153101.

▶ The Ongoing Telmisartan Alone and in Combination with Ramipril Global End Point Trial (ONTARGET) and the Telmisartan Randomized Assessment Study in ACE (Angiotensin-Converting Enzyme) Intolerant Subjects with Cardiovascular Disease (TRANSCEND) trials[1,2] contain baseline and follow-up data on both albuminuria and cognitive function. The authors used multivariable adjusted regression analysis to determine the association between albumin excretion and the cognitive function as measured by the Mini-Mental State Examination score in 28 384 participants with vascular disease or diabetes. This is the first large prospective, cross-sectional study to report a graded association between albuminuria as a marker of microvascular disease and cognitive decline. Interestingly, the association was found to be independent of cardiovascular and either incident or prevalent renal disease. As shown in Fig 2, the odds ratio of developing a decrease in cognitive function tracked with micro- and macroalbuminuria and the findings suggest that albuminuria and cognitive decline are related to alterations in microvascular pathophysiology.

This study extends the observations made by the previous Atherosclerosis Risk in Communities Study 3,[3] which suggested that any form of retinopathy (retinal vessels share common physiologic characteristics with cerebral arterioles) is associated with an increased risk of cognitive impairment, and the

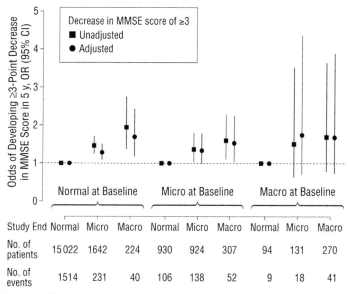

FIGURE 2.—Odds ratios (ORs) and 95% confidence intervals (CIs) of developing a 3-point or greater decrease in Mini-Mental State Examination (MMSE) score during 5 years categorized by baseline normoalbuminuria (normal), microalbuminuria (micro), and macroalbuminuria (macro) and the change in albuminuria status during 5 years of follow-up. (Reprinted from Barzilay JI, for the ONTARGET and TRANSCEND Investigators. Albuminuria and decline in cognitive function: the ONTARGET/TRANSCEND studies. *Arch Intern Med.* 2011;171:142-150, with permission from the American Medical Association.)

Cardiovascular Health Study 4,[4] which demonstrated that the risk of cognitive impairment and dementia increase by 10% and 22% respectively with each doubling of the urine albumin to creatinine excretion ratio. Of great interest was the finding that participants with baseline macroalbuminuria who were treated with either ACEi or angiotensin receptor blocker therapy had a lower odds ratio of cognitive decline than did patients treated with placebo.

Of course, this study cannot prove causality, and the nonrandomized, observational nature of the analysis, together with the high risk of vascular disease among the participants of the ONTARGET and TRANSCEND trials, suggest that the results need to be confirmed in other populations, perhaps using more sensitive studies of cognitive function. However, the results do suggest that microvascular disease in 1 organ bed raises the possibility of disease elsewhere. They also suggest that patients with microalbuminuria might benefit from baseline and serial cognitive assessments, with the possibility of early intervention as more refined treatments become available.

R. Garrick, MD

References

1. Mann JF, Schmieder RE, Dyal L, et al. TRANSCEND (Telmisartan Randomised Assessment Study in ACE Intolerant Subjects With Cardiovascular Disease)

Investigators. Effect of telmisartan on renal outcomes: a randomized trial. *Ann Intern Med.* 2009;151:1-10.

2. Mann JF, Schmieder RE, McQueen M, et al. ONTARGET Investigators. Renal outcomes with telmisartan, ramipril, or both, in people at high vascular risk (the ONTARGET Study): a multicentre, randomised, double-blind, controlled trial. *Lancet.* 2008;372:547-553.

3. Wong TY, Klein R, Sharrett AR, et al. Retinal microvascular abnormalities and cognitive impairment in middle-aged persons: the Atherosclerosis Risk in Communities Study. *Stroke.* 2002;33:1487-1492.

4. Barzilay JI, Fitzpatrick AL, Luchsinger J, et al. Albuminuria and dementia in the elderly: a community study. *Am J Kidney Dis.* 2008;52:216-226.

30 Clinical Nephrology

Randomized Clinical Trial of Long-Acting Somatostatin for Autosomal Dominant Polycystic Kidney and Liver Disease
Hogan MC, Masyuk TV, Page LJ, et al (Mayo Clinic College of Medicine, Rochester, MN)
J Am Soc Nephrol 21:1052-1061, 2010

There are no proven, effective therapies for polycystic kidney disease (PKD) or polycystic liver disease (PLD). We enrolled 42 patients with severe PLD resulting from autosomal dominant PKD (ADPKD) or autosomal dominant PLD (ADPLD) in a randomized, double-blind, placebo-controlled trial of octreotide, a long-acting somatostatin analogue. We randomly assigned 42 patients in a 2:1 ratio to octreotide LAR depot (up to 40 mg every 28 ± 5 days) or placebo for 1 year. The primary end point was percent change in liver volume from baseline to 1 year, measured by MRI. Secondary end points were changes in total kidney volume, GFR, quality of life, safety, vital signs, and clinical laboratory tests. Thirty-four patients had ADPKD, and eight had ADPLD. Liver volume decreased by 4.95% ± 6.77% in the octreotide group but remained practically unchanged (+0.92% ± 8.33%) in the placebo group ($P = 0.048$). Among patients with ADPKD, total kidney volume remained practically unchanged (+0.25% ± 7.53%) in the octreotide group but increased by 8.61% ± 10.07% in the placebo group ($P = 0.045$). Changes in GFR were similar in both groups. Octreotide was well tolerated; treated individuals reported an improved perception of bodily pain and physical activity. In summary, octreotide slowed the progressive increase in liver volume and total kidney volume, improved health perception among patients with PLD, and had an acceptable side effect profile.

▶ The prevalence of autosomal dominant polycystic kidney disease is 1 in 400 to 1 in 1000 live births and in many patients is characterized by progressive renal failure. In all patients it is characterized by enlarged cystic kidneys that pose a risk for infection, bleeding, and painful expansion. Cystic expansion can involve other organs, including the liver, and although these cysts do not typically lead to hepatic failure, they can cause pain and are a source of potential bleeding and infection. There continues to be a search for medications to slow the progression of cyst growth and renal impairment. This study is a randomized, double-blind, placebo-controlled trial of octreotide, a long-acting somatostatin analog, and is focused on the possibility that somatostatin can slow the progression of both hepatic and renal cysts.

Somatostatin blocks vasopressin-induced intracellular cAMP generation in the distal nephron, preventing cystic fluid accumulation. Although V2 receptors are not expressed on the liver, the long-acting somatostatin analog, octreotide, acts on G protein—coupled receptors to inhibit cAMP signaling in cholangiocytes and may thereby potentially slow the growth of both liver and kidney cysts.

A prior pilot study[1] suggested that this agent was both safe and efficacious, and the current octreotide study extends those earlier short-term observations. The findings by Hogan and colleagues are encouraging and demonstrated that kidney volume in response to octreotide remained stable, whereas cyst size increased in the placebo groups. The liver cysts were reduced in size in the octreotide group. Glomerular filtration rate (GFR) did not change significantly in either group, and hepatic function was stable. Plasma glucose increased, but no patient developed diabetes.

A 3-year study sponsored by the National Institutes of Health is now under way. It will be interesting to see whether there will be greater reno-protection (as measured by GFR and renal volume) with longer-term octreotide use. Longer-term follow-up will allow better assessment of glucose stability as well.

M. Brogan, MD

Reference

1. Ruggenenti P, Remuzzi A, Ondei P, et al. Safety and efficacy of long-acting soma-tostostatin treatment in autosmal-dominant polycystic kidney disease. *Kidney Int.* 2005;68:206-216.

Sirolimus Therapy to Halt the Progression of ADPKD
Perico N, Antiga L, Caroli A, et al (Mario Negri Inst for Pharmacological Res, Bergamo, Italy; et al)
J Am Soc Nephrol 21:1031-1040, 2010

Activation of mammalian target of rapamycin (mTOR) pathways may contribute to uncontrolled cell proliferation and secondary cyst growth in patients with autosomal dominant polycystic kidney disease (ADPKD). To assess the effects of mTOR inhibition on disease progression, we performed a randomized, crossover study (The SIRENA Study) comparing a 6-month treatment with sirolimus or conventional therapy alone on the growth of kidney volume and its compartments in 21 patients with ADPKD and GFR $\geq$40 ml/min per 1.73 m^2. In 10 of the 15 patients who completed the study, aphthous stomatitis complicated sirolimus treatment but was effectively controlled by topical therapy. Compared with pretreatment, posttreatment mean total kidney volume increased less on sirolimus (46 ± 81 ml; $P = 0.047$) than on conventional therapy (70 ± 72 ml; $P = 0.002$), but we did not detect a difference between the two treatments ($P = 0.45$). Cyst volume was stable on sirolimus and increased by 55 ± 75 ml ($P = 0.013$) on conventional therapy, whereas parenchymal volume increased by 26 ± 30 ml ($P = 0.005$) on sirolimus and was stable on conventional therapy. Percentage changes in cyst and parenchyma volumes were significantly different between the two treatment periods. Sirolimus had no appreciable effects on intermediate volume and GFR. Albuminuria and proteinuria marginally but significantly increased during sirolimus treatment. In summary, sirolimus halted cyst growth and increased parenchymal volume in patients with ADPKD. Whether these effects translate into improved long-term outcomes requires further investigation.

▶ This proof-of-concept study is included because Type 1 autosomal dominant polycystic kidney disease (ADPKD) is the most common form of inherited kidney injury and is always progressive. Animal studies have demonstrated that the mammalian target of rapamycin (mTOR) pathway can contribute to cell proliferation cyst growth in ADPKD.[1,2] This small prospective randomized crossover clinical trial in adults with ADPKD demonstrated that 6 months of treatment with immunosuppressive agent sirolimus resulted in the stabilization of cyst volume and halted cyst growth. Interesting and surprising was the finding that renal parenchymal volume increased in patients receiving sirolimus therapy but not in those receiving conventional therapy (which consisted of antihypertensives in 10 patients and diuretic therapy in 3 patients). Although it was postulated that the increase in parenchymal volume may have been related to parenchymal expansion presumably related to a reduction of the mass effect of the surrounding cysts, the exact cause of this observation will require further study.

A secondary aim of the trial was to evaluate the safety profile of sirolimus in the setting of polycystic kidney disease. One concern was the development of stomatitis in 10 patients, which is more common than is typically seen with transplant patients and was thought to be related to the lack of concomitant steroid therapy. Significant bone-marrow toxicity and changes in renal function were not observed, but lipid levels, urinary protein, and albumin excretion and liver function studies were increased in patients on sirolimus during this short-term trial. The small sample size did not permit formal dose response evaluation, but the findings did suggest that a minimum dose of sirolimus of 0.049 mg/kg body weight would be required for stabilization and reduction of cyst volume, and this will be useful in the design of future studies. The findings are exciting and suggest that sirolimus may halt the progression of ADPKD and that appropriately powered, long-term efficacy and safety trials of sirolimus therapy in PKD are warranted.

R. Garrick, MD

References

1. Shillingford JM, Murcia NS, Larson CH, et al. The mTOR pathway is regulated by polycystin-1, and its inhibition reverses renal cystogenesis in polycystic kidney disease. *Proc Natl Acad Sci U S A.* 2006;103:5466-5471.
2. Wahl PR, Serra AL, Le Hir M, Molle KD, Hall MN, Wüthrich RP. Inhibition of mTOR with sirolimus slows disease progression in Han: SPRD rats with autosomal dominant polycystic kidney disease (ADPKD). *Nephrol Dial Transplant.* 2006;21:598-604.

Low Socioeconomic Status Associates with Higher Serum Phosphate Irrespective of Race

Gutiérrez OM, on behalf of the CRIC Study Group (Univ of Miami Miller School of Medicine, FL; et al)

J Am Soc Nephrol 21:1953-1960, 2010

Hyperphosphatemia, which associates with adverse outcomes in CKD, is more common among blacks than whites for unclear reasons. Low socioeconomic status may explain this association because poverty both disproportionately affects racial and ethnic minorities and promotes excess intake of relatively inexpensive processed and fast foods enriched with highly absorbable phosphorus additives. We performed a cross-sectional analysis of race, socioeconomic status, and serum phosphate among 2879 participants in the Chronic Renal Insufficiency Cohort Study. Participants with the lowest incomes or who were unemployed had higher serum phosphate concentrations than participants with the highest incomes or who were employed ($P < 0.001$). Although we also observed differences in serum phosphate levels by race, income modified this relationship: Blacks had 0.11 to 0.13 mg/dl higher serum phosphate than whites in the highest income groups but there was no difference by race in the lowest income group. In addition, compared with whites with the highest income, both blacks and whites with the lowest incomes had more than twice the likelihood of hyperphosphatemia in multivariable-adjusted analysis. In conclusion, low socioeconomic status associates with higher serum phosphate concentrations irrespective of race. Given the association between higher levels of serum phosphate and cardiovascular disease, further studies will need to determine whether excess serum phosphate may explain disparities in kidney disease outcomes among minority populations and the poor.

▶ The findings of this study are particularly interesting when juxtaposed with the study (to follow) by Cavanaugh et al regarding health care literacy and mortality in end-stage renal disease. In that study, low health care literacy as defined by the REALM tool was associated with an increased mortality. No difference was found in baseline serum electrolytes among patients with varying degrees of literacy. In this study, the authors performed a cross-sectional analysis by race, socioeconomic status, and serum phosphate among 2879 participants in the Chronic Renal Insufficiency Cohort study. Interestingly, participants with the lowest incomes and the unemployed had the highest serum phosphate concentrations when compared with participants who are either employed or had higher incomes. The difference in serum phosphate level by race was modified by income.

Increased serum phosphate levels are associated with increased mortality in patients with cardiovascular disease and kidney disease.[1,2] Multiple studies have suggested that hyperphosphatemia can promote both vascular calcification and endothelial dysfunction, and a causal link between elevated serum phosphorus level and adverse health outcomes has been suggested.[3,4] Given the data regarding the impact of serum phosphate on mortality, the finding that hyperphosphatemia tracks with both socioeconomic class and income are particularly noteworthy. In patients with chronic kidney disease, dietary phosphate intake directly impacts serum phosphate levels. Inexpensive, highly processed foods, especially "fast foods," are often high in phosphate. These data, coupled with the data regarding health care literacy and mortality, suggest that communication tools regarding dietary phosphate sources should be adjusted for the level of health care literacy.

R. Garrick, MD

References

1. Block GA, Klassen PS, Lazarus JM, Ofsthun N, Lowrie EG, Chertow GM. Mineral metabolism, mortality, and morbidity in maintenance hemodialysis. *J Am Soc Nephrol.* 2004;15:2208-2218.
2. Foley RN, Collins AJ, Herzog CA, Ishani A, Kalra PA. Serum phosphorus levels associate with coronary atherosclerosis in young adults. *J Am Soc Nephrol.* 2009;20:397-404.
3. Tonelli M, Sacks F, Pfeffer M, Gao Z, Curhan G. Relation between serum phosphate level and cardiovascular event rate in people with coronary disease. *Circulation.* 2005;112:2627-2633.
4. Giachelli CM, Jono S, Shioi A, Nishizawa Y, Mori K, Morii H. Vascular calcification and inorganic phosphate. *Am J Kidney Dis.* 2001;38:S34-S37.

Increased Fructose Associates with Elevated Blood Pressure
Jalal DI, Smits G, Johnson RJ, et al (Univ of Colorado Denver Health Sciences Ctr, Aurora)
J Am Soc Nephrol 21:1543-1549, 2010

The recent increase in fructose consumption in industrialized nations mirrors the rise in the prevalence of hypertension, but epidemiologic studies have inconsistently linked these observations. We investigated whether increased fructose intake from added sugars associates with an increased risk for higher BP levels in US adults without a history of hypertension. We conducted a cross-sectional analysis using the data collected from the National Health and Nutrition Examination Survey (NHANES 2003 to 2006) involving 4528 adults without a history of hypertension. Median fructose intake was 74 g/d, corresponding to 2.5 sugary soft drinks each day. After adjustment for demographics; comorbidities; physical activity; total kilocalorie intake; and dietary confounders such as total carbohydrate, alcohol, salt, and vitamin C intake, an increased fructose intake of ≥74 g/d independently and significantly associated with higher odds of elevated BP levels: It led to a 26, 30, and 77% higher risk for BP cutoffs of ≥135/85, ≥140/90, and ≥160/100 mmHg, respectively. These results suggest that high fructose intake, in the form of added sugar, independently associates with higher BP levels among US adults without a history of hypertension.

▶ Fructose consumption (especially in the form of high-fructose corn syrup) has been linked to the metabolic syndrome, abnormalities of oxygen radicals, and changes in uric acid metabolism. The current study is extremely interesting because it suggests that alterations in dietary fructose intake may be a modifiable risk factor for the control of hypertension. Prior animal studies suggested that fructose could raise blood pressure via stimulation of uric acid production, inhibition of endothelial nitric oxide synthase, stimulation of the sympathetic nervous system, or by stimulation of gastrointestinal sodium transport.[1-4] This cross-sectional study, drawn from the National Health and Nutrition Examination Survey (2003 to 2006), involved 4528 adults with no known history of hypertension in whom direct blood pressure determinations were obtained and fructose intake was determined by diet questionnaire. After adjustment for several variables, a fructose intake of greater than 74 g per day (an average of 2.5 sugared soft drinks) increased the odds for the presence of hypertension. The study has limitations in that it was a cross-sectional analysis and relied on dietary recall data; however, other important dietary factors, such as sodium intake and body weight, were available, as were specific blood pressure recordings. Although not establishing causality, the findings are particularly intriguing and lend credence to the concept that a simple reduction in dietary fructose intake may improve blood pressure and cardiovascular health.

M. Brogan, MD

References

1. Glushakova O, Kosugi T, Roncal C, et al. Fructose induces the inflammatory molecule ICAM-1 in endothelial cells. *J Am Soc Nephrol.* 2008;19:1712-1720.
2. Zhao CX, Xu X, Cui Y, et al. Increased endothelial nitric-oxide synthase expression reduces hypertension and hyperinsulinemia in fructose-treated rats. *J Pharmacol Exp Ther.* 2009;328:610-620.
3. Brito JO, Ponciano K, Figueroa D, et al. Parasympathetic dysfunction is associated with insulin resistance in fructose-fed female rats. *Braz J Med Biol Res.* 2008;41: 804-808.
4. Singh AK, Amlal H, Haas PJ, et al. Fructose-induced hypertension: essential role of chloride and fructose absorbing transporters PAT1 and Glut5. *Kidney Int.* 2008; 74:438-447.

Low Health Literacy Associates with Increased Mortality in ESRD
Cavanaugh KL, Wingard RL, Hakim RM, et al (Vanderbilt Univ Med Ctr, Nashville, TN; et al)
J Am Soc Nephrol 21:1979-1985, 2010

Limited health literacy is common in the United States and associates with poor clinical outcomes. Little is known about the effect of health literacy in patients with advanced kidney disease. In this prospective cohort study we describe the prevalence of limited health literacy and examine its association with the risk for mortality in hemodialysis patients. We enrolled 480 incident chronic hemodialysis patients from 77 dialysis clinics between 2005 and 2007 and followed them until April 2008. Measured using the Rapid Estimate of Adult Literacy in Medicine, 32% of patients had limited (<9th grade reading level) and 68% had adequate health literacy (≥9th grade reading level). Limited health literacy was more likely in patients who were male and non-white and who had fewer years of education. Compared with adequate literacy, limited health literacy associated with a higher risk for death (HR 1.54; 95% CI 1.01 to 2.36) even after adjustment for age, sex, race, and diabetes. In summary, limited health literacy is common and associates with higher mortality in chronic hemodialysis patients. Addressing health literacy may improve survival for these patients.

▶ The effect of health care disparities on clinical outcomes has been increasingly recognized.[1] Little information is available regarding how, or if, health care literacy affects patients with advanced kidney disease. This is the first study to directly evaluate the effects of health care literacy on mortality risk among incident dialysis patients. Using the Rapid Estimate of the Adult Literacy in Medicine (REALM) tool, 480 incident chronic hemodialysis patients were assessed within 1 month of initiation of hemodialysis. Patients were drawn from 77 dialysis clinics and were enrolled between 2005 and 2007 and followed until 2008. The authors demonstrated that almost a third of the patients had a less than ninth-grade reading level. This limited literacy was more common in non-white male patients with fewer years of formal education. Importantly, the authors found that there was a significant difference in survival rates among patients with poor health care literacy, with a risk of death 54% higher than among patients with adequate literacy skills (hazard ratio 1.54, 95% confidence interval 1.04-2.28, $P = .013$). This finding persisted after adjustments for multiple comorbidities including sex, race, diabetes, and age. The authors sought to determine whether specific outcomes tracked with literacy and although there was no difference in dialysis adequacy, measurements of anemia, or measurements of bone health (such as calcium phosphate and parathyroid hormone), baseline serum albumin levels were lower in patients with lower levels of health care literacy.

A limitation of the study is that there was no specific measurement of cognitive function; however, prior studies in other patient populations have suggested that cognitive function and health literacy are independently associated with mortality risk.[2] In addition, whether health care literacy tracks with other comorbid conditions that may have had a confounding influence on mortality cannot be determined by this study. The finding that mortality was increased in incident dialysis patients based on their underlying health care literacy does suggest opportunities for mitigation of risk. Oral and written instructions and treatment guidelines should be appropriately crafted and screened by literacy experts so that, at the very least, we are confident that patients understand what we are trying to communicate. Steps such as these have been suggested to improve outcomes in other disease settings, such as diabetes and heart failure,[3,4] and hopefully additional studies will prove that the same holds true for patients with advanced kidney disease.

R. Garrick, MD

References

1. Dewalt DA, Berkman ND, Sheridan S, Lohr KN, Pignone MP. Literacy and health outcomes: a systematic review of the literature. *J Gen Intern Med.* 2004;19: 1228-1239.

2. Baker DW, Wolf MS, Feinglass J, Thompson JA. Health literacy, cognitive abilities, and mortality among elderly persons. *J Gen Intern Med.* 2008;23:723-726.
3. Cavanaugh K, Wallston KA, Gebretsadik T, et al. Addressing literacy and numeracy to improve diabetes care: two randomized controlled trials. *Diabetes Care.* 2009;32:2149-2155.
4. DeWalt DA, Malone RM, Bryant ME, et al. A heart failure self-management program for patients of all literacy levels: a randomized, controlled trial [ISRCTN11535170]. *BMC Health Serv Res.* 2006;6:30.

CKD Awareness and Blood Pressure Control in the Primary Care Hypertensive Population

Ravera M, Noberasco G, Weiss U, et al (Univ of Genoa, Italy; Italian College of General Practitioners, Florence, Italy)
Am J Kidney Dis 57:71-77, 2011

Background.—Chronic kidney disease (CKD) is associated with poor renal and cardiovascular outcomes, and early identification largely depends on general practitioners' (GPs') awareness of it. To date, no study has evaluated CKD prevalence in patients with hypertension in primary care.

Study Design.—Cross-sectional evaluation of the Italian GPs' database.

Setting & Participants.—39,525 patients with hypertension representative of the Italian hypertensive population followed up by GPs in 2005.

Factor.—Estimated glomerular filtration rate (eGFR); eGFR <60 mL/min/1.73 m^2 was defined as CKD.

Outcomes.—GPs' awareness of CKD assessed using *International Classification of Diseases, Ninth Revision, Clinical Modification* diagnostic codes for CKD, and blood pressure (BP) control.

Measurements.—Data concerning serum creatinine levels, BPs, and antihypertensive medications were obtained for each patient from the GPs' database; eGFR was calculated according to the 4-variable Modification of Diet in Renal Disease (MDRD) Study equation.

Results.—CKD prevalence was 23%, but kidney disease was diagnosed by GPs in only 3.9% of patients. BP control was inadequate in patients with CKD and those with eGFR >60 mL/min/1.73 m^2, with only 44% of patients reaching a BP target <140/90 mm Hg and 11% achieving <130/80 mm Hg. Patients with eGFR <60 mL/min/1.73 m^2 whose GPs were aware of CKD were more likely to reach recommended BP target values (OR, 1.35; 95% CI, 1.15-1.59; *P* < 0.001).

Limitations.—The prevalence of decreased eGFR may be overestimated because of the lack of creatinine calibration. Proteinuria data were not available.

Conclusions.—Awareness of CKD by GPs is critical for achieving the recommended guideline BP targets. However, awareness of CKD by GPs is still far too low, highlighting the need to systematically adopt eGFR for more accurate identification of CKD in high-risk populations.

▶ There is an old business adage sometimes attributed to the statistician W. Edwards Deming, which states that "You can't manage what you don't measure." Ravera et al have shown in this article that this adage is equally pertinent in the treatment of chronic kidney disease.

This cross-sectional observational study from the Italian Health Search Database found that only 14% of patients with impaired estimated glomerular filtration rates (eGFR) based on measured plasma creatinine levels were given a diagnosis of chronic kidney disease (CKD) by their general practitioner (GP). Almost 25% of patients with eGFR < 30 cc/min failed to be identified as having CKD. Even worse, a full 60% of these hypertensive patients never even had their plasma creatinine measured! Not surprisingly, the cohort of correctly diagnosed patients had a 73% higher likelihood of achieving target blood pressure (BP) control. Specifically, the correctly diagnosed patient group had a significantly higher likelihood of using 3 or more agents for BP control.

These findings are disturbing because these patients were all known to be hypertensive and, on this basis, were all clearly at increased risk for the development and/or progression of CKD.[1] In a regression analysis, the improvement in BP control seemed to be solely correlated with the GP's awareness of CKD. Not even dyslipidemia or diabetes was similarly correlated with worsened BP control.

This study may be affected by some selection bias because doctors who check creatinine levels and appropriately diagnose their patients are presumed to be more fastidious in treating patients overall. But it seems to lay bare some opportunities for improvement and the need for practitioners to correctly assess the common predictors of CKD and convincingly demonstrates that such awareness improves the GP's ability to carefully modify the risks.

This study should serve as a reminder for GPs, both abroad and in the United States, to measure the plasma creatinine levels of their hypertensive patients and then to appropriately diagnose CKD when present, lest they fail to adequately manage their patients' risk for progression.

M. Klein, MD, JD

Reference

1. Perry HM Jr, Miller JP, Fornoff JR, et al. Early predictors of 15-year end-stage renal disease in hypertensive patients. *Hypertension.* 1995;25:587-594.

Quality of Patient-Physician Discussions About CKD in Primary Care: A Cross-sectional Study
Greer RC, Cooper LA, Crews DC, et al (Johns Hopkins Univ School of Medicine, Baltimore, MD; et al)
Am J Kidney Dis 57:583-591, 2011

Background.—The quality of patient-physician discussions about chronic kidney disease (CKD) in primary care has not been studied previously.

Study Design.—Cross-sectional study.

Settings & Participants.—We audiotaped encounters between 236 patients with hypertension and their primary care physicians (n = 40).

Predictors.—Patient, physician, and encounter characteristics.

Outcomes & Measurements.—We described the occurrence and characteristics (content, use of technical terms, and physician assessment of patient comprehension of new concepts) of CKD discussions. We assessed patient and physician characteristics associated with CKD discussion occurrence.

Results.—Many patients (mean age, 59 years) had uncontrolled hypertension (51%), diabetes (44%), and/or 3 or more comorbid conditions (51%). Most primary care physicians practiced (52%) fewer than 10 years. CKD discussions occurred in few (26%; n = 61) encounters, with content focused on laboratory assessment (89%), risk-factor treatment (28%), and causes (26%) of CKD. In encounters that included a CKD discussion, physicians used technical terms (28%; n = 17) and rarely assessed patients' comprehension (2%; n = 1). CKD discussions were statistically significantly less common in visits of patients with some (vs no) college education (OR, 0.23; 95% CI, 0.09-0.56), with 3 or more (vs fewer) comorbid conditions (OR, 0.49; 95% CI, 0.25-0.96), and who saw physicians with more (vs fewer) than 10 years of practice experience (OR, 0.41; 95% CI, 0.21-0.80). CKD discussions were more common during longer encounters (OR, 1.31; 95% CI, 1.04-1.65) and encounters in which diabetes was (vs was not) discussed (OR, 2.87; 95% CI, 1.22-6.77).

Limitations.—Generalizability of our findings may be limited.

Conclusions.—Patient-physician discussions about CKD in high-risk primary care patients were infrequent. Physicians used technical terms and infrequently assessed patients' understanding of new CKD concepts. Efforts to improve the frequency and content of patient-physician CKD discussions in primary care could improve patients' clinical outcomes.

▶ The new paradigm of medical care, suggested by the Accountable Care Model, anticipates that patients with chronic kidney disease (CKD) may not be primarily cared for by specialists with training in kidney disease, but rather will typically be cared for by primary care providers with specialists only selectively involved until the later stages of disease progression. Thus, this article is particularly timely, as it is the first article to assess in a controlled fashion the frequency and content of CKD discussions between patients and primary care providers. Greer and colleagues assessed patient-provider interaction among patients with underlying hypertension, many of whom had other comorbid conditions such as diabetes. The results suggest that despite the presence of high-risk comorbidities, physician discussions regarding progressive kidney disease occurred infrequently. In addition, physicians often used technical terms and only infrequently assessed patients' understanding of the conversation or their understanding the risk of developing progressive kidney disease. The data demonstrate that most encounters focused on laboratory assessment and that overall, less attention was given to modifiable risk factors as they apply to progressive kidney injury. Prior studies[1,2] have suggested that primary care physicians are not always comfortable discussing issues related to kidney disease. Although not specifically addressed here, it is possible that factors such as this influenced the results of the current study. The findings demonstrate that as new paradigms for health care delivery are developed, the actual impact on patient care and clinical outcomes will need to be simultaneously assessed. In addition, the findings suggest that the use of specific toolkits and other related standardized patient education material would likely be of benefit.

R. Garrick, MD

References

1. Fox CH, Brooks A, Zayas LE, McClellan W, Murray B. Primary care physicians' knowledge and practice patterns in the treatment of chronic kidney disease: an Upstate New York Practice-based Research Network (UNYNET) study. *J Am Board Fam Med.* 2006;19:54-61.
2. Agrawal V, Ghosh AK, Barnes MA, McCullough PA. Awareness and knowledge of clinical practice guidelines for CKD among internal medicine residents: a national online survey. *Am J Kidney Dis.* 2008;52:1061-1069.

Diuretic Strategies in Patients with Acute Decompensated Heart Failure

Felker GM, for the NHLBI Heart Failure Clinical Research Network (Duke Univ School of Medicine and Duke Heart Ctr, Durham, NC; et al)
N Engl J Med 364:797-805, 2011

Background.—Loop diuretics are an essential component of therapy for patients with acute decompensated heart failure, but there are few prospective data to guide their use.

Methods.—In a prospective, double-blind, randomized trial, we assigned 308 patients with acute decompensated heart failure to receive furosemide administered intravenously by means of either a bolus every 12 hours or continuous infusion and at either a low dose (equivalent to the patient's previous oral dose) or a high dose (2.5 times the previous oral dose). The protocol allowed specified dose adjustments after 48 hours. The coprimary end points were patients' global assessment of symptoms, quantified as the area under the curve (AUC) of the score on a visual-analogue scale over the course of 72 hours, and the change in the serum creatinine level from baseline to 72 hours.

Results.—In the comparison of bolus with continuous infusion, there was no significant difference in patients' global assessment of symptoms (mean AUC, 4236 ± 1440 and 4373 ± 1404, respectively; $P = 0.47$) or in the mean change in the creatinine level (0.05 ± 0.3 mg per deciliter [4.4 ± 26.5 μmol per liter] and 0.07 ± 0.3 mg per deciliter [6.2 ± 26.5 μmol per liter], respectively; $P = 0.45$). In the comparison of the high-dose strategy with the low-dose strategy, there was a nonsignificant trend toward greater improvement in patients' global assessment of symptoms in the high-dose group (mean AUC, 4430 ± 1401 vs. 4171 ± 1436; $P = 0.06$). There was no significant difference between these groups in the mean change in the creatinine level (0.08 ± 0.3 mg per deciliter [7.1 ± 26.5 μmol per liter] with the high-dose strategy and 0.04 ± 0.3 mg per deciliter [3.5 ± 26.5 μmol per liter] with the low-dose strategy, $P = 0.21$). The high-dose strategy was associated with greater diuresis and more favorable outcomes in some secondary measures but also with transient worsening of renal function.

Conclusions.—Among patients with acute decompensated heart failure, there were no significant differences in patients' global assessment of symptoms or in the change in renal function when diuretic therapy was administered by bolus as compared with continuous infusion or at a high dose as compared with a low dose. (Funded by the National Heart, Lung, and Blood Institute; ClinicalTrials.gov number, NCT00577135.)

▶ Although loop diuretics are nearly universally prescribed for the treatment of acute decompensated congestive heart failure (ADCHF), there are few data to guide their use. Most admissions for ADCHF are because of congestion and volume overload, so ethical considerations have prevented good placebo-controlled trials of their use. The use of high-dose furosemide has been found to be deleterious in some studies,[1] but it is not clear whether this merely reflects the selection bias of sicker patients who require more aggressive therapy in the first place. Nevertheless, only small trials of varying quality using varied dosing protocols have been conducted. To date, no dosing strategy has consistently been shown to be superior. This trial evaluated whether higher doses lead to improved outcomes, and whether continuous infusion is preferable to bolus injection.

This double-blind randomized trial, called the Diuretic Optimization Strategies Evaluation (DOSE) trial, examined these variables for both efficacy and adverse outcomes. The study used a 2 × 2 factorial design to examine low-dose furosemide (intravenous [IV] dose equal to prior oral [PO] dose) versus high-dose furosemide (IV dose at 2.5 times the prior PO dose), as well as twice-daily dosing versus continuous infusion in 308 patients with acute heart failure.

The patients receiving bolus treatment were nearly twice as likely to require a dose increase in the first 48 hours, and they required a higher median total dose of drug over the 72 hours of treatment. There were no differences, however, in the primary efficacy end point of the patient-reported global assessment of symptoms (GAS) between the 2 dosing strategies, or in renal side effects, as determined by serum creatinine and cystatin-C at 60 days. Not surprisingly, those in the low-dose group were more likely to require a dose increase and, by design, had overall lower doses administered during the trial.

Again, there were no significant differences in the GAS, but there was significant greater net fluid loss and relief from dyspnea in the high-dose group. There was significant short-term worsening of renal function in the high-dose group, but this difference did not persist past 60 days.

That the continuous-infusion arm had no increase in diuresis over the intermittent-dosing arm seems to contradict some prior evidence that continuous infusion of furosemide results in greater diuresis and fewer renal complications[2]; however, this study excluded the sickest patients who had low blood pressure, renal failure, or required inotropic support. Furthermore, the GAS may not be a sufficiently sensitive test because it uses the area under the curve of a visual analog scale.

There appeared to be no differences between the different doses and the different rates of administration affecting the primary end points. But there may still be some evidence here to support the use of higher doses of loop diuretics, at least insofar as it may improve subjective symptoms and produce greater volume excretion, although there may be a temporary worsening of renal function at the higher doses. Overall, there appeared to be little benefit from continuous infusion versus bolus dosing when looking at the primary end points. Whether adding a bolus prior to infusion, as is often done in clinical practice, would have made a difference was not addressed by these investigators.

M. Klein, MD, JD

References

1. Felker GM, O'Connor GM, Braunwald E. Loop diuretics in acute decompensated heart failure: necessary? Evil? A necessary evil? *Circ Heart Fail*. 2009;2:56-62.
2. Salvador DR, Rey NR, Ramos GC, Punzalan FE. Continuous infusion versus bolus injection of loop diuretics in congestive heart failure. *Cochrane Database Syst Rev*. 2005;(3). CD003178.

Got Calcium? Welcome to the Calcium-Alkali Syndrome

Patel AM, Goldfarb S (Univ of Pennsylvania School of Medicine, Philadelphia)
J Am Soc Nephrol 21:1440-1443, 2010

We recommend changing the name of the milk-alkali syndrome to the calcium-alkali syndrome, because the new terminology better reflects the shifting epidemiology and understanding of this disorder. The calcium-alkali syndrome is now the third most common cause of hospital admission for hypercalcemia, and those at greatest risk are postmenopausal or pregnant women. The incidence of the calcium-alkali syndrome is growing in large part as a result of the widespread use of over-the-counter calcium and vitamin D supplements. Advertising for treatment or prevention of osteoporosis has long encouraged this use. Intricate mechanisms mediating the calcium-alkali syndrome depend on interplay among intestine, kidney, and bone. New insights regarding its pathogenesis focus on the key role of calcium-sensing receptors and TRPV5 channels in the modulation of renal calcium excretion. Restoring extracellular blood volume, increasing GFR and calcium excretion, and discontinuing calcium supplementation provide best treatment.

▶ All practitioners should be aware of this syndrome, which has supplanted the prior hypercalcemia syndrome known as the milk-alkali syndrome. As noted by the authors, hypercalcemia, related to overabundance of calcium intake, is estimated to have an incidence of 8% to 38%[1,2] and is now the third most common cause of hospitalizations related to hypercalcemia. Prior to the advent of H-2 blockers, the etiology of the milk-alkali syndrome was linked to the Sippy diet, which was a standard therapy for peptic ulcer disease. The Sippy diet consisted of milk, eggs, and cream, taken on the hour, and sodium bicarbonate, bismuth subcarbonate, and calcium-magnesium taken on the half hour.[3] Peptic ulcer disease and the milk-alkali syndrome related to the Sippy diet were more common in men.

TABLE 1.—Amount of Elemental Calcium in Various Supplements

Type	Trade Name	Elemental Calcium (mg)	Vitamin D (IU)
Calcium carbonate	Caltrate	600	400
	Centrum	200	400
	Centrum Ultra Women's	500	800
	Rolaids Extra Strength	471	
	Os-Cal	500	
	Tums	200	
	Tums Ultra	400	
	Viactiv	500	
Calcium citrate	Citracal Regular with Vitamin D	250	200
Calcium acetate	Phoslo	167	

The current generation's syndrome is more common in patients with chronic renal disease on dialysis, patients with eating disorders, pregnancy, and post-menopausal women taking high amounts of calcium to ward off osteoporosis. The classic features of the calcium-alkali syndrome include a history of excessive ingestion of calcium and often absorbable alkali, which together produce a triad of hypercalcemia, metabolic alkalosis, and varying degrees of renal insufficiency. Unlike the prior milk-alkali syndrome, in which the phosphate content of the Sippy diet led to hyperphosphatemia, in the calcium-alkali syndrome, the phosphate-binding effects of the ingested calcium often lead to hypophosphatemia.

The calcium-alkali syndrome is usually associated with a calcium intake in the range of 4 g/d; however, it has been reported with much lower levels (1-2 g/d) of calcium use. Table 1 demonstrates that these levels of calcium intake can be easily achieved with the use of over-the-counter supplements alone or with the use of supplements together with the ingestion of readily available (and heavily advertised) calcium-fortified foods and juices. Once diagnosed, the syndrome is treated with saline hydration (to reduce calcium reabsorption and repair the volume depletion related to hypercalcemia) and with dietary counseling, which should aim to maintain the daily calcium intake in the 1- to 1.5-g range.

R. Garrick, MD

References

1. Picolos MK, Lavis VR, Orlander PR. Milk-alkali syndrome is a major cause of hypercalcemia among non-end-stage renal disease (non-ESRD) inpatients. *Clin Endocrinol (Oxf)*. 2005;63:566-576.
2. Beall DP, Scofield RH. Milk-alkali syndrome associated with calcium carbonate consumption. Report of 7 patients with parathyroid hormone levels and an estimate of prevalence among patients hospitalized with hypercalcemia. *Medicine (Baltimore)*. 1995;74:89-96.
3. Sippy BW. Gastric and duodenal ulcer: Medical cure by efficient removal of gastric juice corrosion. *JAMA*. 1983;250:2192-2197.

Bevacizumab Increases Risk for Severe Proteinuria in Cancer Patients
Wu S, Kim C, Baer L, et al (Stony Brook Univ Med Ctr, NY; et al)
J Am Soc Nephrol 21:1381-1389, 2010

Treatment with the chemotherapeutic agent bevacizumab, a humanized mAb that neutralizes vascular endothelial growth factor, can lead to proteinuria and renal damage. The risk factors and clinical outcomes of renal adverse events are not well understood. We performed a systematic review and meta-analysis of published randomized, controlled trials to assess the overall risk for severe proteinuria with bevacizumab. We analyzed data from 16 studies comprising 12,268 patients with a variety of tumors. The incidence of high-grade (grade 3 or 4) proteinuria with bevacizumab was 2.2% (95% confidence interval [CI] 1.2 to 4.3%). Compared with chemotherapy alone, bevacizumab combined with chemotherapy significantly increased the risk for high-grade proteinuria (relative risk 4.79; 95% CI 2.71 to 8.46) and nephrotic syndrome (relative risk 7.78; 95% CI 1.80 to 33.62); higher dosages of bevacizumab associated with increased risk for proteinuria. Regarding tumor type, renal cell carcinoma associated with the highest risk (cumulative incidence 10.2%). We did not detect a significant difference between platinum- and non–platinum-based concurrent chemotherapy with regard to risk for high-grade proteinuria ($P = 0.39$). In conclusion, the addition of bevacizumab to chemotherapy significantly increases the risk for high-grade proteinuria and nephrotic syndrome.

▶ Previous studies[1] have highlighted the role of the tumor angiogenesis factor vascular endothelial growth factor (VEGF) in endothelial function in the setting of chronic kidney disease (CKD). The demonstration that bevacizumab, a humanized antibody that neutralizes VEGF, is useful for the treatment of many cancers, including colon, lung, breast, brain, and kidney, has resulted in its widespread clinical use. With increased use, it has become apparent that the drug can be associated with multiple renal side effects. The present meta-analysis study surveyed 12 268 patients drawn from 16 randomized controlled trials. Bevacizumab was given to 6482 patients and compared with 5786 controls. Proteinuria was not noted as a baseline finding in any of the patients, and all had "adequate" baseline renal, hepatic, and hematologic function. The meta-analysis demonstrated that proteinuria occurred in approximately 13% of the patients, and approximately 2% of the population developed high-grade proteinuria (urine protein > 3.5 g per 24 hours, dipstick of 4+, or nephrotic syndrome). Proteinuria occurred most commonly in patients being treated for renal cell cancer, and the development of severe proteinuria appeared to be dose related. Given the frequency and potential seriousness of this complication, it is now recommended that the agent be discontinued if the urinary protein exceeds 2 g per day.

R. Garrick, MD

Reference

1. Di Marco GS, Reuter S, Hillebrand U, et al. The soluble VEGF receptor sFlt1 contributes to endothelial dysfunction in CKD. *J Am Soc Nephrol.* 2009;20: 2235-2245.

Plasma Resistin Levels Associate with Risk For Hypertension among Nondiabetic Women

Zhang L, Curhan GC, Forman JP (Brigham and Women's Hosp and Harvard Med School, Boston, MA)

J Am Soc Nephrol 21:1185-1191, 2010

Emerging evidence suggests a role for resistin in inflammation and vascular dysfunction, which may contribute to the pathogenesis of hypertension, but the association between resistin levels and incident hypertension is unknown. We examined the association between plasma resistin levels and the risk for incident hypertension among 872 women without a history of hypertension or diabetes from the Nurses' Health Study. We identified 361 incident cases of hypertension during 14 years of follow-up. After adjustment for potential confounders, resistin levels in the highest tertile conferred a 75% higher risk for hypertension than the lowest tertile (relative risk [RR] 1.75; 95% confidence interval [CI] 1.19 to 2.56). Further adjustment for other adipokines did not change the RR substantially. In stratified analysis, resistin levels in the highest tertile significantly increased the risk for hypertension among women aged ≥55 years (adjusted RR 2.40; 95% CI 1.55 to 3.73) but not among women aged <55 years (adjusted RR 0.64; 95% CI 0.25 to 1.62). In a subset analysis of 362 women who also had measurements of inflammatory and endothelial biomarkers, plasma resistin levels significantly correlated with IL-6, soluble TNF receptor 2, intercellular adhesion molecule 1, vascular adhesion molecule 1, and E-selectin after controlling for age and body mass index. After further adjustment for these biomarkers and C-reactive protein, resistin levels remained significantly associated with incident hypertension. In conclusion, higher plasma resistin levels independently associate with an increased risk for incident hypertension among women without diabetes.

▶ Essential hypertension remains a leading cause of cardiovascular and renal morbidity. The etiology of this disease remains multifactorial and incompletely understood. Resistin, a polypeptide found mainly in adipose tissue of rodents, was initially thought to provide a link between obesity and insulin resistance.[1] But its nearly exclusive expression by inflammatory cells in humans suggests a role for resistin in inflammatory states. It has been shown both in vitro and in vivo in animal models to stimulate proinflammatory cytokines. Because hypertension has been hypothesized to be an inflammatory disorder,[2] the role of resistin in this disorder has attracted much interest. Some data exist suggesting a correlation between plasma resistin (PR) levels and the risk of hypertension.[3] This study examined the value of PR levels in predicting the incidence of hypertension. The investigators evaluated control subjects in a nested case-control diabetes study taken from the Nurses Health Study cohort in which 872 normotensive nondiabetic women were followed up for 14 years. Secondary analysis of inflammatory markers was performed on 362 participants who had plasma and other biomarkers measured. In the primary analysis, the PR levels and other adipokines were evaluated and stratified by tertile of resistin.

The investigators discovered that the higher PR levels were found in the younger, more sedentary women with higher body mass index (BMI). Smoking was also associated with higher PR levels. Although other adipokine levels were elevated in the women with higher PR, this correlation did not persist after adjustment for BMI. The relative risk of incident hypertension for the highest tertile of PR was 1.79. This elevated risk was most pronounced in the subjects older than 55 years. There was no correlation between BMI and the risk of incident hypertension irrespective of the tertile of PR.

In the secondary analysis, the investigators found significant correlations between PR and other biomarkers of endothelial dysfunction, such as interleukin-6, tumor necrosis factor R2, intercellular adhesion molecule 1, vascular adhesion molecule 1, and E selectin. A significant correlation of PR and C-reactive protein was not found after controlling for BMI and age. However, as shown in Fig 1 in the original article, the relationship between PR and hypertension persisted even when evaluating all these biomarkers in multivariate analysis, suggesting that other unmeasured factors may be contributing to the correlation of resistin to incident hypertension.

This study is the first prospective study to make this connection between plasma resistin and incident hypertension. The correlation with other inflammatory markers suggests a possible causative role. Further studies could lead to new avenues of therapy for essential hypertension.

M. Klein, MD, JD

References

1. Lazar MA. Resistin- and Obesity-associated metabolic diseases. *Horm Metab Res.* 2007;39:710-716.
2. Sesso HD, Buring JE, Rifai N, Blake GJ, Gaziano JM, Ridker PM. C-reactive protein and the risk of developing hypertension. *JAMA.* 2003;290:2945-2951.
3. Takata Y, Osawa H, Kurata M, et al. Hyperresistinemia is associated with coexistence of hypertension and type 2 diabetes. *Hypertension.* 2008;51:534-539.

31 Chronic Kidney Disease and Clinical Nephrology

Regional Variation in Health Care Intensity and Treatment Practices for End-stage Renal Disease in Older Adults
O'Hare AM, Rodriguez RA, Hailpern SM, et al (Univ of Washington, Seattle; Epidemiologist, Katonah, NY; et al)
JAMA 304:180-186, 2010

Context.—An increasing number of older adults are being treated for end-stage renal disease (ESRD) with long-term dialysis.

Objectives.—To determine how ESRD treatment practices for older adults vary across regions with differing end-of-life intensity of care.

Design, Setting, and Participants.—Retrospective observational study using a national ESRD registry to identify a cohort of 41 420 adults (of white or black race), aged 65 years or older, who started long-term dialysis or received a kidney transplant between June 1, 2005, and May 31, 2006. Regional end-of-life intensity of care was defined using an index from the Dartmouth Atlas of Healthcare.

Main Outcome Measures.—Incidence of treated ESRD (dialysis or transplant), preparedness for ESRD (under the care of a nephrologist, having a fistula [vs graft or catheter] at time of hemodialysis initiation), and end-of-life care practices.

Results.—Among whites, the incidence of ESRD was progressively higher in regions with greater intensity of care and this trend was most pronounced at older ages. Among blacks, a similar relationship was present only at advanced ages (men aged ≥80 years and women aged ≥85 years). Patients living in regions in the highest compared with lowest quintile of end-of-life intensity of care were less likely to be under the care of a nephrologist before the onset of ESRD (62.3% [95% confidence interval {CI}, 61.3%-63.3%] vs 71.1% [95% CI, 69.9%-72.2%], respectively) and less likely to have a fistula (vs graft or catheter) at the time of hemodialysis initiation (11.2% [95% CI, 10.6%-11.8%] vs 16.9% [95% CI, 15.9%-17.8%]). Among patients who died within 2 years of ESRD onset (n=21 190), those living in regions in the highest compared with lowest quintile of end-of-life intensity of care were less likely to have discontinued dialysis before death (22.2% [95%

CI, 21.1%-23.4%] vs 44.3% [95% CI, 42.5%-46.1%], respectively), less likely to have received hospice care (20.7% [95% CI, 19.5%-21.9%] vs 33.5% [95% CI, 31.7%-35.4%]), and more likely to have died in the hospital (67.8% [95% CI, 66.5%-69.1%] vs 50.3% [95% CI, 48.5%-52.1%]). These differences persisted in adjusted analyses.

Conclusion.—There are pronounced regional differences in treatment practices for ESRD in older adults that are not explained by differences in patient characteristics.

▶ Most dialysis patients are now older than 65 years,[1] and the care of these patients, who have multiple comorbidities, has become increasingly complex. Available data regarding other disease conditions[2] suggests that there is wide geographic variability in Medicare spending across the United States. The authors sought to assess if regional variations exist that might influence the delivery of dialysis care. The findings are significant because as outcome-based comparative effectiveness research methodology becomes more advanced, it will be especially important for us to understand how elements independent of basic clinical medicine influence clinical decisions and patient outcomes. The authors used the national End-Stage Renal Disease (ESRD) registry to identify a cohort of 41 420 adult patients age 65 years or older who initiated long-term dialysis or received the renal transplant between June 2005 and May 2006. The main outcome measurements included the measures taken to prepare for the initiation of dialysis therapy and practice patterns regarding end-of-life care.

The results are quite interesting, as they suggest that regional patterns influence end-of-life decisions and treatment practices and that these issues appear to be independent of the patient's condition and comorbid factors. The hospital referrals in areas with the highest end-of-life expenditure index were more likely to include metropolitan areas and had the highest density of specialists, including nephrologists and vascular surgeons, and had the greatest number of acute care hospital beds. Somewhat surprising was that despite the availability of specialists, some geographic regions with higher intensity of end-of-life care have a higher incidence of ESRD but less preparedness for the initiation of dialysis. In addition, patients living in the high-intensity care areas were less likely to have discontinued dialysis and less likely to receive hospice care; they were more likely to have died in a hospital setting compared with patients in lower intensity-of-care regions.

The authors conclude that there is "substantial unexplained regional variation in the care of older adults with end-stage renal disease, both prior to ESRD onset and prior to death." There are many possible explanations for these regional differences, and as a community of health care providers, we should take steps to better understand how these factors influence our care patterns and our ability to engage in shared decision making with our patients. For this to be effectively accomplished, constructive physician and patient education is required, and The Renal Physicians Association's clinical practice guidelines regarding shared decision making in the initiation and withdrawal from dialysis may offer useful clinical guidance.[2]

R. Garrick, MD

References

1. US Renal Data System. *USRDS 2010 Annual Data Report: Atlas of Chronic Kidney Disease and End-Stage Renal Disease in the United States.* Bethesda, MD: National Institutes of Health, National Institute of Diabetes and Digestive and Kidney Diseases; 2010. http://www.usrds.org/adr.htm. Accessed April 21, 2011.
2. *Shared Decision-Making in the Appropriate Initiation Withdrawal of Dialysis. Clinical Practice Guideline.* 2nd ed. Rockville, MD: Renal Physicians Association; 2010.

A Randomized, Controlled Trial of Early versus Late Initiation of Dialysis
Cooper BA, for the IDEAL Study (Royal North Shore Hosp, Sydney, Australia; et al)
N Engl J Med 363:609-619, 2010

Background.—In clinical practice, there is considerable variation in the timing of the initiation of maintenance dialysis for patients with stage V chronic kidney disease, with a worldwide trend toward early initiation. In this study, conducted at 32 centers in Australia and New Zealand, we examined whether the timing of the initiation of maintenance dialysis influenced survival among patients with chronic kidney disease.

Methods.—We randomly assigned patients 18 years of age or older with progressive chronic kidney disease and an estimated glomerular filtration rate (GFR) between 10.0 and 15.0 ml per minute per 1.73 m² of body-surface area (calculated with the use of the Cockcroft—Gault equation) to planned initiation of dialysis when the estimated GFR was 10.0 to 14.0 ml per minute (early start) or when the estimated GFR was 5.0 to 7.0 ml per minute (late start). The primary outcome was death from any cause.

Results.—Between July 2000 and November 2008, a total of 828 adults (mean age, 60.4 years; 542 men and 286 women; 355 with diabetes) underwent randomization, with a median time to the initiation of dialysis of 1.80 months (95% confidence interval [CI], 1.60 to 2.23) in the early-start group and 7.40 months (95% CI, 6.23 to 8.27) in the late-start group. A total of 75.9% of the patients in the late-start group initiated dialysis when the estimated GFR was above the target of 7.0 ml per minute, owing to the development of symptoms. During a median follow-up period of 3.59 years, 152 of 404 patients in the early-start group (37.6%) and 155 of 424 in the late-start group (36.6%) died (hazard ratio with early initiation, 1.04; 95% CI, 0.83 to 1.30; P = 0.75). There was no significant difference between the groups in the frequency of adverse events (cardiovascular events, infections, or complications of dialysis).

Conclusions.—In this study, planned early initiation of dialysis in patients with stage V chronic kidney disease was not associated with an improvement in survival or clinical outcomes. (Funded by the National

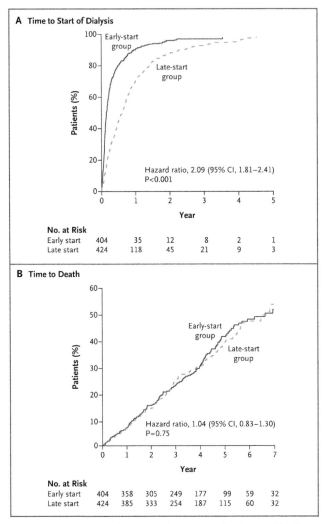

FIGURE 2.—Kaplan—Meier Curves for Time to the Initiation of Dialysis and for Time to Death. The data for time to the initiation of dialysis (Panel A) were censored at the time of death, transplantation, or withdrawal of consent or at the time a patient transferred to a nonparticipating hospital, emigrated, or could not be contacted. The curves for time to death (Panel B) are truncated at 7 years of follow-up and a cumulative hazard of 60%. (Reprinted from Cooper BA, for the IDEAL Study. A randomized, controlled trial of early versus late initiation of dialysis. *N Engl J Med.* 2010;363:609-619. © 2010 Massachusetts Medical Society.)

Health and Medical Research Council of Australia and others; Australian New Zealand Clinical Trials Registry number, 12609000266268.)

▶ Most dialysis patients are now over the age of 65[1] and have a number of comorbid conditions. The study by Cooper and colleagues is important because it is the first randomized controlled trial to evaluate the glomerular filtration rate versus the timing of the initiation of dialysis. The results show that a great deal of judgment is necessary for determining if and when to initiate dialysis in patients with stage V kidney disease. Patients were eligible for inclusion if they had progressive chronic kidney disease and a glomerular filtration rate (GFR) between 10 and 15 mL/min/ 1.73 m^2. Of the 828 adults enrolled, 355 had diabetes. The study evaluated whether planned initiation of dialysis based on a GFR of 10 to 14 mL/min achieved a better outcome than did continuing medical management until the estimated GFR was between 5 and 7 mL/min. The primary outcome was death from any cause, and secondary outcomes included cardiovascular events, cardiovascular death (nonfatal myocardial infarction, nonfatal stroke, transient ischemic attack, or new onset angina), infectious events, and complications of dialysis (Fig 2). All patients received dietary advice, and attention was given to the management of anemia, hyperphosphatemia, and hypertension. The data demonstrated that early planned initiation of dialysis in stage V chronic kidney disease did not result in improved survival or clinical outcomes.

All patients received close clinical follow-up, including monitoring of nutritional status. Almost 76% of the patients in the late-start group became symptomatic and required dialysis when the estimated GFR was above the target level of 7 mL/min. The results failed to support the concept that outcomes are improved by initiating dialysis when renal function reaches a particular predetermined level as is currently suggested by several existing guidelines.[2-4] However, it is important to understand that the patients required close clinical follow-up and that a substantial number of the patients did require intervention before reaching the low target GFR. Together, the results demonstrate that as long as close monitoring by appropriately trained physicians is in place, the trend to early-initiation dialysis likely substantially increases the cost of care but does not significantly improve outcomes. These findings may be especially meaningful for elderly patients as they suggest that, provided that close monitoring is ongoing, the complexity of thrice-weekly dialysis may be reasonably delayed without adversely affecting their expected survival.

R. Garrick, MD

References

1. Renal Data System US. *USRDS 2010 Annual Data Report: Atlas of Chronic Kidney Disease and End-Stage Renal Disease in the United States.* Bethesda, MD: National Institutes of Health, National Institute of Diabetes and Digestive and Kidney Diseases; 2010.
2. Hemodialysis Adequacy 2006 Work Group. Clinical practice guidelines for hemodialysis adequacy, update 2006. *Am J Kidney Dis.* 2006;48:S2-S90.
3. Peritoneal Dialysis Adequacy Work Group. Clinical practice guidelines for peritoneal dialysis adequacy. *Am J Kidney Dis.* 2006;48:S98-S129.
4. Kelly J, Stanley M, Harris D. The CARI guidelines. Acceptance into dialysis guidelines. *Nephrology (Carlton).* 2005;10:S46-S60.

Association between estimated glomerular filtration rate at initiation of dialysis and mortality

Clark WF, Na Y, Rosansky SJ, et al (Univ of Western Ontario, London, Ontario, Canada; Canadian Inst for Health Information, Toronto, Ontario, Canada; William Jennings Bryan Dorn VA Hosp, Columbia, SC; et al)
CMAJ 183:47-53, 2011

Background.—Recent studies have reported a trend toward earlier initiation of dialysis (i.e., at higher levels of glomerular filtration rate) and an association between early initiation and increased risk of death. We examined trends in initiation of hemodialysis within Canada and compared the risk of death between patients with early and late initiation of dialysis.

Methods.—The analytic cohort consisted of 25 910 patients at least 18 years of age who initiated hemodialysis, as identified from the Canadian Organ Replacement Register (2001−2007). We defined the initiation of dialysis as early if the estimated glomerular filtration rate was greater than 10.5 mL/min per 1.73 m². We fitted time-dependent proportional-hazards Cox models to compare the risk of death between patients with early and late initiation of dialysis.

Results.—Between 2001 and 2007, mean estimated glomerular filtration rate at initiation of dialysis increased from 9.3 (standard deviation [SD] 5.2) to 10.2 (SD 7.1) ($p < 0.001$), and the proportion of early starts rose from 28% (95% confidence interval [CI] 27%−30%) to 36% (95% CI 34%−37%). Mean glomerular filtration rate was 15.5 (SD 7.7) mL/min per 1.73 m² among those with early initiation and 7.1 (SD 2.0) mL/min per 1.73 m² among those with late initiation. The unadjusted hazard ratio (HR) for mortality with early relative to late initiation was 1.48 (95% CI 1.43−1.54). The HR decreased to 1.18 (95% CI 1.13−1.23) after adjustment for demographic characteristics, serum albumin, primary cause of end-stage renal disease, vascular access type, comorbidities, late referral and transplant status. The mortality differential between early and late initiation per 1000 patient-years narrowed after one year of follow-up, but never crossed and began widening again after 24 months of follow-up. The differences were significant at 6, 12, 30 and 36 months.

Interpretation.—In Canada, dialysis is being initiated at increasingly higher levels of glomerular filtration rate. A higher glomerular filtration rate at initiation of dialysis is associated with an increased risk of death that is not fully explained by differences in baseline characteristics.

▶ This article was included because the addition of the estimated glomerular filtration rate (eGFR) to most standardized laboratory reports has resulted in an increased awareness of kidney disease. This fact, coupled with the 2006 National Kidney Foundation (NKF) guidelines,[1] which suggested that dialysis be considered for patients with an eGFR of < 15 mL/min/1.73 m², has heightened interest in the timing of the initiation of dialysis. Based on data from the Canadian Organ Replacement Register, and using the abbreviated modified diet in renal disease formula (MDRD), the current study examines the timing of the initiation dialysis in 25 901 adult patients between the years 2001 and 2007. The findings of this observational study suggested that the adjusted hazard ratio for mortality was higher following early initiation of dialysis (eGFR rate > 10.5 mL/min/1.73 m^2) compared with those with late initiation dialysis (eGFR < 10.5 mL/min/ 1.73 m^2). This increased hazard ratio persisted after adjustment for demographic characteristics, such as serum albumin level, the vascular access type, delay in referral and multiple comorbidity adjustments, including coronary artery disease, vascular disease, diabetes, hypertension, pulmonary disease, and other underlying disorders, such as malignancy. So, unlike the IDEAL trial, also reviewed here, the current observational study suggests that early initiation of dialysis can be harmful. A few caveats are in order. First, the GFR was based on the MDRD, and other studies, such as those by Grootendorst et al,[2] suggest that this equation has not been fully validated for patients with a glomerular filtration rate of less than 20 ml/min. In addition, even though comorbidities were considered, the impact of those comorbidities on a given patient cannot be directly assessed. Thus, dialysis may have been initiated earlier in patients in whom the underlying comorbidities were associated with greater clinical symptomatology. The authors raise the possibilities that cardiac events related to dialysis itself may have contributed to the increased hazard ratio, but this cannot be answered from observational outcomes. Nonetheless, this interesting registry study, coupled with the results of the randomized controlled IDEAL trial by Cooper and colleagues indicated that the treatment guidelines such as those of the NKF must not be viewed as therapeutic dogma. Rather, until more controlled studies are available, the decision to initiate dialysis must be carefully individualized and include, where possible, a data-driven risk-benefit and outcome analysis with thoughtful dialogue between a well-trained nephrologist and his or her patient.

R. Garrick, MD

References

1. National Kidney Foundation. KDOQI clinical practice guidelines and clinical practice recommendations for 2006 updates: hemodialysis adequacy, peritoneal dialysis adequacy and vascular access. *Am J Kidney Dis.* 2006;48:S1-S322.
2. Grootendorst DC, Michels WM, Richardson JD, et al. The MDRD formula does not reflect GFR in ESRD patients. *Nephrol Dial Transplant.* 2011;26:1932-1937.

Predialysis Nephrology Care of Older Patients Approaching End-stage Renal Disease

Winkelmayer WC, Liu J, Chertow GM, et al (Brigham and Women's Hosp, Boston, MA; Stanford Univ School of Medicine, Palo Alto, CA)
Arch Intern Med 171:1371-1378, 2011

Background.—Little is known about trends in the timing of first nephrology consultation and associated outcomes among older patients initiating dialysis.

Methods.—Data from patients aged 67 years or older who initiated dialysis in the United States between January 1, 1996, and December 31, 2006, were stratified by timing of the earliest identifiable nephrology visit. Trends of earlier nephrology consultation were formally examined in light of concurrently changing case mix and juxtaposed with trends in 1-year mortality rates after initiation of dialysis.

Results.—Among 323 977 older patients initiating dialysis, the proportion of patients receiving nephrology care less than 3 months before initiation of dialysis decreased from 49.6% (in 1996) to 34.7% (in 2006). Patients initiated dialysis with increasingly preserved kidney function, from a mean estimated glomerular filtration rate of 8 mL/min/1.73 m^2 in 1996 to 12 mL/min/1.73 m^2 in 2006. Patients were less anemic in later years, which was partly attributable to increased use of erythropoiesis-stimulating agents, and fewer used peritoneal dialysis as the initial modality. During the same period, crude 1-year mortality rates remained unchanged (annual change in mortality rate, +0.2%; 95% confidence interval, 0% to +0.4%). Adjustment for changes in demographic and comorbidity patterns yielded estimated annual reductions in 1-year mortality rates of 0.9% (95% confidence interval, 0.7% to 1.1%), which were explained only partly by concurrent trends toward earlier nephrology consultation (annual mortality reduction after accounting for timing of nephrology care was attenuated to 0.4% [0.2% to 0.6%]).

Conclusions.—Despite significant trends toward earlier use of nephrology consultation among older patients approaching maintenance dialysis, we observed no material improvement in 1-year survival rates after dialysis initiation during the same time period (Table 1).

▶ At the risk of being viewed as self-serving, I included this article because I think it is important for internists and others to understand the context of the findings. Prior studies have shown that late nephrology referral is associated with lower survival on initiation of dialysis.[1] Other studies, such as the Fistula First initiative,[2] have demonstrated that early referral to a nephrologist increases the use of the fistula, which in turn is associated with improved survival during the initial phases of dialysis as compared with initiation of dialysis with an indwelling catheter. The current findings were drawn from the United States Renal Data System (USRDS) dialysis database and therefore reflect dialysis initiation in patients older than 65 years, and as noted in Table 1, on average, patients had several significant comorbidities, including diabetes, hypertension, congestive heart failure, coronary vascular disease, and cerebral vascular disease. Thus, it is unclear whether the timing of referral would have been expected to have a significant effect on mortality outcome for this elderly population. In addition, it should be appreciated that the staging criteria for chronic kidney disease and estimated glomerular filtration rate—based practice guidelines were not initiated until approximately 2002, and after acceptance, promulgation and clinical implementation required additional time.

A strength of the study is that the use of the USRDS database provides clear data regarding the timing of the referral to a nephrologist, but the study does

TABLE 1.—Characteristics of Older Patients Initiating Treatment for End-stage Renal Disease by Timing of First Nephrologist Consultation[a]

Characteristic	1996 Earlier (>3-24 mo)	1996 Later (≤3 mo)	2001 Earlier (>3-24 mo)	2001 Later (≤ 3 mo)	2006 Earlier (>3-24 mo)	2006 Later (≤3 mo)
Patients	11 983 (50.4)	11 794 (49.6)	15 614 (54.4)	13 083 (45.6)	21 227 (65.3)	11 302 (34.7)
Age, mean (SD), y	74.9 (5.6)	75.6 (5.9)	75.9 (5.9)	76.7 (6.2)	76.6 (6.2)	77.5 (6.5)
Female vs male sex	6024 (50.3)	5832 (49.5)	7744 (49.6)	6588 (50.4)	9910 (46.7)	5546 (49.1)
Race						
White	8825 (73.7)	9236 (78.3)	11 821 (75.7)	10 237 (78.3)	16 275 (76.7)	8915 (78.9)
African American	2810 (23.5)	2263 (19.2)	3355 (21.5)	2466 (18.9)	4220 (19.9)	1986 (17.6)
Asian American	279 (2.3)	198 (1.7)	336 (2.2)	267 (2.0)	607 (2.9)	306 (2.7)
Native American	69 (0.6)	97 (0.8)	102 (0.7)	113 (0.9)	125 (0.6)	92 (0.8)
Medicaid beneficiary, yes vs no	2262 (18.9)	2057 (17.4)	3052 (19.6)	2544 (19.5)	4237 (20.0)	2266 (20.1)
Region						
Northeast	2659 (22.2)	2743 (23.3)	3169 (20.3)	2490 (19.0)	4244 (20.0)	2030 (18.0)
Midwest	2751 (23.0)	3294 (27.9)	3613 (23.1)	3935 (30.1)	5421 (25.5)	3189 (28.2)
West	1585 (13.2)	1538 (13.0)	2033 (13.0)	1806 (13.8)	2915 (13.7)	1771 (15.7)
South	4895 (40.9)	4157 (35.3)	6658 (42.6)	4776 (36.5)	8510 (40.1)	4246 (37.6)
Other	93 (0.8)	62 (0.5)	141 (0.9)	76 (0.6)	137 (0.7)	66 (0.6)
Modality						
Center hemodialysis	9704 (81.0)	9448 (80.1)	13 147 (84.2)	10 722 (82.0)	18 126 (85.4)	9307 (82.4)
Peritoneal dialysis	1185 (9.9)	837 (7.1)	1045 (6.7)	506 (3.9)	1111 (5.2)	259 (2.3)
Undefined or other	1094 (9.1)	1509 (12.8)	1422 (9.1)	1855 (14.2)	1990 (9.4)	1736 (15.4)
Comorbidities						
Diabetes mellitus	7392 (61.7)	6507 (55.1)	10 890 (69.8)	7965 (60.9)	15 624 (73.6)	7195 (63.7)
Hypertension	11 475 (95.8)	10 697 (90.7)	15 278 (97.9)	12 221 (93.4)	20 990 (98.9)	10 688 (94.6)
Heart failure	9065 (75.7)	8692 (73.7)	11 913 (76.3)	9501 (72.6)	15 997 (75.4)	7815 (69.2)
Coronary artery disease	5835 (48.7)	5371 (45.5)	7687 (49.2)	5923 (45.3)	9655 (45.5)	4497 (39.8)
Cerebrovascular disease	3486 (29.1)	3239 (27.5)	4683 (30.0)	3654 (27.9)	6456 (30.4)	3025 (26.8)
Peripheral artery disease	5347 (44.6)	4904 (41.6)	7870 (50.4)	5813 (44.4)	11 735 (55.3)	5079 (44.9)
Chronic obstructive pulmonary disease	3507 (29.3)	3457 (29.3)	5123 (32.8)	4193 (32.1)	7941 (37.4)	3966 (35.1)
Cancer	1604 (13.3)	1701 (14.4)	2451 (15.7)	2248 (17.2)	3501 (16.5)	2072 (18.3)

[a]Data are presented as number (percentage) unless indicated otherwise. Percentages may not total 100 because of rounding.

not mention the frequency or care pattern of the nephrology follow-up. On the other hand, it is also fair to note that some accepted care patterns implemented prior to definitive study (such as therapy with erythropoietin agents and the early initiation of dialysis) have not been shown to necessarily improve outcome in every (or possibly, any) patient group. The findings clearly raise important questions that deserve careful scrutiny and controlled study. Meanwhile, we should also learn from our prior experiences and not generalize these findings to other age and comorbidity groups. Additionally, we should continue those activities such as early fistula placement when appropriate, phosphate control,[3] and blood pressure control[4] as we seek to reduce mortality in this at-risk population.

R. Garrick, MD

References

1. Avorn J, Bohn RL, Levy E, et al. Nephrologist care and mortality in patients with chronic renal insufficiency. *Arch Intern Med.* 2002;162:2002-2006.
2. Amedia CA Jr, Bolton WK, Cordray T, et al. Vascular access for HD: aligning payment with quality. *Semin Dial.* 2011;24:37-40.
3. Eddington H, Hoefield R, Sinha S, et al. Serum phosphate and mortality in patients with chronic kidney disease. *Clin J Am Soc Nephrol.* 2010;5:2251-2257.
4. Weiss JW, Johnson ES, Petrik A, Smith DH, Yang X, Thorp ML. Systolic blood pressure and mortality among older community-dwelling adults with CKD. *Am J Kidney Dis.* 2010;56:1062-1071.

PART FIVE

PULMONARY DISEASE

JAMES A. BARKER, MD

Introduction

Well, 2011 has almost passed us by. It has been another great year for medical literature. I highly encourage you to read all of the enclosed articles with comments from our field. They all have important new discoveries or contributions that we need to know.

Topical Summaries

ASTHMA AND CYSTIC FIBROSIS

For example, in asthma there is a wonderful article on a randomized placebo-controlled study of IV montelukast in the treatment of acute asthma. This showed significant improvement in pulmonary function during the first 2 hours of treatment. Reduction of bronchial constriction was seen in the first 10 minutes and post hoc analysis showed reduction in the need for hospitalization. This is a small study. A larger study will be required. However, this could portend an exciting new breakthrough. There have been few new therapies available in asthma therapy for more than a decade.

Another study showed tiotropium bromide added to an inhaled corticosteroid (ICS) is a step-up alternative to doubling of the ICS or the addition of salmeterol to ICS. Tiotropium improved symptoms in lung functions and equivalents to the addition of salmeterol to ICSs. Many of us are already doing this. I suspect this is already common practice. Now the science is catching up with the practice.

There is another great article on aerobic training showing that airway inflammation drops in asthmatic patients. I really love these nonpharmacologic approaches and, of course, everyone should become more active.

Please see the fifth article on location and duration of treatment of cystic fibrosis exacerbation. This shows that the venue of therapy doesn't matter. This should help many of us feel more comfortable with options for outpatient therapy for exacerbations. It feels like wasted resources to have patients sitting in the hospital only receiving IV antibiotics. This is really a nicely done article with great comments by Dr Willsie.

CHRONIC OBSTRUCTIVE PULMONARY DISEASE

Shu and co-authors from Taiwan demonstrate nicely that inhaled corticosteroids when used in chronic obstructive pulmonary disease (COPD) do have benefits, but they increased risk of tuberculosis in a susceptible population. This is not a trivial risk, either!

Another article by investigators at the University of Alabama showed that lung function in young adults predicts airflow obstruction 20 years later. This is a fascinating article that shows the importance of early detection. If COPD is diagnosed at a young age, there is a chance we can change disease trajectory.

I have become involved with chronic disease management programs or COPD. An article by Rice et al shows just how successful a chronic disease management program can be. This is done in several VA hospitals within their system. I encourage you to read this. COPD is one of the most expensive diseases we have in the United States, and chronic disease management can improve quality of life as well as decrease costs.

LUNG CANCER

Gomez and Sylvestry show the latest on endobronchial ultrasound for diagnosing and staging lung cancer in their very nice article. This has fast become the standard approach, although the literature is just now catching up.

In addition, see the article by Edell and Krier-Morrow about navigational bronchoscopy. This is another high-tech technique that many of our centers are using. It is nice to have more data on how good this is and whether it actually works. Coupled with navigational bronchoscopy can be the placement of fiducial markers to allow stereotactic body radiation for inoperable early stage cancers. Obviously, in our field of Pulmonary Medicine, we are going to have some patients who are just too ill for surgery. These patients can now be cured by respiratory gated high-dose radiation therapy, particularly when coupled with exact markers from the 3D simulation. Timmerman and partners demonstrate the utility of this technique.

Palliative care is steadily improving the quality of life for patients. There is a must-read article by Timmall et al from Massachusetts General Hospital about early palliative care for patients with metastatic small cell lung cancer. Suffice it to say that early palliative care was highly beneficial. I predict that this will become the standard of care soon.

PLEURAL, INTERSTITIAL LUNG, AND PULMONARY VASCULAR DISEASE

Please see the great article on cryptogenic organizing pneumonia (COP) CT findings in 22 patients over time. This is a very useful article since many of us mistakenly believe that COP demonstrates universally round alveolar infiltrates. Reality is different, however; there can actually be a potpourri of findings. The following article studying the use of bosentan to improve hand perfusion in scleroderma was fascinating to me. I've had patients where one therapy would worsen hand ischemia and the other would worsen other findings. An effective therapy is great news for these patients.

In pleural disease, British Thoracic Society guidelines have been released and are really quite useful. They are synopsized here. In addition, bedside ultrasonography is now being used for many things. See the nice article by Hoffman about using bedside ultrasonography in suspected pulmonary embolism.

There has been a movement toward acute embolectomy for massive pulmonary embolism. Please see the article here by Borha et al discussing this. Saleh, Matta, and partners have done us a great service of showing the fact that venous embolism does occur in chronic liver disease. I am sure that many others hold the same ill-conceived view that I do that auto anticoagulation is protective. However, that is not the case. I encourage everyone to read this important article.

COMMUNITY-ACQUIRED PNEUMONIA

Rello et al have some useful lessons for us on why persons with bacteremic pneumococcal pneumonia have worse disease and what may be going on with worsening prognosis in health care—associated pneumonia versus community-acquired pneumonia. Shandra et al have done a nice multi-center analysis of the emergency dept diagnosis of pneumonia.

LUNG TRANSPLANTATION

An important article has been published by Cleveland Clinic investigators about whether lung transplantation should be done on patients who are already on mechanical ventilators. This comes up frequently as families and patients ask for this rescue therapy. This very real scenario is even more apropos now that extracorporeal membrane oxygenation (ECMO) is offered frequently. Unfortunately, it remains unclear as to whether this is really the best thing to do. An accompanying article by Weiss et al is very helpful in identifying who will be long-term survivors. I think this should guide us in a large degree. After all, long-term survival should be the primary goal in a society with limited resources.

SLEEP DISORDERS

Dr Shirley Jones has supplied us with a number of great articles and I encourage you to read all of them. For example, the article by Marin et al about outcomes in patients with COPD and obstructive sleep apnea (OSA) and the overlap syndrome is a must-read for people in pulmonary medicine. These patients are more complex, more ill, require more oxygen, and have more pulmonary hypertension than patients who have one disorder but not both. Similarly, look at the next article about the impact of untreated OSA on type 2 diabetes glucose control. As expected, untreated OSA makes it difficult to have good glucose control.

The article by Losano et al on CPAP therapy on resistant hypertension is an important one as well. We always generalize and tell patients that hypertension will get better with CPAP therapy. This study directly addresses this. A good therapy affect was seen.

A nice article by Bhatta Charjee et al about removing tonsils for childhood OSA is likewise a must-read for those of us who practice sleep medicine and frequently see children. We routinely refer patients for tonsillectomy, and this article addresses results head on. It does show, surprisingly enough, that the results are not as good as we all think. Obviously, this has impact for follow-up of the patients.

CRITICAL CARE MEDICINE

The Critical Care articles are ones that I specifically picked. I believe they are all important for you to read. Each one of them has useful import for daily practice. Airway pressure release ventilation (APRV) is commonly used, but there is little evidence. Maxwell and co-authors have contributed a useful study showing equal efficacy to acute respiratory distress syndrome (ARDS) net low tidal volume technique—at least in patients with trauma induced ARDS/ALI. In addition, the next article to that outlines the horrible experience of H1N1 influenza leading to refractory ARDS and pneumonia.

In short, this has been another great year of reading medical literature and distilling it to share with you all. I hope that you read each and every article and come away refreshed and educated!

James A. Barker, MD

32 Asthma and Cystic Fibrosis

A randomized placebo-controlled study of intravenous montelukast for the treatment of acute asthma
Camargo CA Jr, Gurner DM, Smithline HA, et al (Harvard Med School, Boston, MA; Merck Res Laboratories, Rahway, NJ; Tufts Univ School of Medicine, Springfield, MA; et al)
J Allergy Clin Immunol 125:374-380, 2010

Background.—Current treatments for acute asthma provide inadequate benefit for some patients. Intravenous montelukast may complement existent therapies.

Objective.—To evaluate efficacy of intravenous montelukast as adjunctive therapy for acute asthma.

Methods.—A total of 583 adults with acute asthma were treated with standard care during a $\leq$60-minute screening period. Patients with FEV_1 $\leq$50% predicted were randomly allocated to intravenous montelukast 7 mg (n = 291) or placebo (n = 292) in addition to standard care. This double-blind treatment period lasted until a decision for discharge, hospital admission, or discontinuation from the study. The primary efficacy endpoint was the time-weighted average change in FEV_1 during 60 minutes after drug administration. Secondary endpoints included the time-weighted average change in FEV_1 at various intervals (10-120 minutes) and percentage of patients with treatment failure (defined as hospitalization or lack of decision to discharge by 3 hours postadministration).

Results.—Montelukast significantly increased FEV_1 at 60 minutes postdose; the difference between change from baseline for placebo (least-squares mean of 0.22 L; 95% CI, 0.17, 0.27) and montelukast (0.32 L; 95% CI, 0.27, 0.37) was 0.10 L (95% CI, 0.04, 0.16). Similar improvements in FEV_1-related variables were seen at all time points (all P <.05). Although treatment failure did not differ between groups (OR 0.92; 95% CI, 0.63, 1.34), a prespecified subgroup analysis suggests likely benefit for intravenous montelukast at US sites.

Conclusion.—Intravenous montelukast added to standard care in adults with acute asthma produced significant relief of airway obstruction

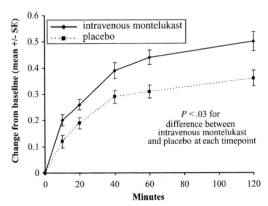

FIGURE 2.—Change from baseline in FEV$_1$ (L) over time (means ± SEs). (Reprinted from Camargo Jr CA, Gurner DM, Smithline HA, et al. A randomized placebo-controlled study of intravenous montelukast for the treatment of acute asthma. *J Allergy Clin Immunol*. 2010;125:374-380, with permission from American Academy of Allergy, Asthma & Immunology.)

throughout the 2 hours after administration, with an onset of action as early as 10 minutes (Fig 2).

▶ Acute asthma exacerbations are a harbinger of poorly controlled asthma and account for large numbers of emergency department visits annually. Significant hospitalizations result from patients whose acute asthma exacerbations fail to respond to standard asthma therapy in the emergency department setting. Hospitalizations related to acute uncontrolled asthma are associated with significant morbidity and mortality. Montelukast, a leukotriene modifier available for some time as an oral agent, has been reported to have potential efficacy in acute asthma.[1] This investigation used montelukast administered intravenously to patients with acute asthma in this double-blinded, randomized, placebo-controlled, multinational study. Demographics of subjects were not statistically different between treated and placebo groups. Fig 2 demonstrates change in forced expiratory volume 1 (FEV$_1$) over time; statistically significant, although not clinically significant, improvements were seen in FEV$_1$ over time with intravenous montelukast. Unfortunately, this did not translate to a reduction in hospitalizations. During post hoc analysis, accounting for site of treatment (international vs US sites), the investigators demonstrated that montelukast therapy was associated with a reduction of the need for hospitalization versus placebo. Reduction in bronchoconstriction was seen in as little as 10 minutes following initiation of intravenous montelukast. This therapy deserves further study, particularly as it relates to optimizing patient selection.

S. K. Willsie, DO

Reference

1. Camargo CA Jr, Smithline HA, Malice MP, Green SA, Reiss TF. A randomized controlled trial of intravenous montelukast in acute asthma. *Am J Respir Crit Care Med*. 2003;167:528-533.

Tiotropium Bromide Step-Up Therapy for Adults with Uncontrolled Asthma

Peters SP, for the National Heart, Lung, and Blood Institute Asthma Clinical Research Network (Wake Forest Univ Health Sciences, Winston-Salem, NC; et al)
N Engl J Med 363:1715-1726, 2010

Background.—Long-acting beta-agonist (LABA) therapy improves symptoms in patients whose asthma is poorly controlled by an inhaled glucocorticoid alone. Alternative treatments for adults with uncontrolled asthma are needed.

Methods.—In a three-way, double-blind, triple-dummy crossover trial involving 210 patients with asthma, we evaluated the addition of tiotropium bromide (a long-acting anticholinergic agent approved for the treatment of chronic obstructive pulmonary disease but not asthma) to an inhaled glucocorticoid, as compared with a doubling of the dose of the inhaled glucocorticoid (primary superiority comparison) or the addition of the LABA salmeterol (secondary noninferiority comparison).

Results.—The use of tiotropium resulted in a superior primary outcome, as compared with a doubling of the dose of an inhaled glucocorticoid, as assessed by measuring the morning peak expiratory flow (PEF), with a mean difference of 25.8 liters per minute (P<0.001) and superiority in most secondary outcomes, including evening PEF, with a difference of 35.3 liters per minute (P<0.001); the proportion of asthmacontrol days, with a difference of 0.079 (P = 0.01); the forced expiratory volume in 1 second (FEV_1) before bronchodilation, with a difference of 0.10 liters (P = 0.004); and daily symptom scores, with a difference of −0.11 points (P<0.001). The addition of tiotropium was also noninferior to the addition of salmeterol for all assessed outcomes and increased the prebronchodilator FEV_1 more than did salmeterol, with a difference of 0.11 liters (P = 0.003).

Conclusions.—When added to an inhaled glucocorticoid, tiotropium improved symptoms and lung function in patients with inadequately controlled asthma. Its effects appeared to be equivalent to those with the addition of salmeterol. (Funded by the National Heart, Lung, and Blood Institute; ClinicalTrials.gov number, NCT00565266.)

▶ Since the Salmeterol Multicenter Asthma Research Trial (SMART) was ended prematurely following an interim analysis that showed an increase in asthma-related deaths and respiratory-related deaths in subjects receiving salmeterol, considerable debate ensued that has led the research community to search for additional therapeutic agents with superior or noninferior efficacy to salmeterol in poorly controlled asthmatics.[1,2] This 3-way, double-blinded, triple dummy crossover trial compared the following therapies: addition of tiotropium bromide (T) to beclomethasone (80 μg twice daily); doubling of beclomethasone dose (DB) (160 μg twice daily); and addition of salmeterol (50 μg twice daily) to beclomethasone (SB) (80 μg twice daily). The primary outcome evaluated was morning peak expiratory flow; secondary outcomes evaluated:

prebronchodilator forced expiratory volume in 1 second (FEV1) and proportion of asthma-free days. Fig 3 in the original article demonstrates primary and secondary outcomes of the study. Tiotropium added to beclomethasone was superior to doubling of the dose of beclomethasone and was noninferior to salmeterol with beclomethasone. Prebronchodilator FEV1 measurements favored T over SB. Given the small number of subjects studied, the results of this study should not be used to change evidence-based guidelines for asthma. Further, large multicenter trials are warranted to ensure that the findings of this study are generalizable and warrant therapeutic change.

S. K. Willsie, DO

References

1. Nelson HS, Weiss ST, Bleecker ER, Yancey SW, Dorinsky PM, SMART Study Group. The Salmeterol Multicenter Asthma Research Trial: a comparison of usual pharmacotherapy for asthma or usual pharmacotherapy plus salmeterol. *Chest.* 2006;129:15-26.
2. Castle W, Fuller R, Hall J, Palmer J. Serevent nationwide surveillance study: comparison of salmeterol with salbutamol in asthmatic patients who require regular bronchodilator treatment. *BMJ.* 1993;306:1034-1037.

Effect of Pregnancy on Maternal Asthma Symptoms and Medication Use
Belanger K, Hellenbrand ME, Holford TR, et al (Yale Univ School of Public Health, New Haven, CT)
Obstet Gynecol 115:559-567, 2010

Objective.—To examine whether factors related to the patient or her treatment influence asthma severity during pregnancy.

Methods.—Symptom and medication data were collected by in-person and telephone interviews. Women were recruited before 24 weeks of gestation through private obstetricians and hospital clinics. Eight hundred seventy-two women had physician-diagnosed asthma, 686 were active asthmatics, and 641 with complete data were analyzed. The Global Initiative for Asthma measured severity. Cumulative logistic regression models for repeated measures assessed changes in asthma severity during each month of pregnancy.

Results.—Two factors had significant and profound effects on the course of asthma: prepregnancy severity and use of medication according to Global Initiative for Asthma guidelines. Although several factors were analyzed (race, age, atopic status, body mass index, parity, fetal sex, and smoking), none were significant risk factors for changes in asthma severity, measured in a clinically important way as a one-step change in Global Initiative for Asthma category. Women with milder asthma received most benefit from appropriate treatment, 62% decreased risk for worsening asthma among those with intermittent asthma (0.38, 95% confidence interval 0.23—0.64) and 52% decreased risk among those with mild persistent asthma (odds ratio 0.48, 95% confidence interval 0.28—0.84). Month or trimester of gestation was not consistently associated with changes in asthma severity.

Conclusion.—Asthma severity during pregnancy is similar to severity in the year before pregnancy, provided patients continue to use their prescribed medication. If women discontinue medication, even mild asthma is likely to become significantly more severe.

▶ Asthma continues to present a therapeutic challenge for providers caring for asthmatic women during pregnancy. Early investigators evaluating the impact of asthma on pregnancy promoted the prediction rule of thirds: one-third of pregnant asthmatics typically get worse during pregnancy, one-third stay the same, and the remaining one-third of asthmatics get better during pregnancy.[1,2] This prospective study of 741 women evaluated the role of prepregnancy asthma severity, race, body mass index, and use of appropriate evidence-based therapy based on severity of asthma on the impact of asthma during pregnancy. Table 2 in the original article demonstrates that 57.5% of subjects were classified prepregnancy as having intermittent asthma; 20.1%, mild persistent asthma; and 22.5%, moderate persistent asthma. Whites were more likely to have moderate/severe asthma than were blacks and Hispanics. Blacks were more likely to have mild persistent asthma, and Hispanics were more likely to have intermittent asthma prepregnancy. Increasing maternal age was associated with a greater likelihood of having moderate persistent asthma. This investigation showed that the protective effect of evidence-based therapy for asthma was greatest in the intermittent asthmatic group; the protective effect was also seen in the mild persistent asthmatic group. Subjects with moderate persistent asthma who were treated according to evidence-based guidelines enjoyed a protective effect, but this did not reach statistical significance. This investigation showed that prepregnancy asthmatic control (1 year immediately preceding pregnancy) and the use of evidence-based therapy for asthma (Global Initiative for Asthma) are 2 factors with the greatest impact on asthma outcomes during pregnancy. The results of this study shed new light on the contribution of asthma to morbidity during pregnancy. Preconception counseling for the purpose of optimizing asthma control, provision of high-quality patient education, and use of evidence-based therapy for asthma should be made a higher priority by health care providers.

S. K. Willsie, DO

References

1. Schatz M, Harden K, Forsythe A, et al. The course of asthma during pregnancy, post partum, and with successive pregnancies: a prospective analysis. *J Allergy Clin Immunol.* 1988;81:509-517.
2. Juniper EF, Newhouse MT. Effect of pregnancy on asthma: a critical appraisal of the literature. In: Schatz M, Zeiger RS, eds. *Asthma and Allergy in Pregnancy.* New York, NY: Dekker; 1993:223-492.

Effects of Aerobic Training on Airway Inflammation in Asthmatic Patients

Mendes FAR, Almeida FM, Cukier A, et al (Univ of São Paulo, Brazil)
Med Sci Sports Exerc 43:197-203, 2011

Purpose.—There is evidence suggesting that physical activity has anti-inflammatory effects in many chronic diseases; however, the role of exercise in airway inflammation in asthma is poorly understood. We aimed to evaluate the effects of an aerobic training program on eosinophil inflammation (primary aim) and nitric oxide (secondary aim) in patients with moderate or severe persistent asthma.

Methods.—Sixty-eight patients randomly assigned to either control (CG) or aerobic training (TG) groups were studied during the period between medical consultations. Patients in the CG (educational program + breathing exercises; $N = 34$) and TG (educational program + breathing exercises + aerobic training; $N = 34$) were examined twice a week during a 3-month period. Before and after the intervention, patients underwent induced sputum, fractional exhaled nitric oxide (FeNO), pulmonary function, and cardiopulmonary exercise testing. Asthma symptom-free days were quantified monthly, and asthma exacerbation was monitored during 3 months of intervention.

Results.—At 3 months, decreases in the total and eosinophil cell counts in induced sputum ($P = 0.004$) and in the levels of FeNO ($P = 0.009$) were observed after intervention only in the TG. The number of asthma symptom-free days and $\dot{V}O_{2max}$ also significantly improved ($P < 0.001$), and lower asthma exacerbation occurred in the TG ($P < 0.01$). In addition, the TG presented a strong positive relationship between baseline FeNO and eosinophil counts as well as their improvement after training ($r = 0.77$ and $r = 0.9$, respectively).

Conclusions.—Aerobic training reduces sputum eosinophil and FeNO in patients with moderate or severe asthma, and these benefits were more significant in subjects with higher levels of inflammation. These results suggest that aerobic training might be useful as an adjuvant therapy in asthmatic patients under optimized medical treatment.

▶ Limited studies have shown protective effect of aerobic exercise in patients with asthma.[1,2] This provocative study of patients with moderate to severe persistent asthma demonstrated reduced airway inflammation (via sputum cell counts, fractional exhaled nitric oxide [FeNO]) and an increase in symptom-free days in patients with asthma randomized to receive aerobic training in addition to education and respiratory exercises undertaken by the control group. Fig 4 in the original article demonstrates asthma-free days, showing statistically significant increase in symptom-free asthma days after 30, 60, and 90 days of aerobic exercise. Fig 3 in the original article displays FeNO levels in the aerobic exercise group versus control group, demonstrating a statistically significant reduction in the aerobic exercise group versus control group. This is one of the first studies to demonstrate reduced airway inflammation following aerobic exercise. Furthermore, large-scale studies are warranted to confirm this effect in a widely diverse asthmatic population.

S. K. Willsie, DO

References

1. Fanelli A, Cabral AL, Neder JA, Martins MA, Carvalho CR. Exercise training on disease control and quality of life in asthmatic children. *Med Sci Sports Exerc.* 2007;39:1474-1480.
2. Neder JA, Nery LE, Silva AC, Cabral AL, Fernandes AL. Short-term effects of aerobic training in the clinical management of moderate to severe asthma in children. *Thorax.* 1999;54:202-206.

Location and Duration of Treatment of Cystic Fibrosis Respiratory Exacerbations Do Not Affect Outcomes

Collaco JM, Green DM, Cutting GR, et al (Johns Hopkins Univ, Baltimore, MD)

Am J Respir Crit Care Med 182:1137-1143, 2010

Rationale.—Individuals with cystic fibrosis (CF) are subject to recurrent respiratory infections (exacerbations) that often require intravenous antibiotic treatment and may result in permanent loss of lung function. The optimal means of delivering therapy remains unclear.

Objectives.—To determine whether duration or venue of intravenous antibiotic administration affect lung function.

Methods.—Data were retrospectively collected on 1,535 subjects recruited by the US CF Twin and Sibling Study from US CF care centers between 2000 and 2007.

Measurements and Main Results.—Long-term decline in FEV_1 after exacerbation was observed regardless of whether antibiotics were administered in the hospital (mean, -3.3 percentage points [95% confidence interval, -3.9 to -2.6]; n = 602 courses of therapy) or at home (mean, -3.5 percentage points [95% confidence interval, -4.5 to -2.5]; n = 232 courses of therapy); this decline was not different by venue using t tests ($P = 0.69$) or regression ($P = 0.91$). No difference in intervals between courses of antibiotics was observed between hospital (median, 119 d [interquartile range, 166]; n = 602) and home (median, 98 d [interquartile range, 155]; n = 232) ($P = 0.29$). Patients with greater drops in FEV_1 with exacerbations had worse long-term decline even if lung function initially recovered with treatment ($P < 0.001$). Examination of FEV_1 measures obtained during treatment for exacerbations indicated that improvement in FEV_1 plateaus after 7–10 days of therapy.

Conclusions.—Intravenous antibiotic therapy for CF respiratory exacerbations administered in the hospital and in the home was found to be equivalent in terms of long-term FEV_1 change and interval between courses of antibiotics. Optimal duration of therapy (7–10 d) may be

TABLE 1.—Demographics

		All	Hospital Only	Home Only	Combination: Hospital and Home	P Value (Hospital vs. Home)*
Data by Subject	Number of subjects	479	261	114	248	—
	Mean courses of antibiotics per subject in dataset	2.7 ± 2.4	—	—	—	—
Data by Therapy Course	Age at most recent FEV_1 (yr) (mean ± SD)	19.4 ± 8.3	18.2 ± 6.5	22.3 ± 9.4	20.4 ± 9.0	<0.0001
	Sex (% male)	47.4	49	34.2	44	0.01
	CFTR (% F508del homozygotes)	49.2 (n = 478)	51.2 (n = 260)	43	48.6 (n = 247)	0.35
	Number of courses	1,278	602	232	444	—
	Age at start of therapy (yr) (mean ± SD)	17.8 ± 8.0	16.2 ± 6.1	22.0 ± 10.0	17.8 ± 8.2	<0.0001
	P. aeruginosa (% positive)	96.4	95.7	97.8	96.6	0.14
	B. cepacia (% positive)	10.6	11.5	9.9	9.9	0.52
	Days treated in hospital (mean ± SD)	—	12.7 ± 5.3	—	6.0 ± 4.3	—
	Days treated at home (mean ± SD)	—	—	18.9 ± 7.4	12.5 ± 5.7	—
	Total days of treatment mean ± SD)	15.8 ± 6.7	12.7 ± 5.3	18.9 ± 7.4	18.5 ± 6.0	<0.0001
	Baseline FEV_1 (mean ± SD)	68.4 ± 22.0	67.4 ± 22.4	65.1 ± 22.1	71.4 ± 21.2	0.17
	Pretherapy FEV_1 (mean ± SD)	60.4 ± 22.0	58.8 ± 22.0	59.5 ± 22.3	63.0 ± 21.5	0.68
	Posttherapy FEV_1 (mean ± SD)	68.7 ± 23.4	67.9 ± 23.3	64.4 ± 23.5	72.0 ± 23.0	0.05
	New baseline FEV_1 (mean ± SD)	64.9 ± 23.3	64.1 ± 23.1	61.5 ± 23.5	67.8 ± 23.3	0.15

*These P values reflect the difference between the hospital and home categories. P values were determined using Student t and chi-square tests.

shorter than current practice. Large prospective studies are needed to answer these essential questions for CF respiratory management (Table 1).

▶ Retrospective data collection from the US Cystic Fibrosis Twin and Sibling study from US cystic fibrosis care centers between 2000 and 2007. Table 1 demonstrates numbers of subjects, numbers treated within the hospital, home, and combination of both; *P* values are given comparing hospital with home. There was no statistical difference in the numbers of exacerbations, which were because of *Pseudomonas aeruginosa* or *Burkholderia cepacia* (*P* > .05). Baseline forced expiratory volume in the first second of expiration (FEV$_1$), pretherapy FEV$_1$, posttherapy FEV$_1$, and new baseline FEV$_1$ did not vary significantly between groups. Fig 4 in the original article details improvement of FEV$_1$ by day of therapy. Pulmonary function tests obtained during therapy demonstrates that improvement occurred until approximately 8 to 10 days of therapy at which time the FEV$_1$ plateaus. Beyond this time period, there was no significant improvement, and actually, there was deterioration of FEV$_1$, despite continued treatment. The venue for intravenous antibiotic therapy for clinician-defined respiratory exacerbation does not affect long-term decline in FEV$_1$; most improvement in lung function appears to occur within the first 8 to 10 days following the initiation of antibiotic therapy.

S. K. Willsie, DO

Effect of VX-770 in Persons with Cystic Fibrosis and the G551D-*CFTR* Mutation

Accurso FJ, Rowe SM, Clancy JP, et al (Univ of Colorado Denver and Children's Hosp, Aurora; Univ of Alabama at Birmingham, AL; et al)
N Engl J Med 363:1991-2003, 2010

Background.—A new approach in the treatment of cystic fibrosis involves improving the function of mutant cystic fibrosis transmembrane conductance regulator (CFTR). VX-770, a CFTR potentiator, has been shown to increase the activity of wild-type and defective cell-surface CFTR in vitro.

Methods.—We randomly assigned 39 adults with cystic fibrosis and at least one G551D-*CFTR* allele to receive oral VX-770 every 12 hours at a dose of 25, 75, or 150 mg or placebo for 14 days (in part 1 of the study) or VX-770 every 12 hours at a dose of 150 or 250 mg or placebo for 28 days (in part 2 of the study).

Results.—At day 28, in the group of subjects who received 150 mg of VX-770, the median change in the nasal potential difference (in response to the administration of a chloride-free isoproterenol solution) from baseline was −3.5 mV (range, −8.3 to 0.5; P = 0.02 for the within-subject comparison, P = 0.13 vs. placebo), and the median change in the level of sweat chloride was −59.5 mmol per liter (range, −66.0 to −19.0; P = 0.008 within-subject, P = 0.02 vs. placebo). The median change from baseline in the percent of predicted forced expiratory volume in 1 second was 8.7% (range, 2.3 to 31.3; P = 0.008 for the within-subject comparison, P = 0.56 vs. placebo).

None of the subjects withdrew from the study. Six severe adverse events occurred in two subjects (diffuse macular rash in one subject and five incidents of elevated blood and urine glucose levels in one subject with diabetes). All severe adverse events resolved without the discontinuation of VX-770.

Conclusions.—This study to evaluate the safety and adverse-event profile of VX-770 showed that VX-770 was associated with within-subject improvements in CFTR and lung function. These findings provide support for further studies of pharmacologic potentiation of CFTR as a means to treat cystic fibrosis. (Funded by Vertex Pharmaceuticals and others; ClinicalTrials.gov number, NCT00457821.)

▶ Despite advances in antibiotic therapy and improved rescue therapy for subjects with cystic fibrosis with chest infections, this multisystem disease continues to cause considerable morbidity and mortality.[1] One of the newer approaches to this disease involves direct targeting of the genetic defect in order to improve the function of the cystic fibrosis transmembrane conductance regulator (CFTR).[2,3] VX-770, known to be a CFTR potentiator,[4] was studied in a randomized, double-blind, placebo-controlled, multicenter study involving patients with cystic fibrosis who had at least on G551D-*CFTR* allele. Subjects took oral VX-770 every 12 hours at doses that ranged from 25 to 150 mg versus placebo for 14 days or doses of 150 or 250 mg versus placebo for 28 days. Fig 2 in the original article demonstrates changes in sweat chloride by dose and days of treatment, and Fig 3 in the original article delineates changes in pulmonary function with treatment. Though no significant differences were seen between VX-770 and placebo groups, significant within-subject improvement was seen, particularly related to respiratory (nasal potential difference), nonrespiratory (sweat chloride concentrations), and improved pulmonary function. In general, the investigational agent was well tolerated in comparison to placebo. Further studies are needed to evaluate VX-770 as a viable therapeutic option for patients with cystic fibrosis.

S. K. Willsie, DO

References

1. Sawicki GS, Sellers DE, Robinson WM. High treatment burden in adults with cystic fibrosis: challenges to disease self-management. *J Cyst Fibros.* 2009;8:91-96.
2. Amaral MD, Kunzelmann K. Molecular targeting of CFTR as a therapeutic approach to cystic fibrosis. *Trends Pharmacol Sci.* 2007;28:334-341.
3. Yang Y, Devor DC, Engelhardt JF, et al. Molecular basis of defective anion transport in L cells expressing recombinant forms of CFTR. *Hum Mol Genet.* 1993;2:1253-1261.
4. Van Goor F, Hadida S, Grootenhuis PD, et al. Rescue of CF airway epithelial cell function in vitro by a CFTR potentiator, VX-770. *Proc Natl Acad Sci U S A.* 2009;106:18825-18830.

33 Chronic Obstructive Pulmonary Disease

Use of High-Dose Inhaled Corticosteroids is Associated With Pulmonary Tuberculosis in Patients With Chronic Obstructive Pulmonary Disease
Shu C-C, the Taiwan Anti-Mycobacteria Investigation (TAMI) Group (Natl Taiwan Univ Hosp, Taipei; et al)
Medicine 89:53-61, 2010

The use of high-dose inhaled corticosteroids (ICS) in patients with chronic obstructive pulmonary disease (COPD) has recently been shown to increase the incidence of pneumonia. However, to our knowledge, the impact of high-dose ICS on pulmonary tuberculosis (TB) has never been investigated. To study that impact, we conducted a retrospective study including patients aged more than 40 years old with irreversible airflow limitation between August 2000 and July 2008 in a medical center in Taiwan.

Of the 36,684 patients who underwent pulmonary function testing, we included 554 patients. Among them, patients using high-dose ICS (equivalent to >500 µg/d of fluticasone) were more likely to have more severe COPD and receive oral corticosteroids than those using medium-dose, low-dose, or no ICS. Sixteen (3%) patients developed active pulmonary TB within a follow-up of 25,544 person-months. Multivariate Cox regression analysis revealed that the use of high-dose ICS, the use of 10 mg or more of prednisolone per day, and prior pulmonary TB were independent risk factors for the development of active pulmonary TB. Chest radiography and sputum smear/culture for *Mycobacterium tuberculosis* should be performed before initiating high-dose ICS and regularly thereafter.

▶ Since inhaled corticosteroids (ICS) were shown to decrease exacerbations in patients with severe chronic obstructive pulmonary disease (COPD), their use as a maintenance treatment has increased dramatically. In fact, the most widely used clinical practice guideline around the management of COPD, the Global Obstructive Lung Disease guideline, recommends a combination of inhaled corticosteroid therapy and inhaled bronchodilator therapy for patients with COPD with severe disease and repeated exacerbations.[1] This approach, while potentially decreasing the morbidity from exacerbations, is not without its side effects. Already, articles have been published documenting, mostly incidentally, increases in the rates of pneumonia in patients treated chronically with ICS.

Recently, it has been documented that this risk occurs even in newly diagnosed patients placed on ICS.[2] Since corticosteroids are immunosuppressive, this should not be a surprise. In this study, 3% of 554 patients with fixed airflow obstruction in a Taiwanese clinic developed active tuberculosis over a period of follow-up of at least 6 months (but a mean of 40-50 months); those on oral steroids or high-dose ICS were at greatest risk and developed the disease at a median of about 20 months. The authors make a general recommendation that patients being placed on high-dose ICS have routine chest X-ray and sputum smear/culture before being started on the drug and regularly thereafter. This may be reasonable in populations with high rates of tuberculosis, but it is not a cost-effective approach in general. However, it is important for clinicians caring for COPD patients on ICS to be aware of this risk and to consider tuberculosis in any atypical presentation of pneumonia.

J. R. Maurer, MD, MBA

References

1. Guidelines and Resources. Available at: <http://www.goldcopd.com>. Accessed August 15, 2010.
2. Joo MJ, Au DH, Fitzgibbon ML, Lee TA. Inhaled corticosteroids and risk of pneumonia in newly diagnosed COPD. *Respir Med.* 2010;104:246-252.

Lung Function in Young Adults Predicts Airflow Obstruction 20 Years Later
Kalhan R, Arynchyn A, Colangelo LA, et al (Northwestern Univ, Chicago, IL; Univ of Alabama at Birmingham; et al)
Am J Med 123:468.e1-468.e7, 2010

Objective.—The burden of obstructive lung disease is increasing, yet there are limited data on its natural history in young adults. To determine in a prospective cohort of generally healthy young adults the influence of early adult lung function on the presence of airflow obstruction in middle age.

Methods.—A longitudinal study was performed of 2496 adults who were 18 to 30 years of age at entry, did not report having asthma, and returned at year 20. Airflow obstruction was defined as a forced expiratory volume in 1 second/forced vital capacity ratio less than the lower limit of normal.

Results.—Airflow obstruction was present in 6.9% and 7.8% of participants at years 0 and 20, respectively. Less than 10% of participants with airflow obstruction self-reported chronic obstructive pulmonary disease. In cross-sectional analyses, airflow obstruction was associated with less education, smoking, and self-reported chronic obstructive pulmonary disease. Low forced expiratory volume in 1 second, forced expiratory volume in 1 second/forced vital capacity ratio, and airflow obstruction in young adults were associated with low lung function and airflow obstruction 20 years later. Of those with airflow obstruction at year 0, 52% had airflow obstruction 20 years later. The forced expiratory volume in 1 second/forced vital capacity at year 0 was highly predictive of airflow obstruction 20 years later (c-statistic 0.91; 95% confidence interval, 0.89-0.93). The effect of cigarette smoking on lung function decline with age was most evident in young adults with preexisting airflow obstruction.

Conclusion.—Airflow obstruction is mostly unrecognized in young and middle-aged adults. Low forced expiratory volume in 1 second, low forced expiratory volume in 1 second/forced vital capacity ratio, airflow obstruction in young adults, and smoking are highly predictive of low lung function and airflow obstruction in middle age.

▶ The population used for this report is from the Coronary Artery Risk Development in Young Adults longitudinal study that in 1985 to 1986 enrolled healthy young adults who did not have known asthma or other airway disease.[1] Lung function was measured at entry, during the study, and after 20 years. Most of the studies of lung function done to date in young adults have either had relatively short follow-up times or have just been cross-sectional. While a correlation has been shown between pulmonary symptoms in early adult life and later development of obstructive airways disease,[2] the long-term outcome or predictive value of asymptomatic obstruction detected early in life has not been previously reported. Currently, spirometry screening for patients who do not report symptoms suggestive of lung disease is not recommended, as it is not cost-effective. However, this study is provocative in that it suggests that lung function abnormalities picked up in early adult life tend to persist. This information would be very valuable for patients to know as they could be counseled to avoid behaviors or occupations that might exacerbate their underlying lung disease.

J. R. Maurer, MD, MBA

References

1. Friedman GD, Cutter GR, Donahue RP, et al. CARDIA: study design, recruitment, and some characteristics of the examined subjects. *J Clin Epidemiol.* 1988;41:1105-1116.
2. de Marco R, Accordini S, Cerveri I, et al. Incidence of chronic obstructive pulmonary disease in a cohort of young adults according to the presence of chronic cough and phlegm. *Am J Respir Crit Care Med.* 2007;175:32-39.

Disease Management Program for Chronic Obstructive Pulmonary Disease: A Randomized Controlled Trial

Rice KL, Dewan N, Bloomfield HE, et al (VA Med Ctr, Minneapolis, MN; VA Med Ctr, Omaha, NE; Univ of Minnesota, Minneapolis; et al)
Am J Respir Crit Care Med 182:890-896, 2010

Rationale.—The effect of disease management for chronic obstructive pulmonary disease (COPD) is not well established.

Objectives.—To determine whether a simplified disease management program reduces hospital admissions and emergency department (ED) visits due to COPD.

Methods.—We performed a randomized, adjudicator-blinded, controlled, 1-year trial at five Veterans Affairs medical centers of 743 patients with severe COPD and one or more of the following during the previous year: hospital admission or ED visit for COPD, chronic home oxygen use, or course of systemic corticosteroids for COPD. Control group patients received usual care. Intervention group patients received a single 1- to 1.5-hour education session, an action plan for self-treatment of exacerbations, and monthly follow-up calls from a case manager.

Measurements and Main Results.—We determined the combined number of COPD-related hospitalizations and ED visits per patient. Secondary outcomes included hospitalizations and ED visits for all causes, respiratory medication use, mortality, and change in Saint George's Respiratory Questionnaire. After 1 year, the mean cumulative frequency of COPD-related hospitalizations and ED visits was 0.82 per patient in usual care and 0.48 per patient in disease management (difference, 0.34; 95% confidence interval, 0.15–0.52; $P < 0.001$). Disease management reduced hospitalizations for cardiac or pulmonary conditions other than COPD by 49%, hospitalizations for all causes by 28%, and ED visits for all causes by 27% ($P < 0.05$ for all).

Conclusions.—A relatively simple disease management program reduced hospitalizations and ED visits for COPD.

Clinical trial registered with www.clinicaltrials.gov (NCT00126776).

▶ Patients with chronic obstructive pulmonary disorder (COPD) have nearly 750 000 inpatient admissions and 500 000 emergency room visits in the United States per year, accounting for more than $20 billion per year in direct health care costs.[1] Combined with other common diseases such as asthma, diabetes, coronary disease, and heart failure, the health care cost burden of these chronic illnesses is excessive, growing, and unsustainable. Approaches to containing these costs and improving quality of life have included disease management programs like those studied here. Briefly, these are programs designed to reduce the use of health care resources by teaching people and assisting them in better caring for themselves through a better understanding of their conditions (Fig 2 in the original article). One might expect this to reduce acute care costs. Disease management programs such as the one reported here have often been hard to assess in that it often takes an extended period of time to show reductions in health care costs in patients with chronic diseases who have multiple ongoing maintenance costs, in addition to their intermittent acute care costs. In addition, many studies have not used randomized studies that apply the disease management intervention to only part of the study participants. Thus, this is a particularly welcome study because it used a robust methodology for the study, and it also used relatively easy interventions, which should be able to be replicated across other groups of patients with COPD. Because it is crucial to not only contain health care costs but also to help those with chronic conditions take more ownership of their conditions and live more fulfilling lives, we applaud this study and hope to see robust disease management programs implemented across many more chronic populations.

J. R. Maurer, MD, MBA

Reference

1. Foster TS, Miller JD, Marton JP, Caloyeras JP, Russell MW, Menzin J. Assessment of the economic burden of COPD in the U.S.: a review and synthesis of the literature. *COPD*. 2006;3:211-218.

34 Lung Cancer

Endobronchial Ultrasound for the Diagnosis and Staging of Lung Cancer
Gomez M, Silvestri GA (Med Univ of South Carolina, Charleston)
Proc Am Thorac Soc 6:180-186, 2009

The diagnosis of indeterminate mediastinal lymph nodes, masses, and peripheral pulmonary nodules constitutes a significant challenge. Options for tissue diagnoses include computed tomography—guided percutaneous biopsy, transbronchial fine-needle aspiration, mediastinoscopy, left anterior mediastinotomy, or video-assisted thoracoscopic surgery; however, these approaches have both advantages and limitations in terms of tissue yield, safety profile, and cost. Endobronchial ultrasound (EBUS) is a new minimally invasive technique that expands the view of the bronchoscopist beyond the lumen of the airway. There are two EBUS systems currently available. The radial probe EBUS allows for evaluation of central airways, accurate definition of airway invasion, and facilitates the diagnosis of peripheral lung lesions. Linear EBUS guides transbronchial needle aspiration of hilar and mediastinal lymph nodes, improving diagnostic yield. This article will review the principles and clinical applications of EBUS, and will highlight the role of this new technology in the diagnosis and staging of lung cancer (Table 2).

▶ Endobronchial ultrasound (EBUS) was introduced in the early 1990s. EBUS is minimally invasive and safe, and a growing evidence base supports its high accuracy. Though it is not a new technology, widespread availability and usage have been relatively slow, related in part to equipment cost, the need for specialized training, and uncertainties in reimbursement. This article by Gomez and Silvestri reviews the 2 types of EBUS and their clinical applications. Radial EBUS is typically used to assess tumor invasion into a bronchus and guide biopsies of peripheral nodules. Radial EBUS can be performed with 2 different types of probes: a standard probe for airway evaluation from the trachea to the level of subsegmental bronchi and an ultraminiature probe for detection of peripheral lesions. Linear (or convex probe) EBUS is most often used to sample lymph nodes in the mediastinum and typically performed in patients with known or suspected lung cancer. This function is the most common application of EBUS at the present time. The authors present a pooled analysis of 12 studies evaluating EBUS in mediastinal staging, outlined in Table 2. Overall, weighted sensitivity was 93%, specificity was 100%, and false-negative rate was 9%. Of note, 10 of the 12 studies were performed in patients with high prevalence of mediastinal cancer involvement (55%-98%), but the other 2 studies were performed in patients with no evidence on

TABLE 2.—Endobronchial Ultrasound-Guided Transbronchial Needle Aspiration Of The Mediastinum In Lung Cancer

Study/Year	Patients	Technique	Sensitivity %	Specificity %	FP %	FN %	Cancer %
Vincent/2008 (50)	152	RT-22 ga	99	100	0	1	74
Herth/2008 (42)*	100	RT-22 ga	89	100	0	1	9
Bauwens/2008 (41)†	106	RT-22 ga	95	97	0	3	55
Koh/2008 (46)	16	Rad-21 ga	83	100	0	13	63
Herth/2006 (43)	502	RT-22 ga	94	100	0	89‡	98
Herth/2006 (44)	100	RT-22 ga	94	100	0	1	17
Plat/2006 (47)	33	Rad-histo	93	100	0	25	82
Yasufuku/2005 (51)	108	RT-22 ga	95	100	0	11	69
Vilman/2005 (49)	31	RT-22 ga	85	100	0	28	65
Rintoul/2005 (48)	20	RT-22 ga	79	100	0	30	70
Kanoh/2005 (45)	54	Rad-19 ga	86	100	0	37	81
Yasufuku/2004 (52)	70	RT-22 ga	95	100	0	10	67
Summary	1292		93	100	0	9	63

Definition of abbreviations: Rad = radial probe; RT = real time.
Reprinted by permission from Reference 36.
*Nodes < 1 cm, negative mediastinal activity in PET scan.
†Increased activity in mediastinum in PET scan.
‡Excluded from calculations because NPV is less reliable with a prevalence of > 90%.

imaging studies of mediastinal adenopathy and prevalence of malignant involvement of only 9% and 17%.[1,2] EBUS performed remarkably well in these patients, with sensitivity of 89% and 94%, specificity of 99%, and false-negative rate of only 1%. It is clear that, in trained hands, EBUS is highly accurate as well as being minimally invasive and safe and offers an efficient alternative to mediastinoscopy.

L. T. Tanoue, MD

References

1. Herth FJ, Eberhardt R, Krasnik M, Ernst A. Endobronchial ultrasound-guided transbronchial needle aspiration of lymph nodes in the radiologically and positron emission tomography-normal mediastinum in patients with lung cancer. *Chest.* 2008;133:887-891.
2. Herth FJ, Ernst A, Eberhardt R, Vilmann P, Dienemann H, Krasnik M. Endobronchial ultrasound-guided transbronchial needle aspiration of lymph nodes in the radiologically normal mediastinum. *Eur Respir J.* 2006;28:910-914.

Navigational Bronchoscopy: Overview of Technology and Practical Considerations—New Current Procedural Terminology Codes Effective 2010

Edell E, Krier-Morrow D (Mayo Clinic, Rochester, MN; Diane Krier-Morrow and Associates, Inc, Evanston, IL)
Chest 137:450-454, 2010

Navigational bronchoscopy provides a three-dimensional virtual "roadmap" that enables a physician to maneuver through multiple branches of the bronchial tree to reach targeted lesions in distal regions of the lung. It is designed to be used with a standard bronchoscope to facilitate obtaining tissue samples and for placing radiosurgical or dye markers. This article overviews this technology and the Current Procedural Terminology codes that have been created for its use.

▶ Navigational bronchoscopy is a minimally invasive technique that allows the bronchoscopist-guided access to peripheral areas of the lung. This requires (1) planning software to convert CT scan images into 3-dimensional reconstruction with virtual images of the airways, (2) a steerable sensor probe able to flexibly perform the procedure, and (3) an electromagnetic navigational system consisting of an electromagnetic board and a field generator connected to a computer loaded with the planning software. This is an expensive technology, both as an initial investment and for the single-use probes. As it is new, reimbursement has been very limited, but new current procedural terminology codes were assigned this year. The role of navigational bronchoscopy is most promising in its ability to reliably guide biopsies of peripheral lung lesions, though there are no studies comparing it with conventional flexible bronchoscopy. Anticipating that routine chest CT imaging may become widespread if CT screening for lung cancer is approved, and in that setting many patients will be diagnosed with small peripheral pulmonary nodules, there may in the future be an important role for this new technology.

L. T. Tanoue, MD

Stereotactic Body Radiation Therapy for Inoperable Early Stage Lung Cancer

Timmerman R, Paulus R, Galvin J, et al (Univ of Texas Southwestern Med Ctr, Dallas; Radiation Therapy Oncology Group, Philadelphia, PA; Thomas Jefferson Univ, Philadelphia, PA; et al)
JAMA 303:1070-1076, 2010

Context.—Patients with early stage but medically inoperable lung cancer have a poor rate of primary tumor control (30%-40%) and a high rate of mortality (3-year survival, 20%-35%) with current management.

Objective.—To evaluate the toxicity and efficacy of stereotactic body radiation therapy in a high-risk population of patients with early stage but medically inoperable lung cancer.

Design, Setting, and Patients.—Phase 2 North American multicenter study of patients aged 18 years or older with biopsy-proven peripheral T1-T2N0M0 non—small cell tumors (measuring <5 cm in diameter) and medical conditions precluding surgical treatment. The prescription dose was 18 Gy per fraction × 3 fractions (54 Gy total) with entire treatment lasting between 1½ and 2 weeks. The study opened May 26, 2004, and closed October 13, 2006; data were analyzed through August 31, 2009.

Main Outcome Measures.—The primary end point was 2-year actuarial primary tumor control; secondary end points were disease-free survival (ie, primary tumor, involved lobe, regional, and disseminated recurrence), treatment-related toxicity, and overall survival.

Results.—A total of 59 patients accrued, of which 55 were evaluable (44 patients with T1 tumors and 11 patients with T2 tumors) with a median follow-up of 34.4 months (range, 4.8-49.9 months). Only 1 patient had a primary tumor failure; the estimated 3-year primary tumor control rate was 97.6% (95% confidence interval [CI], 84.3%-99.7%). Three patients had recurrence within the involved lobe; the 3-year primary tumor and involved lobe (local) control rate was 90.6% (95% CI, 76.0%-96.5%). Two patients experienced regional failure; the local-regional control rate was 87.2% (95% CI, 71.0%-94.7%). Eleven patients experienced disseminated recurrence; the 3-year rate of disseminated failure was 22.1% (95% CI, 12.3%-37.8%). The rates for disease-free survival and overall survival at 3 years were 48.3% (95% CI, 34.4%-60.8%) and 55.8% (95% CI, 41.6%-67.9%), respectively. The median overall survival was 48.1 months (95% CI, 29.6 months to not reached). Protocol-specified treatment-related grade 3 adverse events were reported in 7 patients (12.7%; 95% CI, 9.6%-15.8%); grade 4 adverse events were reported in 2 patients (3.6%; 95% CI, 2.7%-4.5%). No grade 5 adverse events were reported.

Conclusion.—Patients with inoperable non–small cell lung cancer who received stereotactic body radiation therapy had a survival rate of 55.8% at 3 years, high rates of local tumor control, and moderate treatment-related morbidity.

▶ Medically inoperable patients with early-stage non–small cell lung cancer (NSCLC) are typically treated with radiation therapy (RT). Conventional RT in this setting involves up to 30 outpatient radiation treatments spread over a number of weeks. While associated with better outcomes than supportive care alone, conventional RT is known to have relatively poor long-term control of the primary tumor and yields a 2-year survival of approximately 40% at best.[1,2] Stereotactic body RT (SBRT) is a new technology that delivers RT in high doses using small highly focused beams and is completed in a few treatments. In this report, Timmerman and colleagues report the 3-year results of the Radiation Therapy Oncology Group (RTOG) multicenter trial evaluating SBRT in medically inoperable early-stage NSCLC. All patients in the study had T1 or T2 primary tumors (< 5 cm) located more than 2 cm from the trachea, carina, and major lobar bronchi (ie, not central tumors) and were N0M0 by CT and positron emission tomography scanning. All patients underwent extensive SBRT planning, including control of tumor motion related to breathing, and received a total dose of 60 Gy divided in 3 fractions. At 3 years of follow-up, primary tumor control was 97.6%. Survival results are demonstrated in the figure in the original article. Overall 3-year survival in the entire group was 55.8%; in patients with T1 tumors, median disease-free survival was 36.1 months, and median overall survival had not been reached at the 3-year follow-up. Disseminated recurrence occurred in 22.1% of patients, suggesting that occult tumor existed at the time of SBRT that had not been detected by the noninvasive staging techniques. These results are superior to primary tumor control and survival rates achieved with conventional RT. SBRT requires meticulous planning by a multidisciplinary team of radiation oncologists and medical physicists and is not yet widely available. Side effects include fatigue, chest pain, gastrointestinal complaints, and dyspnea. Based on these results as well as other single institution reports, it appears that SBRT will have an important role in the treatment of medically inoperable patients with early-stage lung cancer. A clinical trial jointly sponsored by the American College of Surgeons Oncology Group and the RTOG comparing SBRT with sublobar surgical resection in high-risk (unable to tolerate lobectomy) patients with early-stage NSCLC is currently in progress.

L. T. Tanoue, MD

References

1. Kaskowitz L, Graham MV, Emami B, Halverson KJ, Rush C. Radiation therapy alone for stage I non-small cell lung cancer. *Int J Radiat Oncol Biol Phys.* 1993; 27:517-523.
2. Haffty BG, Goldberg NB, Gerstley J, Fischer DB, Peschel RE. Results of radical radiation therapy in clinical stage I, technically operable non-small cell lung cancer. *Int J Radiat Oncol Biol Phys.* 1988;15:69-73.

Early Palliative Care for Patients with Metastatic Non–Small-Cell Lung Cancer

Temel JS, Greer JA, Muzikansky A, et al (Massachusetts General Hosp, Boston; et al)
N Engl J Med 363:733-742, 2010

Background.—Patients with metastatic non–small-cell lung cancer have a substantial symptom burden and may receive aggressive care at the end of life. We examined the effect of introducing palliative care early after diagnosis on patient-reported outcomes and end-of-life care among ambulatory patients with newly diagnosed disease.

Methods.—We randomly assigned patients with newly diagnosed metastatic non–small-cell lung cancer to receive either early palliative care integrated with standard oncologic care or standard oncologic care alone. Quality of life and mood were assessed at baseline and at 12 weeks with the use of the Functional Assessment of Cancer Therapy–Lung (FACT-L) scale and the Hospital Anxiety and Depression Scale, respectively. The primary outcome was the change in the quality of life at 12 weeks. Data on end-of-life care were collected from electronic medical records.

Results.—Of the 151 patients who underwent randomization, 27 died by 12 weeks and 107 (86% of the remaining patients) completed assessments. Patients assigned to early palliative care had a better quality of life than did patients assigned to standard care (mean score on the FACT-L scale [in which scores range from 0 to 136, with higher scores indicating better quality of life], 98.0 vs. 91.5; P = 0.03). In addition, fewer patients in the palliative care group than in the standard care group had depressive symptoms (16% vs. 38%, P = 0.01). Despite the fact that fewer patients in the early palliative care group than in the standard care group received aggressive end-of-life care (33% vs. 54%, P = 0.05), median survival was longer among patients receiving early palliative care (11.6 months vs. 8.9 months, P = 0.02).

Conclusions.—Among patients with metastatic non–small-cell lung cancer, early palliative care led to significant improvements in both quality of life and mood. As compared with patients receiving standard care, patients receiving early palliative care had less aggressive care at the end of life but longer survival. (Funded by an American Society of Clinical Oncology Career Development Award and philanthropic gifts; ClinicalTrials.gov number, NCT01038271.)

▶ There is broad acknowledgment that palliative care is typically delivered late, perhaps too late, in the disease process of cancer or any other illness, yet there is also general acknowledgment that good palliation improves quality of life. This provocative study by Temel and colleagues evaluated the effect of early palliative intervention integrated with standard oncologic care in patients with stage IV non–small-cell lung cancer, compared with standard oncologic care with introduction of palliative care at the discretion of the treating physician. Because the anticipated median survival of patients with metastatic lung cancer is approximately 1 year at best, these patients can be anticipated within a short time after diagnosis to develop impaired quality of life related to physical and psychological symptoms with disease progression as well as to complications of treatment. Palliative care in this study was delivered by a dedicated team of trained health care professionals. Patients in the palliative care intervention arm had better outcomes as measured by a standardized lung cancer quality of life scale, with fewer depressive symptoms. What was particularly remarkable is that median survival was longer in the intervention group by 2.7 months, as demonstrated in Fig 3 in the original article. This magnitude of benefit, while it may seem small on an absolute scale, is equivalent to the benefit obtained with intervention with standard first-line chemotherapy or with the addition of bevacizumab to chemotherapy in patients with stage IV adenocarcinoma of the lung, and so in the realm of lung cancer, care is quite significant.[1,2] The etiology of this improvement in survival is not clear, though presumably a number of factors are contributing that relate to the alleviation of suffering from physical pain and the avoidance of depression. The message is very clear that early intervention with palliative care should be part of the comprehensive care plan for patients with lung cancer.

L. T. Tanoue, MD

References

1. Schiller JH, Harrington D, Belani CP, et al. Comparison of four chemotherapy regimens for advanced non-small-cell lung cancer. *N Engl J Med.* 2002;346:92-98.
2. Sandler A, Gray R, Perry MC, et al. Paclitaxel-carboplatin alone or with bevacizumab for non-small-cell lung cancer. *N Engl J Med.* 2006;355:2542-2550.

Smoking as a Factor in Causing Lung Cancer
Bach PB (Memorial Sloan-Kettering Cancer Ctr, NY)
JAMA 301:539-541, 2009

Tobacco Smoking as a Possible Etiologic Factor in Bronchiogenic Carcinoma: A Study of Six Hundred and Eighty-Four Proved Cases
Ernest L. Wynder and Evarts A. Graham, MD
JAMA. 1950;143(4):329-336.
In this case-control study, the investigators compared the smoking histories of individuals with lung cancer and without lung cancer. Participants were matched for age and several dimensions of smoking history were ascertained through a standardized set of questionnaires (including age at initiation and cessation, and average amount smoked per day of cigarettes, cigars, or with a pipe). Each individual's occupational history and history of prior lung disease was captured to control for possible confounders. The investigators found that individuals with lung cancer had a more extensive smoking history than individuals without lung cancer.

▶ As part of the *JAMA* Classics series, this is a review of the classic 1950 report by Wynder and Graham linking cigarette smoking to lung cancer.[1] Any physician who has not read the original article or the analysis by Doll and Hill that same year should do so.[2] These studies elegantly and simply establish the causal link between smoking and lung cancer, though a formal acknowledgment by the US Surgeon General of the relationship would not be forthcoming until 1964.[3] A half century later, with 20% of American adults habitually smoking, we are still not successful in efforts at limiting cigarette consumption and have made minimal inroads in limiting the health consequences of smoking. This commentary by Bach outlines some highlights and failures of tobacco control policy and offers some suggestions for the future.

L. T. Tanoue, MD

References

1. Wynder EL, Graham EA. Tobacco smoking as a possible etiologic factor in bronchiogenic carcinoma; a study of 684 proved cases. *JAMA.* 1950;143:329-336.
2. Doll R, Hill AB. Smoking and carcinoma of the lung; preliminary report. *Br Med J.* 1950;2:739-748.
3. US Public Health Service. *Smoking and health. Report of the Advisory committee to the Surgeon General of the Public Health Service.* Publication No. 1103. Washington, DC: US Department of Health, Education, and Welfare, Public Health Service; 1964.

Influence of smoking cessation after diagnosis of early stage lung cancer on prognosis: systematic review of observational studies with meta-analysis

Parsons A, Daley A, Begh R, et al (Univ of Birmingham, Edgbaston)
BMJ 340:b5569, 2010

Objective.—To systematically review the evidence that smoking cessation after diagnosis of a primary lung tumour affects prognosis.

Design.—Systematic review with meta-analysis.

Data Sources.—CINAHL (from 1981), Embase (from 1980), Medline (from 1966), Web of Science (from 1966), CENTRAL (from 1977) to December 2008, and reference lists of included studies.

Study Selection.—Randomised controlled trials or observational longitudinal studies that measured the effect of quitting smoking after diagnosis of lung cancer on prognostic outcomes, regardless of stage at presentation or tumour histology, were included.

Data Extraction.—Two researchers independently identified studies for inclusion and extracted data. Estimates were combined by using a random effects model, and the I^2 statistic was used to examine heterogeneity. Life tables were used to model five year survival for early stage nonsmall cell lung cancer and limited stage small cell lung cancer, using death rates for continuing smokers and quitters obtained from this review.

Results.—In 9/10 included studies, most patients studied were diagnosed as having an early stage lung tumour. Continued smoking was associated with a significantly increased risk of all cause mortality (hazard ratio 2.94, 95% confidence interval 1.15 to 7.54) and recurrence (1.86, 1.01 to 3.41) in early stage non-small cell lung cancer and of all cause mortality (1.86, 1.33 to 2.59), development of a second primary tumour (4.31, 1.09 to 16.98), and recurrence (1.26, 1.06 to 1.50) in limited stage small cell lung cancer. No study contained data on the effect of quitting smoking on cancer specific mortality or on development of a second primary tumour in nonsmall cell lung cancer. Life table modelling on the basis of these data estimated 33% five year survival in 65 year old patients with early stage non-small cell lung cancer who continued to smoke compared with 70% in those who quit smoking. In limited stage small cell lung cancer, an estimated 29% of continuing smokers would survive for five years compared with 63% of quitters on the basis of the data from this review.

Conclusions.—This review provides preliminary evidence that smoking cessation after diagnosis of early stage lung cancer improves prognostic outcomes. From life table modelling, the estimated number of deaths prevented is larger than would be expected from reduction of cardiorespiratory deaths after smoking cessation, so most of the mortality gain is likely to be due to reduced cancer progression. These findings indicate

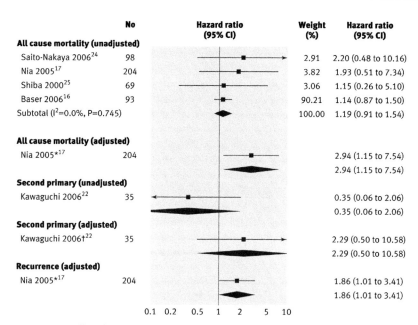

FIGURE 2.—Effect of continued smoking on all cause mortality and recurrence in non-small cell lung cancer. Weights are from random effects analysis. *Adjusted for age, sex, type of operation, histology, postoperative radiotherapy, N status, T status, and previous malignancies. †Adjusted for sex, histology, and cumulative smoking. (Reprinted from Parsons A, Daley A, Begh R, et al. Influence of smoking cessation after diagnosis of early stage lung cancer on prognosis: systematic review of observational studies with meta-analysis. *BMJ.* 2010;340:b5569, reproduced with permission from the BMJ Publishing Group Ltd.)

that offering smoking cessation treatment to patients presenting with early stage lung cancer may be beneficial (Figs 2 and 3).

▶ Ninety percent of lung cancer cases are attributable to cigarette smoking in countries where cigarette smoking is common.[1] Lifelong smokers incur on average a 20-fold increase in lung cancer risk compared with people who have never smoked, and by the age of 75 years, a cumulative risk of approximately 16% is observed.[2,3] It is well recognized that smoking cessation at any age reduces the risk of lung cancer.[3] It is perhaps less appreciated that smoking cessation after lung cancer diagnosis and treatment may be associated with better outcomes. A remarkable percentage of individuals, as many as 60%, continue to smoke after treatment of lung cancer.[4] In this systematic review with meta-analysis, 10 longitudinal observational studies measuring the effect of smoking cessation after lung cancer diagnosis on clinical outcomes were identified and combined. Most patients in these studies had early-stage cancer. The results of the meta-analysis are shown in Figs 2 and 3. The risk of all primary outcomes measures—all-cause mortality and cancer recurrence in early-stage non—small cell lung cancer and all-cause mortality, cancer recurrence, and development of a second primary tumor in limited-stage small cell

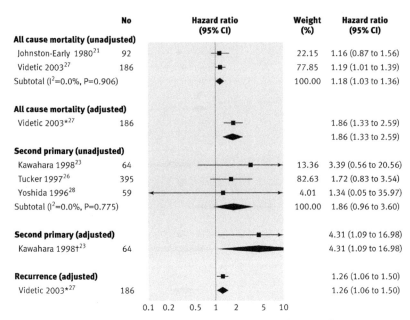

	No	Hazard ratio (95% CI)	Weight (%)	Hazard ratio (95% CI)
All cause mortality (unadjusted)				
Johnston-Early 1980[21]	92		22.15	1.16 (0.87 to 1.56)
Videtic 2003[27]	186		77.85	1.19 (1.01 to 1.39)
Subtotal (I²=0.0%, P=0.906)			100.00	1.18 (1.03 to 1.36)
All cause mortality (adjusted)				
Videtic 2003*[27]	186			1.86 (1.33 to 2.59)
				1.86 (1.33 to 2.59)
Second primary (unadjusted)				
Kawahara 1998[23]	64		13.36	3.39 (0.56 to 20.56)
Tucker 1997[26]	395		82.63	1.72 (0.83 to 3.54)
Yoshida 1996[28]	59		4.01	1.34 (0.05 to 35.97)
Subtotal (I²=0.0%, P=0.775)			100.00	1.86 (0.96 to 3.60)
Second primary (adjusted)				4.31 (1.09 to 16.98)
Kawahara 1998†[23]	64			4.31 (1.09 to 16.98)
Recurrence (adjusted)				1.26 (1.06 to 1.50)
Videtic 2003*[27]	186			1.26 (1.06 to 1.50)

0.1 0.2   0.5   1   2   5 10

FIGURE 3.—Effect of continued smoking on all cause mortality, development of a second primary, or recurrence in small cell lung cancer. Weights are from random effects analysis. *Adjusted for sex, age, and volume of limited disease. †Adjusted for sex, age, performance status, etoposide, radiotherapy, and cumulative smoking. (Reprinted from Parsons A, Daley A, Begh R, et al. Influence of smoking cessation after diagnosis of early stage lung cancer on prognosis: systematic review of observational studies with meta-analysis. *BMJ.* 2010;340:b5569, reproduced with permission from the BMJ Publishing Group Ltd.)

lung cancer—were increased in patients who continued to smoke after treatment. These data suggest that continued exposure to tobacco smoke has a significant effect on the biologic behavior of early-stage lung cancers and also clearly argue against a nihilistic approach to smoking cessation after lung cancer diagnosis.

L. T. Tanoue, MD

References

1. Peto R. *Mortality from smoking in developed countries 1950–2000: indirect estimates from national vital statistics.* New York, NY: Oxford University Press; 1994.
2. Alberg AJ, Ford JG, Samet JM. Epidemiology of lung cancer: ACCP evidence-based clinical practice guidelines (2nd edition). *Chest.* 2007;132:29S-55S.
3. Peto R, Darby S, Deo H, Silcocks P, Whitley E, Doll R. Smoking, smoking cessation, and lung cancer in the UK since 1950: combination of national statistics with two case-control studies. *BMJ.* 2000;321:323-329.
4. Pinto BM, Trunzo JJ. Health behaviors during and after a cancer diagnosis. *Cancer.* 2005;104:2614-2623.

35 Pleural, Interstitial Lung, and Pulmonary Vascular Disease

Management of pleural infection in adults: British Thoracic Society pleural disease guideline 2010
Davies HE, on behalf of the BTS Pleural Disease Guideline Group (Oxford Radcliffe Hosp, UK; et al)
Thorax 65:ii41-ii53, 2010

Background.—Prompt evaluation and therapeutic intervention for pleural infection can reduce morbidity, mortality, and healthcare costs for this common clinical problem. Guidelines were developed from a peer-reviewed systematic literature review and expert opinion of the preferred management.

Considerations.—The care of all patients who require chest tube drainage for a pleural infection should be directed by a chest physician or thoracic surgeon. The clinician should ensure that patients with pleural infection are adequately nourished. These patients are at high risk for developing venous thromboembolism, so adequate thrombosis prophylaxis with heparin is advisable unless contraindicated. If patients with pneumonia progress to ongoing sepsis and elevated C reactive protein levels within 3 days, pleural infection is a possibility and blood cultures for aerobic and anaerobic bacteria are recommended. If pleural effusion accompanies sepsis or pneumonic illness, diagnostic pleural fluid sampling is needed. The pH of pleural fluid is measured in all nonpurulent effusions when pleural infection is suspected. If such data cannot be obtained, the pleural fluid glucose level should be assessed.

Management.—Patients with purulent or turbid/cloudy pleural fluid should be managed with prompt pleural space chest tube drainage. Samples are tested using Gram stain and/or culture to determine if the infection is established. Chest tube drainage is indicated for patients whose samples contain pathogenic organisms and those whose pleural fluid pH exceeds 7.2. Antibiotics alone may be sufficient for patients whose parapneumonic effusions do not meet these criteria. Patient review, repeat pleural fluid sampling, and chest tube drainage are advised for patients whose clinical progress is poor. Early chest tube drainage aids patients with a loculated pleural collection. To relieve symptoms, large nonpurulent effusions are drained by aspiration or chest tube.

If chest tube drainage is chosen, usually a small-bore catheter (10 to 14 F) is used, but no specific size is considered optimal. Small-bore flexible catheters require regular flushing to avoid catheter blockage. Chest tubes placement is guided by imaging.

Antibiotics include agents targeted to treat the bacterial profile of modern pleural infection and consider local antibiotic policies and resistance patterns. All patients except those with culture-proven pneumococcal infection need antibiotics directed at anaerobic infection. Unless objective evidence reveals a high clinical index of suspicion for atypical pathogens, macrolide antibiotics are not indicated. Bacterial culture results and advice from a microbiologist should guide antibiotic choice. Pleural space penetration is quite adequate with penicillins, pencillins plus β-lactamase inhibitors, metronidazole, and cephalosporins. Aminoglycosides are avoided. With negative bacterial cultures, antibiotics must cover both common community-acquired bacterial pathogens and anaerobic organisms. Empirical antibiotic therapy for hospital-acquired empyema includes coverage for anaerobic organisms and methicillin-resistant *Staphylococcus aureus* (MRSA). Once sepsis improves both clinically and objectively, oral therapy can be substituted for intravenous antibiotics. There is no indication for intrapleural antibiotics, and intrapleural fibrinolytics are not routinely needed. Antibiotics can be given for an extended time on an outpatient basis.

Chest drains are removed once radiographs show successful pleural drainage. If sepsis or a residual pleural collection persists, additional radiographic imaging is needed, along with a thoracic surgical consultation.

Surgery is needed for patients with persistent sepsis and pleural collection despite chest tube drainage and antibiotic therapy. A thoracic surgical consultation is also helpful, allowing better assessment of the suitability for anesthesia. Among the less radical approaches are rib resection and placement of a large-bore drain, particularly useful in frail patients. Sometimes these less invasive procedures are accomplished under local or epidural anesthesia. If effusion drainage is ineffective and sepsis persists in patients who cannot tolerate general anesthesia, reimaging of the thorax, and placement of a small-bore catheter under image guidance, the thoracic surgeon may choose to use a larger-bore chest tube or an intrapleural fibrinolytic. Some patients may benefit from palliative treatment and active symptom control measures. Bronchoscopy is needed only when there is a high index of suspicion of bronchial obstruction.

Conclusions.—Outpatient follow-up is needed for all patients who develop empyema and pleural infection. With prompt treatment, the long-term survival of patients with pleural infection is good. However, long-term sequelae associated with pleural empyema include residual

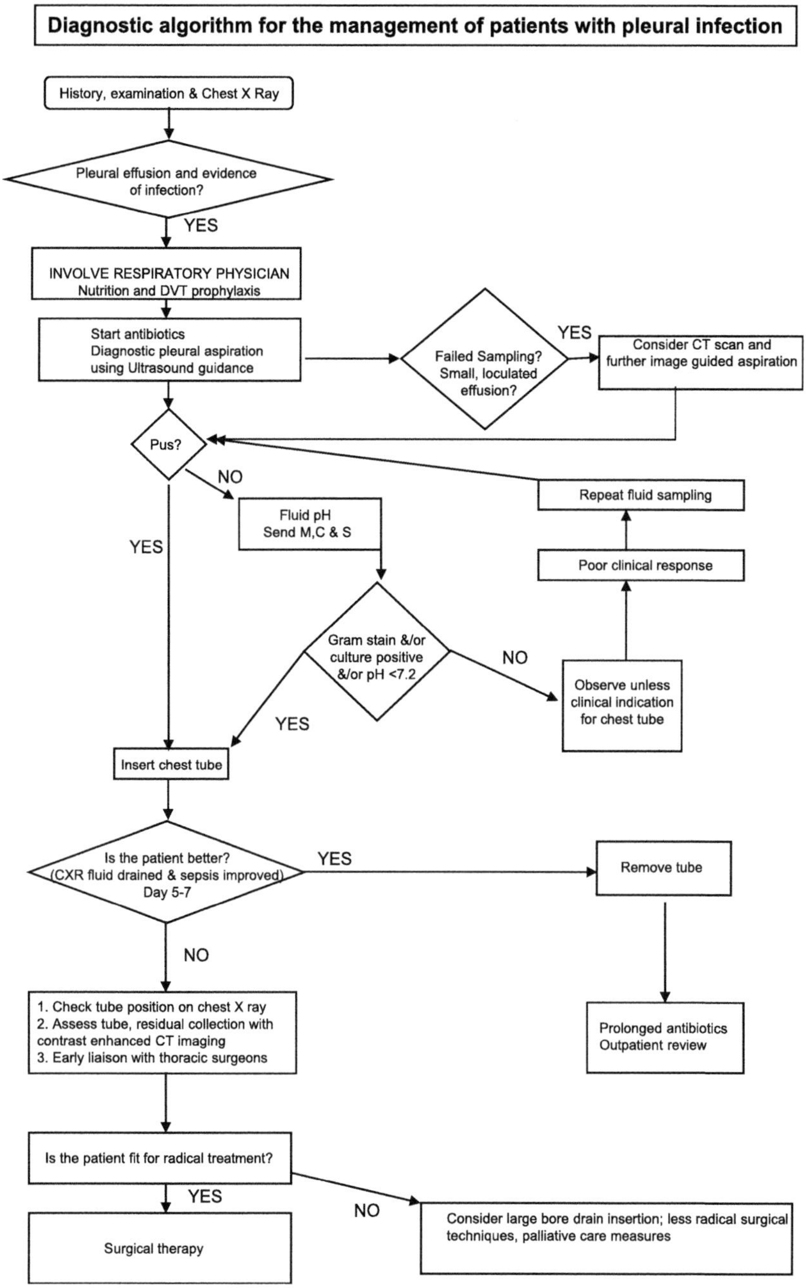

FIGURE 1.—Flow diagram describing the management of pleural infection. (Reprinted from Davies HE, on behalf of the BTS Pleural Disease Guideline Group, Management of pleural infection in adults: British Thoracic Society pleural disease guideline 2010. *Thorax*. 2010;65:ii41-ii53, and reproduced/amended with permission from the BMJ Publishing Group.)

pleural thickening. Patients with pyothorax present for over 20 years may rarely develop pleural lymphoma (Fig 1).

▶ These are new guidelines for treating pleural infection. I suggest every pulmonologist go over the Web site since access is free. There is always a debate on how big a catheter to place and when to place it for infected pleural effusions. According to British Thoracic Society, the catheter size could be as small as 10 to 14 F and needs frequent flushing. The other point is to put a chest tube in if only the Gram stain is positive even if the effusion does not look complicated.

M. Ali Raza, MD, FCCP, DABSM

Cryptogenic Organizing Pneumonia: Serial High-Resolution CT Findings in 22 Patients
Lee JW, Lee KS, Lee HY, et al (Sungkyunkwan Univ School of Medicine, Seoul, Republic of Korea)
AJR Am J Roentgenol 195:916-922, 2010

Objective.—We conducted a review of serial high-resolution CT (HRCT) findings of cryptogenic organizing pneumonia (COP).

Materials and Methods.—Over the course of 14 years, we saw 32 patients with biopsy-confirmed COP. Serial HRCT scans were available for only 22 patients (seven men and 15 women; mean age, 52 years; median follow-up period, 8 months; range, 5—135 months). Serial CT scans were evaluated by two chest radiologists who reached a conclusion by consensus. Overall changes in disease extent were classified as cured, improved (i.e., ≥10% decrease in extent), not changed, or progressed (i.e., ≥10% increase in extent). When there were remaining abnormalities, the final follow-up CT images were analyzed to express observers' ideas regarding what type of interstitial lung disease the images most likely suggested.

Results.—The two most common patterns of lung abnormality on initial scans were ground-glass opacification (86% of patients [19/22]) and consolidation (77% of patients [17/22]), distributed along the bronchovascular bundles or subpleural lungs in 13 patients (59%). In six patients (27%), the disease disappeared completely; in 15 patients (68%), the disease was decreased in extent; and in one patient (5%), no change in extent was detected on follow-up CT. When lesions remained, the final follow-up CT findings were reminiscent of fibrotic nonspecific interstitial pneumonia in 10 of 16 patients (63%).

Conclusion.—Although COP is a disease with a generally good prognosis, most patients (73%) with COP have some remaining disease seen on follow-up CT scans, and, in such cases, the lesions generally resemble a fibrotic nonspecific interstitial pneumonia pattern.

▶ I included this retrospective study with its limitations of being small sample size to press on the following points:

1. Long-term follow-up shows complete resolution of the cryptogenic organizing pneumonia in only 27%, a lower number than that previously described.
2. The patients who are going to resolve versus who will not get complete resolution have more restrictive disease (forced vital capacity 93 ± 7.2% vs 58 ± 16.2% predicted) and lower single-breath carbon monoxide diffusing capacity of the lung (86 ± 15.8% vs 65 ± 14.2% predicted).
3. There is no evidence of any crucial decline in pulmonary function tests after initial assessment in any of the patients with the right treatment.
4. If reticulation is the initial picture on high-resolution CT, then the patients are less likely to respond to therapy.
5. The relapse rate is about 10%.[1,2]

M. Ali Raza, MD, FCCP, DABSM

References

1. Cordier JF, Loire R, Brune J. Idiopathic bronchiolitis obliterans organizing pneumonia: definition of characteristic clinical profiles in a series of 16 patients. *Chest.* 1989;96:999-1004.
2. Epler GR, Colby TV, McLoud TC, Carrington CB, Gaensler EA. Bronchiolitis obliterans organizing pneumonia. *N Engl J Med.* 1985;312:152-158.

Bedside Transthoracic Sonography in Suspected Pulmonary Embolism: A New Tool for Emergency Physicians

Hoffmann B, Gullett JP (Johns Hopkins Univ, Baltimore, MD; Johns Hopkins Bayview Med Ctr, Baltimore, MD)
Acad Emerg Med 17:e88-e93, 2010

Background.—The signs and symptoms of pulmonary embolism (PE) are nonspecific, making it difficult to diagnose without a high index of suspicion. Technical advances including D-dimer and multidetector-row computed tomography (MDCT) scan have increased detection rates, especially for segmental and subsegmental PE, but with lower specificity. MDCT drawbacks include not being widely available; not being feasible for all patients who require a PE workup, particularly unstable patients; exposing patients to radiation; and requiring more time than bedside ultrasound (US). Bedside pulmonary US has successfully diagnosed pneumothorax, pleural effusion, pneumonia, lung edema, and PE. Little information exists on the use of bedside US in emergency department (ED) settings. Three patients were diagnosed provisionally using chest/pulmonary US and confirmed using MDCT.

Case Reports.—Case 1: Woman, 21, came to the ED complaining of several days of severe and worsening chest pain that disturbed her sleep. Symptoms began about 24 hours after an elective surgical abortion at gestational age 8 2/7 weeks. She smoked but had no other known risk factors for PE. The pain was located inferior to the right breast and was accompanied by palpitations, periodic shortness of breath, and cough with minor hemoptysis the day she came for treatment. Her vital signs were blood pressure 127/81 mm Hg, heart rate 109 beats/min, respirations 18 breaths/min, oxygen saturation 100% on room air, and temperature 38.2°C. Respirations increased and pain worsened when she spoke. Heart tones were normal with coarse rhonchi over the right lung and diminished breath sounds over the right lung base. Chest pain was reproducible on chest wall palpation of the right lower chest. Focused bedside US showed the right lower lung had multiple wedge-shaped hypodense parenchymal defects at the lung periphery with localized and basal effusion. Doppler US showed no perfusion of the edematous lung tissue. PE with lung infarction was diagnosed.

Case 2: Woman, 65, had a past history of hypertension and stroke and came for treatment of sudden-onset sharp chest pain worsening with deep breathing. Her blood pressure was 168/69 mm Hg, heart rate 69 beats/min, respirations 18 breaths/min, and oxygen saturation 99% on 2 L of oxygen by nasal cannula. Her lungs were clear and she had a regular heart rate and rhythm with no murmurs or rubs. Chest x-ray was negative, but sonography showed several subtle wedge-shaped or rounded hypodense parenchymal areas adjacent to the pleural space, suggesting PE. Transthoracic US found large areas of normal lung. A contrast-enhanced MDCT with PE protocol revealed bilateral PE.

Case 3: Man, 52, came to the ED with chest pain and shortness of breath while walking to work. He felt diaphoretic and febrile. His blood pressure was 153/87 mm Hg, heart rate 132 beats/min (tachycardic), and respirations 20 breaths/min (mildly tachypneic). Initial oxygen saturation on room air was 83%, but this improved to 96% on 3 L of oxygen by nasal cannula. On auscultation he had a regular heart rate with no murmurs, coarse breath sounds bilaterally, and chest pain on deep breathing. Focused bedside sonography found no pneumothorax but multiple small wedge-shaped parenchymal defects at the lung periphery with localized pleural effusion, suggesting multiple PE.

Conclusions.—Using bedside US of the thorax and heart may improve the assessment of patients with suspected PE. This approach may be especially useful for patients in an intermediate risk group or when D-dimer and chest CT are not available or feasible. The effectiveness of US for adults and children and the possible inclusion of this modality into clinical decision-making algorithms will need to be assessed through large multicenter studies. Transthoracic US for the diagnosis of PE in the ED should

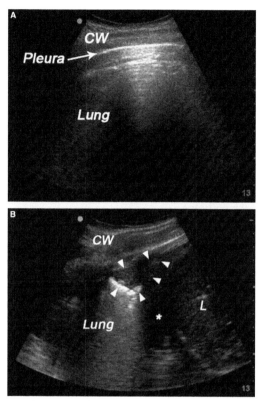

FIGURE 1.—(A) TUS showing normal left lung. The transducer is placed at the left mid-axillary line above the diaphragm parallel to the fourth intercostal space. The pleura is identified as a bright hyperechoic line. (B) The transducer is placed in the right coronal plane at the level of the diaphragm. The lung parenchyma is seen with a pleural-based, wedge-shaped, parenchymal hypodense area (white arrowheads) marking the visible area of lung infarction. There is strong posterior enhancement and parenchymal consolidation (white hyperdense area central to the peripheral defect). *Pleural effusion between liver (L) and right lung. CW = chest wall; TUS = transthoracic ultrasound. (Reprinted from Hoffmann B, Gullett JP. Bedside transthoracic sonography in suspected pulmonary embolism: a new tool for emergency physicians. *Acad Emerg Med.* 2010;17:e88-e93, with permission from the Society for Academic Emergency Medicine.)

be considered, especially for patients who have contraindications for CT radiation exposure or contrast application (Fig 1).

▶ Ultrasound used at bedside in the critical care areas and emergency room is becoming a norm now. It has a great advantage in timely and accurate assessment of the clinical condition. Ultrasound of the lung has not been catching fame, but I believe in the right clinical context, it has a great role to play, and this study is a great example of that. I am sure that this scenario has happened to all of us as described in the cases, and at least in few instances, we have overlooked the possibility of pulmonary embolism because the patient is pregnant and infiltrates are shown with fever and high white blood cell count. I am including this article so that all of us know about the future application of bedside ultrasound when it is at its prime in the coming years.

M. Ali Raza, MD, FCCP, DABSM

Early and Late Clinical Outcomes of Pulmonary Embolectomy for Acute Massive Pulmonary Embolism

Vohra HA, Whistance RN, Mattam K, et al (Southampton Univ Hosps NHS Trust, UK)
Ann Thorac Surg 90:1747-1752, 2010

Background.—The aim of this study was to investigate the early and late outcomes of patients undergoing pulmonary embolectomy for acute massive pulmonary embolus.

Methods.—Twenty-one patients (15 male, 6 female) underwent pulmonary embolectomy at our institution between March 2001 and July 2010. The median age was 55 years (range, 24 to 70 years). Of these, 9 patients presented with out-of-hospital cardiac arrest and 8 presented with New York Heart Association class III or IV. Sixteen patients underwent preoperative transthoracic echocardiography, which showed evidence of right ventricular dilatation in all, whereas in 14 patients (66.6%) pulmonary artery pressures were significantly elevated with moderate to severe tricuspid regurgitation. The median preoperative Euroscore was 9 (range, 3 to 16), and 11 patients (52.1%) received systemic thrombolysis preoperatively. There were 6 salvage (28.5%), 10 emergency (47.6%), and 5 urgent (23.8%) procedures. Concomitant procedures were performed in 3 patients (14.2%), and surgery was performed without the use of cardiopulmonary bypass in 3 patients (14.2%). The median follow-up was 38 months (range, 0 to 114 months).

Results.—The in-hospital mortality was 19% (n = 4). Postoperative complications included stroke (n = 3, 14.2%), lower respiratory tract infection (n = 6, 28.5%), wound infection (n = 3, 14.2%), acute renal failure requiring hemofiltration (n = 4, 19%), and supraventricular tachyarrhythmias (n = 4, 19%). At discharge, transthoracic echocardiography showed mild to moderate right ventricular dysfunction and dilatation in 11 survivors (64.7%). Two patients died during follow-up, and actuarial survival at 5 years was 76.9% ± 10.1% and at 8 years was 51.2% ± 22.0%. At final follow-up, 11 of the 15 survivors (73.3%) were New York Heart Association class I, and no patients required further intervention.

Conclusions.—Patients who undergo surgery for massive pulmonary embolism have an acceptable outcome despite being high-risk.

▶ I am including this article to show that except for 1 or 2 large centers, who have exceptionally low rates of morbidity and mortality associated with thromboendarterectomy, there is at least 20% mortality associated with this procedure in major centers. This may also be related to low number of cases done and only taking cases who are in impending arrest. This treatment is still much better than thrombolytics used for patients with unstable pulmonary embolism, which is close to 40%. There is another approach that minimizes the mortality to even lower 6%, showed by Leacche et al,[1,2] where they take all patients with large central clot burden and impending right ventricular failure for operation.

M. Ali Raza, MD, FCCP, DABSM

References

1. Leacche M, Unic D, Goldhabe SZ, et al. Modern surgical treatment of massive pulmonary embolism: results of 47 consecutive patients after rapid diagnosis and aggressive surgical approach. *J Thorac Cardiovasc Surg.* 2005;129:1018-1023.
2. Kadner A, Schmidli J, Schönhoff F, et al. Excellent outcome after surgical treatment of massive pulmonary embolism in critically ill patients. *J Thorac Cardiovasc Surg.* 2008;136:448-451.

Bosentan Improves Skin Perfusion of Hands in Patients with Systemic Sclerosis with Pulmonary Arterial Hypertension

Rosato E, Molinaro I, Borghese F, et al (Sapienza Univ of Rome, Italy)
J Rheumatol 37:2531-2539, 2010

Objective.—Our aim was to investigate effects of bosentan on hand perfusion in patients with systemic sclerosis (SSc) with pulmonary arterial hypertension (PAH), using laser Doppler perfusion imaging (LDPI).

Methods.—We enrolled 30 SSc patients with PAH, 30 SSc patients without PAH, and 30 healthy controls. In SSc patients and healthy controls at baseline, skin blood flow of the dorsum of the hands was determined with a Lisca laser Doppler perfusion imager. The dorsal surface of the hands was divided into 3 regions of interest (ROI). ROI 1 included 3 fingers of the hand from the second to the fourth distally to the proximal interphalangeal finger joint. ROI 2 included the area between the proximal interphalangeal and the metacarpophalangeal joint. ROI 3 included only the dorsal surface of the hand without the fingers. LDPI was repeated in SSc patients and controls after 4, 8, and 16 weeks of treatment. In SSc patients, nailfold videocapillaroscopy and Raynaud Condition Score (RCS) were performed at baseline and at 4, 8, and 16 weeks.

Results.—SSc patients with PAH enrolled in the study received treatment with bosentan as standard care for PAH. In these patients with PAH, after 8 and 16 weeks of treatment, bosentan improved minimum, mean, and maximum perfusion and the perfusion proximal-distal gradient. Bosentan seems to be most effective in patients with the early and active capillaroscopic pattern than in patients with the late pattern. Bosentan improved skin blood flow principally in the ROI 1 compared to the ROI 2 and ROI 3. Bosentan restored the perfusion proximal-distal gradient in 57% of SSc patients with the early capillaroscopic pattern. No significant differences from baseline were observed in the RCS in SSc patients with PAH.

Conclusion.—Bosentan improved skin perfusion in SSc patients with PAH, although it did not ameliorate symptoms of Raynaud's phenomenon. Skin blood perfusion increased in SSc patients with PAH, particularly in the skin region distal to the proximal interphalangeal joint, and in patients with the early/active capillaroscopic pattern. Double-blind randomized clinical trials are needed to evaluate the effects of bosentan on skin perfusion of SSc patients without PAH and with active digital ulcers.

▶ Bosentan has significant therapeutic advantage in pulmonary arterial hypertension (PAH) and more so in the connective tissue diseases. The above study shows the effect of 62.5 mg and 125 mg doses of bosentan on digital perfusion. These changes were more evident in patients with the early/active capillaroscopic pattern than in patients with the late pattern. Because activation of the endothelin-I system also plays a role in determining endothelial dysfunction in systemic sclerosis, we can suppose that bosentan ameliorates endothelial dysfunction and consequently microcirculatory flow. The study is restricted by its limitations namely, correction for temperature, the open-label approach, the lack of a run-in treatment-free period, the lack of a crossover design, including the diagnosis of PAH in these patients without right heart catheter. I personally believe that endothelin receptor blockers have significant added advantages pertaining to the microvascular remodelling and prevention of microthrombi formation, which is the ultimate cause of end-organ damage and ischemia.

M. Ali Raza, MD, FCCP, DABSM

Venous Thromboembolism with Chronic Liver Disease
Saleh T, Matta F, Alali F, et al (St Joseph Mercy Oakland Hosp, Pontiac, MI; Michigan State Univ, East Lansing)
Am J Med 124:64-68, 2011

Background.—Patients with chronic liver disease have both antithrombotic and prothrombotic coagulation abnormalities. Published data conflict on whether patients with chronic liver disease have a high or low prevalence of venous thromboembolism.

Methods.—The number of patients discharged from hospitals throughout the US with a diagnostic code for chronic alcoholic and chronic nonalcoholic liver disease from 1979 through 2006 was obtained from the National Hospital Discharge Survey. We compared prevalences of venous thromboembolism among patients with chronic alcoholic liver disease and chronic nonalcoholic liver disease.

Results.—Among 4,927,000 hospitalized patients with chronic alcoholic liver disease from 1979-2006, the prevalence of venous thromboembolism was 0.6%, compared with 0.9% among 4,565,000 hospitalized patients with chronic nonalcoholic liver disease.

Conclusion.—The prevalence of venous thromboembolism in hospitalized patients with chronic liver disease, both alcoholic and nonalcoholic, was low. The prevalence of venous thromboembolism was higher in those with chronic non-alcoholic liver disease, but the difference was small and of no clinical consequence. Based on the literature, both showed a lower prevalence of venous thromboembolism than in hospitalized patients with

TABLE 3.—Prevalence of Deep Venous Thrombosis and Venous Thromboembolism in Selected Medical Illnesses

Medical Illness	Prevalence of DVT (%)	Prevalence of VTE (%)	Age Group	Reference (First Author)
Non-alcoholic liver disease	0.6	0.9	≥18 years	Present study
Alcoholic liver disease	0.5	0.6	≥18 years	Present study
Cancer of pancreas	3.9	5.1	All ages	Stein[20]
Cancer of brain	3.7	4.9	All ages	Stein[20]
Myeloproliferative, lymphatic/hematopoietic	3.0	3.4	All ages	Stein[20]
Cancer of stomach	2.2	2.6	All ages	Stein[20]
Obesity	2.0	−	All ages	Stein[21]
Cancer of prostate	1.7	2.2	All ages	Stein[20]
Rheumatoid arthritis	1.6	2.3	All ages	Matta[22]
Cancer of colon	1.5	2.1	All ages	Stein[20]
Ulcerative colitis	1.5	1.9	All ages	Saleh[23]
Nephrotic syndrome	1.5	−	>1 month	Kayali[24]
Hemorrhagic stroke	1.4	1.9	All ages	Skaf[25]
Hypothyroidism	1.4	1.8	All ages	Danescu[26]
Human immunodeficiency virus	1.4	1.7	≥18 years	Matta[27]
Heart failure	1.0	1.6	All ages	Beemath[28]
Crohn disease	1.1	1.2	All ages	Saleh[23]
COPD	1.1	1.6	>20 years	Stein[29]
Diabetes mellitus	1.0	1.4	All ages	Stein[30]
Ischemic stroke	0.7	1.2	All ages	Skaf[25]
Sickle cell disease	0.6	−	All ages	Stein[31]

COPD = chronic obstructive pulmonary disease; DVT = deep venous thrombosis; VTE = venous thromboembolism.
Editor's Note: Please refer to original journal article for full references.

most other medical diseases. It may be that both chronic alcoholic liver disease and chronic nonalcoholic liver disease have protective antithrombotic mechanisms, although the mechanisms differ (Table 3).

► It is always a question of whether to do venous thromboembolism (VTE) prophylaxis for patients with chronic liver disease or not because they are mostly autoanticoagulated.[1] The above study is a big step in alleviating the concern because it agrees with the previous work done on the incidence of pulmonary embolism (PE)/deep venous thrombosis (DVT) in liver cirrhosis. The risk of PE is 0.1% to 0.3% and DVT is 0.5% to 0.6% in the cohort of all patients with chronic liver disease. In our center, we consider it simply by looking at the prothrombin time and international normalized ratio (INR) of the patients with chronic liver disease, and if the INR is more than 2, then we don't give DVT prophylaxis. Prophylaxis is recommended for an INR less than 1.5, and an INR between 1.5 and 2.0 is even more tricky. To date, I don't see a study approving this approach but it makes sense and we have not had a major problem so far. Please remember that it is anecdotal rather than evidence.

The strength of the investigation is the large number of patients identified with alcoholic liver disease and VTE (30 000 patients) and nonalcoholic liver disease[2] with VTE (42 000 patients).

Diversity of the population ranges in terms of age, race, sex, and geographic regions (all 50 states and the District of Columbia), and the extensive duration of observation (28 years).

Limitations include lack of data on the severity of the liver disease, the proportion with ascites, hepatic decompensation, reason for hospitalization, proportion of patients hospitalized more than once, and the basis for the diagnosis of liver disease.

M. Ali Raza, MD, FCCP, DABSM

References

1. Northup PG, McMahon MM, Ruhl AP, et al. Coagulopathy does not fully protect hospitalized cirrhosis patients from peripheral venous thromboembolism. *Am J Gastroenterol*. 2006;101:1524-1528.
2. García-Fuster MJ, Abdilla N, Fabiá MJ, Fernández C, Oliver V, Forner MJ. [Venous thromboembolism and liver cirrhosis]. *Rev Esp Enferm Dig*. 2008;100: 259-262.

Investigation of a unilateral pleural effusion in adults: British Thoracic Society pleural disease guideline 2010

Hooper C, on behalf of the BTS Pleural Guideline Group (Southmead Hosp, Bristol, UK; et al)

Thorax 65:ii4-ii17, 2010

Pleural effusions are a common medical problem with more than 50 recognised causes including disease local to the pleura or underlying lung, systemic conditions, organ dysfunction and drugs.

Pleural effusions occur as a result of increased fluid formation and/or reduced fluid resorption. The precise pathophysiology of fluid accumulation varies according to underlying aetiologies. As the differential diagnosis for a unilateral pleural effusion is wide, a systematic approach to investigation is necessary. The aim is to establish a diagnosis swiftly while minimising unnecessary invasive investigations and facilitating treatment, avoiding the need for repeated therapeutic aspirations when possible.

Since the 2003 guideline, several clinically relevant studies have been published, allowing new recommendations regarding image guidance of pleural procedures with clear benefits to patient comfort and safety, optimum pleural fluid sampling and processing and the particular value of thoracoscopic pleural biopsies. This guideline also includes a review of recent evidence for the use of new biomarkers including N-terminal pro-brain natriuretic peptide (NT-proBNP), mesothelin and surrogate markers of tuberculous pleuritis (Table 1).

▶ British Thoracic Society guidelines are a must read. The updates for unilateral pleural effusion are:

1. Aspiration should not be performed for bilateral effusions in a clinical setting strongly suggestive of a transudate unless there are atypical features or they fail to respond to therapy.
2. An accurate drug history should be taken during clinical assessment.
3. Ultrasound detects pleural fluid septations with greater sensitivity than CT.

TABLE 1.—Pleural Fluid Tests and Sample Collection Guidance

Test	Notes
Recommended tests for all sampled pleural effusions	
Biochemistry: LDH and protein	2—5 ml in plain container or serum blood collection tube depending on local policy. Blood should be sent simultaneously to biochemistry for total protein and LDH so that Light's criteria can be applied
Microscopy and culture (MC and S)	5 ml in plain container. If pleural infection is particularly suspected, a further 5 ml in both anaerobic and aerobic blood culture bottles should be sent
Cytological examination and differential cell count	Maximum volume from remaining available sample in a plain universal container. Refrigerate if delay in processing anticipated (eg, out of hours)
Other tests sent only in selected cases as described in the text	
pH	In non-purulent effusions when pleural infection is suspected. 0.5—1 ml drawn up into a heparinised blood gas syringe immediately after aspiration. The syringe should be capped to avoid exposure to air. Processed using a ward arterial blood gas machine
Glucose	Occasionally useful in diagnosis of rheumatoid effusion. 1—2 ml in fluoride oxalate tube sent to biochemistry
Acid-fast bacilli and TB culture	When there is clinical suspicion of TB pleuritis. Request with MC and S. 5 ml sample in plain container
Triglycerides and cholesterol	To distinguish chylothorax from pseudochylothorax in milky effusions. Can usually be requested with routine biochemistry (LDH, protein) using the same sample
Amylase	Occasionally useful in suspected pancreatitis-related effusion. Can usually be requested with routine biochemistry
Haematocrit	Diagnosis of haemothorax. 1—2 ml sample in EDTA container sent to haematology

LDH, lactate dehydrogenase; PH, pulmonary hypertension; TB, tuberculosis.

4. The appearance of the pleural fluid and any odor should be recorded.

5. *N*-terminal probrain natriuretic peptide levels in blood and pleural fluid correlate closely, and the measurement of both has been shown in several series to be effective in discriminating transudates associated with congestive heart failure from other transudative or exudative causes. The cutoff value of these studies varies from 600 to 4000 pg/mL (with 1500 pg/mL being most commonly used).

6. There is no significant increase in cytology yield after 2 samples.

M. Ali Raza, MD, FCCP, DABSM

Management of a malignant pleural effusion: British Thoracic Society pleural disease guideline 2010
Roberts ME, on behalf of the BTS Pleural Disease Guideline Group (Sherwood Forest Hosps NHS Foundation Trust, UK; et al)
Thorax 65:ii32-ii40, 2010

Background.—Finding malignant cells in pleural fluid and/or parietal pleura indicates a disseminated or advanced disease and reduced life expectancy in patients who have cancer. The management of malignant pleural effusion was outlined.

Clinical Presentation.—Most malignant effusions produce symptoms. If the pleural effusions are massive, with complete or almost complete opacification of a hemithorax on the chest x-ray, malignancy is the most common cause.

Management.—Asymptomatic patients who have a known tumor type can be observed. Symptomatic malignant effusions prompt consultation with the respiratory team and/or respiratory multidisciplinary team. If pleural effusions are treated by aspiration alone, recurrence of effusion within 1 month is likely. If the patient's life expectancy exceeds 1 month, aspiration is not recommended. Caution is needed if more than 1.5 L is removed in a single episode. Except in patients with short life expectancies, small-bore chest tubes and pleurodesis are preferred to repeat aspiration. Pleurodesis after intercostal drainage prevents recurrence except with significant trapped lung.

For effusion drainage plus pleurodesis, small-bore (10 to 14 F) intercostal catheters are chosen initially. For large pleural effusions, controlled drainage will reduce the risk of re-expansion pulmonary edema. If only partial pleural apposition can be done, chemical pleurodesis may provide relief of symptoms. If pleural apposition is not possible in a patient with symptoms, an indwelling pleural catheter is more efficacious than repeat aspiration. Radiographic confirmation of effusion drainage and lung re-expansion should be immediately followed by pleurodesis. Usually suction to help pleural drainage is unnecessary, but if used, a high-volume low-pressure system is needed.

Because intrapleural administration of sclerosing agents can be painful, 3 mg/kg of lidocaine (maximum 250 mg) is given intrapleurally just before the sclerosant is given. The use of premedication can alleviate both anxiety and pain associated with pleurodesis. The most effective sclerosant available is talc. Graded talc is preferred to ungraded talc because of the lower risk of arterial hypoxemia. Either a slurry or insufflation can be used. An alternative to talc is bleomycin, which has modest efficacy. Sclerosant administration can be complicated by pleuritic chest pain and fever. After intrapleural instillation of sclerosant, it is not necessary to rotate the patient. The intercostal tube is clamped for 1 hour after administering the sclerosant. The tube is removed within 24 to 48 hours if fluid drainage is not excessive (less than 250 mg/day).

In patients with proven or suspected mesothelioma, prophylactic radiotherapy may be used at the site of thoracoscopy, surgery, or insertion of a large-bore chest tube. However, for pleural aspiration or biopsy, such prophylaxis is not needed. For the relief of distressing dyspnea caused by multiloculated malignant effusion resistant to simple drainage, fibrinolytic drugs can be instilled intrapleurally.

Thoracoscopy is recommended to diagnose suspected malignant pleural effusion and for drainage and pleurodesis of known malignant pleural effusion in patients with good performance status. To control recurrent malignant pleural effusion, thoracoscopic talc poudrage may be helpful. Thorascopy is safe and has low complication rates. To control recurrent and symptomatic malignant effusions, ambulatory indwelling pleural catheters may be useful. Pleurectomy cannot be recommended as an alternative to pleurodesis or an indwelling pleural catheter in patients with recurrent effusions or trapped lung.

Conclusions.—Lung cancer is the most common metastatic tumor (50% to 65% of cases) to the pleura in men and breast tissue in women, followed by lymphomas and tumors of the genitourinary tract and gastrointestinal tract (25% of cases). The primary is unknown in 7% to 15% of malignant pleural effusions. The clinical characteristics of pleural fluid have not yet

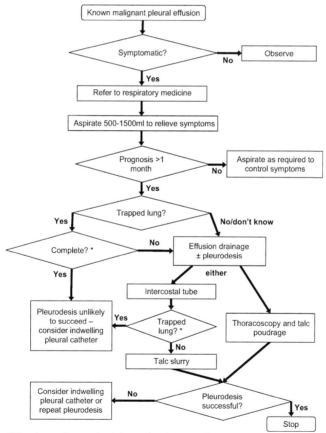

* There is no evidence as to what proportion of unapposed pleura prevents pleurodesis. We suggest that <50% pleural apposition is unlikely to lead to successful pleurodesis

FIGURE 1.—Management algorithm for malignant pleural effusion. (Reprinted from Roberts ME, on behalf of the BTS Pleural Disease Guideline Group. Management of a malignant pleural effusion: British Thoracic Society pleural disease guideline 2010. *Thorax.* 2010;65:ii32-ii40, and reproduced/amended with permission from the BMJ Publishing Group.)

TABLE 1.—Primary Tumour Site in Patients with Malignant Pleural Effusion

Primary Tumour Site	Salyer[14] (n=95)	Chernow[1] (n=96)	Johnston[13] (n=472)	Sears[4] (n=592)	Hsu[12] (n=785)	Total (%)
Lung	42	32	168	112	410	764 (37.5)
Breast	11	20	70	141	101	343 (16.8)
Lymphoma	11	—	75	92	56	234 (11.5)
Gastrointestinal	—	13	28	32	68	141 (6.9)
Genitourinary	—	13	57	51	70	191 (9.4)
Other	14	5	26	88	15	148 (7.8)
Unknown primary	17	13	48	76	65	219 (10.7)

Editor's Note: Please refer to original journal article for full references.

been shown to correlate with survival. Guidelines for the management of malignant pleural effusions were offered (Fig 1, Table 1).

▶ I would encourage all pulmonologists to review the guidelines. New information is summarized as follows:

1. No need to only aspirate pleural effusion in patients with life expectancy of > 1 month. Better to drain it with chest tube.
2. Size 10 to 14 F catheters are good enough as an initial choice for drainage and pleurodesis.
3. In cases of trapped lung, indwelling pleural catheters have a role.
4. Suction to aid pleurodesis is not necessary.
5. Graded talc is the sclerosing agent of choice.
6. For suspected mesothelioma, biopsy or drainage of effusion is not proven to be associated with seeding of chest wall but should be radiated before any other major intervention.
7. Chest tube can be removed if drainage is < 250 mL/d.
8. Recurrent pleural effusion with good performance status should be treated with thoracoscopy. Please review Fig 1.

M. Ali Raza, MD, FCCP, DABSM

36 Community-Acquired Pneumonia

Why Mortality Is Increased in Health-Care-Associated Pneumonia: Lessons From Pneumococcal Bacteremic Pneumonia
Rello J, for the PROCORNEU Study Group (Joan XXIII Univ Hosp, Tarragona, Spain; et al)
Chest 137:1138-1144, 2010

Background.—A cohort of patients with bacteremic *Streptococcus pneumoniae* pneumonia was reviewed to assess why mortality is higher in health-care-associated pneumonia (HCAP) than in community-acquired pneumonia (CAP).

Methods.—A prospective cohort of all adult patients with bacteremic pneumococcal pneumonia attended at the ED was used.

Results.—One hundred eighty-four cases were classified as CAP and 44 (19%) as HCAP. Fifty-two (23%) were admitted to the ICU. Three (1.5%) isolates were resistant to β-lactams, and only two patients received inappropriate therapy. The CAP cohort was significantly younger (median age 68 years, interquartile range [IQR] 42-78 vs 77 years, IQR 67-82, $P < .001$). The HCAP cohort presented a higher Charlson index (2.81 ± 1.9 vs 1.23 ± 1.42, $P < .001$) and had higher severity of illness at admission (altered mental status, respiratory rate > 30/min, Pao_2 /Fio_2 <250, and multi-lobar involvement). HCAP patients had a lower rate of ICU admission (11.3% vs 25.5%, $P < .05$), and a trend toward lower mechanical ventilation (9% vs 19%, $P = .17$) and vasopressor use (9% vs 18.4%, $P = .17$) were documented. More patients in the HCAP cohort presented with a pneumonia severity index score >90 (class IV-V, 95% vs 65%, $P < .001$), and 30-day mortality was significantly higher (29.5% vs 7.6%, $P < .001$). A multivariable regression logistic analysis adjusting for underlying conditions and variables related to severity of illness confirmed that HCAP is an independent variable associated with increased mortality (odds ratio = 5.56; 95% CI, 1.86-16.5).

Conclusions.—Pneumococcal HCAP presents excess mortality, which is independent of bacterial susceptibility. Differences in outcomes were probably due to differences in age, comorbidities, and criteria for ICU admission rather than to therapeutic decisions.

▶ Health care—associated pneumonia (HCAP) has been defined as a subset of pneumonia that occurs in people who have had some ongoing relationship with health care institutions so that they are likely to have had some exposure to resistant or more aggressive organisms than the usual causes of community-acquired pneumonia (CAP). The characteristics of HCAP are still being defined. For instance, as the authors note, it is not yet clear whether the poor outcomes of patients with HCAP are because of comorbidities or a higher rate of antibiotic-resistant bacteria that do not respond to the usual empiric treatment regimens. The point of this study was to try to address some of these issues. To do this the authors decided to concentrate on bacteremic pneumococcal pneumonia in a cohort of all patients presenting to an emergency department with pneumonia over an 8.5-year period. While they were prospectively identified with pneumonia, they were retrospectively assigned a designation of HCAP versus routine CAP. Approximately one-fifth of the patients were classified into this group. Patients with HCAP had higher death rates but lower use of ICUs and more frequently had advance directives around limits on therapy. Only 2 patients, 1 in each group, received inappropriate therapy for their isolate. The patients with HCAP were indeed older, had more comorbidities, and appeared generally sicker. The authors state that the higher mortality in HCAP was possibly because of the decision of the physician and patient to limit the extent of support. Whether the use of ICU care would have affected 30-day mortality is questionable. It certainly would have been much more expensive.

J. R. Maurer, MD, MBA

A multicenter analysis of the ED diagnosis of pneumonia
Chandra A, Nicks B, Maniago E, et al (Duke Univ Med Ctr Durham, NC; Wake Forest Univ Baptist Med Ctr, Winston Salem, NC; Staten Island Univ Hosp, NY)
Am J Emerg Med 28:862-865, 2010

Objectives.—The objective of this study was to describe the prevalence of pneumonia-like signs and symptoms in patients admitted from the emergency department (ED) with a diagnosis of community acquired pneumonia (CAP) but subsequently discharged from the hospital with a nonpneumonia diagnosis.

Methods.—A retrospective, structured, chart review of ED patients with CAP at 3 academic hospitals was performed by trained extractors on all adult patients admitted for CAP. Demographic data, Pneumonia Patient Outcomes Research Team scores, and discharge diagnosis data (*International Classification of Diseases, Ninth Revision* [ICD-9] codes) were extracted using a predetermined case report form.

Results.—A total of 800 patients were admitted from the ED with a diagnosis of CAP from the 3 hospitals, and 219 (27.3%; 95% confidence interval [CI], 24-31) ultimately had a nonpneumonia diagnosis upon discharge. Characteristics of this group included a mean age of 62.6 years, 50% female, and a history of congestive heart failure (CHF) (14%) or cancer (12%). After excluding patients with missing data, 123 patients (65%) had an abnormal chest x-ray, and 13% had abnormal oxygen saturation. Cough, sputum production, fever, tachypnea, or leukocytosis were present in 91.5% of this cohort, and 63.8% had at least 2 of these findings. Twenty alternate *ICD-9*s were identified, including non-CAP pulmonary disease (18%; 95% CI, 13-24), renal disease (16%; 95% CI, 13-19), other infections (9%; 95% CI, 7-11), cardiovascular diseases (3%; 95% CI, 2-4), and other miscellaneous diagnosis (28%; 95% CI, 25-31).

Conclusions.—Our data suggest that the ED diagnosis of CAP frequently differs from the discharge diagnosis. This may be due to the fact that a diagnosis of CAP relies on a combination of potentially nonspecific clinical and radiographic features. New diagnostic approaches and tools with better specificity are needed to improve ED diagnosis of CAP.

▶ Data collected from large content management system databases have resulted in the development of quality standards for the acute management of community-acquired pneumonia.[1] One of the most controversial of these standards has been the timing of delivery of the first dose of antibiotic treatment. Because database analysis showed that patients receiving antibiotics early (typically within 4 hours of presentation) had lower mortality rates, antibiotic timing became a critical quality measure. This has led to concerns around several issues. First, clinicians note that patients, especially elderly patients, with congestive heart failure or other conditions may be given unnecessary (and potentially harmful) antibiotics. Second, there is a concern that with the emphasis on early antibiotics, other diagnoses may be overlooked or delayed to the patient's detriment. Third, overuse of antibiotics is both costly and may increase antibiotic resistance. Fourth, there is concern that the use of a retrospective database to inform widespread, prospective, acute care may be treacherous. This study is the latest and a multicenter study that suggests that an emergency room diagnosis of community-acquired pneumonia is wrong at least one-quarter of the time and that currently used signs, symptoms, and tests often do not adequately separate pneumonia from other conditions. I agree with the authors that increased research into more specific means of diagnosis are urgently needed as are studies looking at varied timing of first antibiotic administration.

J. R. Maurer, MD, MBA

Reference

1. Houck PM, Bratzler DW, Nsa W, Ma A, Bartlett JG. Timing of antibiotic administration and outcomes for Medicare patients hospitalized with community-acquired pneumonia. *Arch Intern Med.* 2004;164:637-644.

37 Lung Transplantation

Should lung transplantation be performed for patients on mechanical respiratory support? The US experience
Mason DP, Thuita L, Nowicki ER, et al (Cleveland Clinic, OH)
J Thorac Cardiovasc Surg 139:765-773, 2010

Objective.—The study objectives were to (1) compare survival after lung transplantation in patients requiring pretransplant mechanical ventilation or extracorporeal membrane oxygenation with that of patients not requiring mechanical support and (2) identify risk factors for mortality.

Methods.—Data were obtained from the United Network for Organ Sharing for lung transplantation from October 1987 to January 2008. A total of 15,934 primary transplants were performed: 586 in patients on mechanical ventilation and 51 in patients on extracorporeal membrane oxygenation. Differences between nonsupport patients and those on mechanical ventilation or extracorporeal membrane oxygenation support were expressed as 2 propensity scores for use in comparing risk-adjusted survival.

Results.—Unadjusted survival at 1, 6, 12, and 24 months was 83%, 67%, 62%, and 57% for mechanical ventilation, respectively; 72%, 53%, 50%, and 45% for extracorporeal membrane oxygenation, respectively; and 93%, 85%, 79%, and 70% for unsupported patients, respectively ($P < .0001$). Recipients on mechanical ventilation were younger, had lower forced vital capacity, and had diagnoses other than emphysema. Recipients on extracorporeal membrane oxygenation were also younger, had higher body mass index, and had diagnoses other than cystic fibrosis/bronchiectasis. Once these variables, transplant year, and propensity for mechanical support were accounted for, survival remained worse after lung transplantation for patients on mechanical ventilation and extracorporeal membrane oxygenation.

Conclusion.—Although survival after lung transplantation is markedly worse when preoperative mechanical support is necessary, it is not dismal. Thus, additional risk factors for mortality should be considered when selecting patients for lung transplantation to maximize survival. Reduced survival for this high-risk population raises the important issue of balancing maximal individual patient survival against benefit to the maximum number of patients.

▶ At its most extreme in terms of prioritizing the sickest patients for lung transplant, the Lung Allocation Score model introduced in 2005 as the means of allocation of donor lungs to waiting recipients identifies those patients on mechanical ventilation or extracorporeal membrane oxygenation (ECMO) at the top of the waitlist (receive the highest scores). But what are the outcomes of these patients? Like the more generic article by Russo et al (included in this section), clearly the sickest patients have the worst outcomes. This particular study, using the same United Network for Organ Sharing database as the Russo et al study, broke down the sickest patients into those on mechanical ventilation and those on ECMO. Overall, these were younger patients than the overall transplant population (mean age 38-39 years) and most had diagnoses of either pulmonary fibrosis or cystic fibrosis. Nevertheless, the survivals, especially in the early posttransplant period and especially on patients supported by ECMO, were significantly worse than unsupported patients. In addition, the medical resources consumed are highest in the ECMO group, which had the lowest survivals. This again highlights the ethical issue, as the authors note, of "balancing maximal individual patient survival against benefit to the maximum number of patients," an issue that requires careful thought and fairness and will not be easy to resolve.

J. R. Maurer, MD, MBA

Factors indicative of long-term survival after lung transplantation: A review of 836 10-year survivors
Weiss ES, Allen JG, Merlo CA, et al (The Johns Hopkins Med Insts, Baltimore, MD)
J Heart Lung Transplant 29:240-246, 2010

Introduction.—Despite 20 years of lung transplantation (LTx), factors influencing long-term survival remain largely unknown. The United Network for Organ Sharing (UNOS) data set provides an opportunity to examine long-term LTx survivors.

Methods.—We conducted a case-control study embedded within the prospectively collected UNOS LTx cohort to identify 836 adults from 1987 to 1997 who survived ≥10 years after first LTx. LTx patients within the same era and surviving 1 to 5 years served as controls. Multivariable logistic regression with incorporation of spline terms evaluated the odds of being a 10-year survivor. Two separate models were constructed. Model A incorporated pre-operative, operative, and donor-specific factors. Model B incorporated the factors used in Model A with post-operative covariates. Additional outcomes evaluated included hospitalizations for infection, rejection, and bronchiolitis obliterans.

Results.—Of 4,818 LTx patients from 1987 to 1997, 836 (17.3%) survived ≥10 years with a mean follow-up of 148.8 ± 21.6 months. Mean follow-up for 1,657 controls was 34.0 ± 13.9 months. The distribution of 10-year survivors by disease was cystic fibrosis, 170 (20%); chronic obstructive pulmonary disease, 254 (30%); and idiopathic pulmonary fibrosis, 92 (11%). On multivariable logistic regression, significant factors influencing 10-year survival included age ≤35 years (odds ratio [OR] 1.07,

95% confidence interval [CI], 1.03−1.11; $p = 0.01$), bilateral LTx (OR. 1.71; 95% CI, 1.25−2.34; $p = 0.001$), and hospitalizations for infections (OR, 1.40; 95% CI, 1.27−1.54; $p < 0.001$) and for rejection (OR, 0.55; 95% CI, 0.48−0.65; $p < 0.001$).

Conclusions.—Examination of a cohort of long-term LTx survivors in the UNOS data set indicates that bilateral LTx and fewer hospitalizations for rejection may portend improved long-term survival after LTx.

▶ Are there specific characteristics or events around or after transplant that impact long-term survival? Or is it mostly luck? We have not previously had enough patients in the 10-year survival group to learn about this. For this study 10-year survivors (transplanted between 1987 and 1997) were compared with a control group of patients who were transplanted during the same 10-year period but survived only 1 to 5 years. Interestingly, the number of 10-year survivors increased dramatically between 1987 and 1990 but remained constant for the next 7 years. More than 60% of 10-year survivors had bronchiolitis obliterans syndrome (BOS) compared with about 45% of the controls; however, the controls died more often of BOS. Ten-year survivors were more likely to die of nonspecific respiratory failure or malignancy. Possibly, the most important finding in this analysis was the significant impact of bilateral transplant. In patients surviving at least a year, the impact of receiving a bilateral transplant instead of a unilateral transplant was to double the odds of surviving for 10 years. While many centers have routinely adopted bilateral transplant for most candidates for a variety of reasons, this objective finding suggests substantial utility to this approach and may have implications for overall lung transplant policy decisions.

J. R. Maurer, MD, MBA

38 Sleep Disorders

Outcomes in Patients with Chronic Obstructive Pulmonary Disease and Obstructive Sleep Apnea: The Overlap Syndrome

Marin JM, Soriano JB, Carrizo SJ, et al (Hospital Universitario Miguel Servet and Instituto Aragones de Ciencias de la Salud, Zaragoza, Spain; CIBER in Respiratory Diseases (CIBERES), Madrid, Spain; et al)
Am J Respir Crit Care Med 182:325-331, 2010

Rationale.—Patients with chronic obstructive pulmonary disease (COPD) and obstructive sleep apnea (OSA) (overlap syndrome) are more likely to develop pulmonary hypertension than patients with either condition alone.

Objectives.—To assess the relation of overlap syndrome to mortality and first-time hospitalization because of COPD exacerbation and the effect of continuous positive airway pressure (CPAP) on these major outcomes.

Methods.—We included 228 patients with overlap syndrome treated with CPAP, 213 patients with overlap syndrome not treated with CPAP, and 210 patients with COPD without OSA. All were free of heart failure, myocardial infarction, or stroke. Median follow-up was 9.4 years (range, 3.3−12.7). End points were all-cause mortality and first-time COPD exacerbation leading to hospitalization.

Measurements and Main Results.—After adjustment for age, sex, body mass index, smoking status, alcohol consumption, comorbidities, severity of COPD, apnea-hypopnea index, and daytime sleepiness, patients with overlap syndrome not treated with CPAP had a higher mortality (relative risk, 1.79; 95% confidence interval, 1.16−2.77) and were more likely to suffer a severe COPD exacerbation leading to hospitalization (relative risk, 1.70; 95% confidence interval, 1.21−2.38) versus the COPD-only group. Patients with overlap syndrome treated with CPAP had no increased risk for either outcome compared with patients with COPD-only.

Conclusions.—The overlap syndrome is associated with an increased risk of death and hospitalization because of COPD exacerbation. CPAP treatment was associated with improved survival and decreased hospitalizations in patients with overlap syndrome.

▶ This is a great study. Investigators longitudinally followed 3 groups of patients: (1) chronic obstructive pulmonary disease (COPD) without obstructive sleep apnea (OSA), (2) COPD with untreated OSA, and (3) COPD with treated OSA. Follow-up occurred for 9 years, and primary outcome was time to death from any cause. Secondary outcome was time to a first severe COPD exacerbation. There are 3 important findings in this study. First, the overlap syndrome is associated with higher mortality compared with COPD alone. Second, treatment of OSA in the overlap syndrome mitigates the increase in mortality. Third, use of continuous positive airway pressure (CPAP) in patients with overlap syndrome reduces COPD exacerbations. Although the exact mechanism is unknown, the authors do suggest some possibilities.

I think that this study has sound implications. We need to evaluate for concomitant OSA in patients with COPD. These patients are more likely to have daytime hypoxemia and higher pulmonary pressures. Furthermore, promotion of use and adherence to CPAP should be emphasized in those patients with the overlap syndrome. The findings in this article can be used to strengthen the support and education of CPAP use in these patients.

S. F. Jones, MD, FCCP, DABSM

Impact of Untreated Obstructive Sleep Apnea on Glucose Control in Type 2 Diabetes

Aronsohn RS, Whitmore H, Van Cauter E, et al (Univ of Chicago, IL)
Am J Respir Crit Care Med 181:507-513, 2010

Rationale.—Obstructive sleep apnea (OSA), a treatable sleep disorder that is associated with alterations in glucose metabolism in individuals without diabetes, is a highly prevalent comorbidity of type 2 diabetes. However, it is not known whether the severity of OSA is a predictor of glycemic control in patients with diabetes.

Objectives.—To determine the impact of OSA on hemoglobin A1c (HbA1c), the major clinical indicator of glycemic control, in patients with type 2 diabetes.

Methods.—We performed polysomnography studies and measured HbA1c in 60 consecutive patients with diabetes recruited from outpatient clinics between February 2007 and August 2009.

Measurements and Main Results.—A total of 77% of patients with diabetes had OSA (apnea–hypopnea index [AHI] ≥5). Increasing OSA severity was associated with poorer glucose control, after controlling for age, sex, race, body mass index, number of diabetes medications, level of exercise, years of diabetes and total sleep time. Compared with patients without OSA, the adjusted mean HbA1c was increased by 1.49% ($P = 0.0028$) in patients with mild OSA, 1.93% ($P = 0.0033$) in patients with moderate OSA, and 3.69% ($P < 0.0001$) in patients with severe OSA ($P < 0.0001$ for linear trend). Measures of OSA severity, including total AHI ($P = 0.004$), rapid eye movement AHI ($P = 0.005$), and the oxygen desaturation index during total and rapid eye movement sleep ($P = 0.005$ and $P = 0.008$, respectively) were positively correlated with increasing HbA1c levels.

Conclusions.—In patients with type 2 diabetes, increasing severity of OSA is associated with poorer glucose control, independent of adiposity and other confounders, with effect sizes comparable to those of widely used hypoglycemic drugs.

▶ The authors set out to examine the association between obstructive sleep apnea (OSA) and hemoglobin A1c (a marker of glycemic control). In a sample of 60 patients with a known diagnosis of diabetes, polysomnography was performed. The findings are interesting in a number of ways. First, 77% of subjects had polysomnography-proven OSA (apnea-hypopnea index [AHI] ≥5). The mean AHI in patients with OSA was 19.2 ± 14.8 versus 2.0 ± 1.2 in subjects who did not have OSA. The high prevalence of OSA in the diabetic population is in stark contrast to the general population, which is reported to be 2% to 4%. Of course, the body mass index of subjects in this study is increased. Second, nearly 90% of patients in this study had *not* been previously evaluated for OSA. Only one-third of the subjects reported snoring; I am unsurprised, since this symptom often elicits further suspicion of OSA on the doctor's part. Nevertheless, I think it is important that we recognize the amount of undiagnosed OSA in this at-risk population. Third—and the biggest finding—is that increasing severity of OSA was associated with poorer glucose control after adjusting for covariates. The difference between adjusted mean hemoglobin A1c in mild, moderate, and severe OSA when compared with those without OSA was 1.49%, 1.93%, and 3.69%, respectively. The authors introduce an interesting idea in the discussion. Because many diabetic medications are associated with side effects of weight gain, this may impact the severity of OSA or promote its development. The authors' work supports the hypothesis that improving OSA would improve glycemic control. One step further... nonpharmacologic treatment of OSA may improve glycemic control. At the present time, a diagnosis of diabetes is not factored into the decision to treat OSA, which is in contrast to hypertension, coronary artery disease, and stroke in which the threshold to treat OSA is lower (AHI ≥ 5 events per hour). With the significance of this work, maybe it should be factored.

S. F. Jones, MD, FCCP, DABSM

Continuous positive airway pressure treatment in sleep apnea patients with resistant hypertension: a randomized, controlled trial
Lozano L, Tovar JL, Sampol G, et al (Hosp Mútua de Terrassa, Spain; Universitat Autònoma de Barcelona (UAB), Spain)
J Hypertens 28:2161-2168, 2010

Objectives.—This controlled trial assessed the effect of continuous positive airway pressure (CPAP) on blood pressure (BP) in patients with obstructive sleep apnea (OSA) and resistant hypertension (RH).

Methods.—We evaluated 96 patients with resistant hypertension, defined as clinic BP at least 140/90 mmHg despite treatment with at least three drugs at adequate doses, including a diuretic. Patients underwent a polysomnography and a 24-h ambulatory BP monitoring (ABPM). They were classified as consulting room or ABPM-confirmed resistant hypertension, according to

24-h BP lower or higher than 125/80 mmHg. Patients with an apnea-hypopnea index at least 15 events/h ($n = 75$) were randomized to receive either CPAP added to conventional treatment ($n = 38$) or conventional medical treatment alone ($n = 37$). ABPM was repeated at 3 months. The main outcome was the change in systolic and diastolic BP.

Results.—Sixty-four patients completed the follow-up. Patients with ABPM-confirmed resistant hypertension treated with CPAP ($n = 20$), unlike those treated with conventional treatment ($n = 21$), showed a decrease in 24-h diastolic BP (-4.9 ± 6.4 vs. 0.1 ± 7.3 mmHg, $P = 0.027$). Patients who used CPAP > 5.8 h showed a greater reduction in daytime diastolic BP {-6.12 mmHg [confidence interval (CI) -1.45; -10.82], $P = 0.004$}, 24-h diastolic BP (-6.98 mmHg [CI -1.86; -12.1], $P = 0.009$) and 24-h systolic BP (-9.71 mmHg [CI -0.20; -19.22], $P = 0.046$). The number of patients with a dipping pattern significantly increased in the CPAP group (51.7% vs. 24.1%, $P = 0.008$).

Conclusion.—In patients with resistant hypertension and OSA, CPAP treatment for 3 months achieves reductions in 24-h BP. This effect is seen in patients with ABPM-confirmed resistant hypertension who use CPAP more than 5.8 h.

▶ Available literature supports that blood pressure reductions can be seen in patients with resistant hypertension who are on multiple medications with use of continuous positive airway pressure (CPAP). The authors of this article performed a randomized controlled trial to evaluate this. Improvements were seen only in patients who had defined resistant hypertension based on 24-hour ambulatory blood pressure monitoring. CPAP generated significant reductions in 24-hour diastolic blood pressure. Additional significant reductions in blood pressure were associated with longer durations of CPAP usage.

The population studied primarily included patients with severe obstructive sleep apnea (mean apnea-hypopnea index 52.67 events per hour). While the degree of blood pressure improvement in patients with resistant hypertension has been questioned (please refer to the article by Pépin et al, which I have also commented on), I believe that this article lends profound strength to the theory that there is an additive role of CPAP to conventional therapy, especially in patients with severe obstructive sleep apnea and resistant hypertension, despite multiple antihypertensive medications.

S. F. Jones, MD, FCCP, DABSM

Adenotonsillectomy Outcomes in Treatment of Obstructive Sleep Apnea in Children: A Multicenter Retrospective Study

Bhattacharjee R, Kheirandish-Gozal L, Spruyt K, et al (Univ of Louisville, KY; et al)
Am J Respir Crit Care Med 182:676-683, 2010

Rationale.—The overall efficacy of adenotonsillectomy (AT) in treatment of obstructive sleep apnea syndrome (OSAS) in children is unknown.

Although success rates are likely lower than previously estimated, factors that promote incomplete resolution of OSAS after AT remain undefined.

Objectives.—To quantify the effect of demographic and clinical confounders known to impact the success of AT in treating OSAS.

Methods.—A multicenter collaborative retrospective review of all nocturnal polysomnograms performed both preoperatively and postoperatively on otherwise healthy children undergoing AT for the diagnosis of OSAS was conducted at six pediatric sleep centers in the United States and two in Europe. Multivariate generalized linear modeling was used to assess contributions of specific demographic factors on the post-AT obstructive apnea-hypopnea index (AHI).

Measurements and Main Results.—Data from 578 children (mean age, 6.9 ± 3.8 yr) were analyzed, of which approximately 50% of included children were obese. AT resulted in a significant AHI reduction from 18.2 ± 21.4 to 4.1 ± 6.4/hour total sleep time ($P < 0.001$). Of the 578 children, only 157 (27.2%) had complete resolution of OSAS (i.e., post-AT AHI <1/h total sleep time). Age and body mass index z-score emerged as the two principal factors contributing to post-AT AHI ($P < 0.001$), with modest contributions by the presence of asthma and magnitude of pre-AT AHI ($P < 0.05$) among nonobese children.

Conclusions.—AT leads to significant improvements in indices of sleep-disordered breathing in children. However, residual disease is present in a large proportion of children after AT, particularly among older (>7 yr) or obese children. In addition, the presence of severe OSAS in nonobese children or of chronic asthma warrants post-AT nocturnal polysomnography, in view of the higher risk for residual OSAS.

▶ Obstructive sleep apnea (OSA) syndrome affects 2% to 3% of children.[1] While most clinicians, in keeping with the American Academy of Pediatrics, recommend adenotonsillectomy as the first line of treatment, we really do not know its efficacy. Traditionally, very high cure rates of 90% or more are cited. These particular authors challenge that exact notion. Many of us have seen children with residual OSA after adenotonsillectomy and have been curious about its risk factors (age, body mass index [BMI], and severity of presurgical OSA). This article examines the success of adenotonsillectomy in children and aims to delineate the factors that may contribute to residual OSA post surgery. The investigators performed a multicenter retrospective review of all nocturnal polysomnograms (preadenotonsillectomy and postadenotonsillectomy) performed in healthy children for OSA. This study included 578 children from 8 centers in the United States and Europe. The authors found that curative rates of adenotonsillectomy are not as good as expected. Though most children had a significant reduction in the severity of OSA with adenotonsillectomy, only 27.2% of children has postoperative apnea-hypopnea index (AHI) <1 per hour, and 21.6% had postoperative AHI > 5 per hour. Examination of risk factors indicates that age > 7 years and increasing BMI were the most predictive of residual OSA. Over half of the children studied meet the criteria for obesity.

Presence of asthma and severity of preoperative OSA were also predictive, though to a lesser degree, particularly in nonobese children.

There is a significant degree of criticism surrounding the methods of this study (retrospective, most patients from 2 of the 8 sites, possible selection bias, and lack of standardization of polysomnographic practices between sites). All of these are addressed by the authors. This article certainly generates thought and suggests which patients may need postoperative polysomnography (age > 7 years, obese, and severity of preoperative AHI or presence of asthma in nonobese children). Until a prospective study is performed, the efficacy of adenotonsillectomy should be refuted.

S. F. Jones, MD, FCCP, DABSM

Reference

1. Mitki T, Pillar G. Absence of positional effect in children with moderate-severe obstructive sleep apnea syndrome. *Harefuah*. 2009;148:300-303.

Acute Care Surgery Performed by Sleep Deprived Residents: Are Outcomes Affected?

Yaghoubian A, Kaji AH, Ishaque B, et al (Harbor-UCLA Med Ctr, Torrance)
J Surg Res 163:192-196, 2010

Background.—The Institute of Medicine recently recommended further reductions in resident duty hours, including a 5-h rest time for on-call residents after 16 h of work. This recommendation was purportedly intended to better protect patients against fatigue-related errors made by physician trainees. Yet no data are available regarding outcomes of operations performed by surgical trainees working without rest beyond 16 h in the current 80-h workweek era.

Methods.—A retrospective review of all laparoscopic cholecystectomies (LC) and appendectomies performed by surgery residents at a public teaching hospital from July 2003 through March 2009. Operations after 10 PM were performed by residents who began their shift at 6 AM and had thus been working 16 or more hours. An outcomes comparison between time periods was conducted for operations performed between 6 AM and 10 PM (daytime) and 10 PM and 6 AM (nighttime). Outcome measures were rates of total complications, bile duct injury, conversion to open operation, length of surgery, and mortality.

Results.—Over the 7-y study period, 2908 LC and 1726 appendectomies were performed. Appendectomies were performed laparoscopically in 73% of cases in patients for both time periods. There were no differences in rates of overall morbidity and mortality for operations when performed in nighttime compared with daytime. On multivariable analysis, there were no differences in outcomes between the two groups.

Conclusion.—The two most commonly performed general surgical operations performed at night by unrested residents have favorable outcomes similar to those performed during the day. Instituting a 5-h rest period at night is unlikely to improve the outcomes for these commonly performed operations.

▶ Changes to the resident duty hours continue to evolve. It is hard to believe that 7 years ago the 80-hour workweek was adopted. Recently, the Institute of Medicine has recommended additional refinement to the resident duty hours with the aim of reducing errors in care because of fatigue. The current recommendation is to allow for a 5-hour rest time for on-call residents after 16 hours of duty. If you serve on resident education and advisory committees, these recommendations have set forth construction of task forces designed to strategize the implementation of these forthcoming changes.

Fatigue-related errors are real. Need we be reminded about national and international catastrophies (Challenger, Valdez, etc) traced back to fatigue? Despite this, there is little available evidence examining outcomes in patient care because of sleep deprivation. The authors performed a retrospective study examining outcomes in patients who underwent cholecystectomy and appendectomy during daytime versus nighttime hours. The authors state that the nighttime surgeries were performed by residents who had started call by 6 AM that morning (16 hours of duty). They report that the predictor of complications was not the time of day in which the surgery was performed but rather patient-related factors (presence of perforation, gender, and age) and length of duration of surgery. The authors make arguments for how the new changes will affect resident education negatively.

Will patient-centered outcomes be improved with reduction in resident duty hours as suggested by the Institute of Medicine? This is not something where we can perform a randomized controlled trial because 1 negative outcome is too many. As the authors discuss, I believe that there may be some downsides but also some positives. I included this article just for some thought provocation.

S. F. Jones, MD, FCCP, DABSM

Consequences of Comorbid Sleep Apnea in the Metabolic Syndrome—Implications for Cardiovascular Risk

Trombetta IC, Somers VK, Maki-Nunes C, et al (Univ of São Paulo Med School, Brazil; Mayo Clinic and Foundation, Rochester, MN)
Sleep 33:1193-1199, 2010

Study Objectives.—Metabolic syndrome (MetSyn) increases overall cardiovascular risk. MetSyn is also strongly associated with obstructive sleep apnea (OSA), and these 2 conditions share similar comorbidities. Whether OSA increases cardiovascular risk in patients with the MetSyn has not been investigated. We examined how the presence of OSA in patients with MetSyn affected hemodynamic and autonomic variables associated with poor cardiovascular outcome.

Design.—Prospective clinical study.

Participants.—We studied 36 patients with MetSyn (ATP-III) divided into 2 groups matched for age and sex: (1) MetSyn+OSA (n = 18) and (2) MetSyn-OSA (n = 18).

Measurements.—OSA was defined by an apnea-hypopnea index (AHI) > 15 events/hour by polysomnography. We recorded muscle sympathetic nerve activity (MSNA - microneurography), heart rate (HR), and blood pressure (BP - Finapres). Baroreflex sensitivity (BRS) was analyzed by spontaneous BP and HR fluctuations.

Results.—MSNA (34 ± 2 vs 28 ± 1 bursts/min, P = 0.02) and mean BP (111 ± 3 vs. 99 ± 2 mm Hg, P = 0.003) were higher in patients with MetSyn+OSA versus patients with MetSyn-OSA. Patients with MetSyn+OSA had lower spontaneous BRS for increases (7.6 ± 0.6 vs 12.2 ± 1.2 msec/mm Hg, P = 0.003) and decreases (7.2 ± 0.6 vs 11.9 ± 1.6 msec/mm Hg, P = 0.01) in BP. MSNA was correlated with AHI (r = 0.48; P = 0.009) and minimum nocturnal oxygen saturation (r = −0.38, P = 0.04).

Conclusion.—Patients with MetSyn and comorbid OSA have higher BP, higher sympathetic drive, and diminished BRS, compared with patients with MetSyn without OSA. These adverse cardiovascular and autonomic consequences of OSA may be associated with poorer outcomes in these patients. Moreover, increased BP and sympathetic drive in patients with MetSyn+OSA may be linked, in part, to impairment of baroreflex gain.

▶ In this prospective case-control study, the authors set out to examine differences in the hemodynamic and autonomic variables in patients with metabolic syndrome and obstructive sleep apnea and compare them with metabolic syndrome patients without obstructive sleep apnea. The authors report that baroreflex sensitivity (spontaneous heart rate and blood pressure fluctuation) was significantly lower in subjects with metabolic syndrome and obstructive sleep apnea. In addition, muscle sympathetic nerve activity and mean blood pressure were higher. Increased sympathetic activity correlated with the severity of the obstructive sleep apnea and the nadir of the oxygen saturation. The authors suggest 2 possible mechanisms for the enhanced sympathetic activation: sleep-related hypoxia or an impaired baroreflex sensitivity. Both plausible mechanisms support the available evidence of increased cardiovascular risk in those with obstructive sleep apnea. It is already known that metabolic syndrome alone is associated with increased cardiovascular risk. This study suggests that those with both conditions may be at an even higher risk. Additional important and much needed areas of research should focus on whether treatment of obstructive sleep apnea reduces the risk in this group and whether increased risk is still seen in those subjects being treated for metabolic syndrome.

S. F. Jones, MD, FCCP, DABSM

39 Critical Care Medicine

A Randomized Prospective Trial of Airway Pressure Release Ventilation and Low Tidal Volume Ventilation in Adult Trauma Patients With Acute Respiratory Failure

Maxwell RA, Green JM, Waldrop J, et al (Univ of Tennessee College of Medicine, Chattanooga; Carolinas Med Ctr, Charlotte, NC; et al)
J Trauma 69:501-511, 2010

Background.—Airway pressure release ventilation (APRV) is a mode of mechanical ventilation, which has demonstrated potential benefits in trauma patients. We therefore sought to compare relevant pulmonary data and safety outcomes of this modality to the recommendations of the Adult Respiratory Distress Syndrome Network.

Methods.—Patients admitted after traumatic injury requiring mechanical ventilation were randomized under a 72-hour waiver of consent to a respiratory protocol for APRV or low tidal volume ventilation (LOVT). Data were collected regarding demographics, Injury Severity Score, oxygenation, ventilation, airway pressure, failure of modality, tracheostomy, ventilator-associated pneumonia, ventilator days, length of stay (LOS), pneumothorax, and mortality.

Results.—Sixty-three patients were enrolled during a 21-month period ending in February 2006. Thirty-one patients were assigned to APRV and 32 to LOVT. Patients were well matched for demographic variables with no differences between groups. Mean Acute Physiology and Chronic Health Evaluation II score was higher for APRV than LOVT (20.5 ± 5.35 vs. 16.9 ± 7.17) with a p value = 0.027. Outcome variables showed no differences between APRV and LOVT for ventilator days (10.49 days ± 7.23 days vs. 8.00 days ± 4.01 days), ICU LOS (16.47 days ± 12.83 days vs. 14.18 days ± 13.26 days), pneumothorax (0% vs. 3.1%), ventilator-associated pneumonia per patient (1.00 ± 0.86 vs. 0.56 ± 0.67), percent receiving tracheostomy (61.3% vs. 65.6%), percent failure of modality (12.9% vs. 15.6%), or percent mortality (6.45% vs. 6.25%).

Conclusions.—For patients sustaining significant trauma requiring mechanical ventilation for greater than 72 hours, APRV seems to have a similar safety profile as the LOVT. Trends for APRV patients to have increased ventilator days, ICU LOS, and ventilator-associated pneumonia may be explained by initial worse physiologic derangement demonstrated by higher Acute Physiology and Chronic Health Evaluation II scores.

▶ I applaud these authors for this very nice study. Airway pressure release ventilation (APRV) is commonly used in adult respiratory distress syndrome (ARDS) and patients with acute lung injury (ALI). Likewise, it is commonly used in patients with trauma. However, there are little data available as to proof of efficacy. The goals of ventilation are clearly different for this mode (pressure targeted, focused on oxygenation, perhaps at the expense of ventilation, and not focused on tidal volume size) as compared with the ARDS Network protocol with which we are all familiar. (Recall that ARDS Network protocol is volume limited with tidal volume 5-6 cc/kg ideal body weight of the patient along with moderate positive and expiratory pressure and high ventilator rate.)

The results of this study are important: there was no difference in any significant parameters such as survival or ventilator days amongst the 2 groups. So at least for patients with trauma with ALI/ARDS, APRV can be considered equally safe and efficacious as to the ARDS Network protocol. Our armamentarium of ventilator strategies can thus be expanded!

The authors noted that CO_2 clearance was better with APRV despite a lower minute ventilation rate. This is a surprise finding and one that I believe should be further investigated. Is it better clearance through the long breath hold? Or is it the dump cycle? Or perhaps is it because the patients can freely breathe throughout any APRV cycle? The physiology questions are intriguing.

J. A. Barker, MD

A 29-Year-Old Female at 33 Weeks' Gestation With Respiratory Failure
Gayle RB, Dorsey DA, Cole MA, et al (William Beaumont Army Med Ctr, El Paso, TX)
Chest 137:1474-1478, 2010

Background.—The influenza A (H1N1) pandemic occurring in the United States between August and November 2009 included 26,315 laboratory-confirmed influenza-associated hospitalizations and 1049 influenza-associated deaths, according to the Centers for Disease Control and Prevention (CDC). Younger patients, age 27 to 44 years, were particularly susceptible, along with pregnant women, who are at a fourfold to fivefold increased risk of severe illness or hospitalization when infected with influenza. A young pregnant patient came for treatment after a syncopal episode associated with rhinorrhea and cough, myalgia, lethargy, fever, and progressive dyspnea.

Case Report.—Woman, 29, at 33 weeks' gestation complained of rhinorrhea, cough, myalgias, lethargy, fever, and progressive dyspnea, for which she was given albuterol, azithromycin, and acetaminophen. With progressive dyspnea and a syncopal episode 2 days later, she was admitted to the hospital. Her coughing produced nonbloody yellowish sputum and her fever was as high as 39.4°C. Her history showed no ill contacts and no chronic medical problems, but she had had breast augmentation and previous dilatation and curettage for a spontaneous abortion with retained products of conception. She did not smoke or use illicit drugs and rarely consumed alcohol.

Physical examination revealed mild tachycardia, heart rate of 114 beats/min, normotension, fever of 38.4°C, tachypnea, and oxygen saturation of 89% while breathing 5 L via nasal cannula. She appeared ill but alert and oriented and had rhonchi and wheezing bilaterally. Her white blood cell count was 4.1×10^3 cells/μL with 89% neutrophils and 9% lymphocytes. Platelet count was 91×10^3 cells/μL. Sodium was 133 mEq/L and potassium 2.8 mEq/L; other blood chemistry values were normal. Mild elevations of aspartate aminotransferase and myoglobin levels were noted. The chest radiograph showed bilateral alveolar infiltrates and a dense region of consolidation in the left hilar area.

The patient's respiratory status grew worse, leading to admission to the intensive care unit (ICU). She was intubated after an arterial blood gas test revealed a pH of 7.44, partial pressure of carbon dioxide (Pco_2) of 25 mm Hg, and partial pressure of oxygen (Po_2) of 61 mm Hg while receiving 100% inspired oxygen fraction (FIO_2) delivered through a non-rebreather mask. Her rapid influenza antigen test was negative, but a real-time reverse transcriptase-polymerase chain reaction (rFT-PCR) test was positive for influenza A (H1N1).

Management included oseltamivar and broad-spectrum antibiotics to guard against possible secondary infection, corticosteroids for fetal lung maturity, and an emergency cesarean section. Airway pressure release ventilation stabilized her hypoxemia for about a week, then refractory hypoxemia developed. High-frequency oscillatory ventilation was begun, along with inhaled nitric oxide, which eventually stabilized her hypoxemic respiratory failure. The patient then developed severe fibrotic acute respiratory distress syndrome (ARDS). Her oxygenation index (OI) was monitored throughout her hospitalization. The prolonged ICU stay was complicated by bilateral pneumothoraces and a methicillin-resistant *Staphylococcus aureus* ventilator-associated pneumonia, but the patient finally recovered and was transferred to a rehabilitation facility. Both patient and baby are now doing well.

Conclusions.—It is important to have a high index of suspicion for influenza A (H1N1) in patients who complain of fever and respiratory distress. The diagnosis of influenza cannot be made on the basis of a rapid influenza diagnostic test, which is unable to distinguish between virus subtypes and has a low sensitivity. rRT-PCR tests are the most sensitive and specific tests currently available but require 48 to 96 hours for processing. Patients who are hospitalized with suspected, probable, or confirmed influenza can be managed effectively with oxeltamivir or zanamivir. ARDS secondary to influenza A (H1N1) often produces severe hypoxemia that requires lung rescue therapies. Pregnant patients with ARDS must be managed with consideration of both the patient and the fetus. A multidisciplinary team, including an intensivist, maternal fetal medicine specialist, anesthesiologist, and neonatologist, will provide optimal care in these cases (Figs 2 and 3).

▶ This case report nicely outlines the severe illness that we just endured in epidemic form, namely H1N1 influenza. As outlined here, there was a predilection for pregnant and otherwise healthy patients. This influenza strain seemed to be particularly pulmonary virulent in some patients, leading to a hemorrhagic process similar to that previously described with *Hantavirus*.

The progression of ventilation that occurred here is identical to what ours would be and, I suspect, to that of most centers. The patient was first treated with acute respiratory distress syndrome NET low VT approach. Next she was changed to airway pressure release ventilation (APRV) when oxygenation worsened and then moved over to high frequency oscillation ventilation when oxygenation did not hold with APRV. She did not progress to the need for extracorporeal membrane oxygenation, but in many centers that was required for survival of these patients.

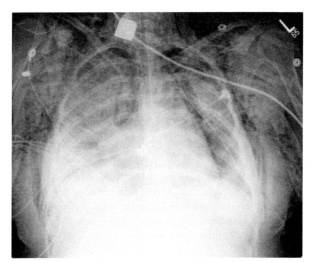

FIGURE 2.—Chest radiograph from hospital day 6 showing dense bilateral alveolar infiltrates with air bronchograms, subcutaneous emphysema, and left thoracostomy tube. (Reprinted from Gayle RB, Dorsey DA, Cole MA, et al. A 29-year-old female at 33 weeks' gestation with respiratory failure. *Chest.* 2010;137:1474-1478.)

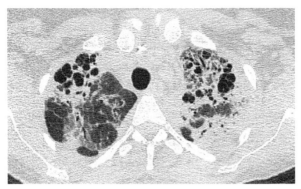

FIGURE 3.—Chest CT scan from late in the hospital course reveals severe bilateral fibrotic changes with traction bronchiectasis and airspace disease. (Reprinted from Gayle RB, Dorsey DA, Cole MA, et al. A 29-year-old female at 33 weeks' gestation with respiratory failure. *Chest*. 2010;137:1474-1478.)

Likewise, it is illustrated that she developed methicillin-resistant *Staphylococcus aureus* pneumonia as a complication. *S aureus* pneumonia is unfortunately a common sequelae of severe influenzae.

Fortunately for our patient here, survival occurred!

Unfortunately, it requires an epidemic such as H1N1 to push us to learn how to improve our armamentarium of preparedness for epidemics as well as to stretch out and improve our acute respiratory distress syndrome care.

J. A. Barker, MD

A 24-Year-Old Pregnant Patient With Diffuse Alveolar Hemorrhage
Venkatram S, Muppuri S, Niazi M, et al (Bronx Lebanon Hosp Ctr, NY)
Chest 138:220-223, 2010

Background.—Choriocarcinoma is a highly aggressive germ cell tumor identifiable by the secretion of Human Chorionic Gonadotropin (HCG) and hematogenous metastasis. It may be seen after a hydatiform mole, spontaneous abortion, or ectopic pregnancy, but also occurs at a rate of 1 in 40,000 term pregnancies. A young pregnant woman was diagnosed with diffuse alveolar hemorrhage (DAH) that was eventually attributed to choriocarcinoma.

Case Report.—Woman, 24, at 33 weeks' gestation was admitted to the hospital complaining of dyspnea of 2 weeks' duration and a mild dry cough. She had experienced multiple spontaneous abortions caused by cervical incompetence, so prophylactic cerclage had been performed during this pregnancy. She reported no chest pain, fever, hemoptysis, night sweats, arthralgias, rash, anorexia, abdominal pain, nausea, vomiting, toxic habits, or travel history. Her tuberculin test 6 months previously was negative. Physical examination showed her heart rate at 125 beats/min, blood pressure

110/65 mm Hg, temperature 36.6°C, and respiratory rate 28 breaths/min. No cardiac abnormalities were noted, nor was there jugular venous distention. Rales were noted bilaterally over the lung bases. Her white blood cell count was 8400 cells/mm^3, hematocrit 24%, and platelet count 219 cells/mm^3. Bilateral diffuse nodular infiltrates were seen on the chest radiograph, but her electrolytes, creatinine, liver function tests, and coagulation profile were normal.

The acute hypoxic respiratory failure was managed in the intensive care unit (ICU) with antibiotics given for suspected community-acquired pneumonia and infective endocarditis. The second day her respiratory status deteriorated, requiring a higher inspired oxygen fraction (FIO$_2$). Worsening pulmonary infiltrates were found on the third day, leading to intubation, after which she developed moderate hemoptysis, requiring emergency fiberoptic bronchoscopy. Blood was oozing diffusely from all lung segments. An elective cesarean section produced a viable fetus. Lavage cleared the fluid, which yielded a negative result on Gram staining and culturing. No malignant cells were found. The patient developed acute respiratory distress syndrome (ARDS), septic shock, and multiple organ failure. β-HCG levels fell from 71,139 to 40,331 IU/L after the infant's delivery. Hemosiderin-laden macrophages were found on a second fiberoptic bronchoscopy for hemoptysis, but cytologic and microbiologic analyses remained negative for pathogens. The patient maintained normal heart function, but remained in critical condition with refractory ARDS, managed with high oxygen concentrations and positive end-expiratory pressure. Doctors were unable to perform a surgical lung biopsy because of her critical state. After 13 days the patient died. Autopsy findings indicated choriocarcinoma.

Conclusions.—Rarely does choriocarcinoma cause DAH in pregnancy, so clinicians must have a high index of suspicion to detect it. The diagnosis should be considered in pregnant patients with nodular pulmonary lesions. β-HCG levels should be followed closely after delivery to ensure they decline as expected. Early diagnosis of choriocarcinoma is possible by inspecting the placenta of postpartum patients with lung nodules, especially when lung biopsy is not possible. High cure rates, even in advanced metastatic disease, are achievable with chemotherapy. Early diagnosis is essential.

▶ I wish I had seen this case report a few months ago! We had an identical case here in Texas. I learned about molar pregnancy during MS3 clerkship many years ago. All I knew was that it was pregnancy dedifferentiated into cancer but one that was curable. Of course, much has changed in 30 years since then. β-human chorionic gonadotropin (β-HCG) is now routinely used as is ultrasound imaging in pregnancy. Likewise, diffuse pulmonary hemorrhage is now much more treatable. However, as is illustrated in this nicely done case report, even being young and vigorously healthy may not prevent mortality in the face of diffuse metastatic malignancy.

Major take-home points I would emphasize from this case:

(1) Think of this possibility in those young women who are fertile.

(2) Consider β-HCG plus ultrasound to confirm pregnancy versus molar pregnancy/cancer. Realize that in both pregnancy and this malignancy that β-HCG may be quite high.

(3) Include metastatic malignancy in the differential diagnosis of patients with diffuse alveolar hemorrhage.

(4) When in doubt, a biopsy is in order.

(5) Diffuse metastatic disease with respiratory failure portends a poor prognosis even in previously healthy patients.

J. A. Barker, MD

3,423 Emergency Tracheal Intubations at a University Hospital: Airway Outcomes and Complications

Martin LD, Mhyre JM, Shanks AM, et al (Univ of Michigan Med School, Ann Arbor)
Anesthesiology 114:42-48, 2011

Background.—There are limited outcome data regarding emergent nonoperative intubation. The current study was undertaken with a large observational dataset to evaluate the incidence of difficult intubation and complication rates and to determine predictors of complications in this setting.

Methods.—Adult nonoperating room emergent intubations at our tertiary care institution from December 5, 2001 to July 6, 2009 were reviewed. Prospectively defined data points included time of day, location, attending physician presence, number of attempts, direct laryngoscopy view, adjuvant use, medications, and complications. At our institution, a senior resident with at least 24 months of anesthesia training is the first responder for all emergent airway requests. The primary outcome was a composite airway complication variable that included aspiration, esophageal intubation, dental injury, or pneumothorax.

Results.—A total of 3,423 emergent nonoperating room airway management cases were identified. The incidence of difficult intubation was 10.3%. Complications occurred in 4.2%: aspiration, 2.8%; esophageal intubation, 1.3%; dental injury, 0.2%; and pneumothorax, 0.1%. A bougie introducer was used in 12.4% of cases. Among 2,284 intubations performed by residents, independent predictors of the composite complication outcome were as follows: three or more intubation attempts (odds ratio, 6.7; 95% CI, 3.2−14.2), grade III or IV view (odds ratio, 1.9;

TABLE 2.—Complications Overall Compared with Complications for Resident-Only Intubations

Complication	All Intubations (n = 3,423)	Senior Residents Only (n = 2,284)	P Value*
Aspiration	95 (2.8)	69 (3.0)	0.57
Esophageal intubation	46 (1.3)	26 (1.1)	0.50
Dental injury	6 (0.2)	4 (0.2)	1.00
Pneumothorax	4 (0.1)	1 (0.04)	0.65
Composite complication[†]	144 (4.2)	96 (4.2)	1.00

Data are given as number (percentage) of each group.
Some patients experienced more than one complication.
*Calculated using the Pearson chi-square or Fisher exact test.
[†]Denotes the total number of patients experiencing a complication.

95% CI, 1.1–3.5), general care floor location (odds ratio, 1.9; 95% CI, 1.2–3.0), and emergency department location (odds ratio, 4.7; 95% CI, 1.1–20.4).

Conclusions.—During emergent nonoperative intubation, specific clinical situations are associated with an increased risk of airway complication and may provide a starting point for allocation of experienced first responders (Table 2).

▶ This is a very useful article. The authors analyzed a very large number of emergent hospital intubations. The conditions were realistic compared with my own experience in teaching hospitals: two-thirds of the intubations were done by upper-level anesthesia residents and one-third had a staff anesthesiologist present. The incidence of complications is higher than I was aware of and should change my practice. In other words, I think I probably should pay much more attention to these high-risk people now after intubations.

The widespread use of many adjunctive techniques is fascinating and demonstrates that the field continues to evolve. Difficult airway techniques are very much in use. (See Fig 1 in the original article for the breakdown.)

Table 2 has probably the most important data outlined. Namely, there is no statistical difference in results or complications when attendings join the upper-level residents in the procedures. Difficult airways are apparently difficult for everyone!

J. A. Barker, MD

Clinical characteristics and outcomes of patients with obstructive sleep apnoea requiring intensive care
Hang LW, Chen W, Liang SJ, et al (China Med Univ Hosp, Taichung, Taiwan)
Anaesth Intensive Care 38:506-512, 2010

We reviewed the clinical characteristics, required intervention and short- and long-term outcomes in obstructive sleep apnoea (OSA) patients requiring intensive care. A retrospective, single-centre, observational cohort study was undertaken in a multidisciplinary teaching medical and surgical intensive care unit. Adult patients with OSA (apnoea-hypopnoea index of 5 or higher) requiring intensive care from January 2000 to January 2005 were included. Thirty-seven OSA patients (age: 58 ± 14 years, male:female 27:10) were admitted due to respiratory (n=12, 32%), cerebrovascular (n=8, 22%), cardiovascular (n=16, 43%) and infectious events (n=1, 2.7%). Comparing the clinical features, polysomnographic data and outcome among these groups, we found that OSA patients admitted due to respiratory events had significantly higher Acute Physiology and Chronic Health Evaluation II scores, lower arterial blood gas pH, higher $PaCO_2$, a higher incidence of respiratory failure (92%) and required non-invasive ventilation after extubation (73%), and higher intensive care unit readmission rates than patients admitted due to cerebrovascular events and cardiovascular events ($P < 0.05$). No difference was found in the in-hospital and long-term mortality rate.

The most common reason for intensive care unit admission in critically ill OSA patients was a cardiovascular event, followed by respiratory and cerebrovascular events. The baseline polysomnographic data of the OSA patients were not correlated with their clinical features and outcomes in the intensive care unit. A more complicated clinical course and higher intensive care unit readmission rate were encountered in OSA patients admitted due to respiratory events. Further studies would be required to evaluate the efficacy of non-invasive ventilation for facilitation of extubation in OSA patients presenting with hypercapnic respiratory failure.

▶ As the population ages and the obesity epidemic widens, it will behoove us to understand this growing (pun intended!) subgroup of patients in the ICU. Obstructive sleep apnea really does appear to predispose people to cardiovascular and cerebrovascular events. Patients with sleep apnea who are admitted to ICU are more ill in general than other patients. Consequently, their respiratory health is more complex. Over 70% require noninvasive ventilation after extubation. This study collates some very useful information.

J. A. Barker, MD

The case against confirmatory tests for determining brain death in adults
Wijdicks EFM (Mayo Clinic, Rochester, MN)
Neurology 75:77-83, 2010

The determination of brain death is based on a comprehensive clinical assessment. A confirmatory test—at least, in adult patients in the United States—is not mandatory, but it typically is used as a safeguard or added when findings on clinical examination are unwontedly incomplete. In other countries, confirmatory tests are mandatory; in many, they are optional. These tests can be divided into those that test the brain's electrical function and those that test cerebral blood flow. A false-positive result (i.e., the test result suggests brain death, but clinically the patient does not meet the criteria) is not common but has been described for tests frequently used to determine brain death. A false-negative result (i.e., the test result suggests intact brain function, but clinically the patient meets the criteria) in one test may result in more confirmatory tests and no resolution when the test results diverge. Also, pathologic studies have shown that considerable areas of viable brain tissue may remain in patients who meet the clinical criteria of brain death, a fact that makes these tests less diagnostic. Confirmatory tests are residua from earlier days of refining comatose states. A comprehensive clinical examination, when performed by skilled examiners, should have perfect diagnostic accuracy (Fig 1).

▶ This is a cogent well-discussed editorial by an authoritative leader in neuro-critical care. I happen to agree with him completely. Performance of unnecessary tests is never helpful and always has the risk of unintended consequences or harmful side effects. The neurologic examination performed by an experienced and competent physician coupled with a simple bedside apnea test is certainly sufficient for this diagnosis. Fig 1 well demonstrates the chaos that can occur when confirmatory tests are added to the mix. I cringe when families ask for an electroencephalogram in an ICU. The chance of electrical interference is so high that electrical silence may not be diagnosed despite its high likelihood.

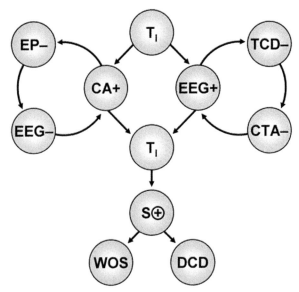

FIGURE 1.—Chaotic approach with confirmatory tests. The chaotic approach uses multiple confirmatory tests when test results do not match the findings on clinical examination. Generally, flow studies are followed by electrical physiologic studies and vice versa. Circles indicate other considered tests. In the worst case scenario, 2–3 tests are used to resolve the discrepancies. CA+ = flow on cerebral angiogram; CTA− = no flow on contrast CT angiogram; DCD = donation after cardiac death criteria met; EEG+ = discernible cortical activity; EP− = absent evoked potentials (brainstem or somatosensory potentials or both); S+ = return of brainstem reflexes (e.g., cough returns); TCD− = no flow identified on transcranial Doppler; T_I = test incomplete or confounded; WOS = withdrawal of support. (Reprinted from Wijdicks EFM. The case against confirmatory tests for determining brain death in adults. *Neurology.* 2010;75:77-83, with permission from AAN Enterprises, Inc.)

I appreciate the candor expressed in this well-thought editorial. Bravo, Dr Wijdicks!

J. A. Barker, MD

Causes and Outcomes of Acute Neuromuscular Respiratory Failure
Serrano MC, Rabinstein AA (Mayo Clinic, Rochester, MN)
Arch Neurol 67:1089-1094, 2010

Objective.—To identify the spectrum of causes, analyze the usefulness of diagnostic tests, and recognize prognostic factors in patients with acute neuromuscular respiratory failure.

Methods.—We evaluated 85 patients admitted to the intensive care unit (ICU) at Mayo Clinic, Rochester, between 2003 and 2009 with acute neuromuscular respiratory failure, defined as a need for mechanical ventilation owing to primary impairment of the peripheral nervous system. Outcome was assessed at hospital discharge and at last follow-up. Poor outcome was defined as a modified Rankin score greater than 3.

Results.—The median age was 66 years; median follow-up, 5 months. The most frequent diagnoses were myasthenia gravis, Guillain-Barré syndrome, myopathies, and amyotrophic lateral sclerosis (27, 12, 12, and 12 patients, respectively). Forty-seven patients (55%) had no known neuromuscular diagnosis before admission, and 36 of them (77%) had poor short-term outcomes. In 10 patients (12%), the diagnosis remained unknown on discharge; only 1 (10%) had regained independent function. Older age was associated with increased mortality during hospitalization. Longer mechanical ventilation times and ICU stays were associated with poor outcome at discharge but not at the last follow-up. Patients without a known neuromuscular diagnosis before admission had longer duration of mechanical ventilation, longer ICU stays, and worse outcomes at discharge. Electromyography was the most useful diagnostic test in patients without previously known neuromuscular diagnoses. The presence of spontaneous activity on needle insertion predicted poor short-term outcome regardless of final diagnosis. Coexistent cardiopulmonary diseases also predicted poor long-term outcome.

Conclusions.—Among patients with neuromuscular respiratory failure, those without known diagnosis before admission have poorer outcomes. Patients whose diagnoses remain unclear at discharge have the highest rates of disability (Tables 1 and 2).

▶ I definitely recommend this article to intensivists who practice in general medical-surgical ICUs. Respiratory failure can occur for myriad reasons. Primary lung disease is not a sine qua non. I have found a number of new cases of amyotrophic lateral sclerosis (ALS) and myasthenia gravis in investigating patients who appear with respiratory failure of apparent neuromuscular cause.

TABLE 1.—Final Diagnoses of Patients Admitted to the ICU With Acute Neuromuscular Respiratory Failure

Final Diagnosis	Patients, No. (%)
Myasthenia	27 (32)
GBS	12 (14)
Myopathies	12 (14)
Dermatomyositis	2
α-sarcoglycanopathy	1
Toxic necrotizing myopathy	1
Hypernatremic myopathy	1
Myotonic dystrophy	1
Myopathy with anti-SRP antibodies	1
Undetermined	5
ALS	12 (14)
Postpolio syndrome	3 (4)
CIDP	2 (2)
West Nile infection polyradiculoneuropathy	2 (2)
Amyloid polyradiculoneuropathy	1 (1)
Kennedy syndrome	1 (1)
Congenital myasthenic syndrome	1 (1)
Pseudocholinesterase deficiency	1 (1)
Myelopathy	1 (1)
Unknown	10 (12)

Abbreviations: ALS, amyotrophic lateral sclerosis; CIDP, chronic inflammatory demyelinating polyradiculoneuropathy; GBS, Guillain-Barré syndrome; ICU, intensive care unit; SRP, signal recognition particle.

TABLE 2.—Final Diagnoses in Patients Without Known Neuromuscular Disease at Admission

Final Diagnosis	Patients, No.
GBS	12
ALS	8
Myasthenia	4
Myopathies	4
Hypernatremic myopathy	1
Toxic necrotizing myopathy	1
Myopathy with anti-SRP antibodies	1
Undetermined	1
CIDP	2
West Nile polyradiculoneuropathy	2
Postpolio syndrome	1
Kennedy disease	1
Pseudocholinesterase deficiency	1
Probable botulism	1
Amyloidosis	1
Unknown	10

Abbreviations: ALS, amyotrophic lateral sclerosis; CIDP, chronic inflammatory demyelinating polyradiculoneuropathy; GBS, Guillain-Barré syndrome; SRP, signal recognition particle.

The authors characterize their experience here in Table 1. Of interest, ALS was the second most common diagnosis in those admitted without a known neurologic diagnosis (Table 2).

The authors herein found electromyography (EMG) as the most useful tool in differentiating these patients and disorders. This is an important pearl. Neurologic colleagues have usually declined to do EMGs in ICUs where I have worked, citing concerns about portable machines and high degrees of electrical interference.

Clearly the experiences at Mayo Clinic will not necessarily mirror other practices. However, I believe this article offers important epidemiologic and prognostic information for all of us who practice in adult medical critical care.

J. A. Barker, MD

40 Cardiac Arrhythmias, Conduction Disturbances, and Electrophysiology

Age as a Risk Factor for Stroke in Atrial Fibrillation Patients: Implications for Thromboprophylaxis
Marinigh R, Lip GYH, Fiotti N, et al (Univ of Birmingham Centre for Cardiovascular Sciences, UK; Univ of Trieste, Italy)
J Am Coll Cardiol 56:827-837, 2010

The prevalence of atrial fibrillation (AF) is related to age and is projected to rise exponentially as the population ages and the prevalence of cardiovascular risk factors increases. The risk of ischemic stroke is significantly increased in AF patients, and there is evidence of a graded increased risk of stroke associated with advancing age. Oral anticoagulation (OAC) is far more effective than antiplatelet agents at reducing stroke risk in patients with AF. Therefore, increasing numbers of elderly patients are candidates for, and could benefit from, the use of anticoagulants. However, elderly people with AF are less likely to receive OAC therapy. This is mainly due to concerns about a higher risk of OAC-associated hemorrhage in the elderly population. Until recently, older patients were under-represented in randomized controlled trials of OAC versus placebo or antiplatelet therapy, and therefore the evidence base for the value of OAC in the elderly population was not known. However, analyses of the available trial data indicate that the expected net clinical benefit of warfarin therapy is highest among patients with the highest untreated risk for stroke, which includes the oldest age category. An important caveat with warfarin treatment is maintenance of a therapeutic international normalized ratio, regardless of the age of the patient, where time in therapeutic range should be ≥65%. Therefore, age alone should not prevent prescription of OAC in elderly patients, given an appropriate stroke and bleeding risk stratification (Tables 3 and 4).

▶ Thromboembolic complications of atrial fibrillation (AF) are associated with significant morbidity and mortality. Both risk of stroke and prevalence of AF

TABLE 3.—Stroke Risk Assessment in AF: CHA$_2$DS$_2$-VASc*

Stroke Risk Factors	Score
Congestive heart failure/LV dysfunction	1
Hypertension	1
Age ≥75 yrs	2
Diabetes mellitus	1
Stroke/TIA/TE	2
Vascular disease (prior MI, PAD, or aortic plaque)	1
Age 65–74 years	1
Sex category (i.e., female sex)	1

The CHA$_2$DS$_2$-VASc schema assesses stroke risk in patients with nonvalvular atrial fibrillation (51).
TE = thromboembolic event; TIA = transient ischemic attack.
*For a CHA$_2$DS$_2$-VASc score >1, such patients are high risk and should have oral anticoagulation (e.g., warfarin); for a CHA$_2$DS$_2$-VASc score = 1, antithrombotic therapy is recommended, either as oral anticoagulation or aspirin 75 to 325 mg daily, but oral anticoagulation is preferred rather than aspirin; for a CHA$_2$DS$_2$-VASc score = 0 ("truly low risk"), either aspirin 75 to 325 mg daily or no antithrombotic therapy can be used, but no antithrombotic therapy may be preferred. Maximum score is 9 (51).

TABLE 4.—Bleeding Risk Assessment in AF: HAS-BLED Bleeding Risk Score

Letter	Clinical Characteristic*	Points Awarded
H	Hypertension	1
A	Abnormal renal and liver function (1 point each)	1 or 2
S	Stroke	1
B	Bleeding	1
L	Labile INRs	1
E	Elderly	1
D	Drugs or alcohol (1 point each)	1 or 2
		Maximum 9 points

*Hypertension is defined as systolic blood pressure >160 mm Hg. Abnormal kidney function is defined as the presence of chronic dialysis or renal transplantation or serum creatinine ≥200 μmol/l. Abnormal liver function is defined as chronic hepatic disease (e.g., cirrhosis) or biochemical evidence of significant hepatic derangement (e.g., bilirubin >2× upper limit of normal, in association with AST/ALT/ALP (aspartate aminotransferase/alanine aminotransferase/alkaline phosphatase) >3× upper limit normal, and so on). Bleeding refers to previous bleeding history and/or predisposition to bleeding (e.g., bleeding diathesis, anemia). LabileINRs (international normalized ratios) refers to unstable/high INRs or poor time in therapeutic range (e.g., <60%). Drugs/alcohol use refers to concomitant use of drugs, such as antiplatelet agents, nonsteroidal anti-inflammatory drugs (65).

increase with age, and older age has consistently been identified as an independent risk for thromboembolic complications of AF. However, reluctance persists to treat older patients with oral anticoagulants (OACs) because of a perceived prohibitive bleeding risk in this population. In this context, Marinigh et al performed a systematic review of published studies evaluating the relationship between age, thromboembolism, and bleeding risk in AF. Twelve of 17 identified studies evaluating the relationship between age and stroke in AF found age to be an independent risk factor for stroke, and a pooled analysis of 5 randomized controlled trials resulted in a relative risk of 1.4 (95% confidence interval [CI], 1.1-1.8) for stroke by increasing decade. This risk was evident in most studies whether patients were dichotomized by a threshold age (eg, > 75 years) or stratified by decade. The newer CHA$_2$DS$_2$-VASc schema also includes age of 65 to 74 years as a risk factor and > 75 years as a high-risk feature, consistent with data that age is a continuous variable for risk (Table 3). Elderly patients also appear to benefit from anticoagulation; a meta-analysis of 11 trials demonstrated a hazard ratio (HR) of 0.36 (95% CI, 0.29-0.45) for warfarin compared with aspirin that was not attenuated with increasing age. However, age has also consistently been shown to be a risk factor for bleeding; 1 recent meta-analysis reporting an HR of 1.6 (95% CI, 1.47-1.77) for major bleeding. Interestingly, the bleeding risk was similar for patients taking warfarin or aspirin. Further stratification of bleeding risk in elderly patients has been demonstrated with several risk prediction models, such as HAS-BLED (Table 4). Importantly, stroke and bleeding risks are affected by time in therapeutic range (TTR) with warfarin. TTR, in turn, has been shown to be affected by a variety of patient-specific factors, many of which are more common in the elderly. Despite this risk, the authors identified 2 analyses evaluating the net clinical benefit (rate of thromboembolic complications minus bleeding complications) of OAC in older patients, and both suggested a significant benefit in this population over antiplatelet therapy. Based on their review, the authors conclude that while elderly patients are at higher risk for bleeding, OAC should be considered given the greater net clinical benefit of stroke prevention in a high-risk population. Although this systematic review reinforces the need for careful consideration of risks of using and avoiding OACs in elderly patients with AF, with an aging population and the recent development of alternative OACs, such as dabigitran and rivaroxaban, this will become an even more frequent and complex issue in clinical practice.

M. R. Gold, MD, PhD

Dabigatran versus Warfarin in Patients with Atrial Fibrillation

Connolly SJ, the RE-LY Steering Committee and Investigators (McMaster Univ and Hamilton Health Sciences, Ontario, Canada; et al)
N Engl J Med 361:1139-1151, 2009

Background.—Warfarin reduces the risk of stroke in patients with atrial fibrillation but increases the risk of hemorrhage and is difficult to use. Dabigatran is a new oral direct thrombin inhibitor.

Methods.—In this noninferiority trial, we randomly assigned 18,113 patients who had atrial fibrillation and a risk of stroke to receive, in a blinded fashion, fixed doses of dabigatran — 110 mg or 150 mg twice daily — or, in an unblinded fashion, adjusted-dose warfarin. The median duration of the follow-up period was 2.0 years. The primary outcome was stroke or systemic embolism.

Results.—Rates of the primary outcome were 1.69% per year in the warfarin group, as compared with 1.53% per year in the group that received 110 mg of dabigatran (relative risk with dabigatran, 0.91; 95% confidence interval [CI], 0.74 to 1.11; P<0.001 for noninferiority) and 1.11% per year in the group that received 150 mg of dabigatran (relative risk, 0.66; 95% CI, 0.53 to 0.82; P<0.001 for superiority). The rate of major bleeding was 3.36% per year in the warfarin group, as compared with 2.71% per year in the group receiving 110 mg of dabigatran (P=0.003) and 3.11% per year in the group receiving 150 mg of dabigatran (P=0.31). The rate of hemorrhagic stroke was 0.38% per year in the warfarin group, as compared with 0.12% per year with 110 mg of dabigatran (P<0.001) and 0.10% per year with 150 mg of dabigatran (P<0.001). The mortality rate was 4.13% per year in the warfarin group, as compared with 3.75% per year with 110 mg of dabigatran (P=0.13) and 3.64% per year with 150 mg of dabigatran (P=0.051).

Conclusions.—In patients with atrial fibrillation, dabigatran given at a dose of 110 mg was associated with rates of stroke and systemic embolism that were similar to those associated with warfarin, as well as lower rates of major hemorrhage. Dabigatran administered at a dose of 150 mg, as compared with warfarin, was associated with lower rates of stroke and systemic embolism but similar rates of major hemorrhage. (ClinicalTrials. gov number, NCT00262600.)

▶ For 60 years warfarin has been the only effective oral anticoagulant for use in venous and selected arterial thrombotic disorders and as a preventive medicine for systemic embolization and stroke in patients with atrial fibrillation. Problems with warfarin include a requirement for laboratory monitoring by prothrombin times, a narrow therapeutic index, a long half-life resulting in a slow onset of therapeutic effect, and a need for parenteral anticoagulation until warfarin becomes effective. In addition, there are numerous interactions with other drugs and foods, such as leafy green vegetables containing vitamin K. Dabigatran etexilate is an oral prodrug that is converted by a serum esterase to dabigatran, a potent competitive thrombin inhibitor. This is the first study establishing dabigatran etexilate as equally or, with the 150-mg dose twice a day (BID), more effective in preventing stroke or systemic emboli in patients with atrial fibrillation without increasing major bleeding and less likely than warfarin to cause hemorrhagic stroke. The first oral direct thrombin inhibitor, ximelagatran, almost a decade ago was effective in arterial and venous thrombotic disorders including atrial fibrillation but with long-term use was found to have hepatotoxicity.

Dabigatran has many advantages over warfarin in that it has a relatively short half-life, obviating the need for parenteral anticoagulation before the drug takes effect, little drug or dietary interactions, and especially no laboratory monitoring. In the 2-year follow-up, there has been no hepatotoxicity beyond that seen with warfarin. Subsequent substudies of this study have shown that the benefits of the 150 mg BID dose at reducing stroke, the 110-mg BID dose at reducing bleeding, and both doses at reducing intracranial bleeding versus warfarin were consistent regardless of the individual center's quality of international normalized ratio control[1] and that both doses were equally effective in those with and without previous stroke or transient ischemic attack.[2]

There are a number of other thrombin inhibitors and other drugs effective at the terminus of the coagulation cascade, such as direct factor Xa inhibitors, the most advanced ones being rivaroxaban and apixaban. Zikria and Ansell have published a very good review of the oral direct thrombin and factor Xa inhibitors.[3] If these initial reports are confirmed by other studies and no important adverse effects are noted on long-term follow-up, these novel oral anticoagulants will be a marked advance in the treatment of arterial and venous thrombotic disorders.

M. D. Cheitlin, MD

References

1. Wallentin L, Yusuf S, Ezekowitz MD, et al. Efficacy and safety of dabigatran compared with warfarin at different levels of international normalised ratio control for stroke prevention in atrial fibrillation: an analysis of the RE-LY trial. *Lancet.* 2010;376:975-983.
2. Diener HC, Connolly SJ, Ezekowitz MD, et al. Dabigatran compared with warfarin in patients with atrial fibrillation and previous transient ischaemic attack or stroke: a subgroup analysis of the RE-LY trial. *Lancet Neurol.* 2010;9:1157-1163.
3. Zikria J, Ansell J. Oral anticoagulation with Factor Xa and thrombin inhibitors: Is there an alternative to warfarin? *Discov Med.* 2009;8:196-203.

Effect of Home Testing of International Normalized Ratio on Clinical Events

Matchar DB, for the THINRS Executive Committee and Site Investigators (Duke Univ Med Ctr, Durham, NC; et al)

N Engl J Med 363:1608-1620, 2010

Background.—Warfarin anticoagulation reduces thromboembolic complications in patients with atrial fibrillation or mechanical heart valves, but effective management is complex, and the international normalized ratio (INR) is often outside the target range. As compared with venous plasma testing, point-of-care INR measuring devices allow greater testing frequency and patient involvement and may improve clinical outcomes.

Methods.—We randomly assigned 2922 patients who were taking warfarin because of mechanical heart valves or atrial fibrillation and who were competent in the use of point-of-care INR devices to either weekly self-testing at home or monthly high-quality testing in a clinic. The primary end point was the time to a first major event (stroke, major bleeding episode, or death).

Results.—The patients were followed for 2.0 to 4.75 years, for a total of 8730 patient-years of follow-up. The time to the first primary event was not significantly longer in the self-testing group than in the clinic-testing group (hazard ratio, 0.88; 95% confidence interval, 0.75 to 1.04; P = 0.14). The two groups had similar rates of clinical outcomes except that the self-testing group reported more minor bleeding episodes. Over the entire follow-up period, the self-testing group had a small but significant improvement in the percentage of time during which the INR was within the target range (absolute difference between groups, 3.8 percentage points; P<0.001). At 2 years of follow-up, the self-testing group also had a small but significant improvement in patient satisfaction with anticoagulation therapy (P = 0.002) and quality of life (P<0.001).

Conclusions.—As compared with monthly high-quality clinic testing, weekly self-testing did not delay the time to a first stroke, major bleeding episode, or death to the extent suggested by prior studies. These results do not support the superiority of self-testing over clinic testing in reducing the risk of stroke, major bleeding episode, and death among patients taking warfarin therapy. (Funded by the Department of Veterans Affairs Cooperative Studies Program; ClinicalTrials.gov number, NCT00032591.)

▶ Anticoagulation with warfarin has been the clinical standard for decades to prevent stroke and other thromboembolic events among patients with mechanical valves and high-risk patients with atrial fibrillation. However, warfarin is one of the more difficult drugs to manage, requiring frequent monitoring of prothrombin time. One potential strategy to simplify regulation of warfarin dosing is to develop point of care management with home international normalized ratio testing. In this prospective randomized study of 2922 patients, this approach was evaluated. Compared with the control group strategy of regular clinic-based monitoring, home monitoring did not reduce embolic events or the primary composite end point of stroke, major bleed, or death (Fig 2 in the original article). The time in the therapeutic range was slightly greater in the home monitoring group, but this was not clinically meaningful. These results reinforce the challenges of warfarin use and the enthusiasm for alternative anticoagulants, such as dabigitran, to simplify patient care and improve outcomes.

M. R. Gold, MD, PhD

Cardiac Resynchronization Therapy in Asymptomatic or Mildly Symptomatic Heart Failure Patients in Relation to Etiology: Results From the REVERSE (REsynchronization reVErses Remodeling in Systolic Left vEntricular Dysfunction) Study
Linde C, on behalf of the REVERSE Study Group (Karolinska Univ Hosp, Stockholm, Sweden; et al)
J Am Coll Cardiol 56:1826-1831, 2010

Objectives.—The purpose of this study was to determine the effects of cardiac resynchronization therapy (CRT) with respect to heart failure etiology among patients in the REVERSE (REsynchronization reVErses Remodeling in Systolic Left vEntricular Dysfunction) study.

Background.—CRT improves outcomes in New York Heart Association functional class III/IV heart failure with wide QRS with a more pronounced effect on left ventricular (LV) reverse remodeling in nonischemic patients.

Methods.—A total of 277 patients with nonischemic heart disease (IHD) and 333 with IHD etiology in New York Heart Association functional class I or II with QRS ≥120 ms and left ventricular ejection fraction ≤40% received a CRT (± implantable cardioverter-defibrillator) and were randomized to CRT-ON or CRT-OFF for 12 months. The primary end point was the percentage of patients worsened by the HF clinical composite response, and multiple prespecified secondary end points were evaluated regarding etiology using univariable and multivariable analysis.

Results.—At baseline, IHD patients were significantly older and had more comorbidities and less dyssynchrony than non-IHD patients. In non-IHD patients, 10% worsened in CRT-ON compared with 19% in CRT-OFF (p = 0.01). In IHD patients, 20% worsened in the CRT-ON compared with 24% in the CRT-OFF group (p = 0.10). Non-IHD patients assigned to CRT-ON improved more in left ventricular end-systolic volume index than IHD patients. Randomization to CRT, left bundle branch block, and wider QRS duration independently predicted response to both end points, whereas non-IHD etiology was an independent predictor only for left ventricular end-systolic volume index.

Conclusions.—This substudy of REVERSE shows that CRT reverses left ventricular remodeling with a more extensive effect on nonischemic

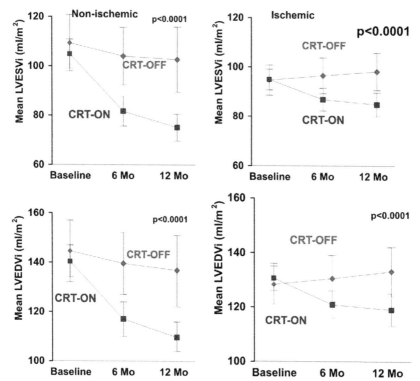

FIGURE 2.—Reverse Remodeling Left Ventricular End-Systolic and End-Diastolic Volume Index In Nonischemic and Ischemic Patients During CRT-ON and -OFF. The p values compare change from baseline to 12 months between cardiac resynchronization therapy (CRT)-ON and -OFF (2-sample *t* test). **Error bars** represent 95% confidence intervals. (Reprinted from the Journal of the American College of Cardiology, Linde C, on behalf of the REVERSE Study Group. Cardiac Resynchronization Therapy in Asymptomatic or Mildly Symptomatic Heart Failure Patients in Relation to Etiology: Results From the REVERSE (REsynchronization reVErses Remodeling in Systolic Left vEntricular Dysfunction) study. *J Am Coll Cardiol.* 2010;56:1826-1831. Copyright 2010, with permission from the American College of Cardiology.)

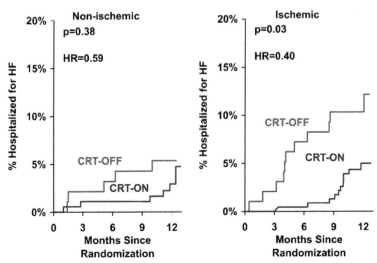

FIGURE 3.—Time to First Heart Failure—Related Hospitalization In Nonischemic and Ischemic Patients During CRT-ON and -OFF, Respectively. CRT = cardiac resynchronization therapy; HF = heart failure; HR = hazard ratio. (Reprinted from the Journal of the American College of Cardiology, Linde C, on behalf of the REVERSE Study Group. Cardiac Resynchronization Therapy in Asymptomatic or Mildly Symptomatic Heart Failure Patients in Relation to Etiology: results from the REVERSE (REsynchronization reVErses Remodeling in Systolic Left vEntricular Dysfunction) study. *J Am Coll Cardiol.* 2010;56:1826-1831. Copyright 2010, with permission from the American College of Cardiology.)

patients. Etiology was, however, not an independent predictor of clinical response. (REsynchronization reVErses Remodeling in Systolic Left vEntricular Dysfunction [REVERSE]; NCT00271154) (Figs 2 and 3).

▶ Controversy exists regarding the relative benefit of cardiac resynchronization therapy (CRT) among patients with ischemic cardiomyopathy (ICM) versus nonischemic cardiomyopathy. This substudy of the Resynchronization Reverses Remodeling in Systolic Left Ventricular Dysfunction trial examined the impact of etiology of cardiomyopathy on the clinical and mechanical benefits of CRT in patients with mild-moderate congestive heart failure (CHF). As depicted in Fig 2, patients with nonischemic heart disease (NIHD) had a larger benefit with respect to left ventricular (LV) remodeling (improved LV end-systolic volume index) compared with ICM; however, this did not correlate with improved clinical benefit, including decreased hospitalizations for CHF or death (Fig 3). The ischemic heart disease (IHD) group had statistically less dyssynchrony compared with the NIHD group, which may explain the lesser extent of reverse remodeling. The results of this study were consistent with those of prior CRT trials, and as noted previously, predictors of response included randomization to CRT-ON, as well as left bundle branch block (LBBB) morphology and QRS width. Etiology of cardiomyopathy (IHD vs NIHD) should not be a determinant in selecting patients for CRT; selecting patients with wide LBBB morphology QRS will likely result in greater remodeling and net clinical benefit.

M. R. Gold, MD, PhD

Heart rate as a risk factor in chronic heart failure (SHIFT): the association between heart rate and outcomes in a randomised placebo-controlled trial
Böhm M, on behalf of the SHIFT Investigators (Universitätsklinikum des Saarlandes, Homburg/Saar, Germany; et al)
Lancet 376:886-894, 2010

Background.—Raised resting heart rate is a marker of cardiovascular risk. We postulated that heart rate is also a risk factor for cardiovascular events in heart failure. In the SHIFT trial, patients with chronic heart failure were treated with the selective heart-rate-lowering agent ivabradine. We aimed to test our hypothesis by investigating the association between heart rate and events in this patient population.

Methods.—We analysed cardiovascular outcomes in the placebo (n=3264) and ivabradine groups (n=3241) of this randomised trial, divided by quintiles of baseline heart rate in the placebo group. The primary composite endpoint was cardiovascular death or hospital admission for worsening heart failure. In the ivabradine group, heart rate achieved at 28 days was also analysed in relation to subsequent outcomes. Analysis adjusted to change in heart rate was used to study heart-rate reduction as mechanism for risk reduction by ivabradine directly.

Findings.—In the placebo group, patients with the highest heart rates (≥87 beats per min [bpm], n=682, 286 events) were at more than twofold higher risk for the primary composite endpoint than were patients with the lowest heart rates (70 to <72 bpm, n=461, 92 events; hazard ratio [HR] 2.34, 95% CI 1.84—2.98, p<0.0001). Risk of primary composite endpoint events increased by 3% with every beat increase from baseline heart rate and 16% for every 5-bpm increase. In the ivabradine group, there was a direct association between heart rate achieved at 28 days and subsequent cardiac outcomes. Patients with heart rates lower than 60 bpm at 28 days on treatment had fewer primary composite endpoint events during the study (n=1192; event rate 17.4%, 95% CI 15.3—19.6) than did patients with higher heart rates. The effect of ivabradine is accounted for by heart-rate reduction, as shown by the neutralisation of the treatment effect after adjustment for change of heart rate at 28 days (HR 0.95, 0.85—1.06, p=0.352).

Interpretation.—Our analysis confirms that high heart rate is a risk factor in heart failure. Selective lowering of heart rates with ivabradine improves cardiovascular outcomes. Heart rate is an important target for treatment of heart failure (Figs 2 and 4).

▶ Heart rate is a predictor of mortality in advanced heart failure (HF). β-Blockers have been shown to improve survival in this population, but it is not clear whether the mechanism is reducing heart rate or blocking other β-adrenergic functions. The Systolic Heart failure treatment with the I_f inhibitor ivabradine Trial (SHIFT) analyzed the effect of the I_f current antagonist, ivabradine, in a population with a chronic HF. A total of 6905 patients with New York Heart Association class II and higher symptoms, left-ventricular ejection fraction of < 35%,

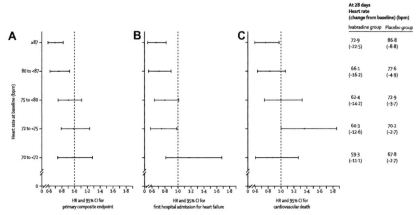

FIGURE 2.—Effect of ivabradine compared with placebo on (A) the primary composite endpoint, (B) first hospital admissions for worsening heart failure, and (C) cardiovascular deaths in the whole patient population, defined by quintiles of baseline heart-rate distribution. Primary composite endpoint includes cardiovascular deaths and hospital admissions for worsening heart failure. Adjusted for β-blocker intake at randomisation, New York Heart Association class, left-ventricular ejection fraction, ischaemic cause, age, systolic blood pressure, and creatinine clearance at baseline. HR=hazard ratio. bpm=beats per min. (Reprinted from Böhm M, on behalf of the SHIFT Investigators. Heart rate as a risk factor in chronic heart failure (SHIFT): The association between heart rate and outcomes in a randomised placebo-controlled trial. *Lancet.* 2010;376:886-894, with permission from Elsevier.)

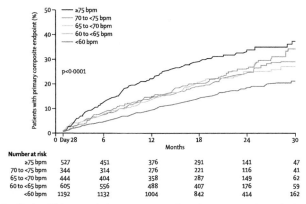

FIGURE 4.—Kaplan-Meier cumulative event curves for primary composite endpoint events in the ivabradine group, according to groups defined by heart rate achieved at 28 days. Data exclude patients reaching primary composite endpoint (cardiovascular death or hospital admission for worsening heart failure) during the first 28 days of follow-up. The log-rank p value is shown for the difference between the Kaplan-Meier curves. (Reprinted from Böhm M, on behalf of the SHIFT Investigators. Heart rate as a risk factor in chronic heart failure (SHIFT): The association between heart rate and outcomes in a randomised placebo-controlled trial. *Lancet.* 2010;376:886-894, with permission from Elsevier.)

and sinus rhythm with rates above 70 beats per minute (bpm) were randomized to placebo or ivabradine and were assessed for cardiovascular death or hospitalization and worsening HF. As a selective bradycardic agent, ivabradine was studied to assess the effect of heart rate control alone on patients with HF.

Baseline heart rate in the placebo group predicted a 2-fold difference in primary outcomes when comparing the highest (>87 bpm) with the lowest (70-72 bpm) quintiles (Fig 2). Ivabradine-treated patients in the lowest on-treatment quintile (<60 bpm) reached significantly fewer primary end points at 28 days compared with those in the highest quintile (>75 bpm). As summarized in Fig 4, the SHIFT demonstrates that ivabradine can improve cardiovascular outcomes by providing rate control alone and baseline heart rate is a modifiable risk factor in population with a chronic HF.

M. R. Gold, MD, PhD

Automated External Defibrillators and Survival After In-Hospital Cardiac Arrest

Chan PS, for the American Heart Association National Registry of Cardiopulmonary Resuscitation (NRCPR) Investigators (Saint Luke's Mid America Heart Inst, Kansas City, MO; et al)
JAMA 304:2129-2136, 2010

Context.—Automated external defibrillators (AEDs) improve survival from out-of-hospital cardiac arrests, but data on their effectiveness in hospitalized patients are limited.

Objective.—To evaluate the association between AED use and survival for in-hospital cardiac arrest.

Design, Setting, and Patients.—Cohort study of 11 695 hospitalized patients with cardiac arrests between January 1, 2000, and August 26, 2008, at 204 US hospitals following the introduction of AEDs on general hospital wards.

Main Outcome Measure.—Survival to hospital discharge by AED use, using multivariable hierarchical regression analyses to adjust for patient factors and hospital site.

Results.—Of 11 695 patients, 9616 (82.2%) had nonshockable rhythms (asystole and pulseless electrical activity) and 2079 (17.8%) had shockable rhythms (ventricular fibrillation and pulseless ventricular tachycardia). AEDs were used in 4515 patients (38.6%). Overall, 2117 patients (18.1%) survived to hospital discharge. Within the entire study population, AED use was associated with a lower rate of survival after in-hospital cardiac arrest compared with no AED use (16.3% vs 19.3%; adjusted rate ratio [RR], 0.85; 95% confidence interval [CI], 0.78-0.92; $P < .001$). Among cardiac arrests due to nonshockable rhythms, AED use was associated with lower survival (10.4% vs 15.4%; adjusted RR, 0.74; 95% CI, 0.65-0.83; $P < .001$). In contrast, for cardiac arrests due to shockable rhythms, AED use was not associated with survival (38.4% vs 39.8%; adjusted RR, 1.00; 95% CI, 0.88-1.13; $P = .99$). These patterns were consistently observed in both monitored and nonmonitored hospital units where AEDs were used, after matching patients to the individual units in each hospital where the cardiac arrest occurred, and with a propensity score analysis.

TABLE 3.—Survival to Discharge[a]

	No. of Survivors/Total No. of Patients (%)		Unadjusted RR (95% CI)	Adjusted RR (95% CI)[b]	P Value
	AED Used	AED Not Used			
All units					
All arrests	734/4515 (16.3)	1383/7180 (19.3)	0.84 (0.78-0.92)	0.85 (0.78-0.92)	<.001
VF and pulseless VT	364/947 (38.4)	450/1132 (39.8)	0.97 (0.87-1.08)	1.00 (0.88-1.13)	.99
Asystole and PEA	370/3568 (10.4)	933/6048 (15.4)	0.67 (0.60-0.75)	0.74 (0.65-0.83)	<.001
Monitored units					
All arrests	488/2104 (23.2)	992/4156 (23.9)	0.97 (0.88-1.07)	0.87 (0.79-0.97)	.01
VF and pulseless VT	286/593 (48.2)	368/804 (45.8)	1.05 (0.94-1.18)	1.03 (0.89-1.18)	.71
Asystole and PEA	202/1511 (13.4)	624/3352 (18.6)	0.72 (0.62-0.83)	0.72 (0.62-0.85)	<.001
Nonmonitored units					
All arrests	246/2411 (10.2)	391/3024 (12.9)	0.79 (0.68-0.92)	0.82 (0.70-0.98)	.03
VF and pulseless VT	78/354 (22.0)	82/328 (25.0)	0.88 (0.67-1.16)	0.93 (0.63-1.36)	.71
Asystole and PEA	168/2057 (8.2)	309/2696 (11.5)	0.71 (0.60-0.85)	0.79 (0.65-0.96)	.02

Abbreviations: AED, automated external defibrillator; CI, confidence interval; PEA, pulseless electrical activity; RR, rate ratio; VF, ventricular fibrillation; VT, ventricular tachycardia.
[a]Crude and adjusted rates of survival to discharge by AED use are presented. Results for the entire cohort and stratified by monitoring status are depicted.
[b]Adjusted for hospital site and patient and hospital factors using hierarchical models.

Conclusion.—Among hospitalized patients with cardiac arrest, use of AEDs was not associated with improved survival (Table 3).

▶ Strategies to improve survival associated with out-of-hospital cardiac arrest have developed over the past decade. Central in most approaches is the increased availability of automated external defibrillators (AEDs). This study evaluates the role of a similar strategy for in-hospital arrest. The cohort study was derived from 550 acute care hospitals with a total patient population of 110 132. The final study sample was 11 695 or 11% of the initial database and included only 204 hospitals (37%). The authors restricted their analysis to this smaller population to improve and ensure that the comparisons of AED use and survival were appropriate and contemporary. In the study population, there was a baseline difference in those with metastatic malignancy, baseline depression, and metabolic abnormality. These were all statistically higher in those with AED usage and may have some effect on survival.

Statistically, this study used multivariable hierarchy regression models to assess the relationship of AED use and survival. A propensity score was used to standardize the care of these patients and ensure balance. By doing this, the results showed a 16.3% decrease in the survival in those using AED versus 19.3% in those in whom it was not used (*P* < .001). In those with treatable arrhythmias, AED use showed a survival of 38.4% compared with 39% for no AED use. Those in whom the AED would not expect to be helped (nontreatable arrhythmias), survival was worse with AED use 10.4% versus 15.5% (*P* < .001), suggesting that AEDs delayed treatment of the underlying cause of arrest.

The limitations of this study may be failure to implement AEDs efficiently from possibly poor training, which would attenuate the benefits. Smaller hospitals had a higher use of AEDs. Clearly, training to evaluate and treat an arrhythmia may have significant effects on survival. One of the most important items noted by the author is the huge increase in use of AEDs. Because 37% of hospitals now have AEDs, and more may be added annually, the effectiveness of their treatment should be established. These results indicate that a prospective randomized controlled study should be performed to evaluate the routine use of AEDs in hospitals.

M. R. Gold, MD, PhD

Chest Compression–Only CPR by Lay Rescuers and Survival From Out-of-Hospital Cardiac Arrest

Bobrow BJ, Spaite DW, Berg RA, et al (Arizona Dept of Health Services, Phoenix; Univ of Arizona, Tucson; Children's Hosp of Philadelphia, PA; et al)
JAMA 304:1447-1454, 2010

Context.—Chest compression—only bystander cardiopulmonary resuscitation (CPR) may be as effective as conventional CPR with rescue breathing for out-of-hospital cardiac arrest.

Objective.—To investigate the survival of patients with out-of-hospital cardiac arrest using compression-only CPR (COCPR) compared with conventional CPR.

Design, Setting, and Patients.—A 5-year prospective observational cohort study of survival in patients at least 18 years old with out-of-hospital cardiac arrest between January 1, 2005, and December 31, 2009, in Arizona. The relationship between layperson bystander CPR and survival to hospital discharge was evaluated using multivariable logistic regression.

Main Outcome Measure.—Survival to hospital discharge.

Results.—Among 5272 adults with out-of-hospital cardiac arrest of cardiac etiology not observed by responding emergency medical personnel, 779 were excluded because bystander CPR was provided by a health care professional or the arrest occurred in a medical facility. A total of 4415 met all inclusion criteria for analysis, including 2900 who received no bystander CPR, 666 who received conventional CPR, and 849 who received COCPR. Rates of survival to hospital discharge were 5.2% (95% confidence interval [CI], 4.4%-6.0%) for the no bystander CPR group, 7.8% (95% CI, 5.8%-9.8%) for conventional CPR, and 13.3% (95% CI, 11.0%-15.6%) for COCPR. The adjusted odds ratio (AOR) for survival for conventional CPR vs no CPR was 0.99 (95% CI, 0.69-1.43), for COCPR vs no CPR, 1.59 (95% CI, 1.18-2.13), and for COCPR vs conventional CPR, 1.60 (95% CI, 1.08-2.35). From 2005 to 2009, lay rescuer CPR increased from 28.2% (95% CI, 24.6%-31.8%) to 39.9% (95% CI, 36.8%-42.9%; $P < .001$); the proportion of CPR that was COCPR increased from 19.6% (95% CI, 13.6%-25.7%) to 75.9% (95% CI, 71.7%-80.1%; $P < .001$). Overall survival increased from 3.7% (95% CI, 2.2%-5.2%) to 9.8% (95% CI, 8.0%-11.6%; $P < .001$).

Conclusion.—Among patients with out-of-hospital cardiac arrest, layperson compression-only CPR was associated with increased survival compared with conventional CPR and no bystander CPR in this setting with public endorsement of chest compression-only CPR.

▶ Though survival of out-of-hospital cardiac arrest is improved with early and effective cardiopulmonary resuscitation (CPR), most patients suffering cardiac arrest do not receive bystander CPR; moreover, the optimal methods for CPR administration continue to evolve. As an alternative to conventional CPR with interruptions for ventilation, compression-only CPR (COCPR) has gained popularity for untrained medical personnel because of its simplicity and focus on effective chest compressions, a principle that has been emphasized as an important component of high-quality CPR.

The authors of this study sought to evaluate the effectiveness of a statewide public campaign to promote COCPR as compared with conventional bystander CPR and no bystander CPR. Following Arizona's statewide dissemination of information promoting COCPR, 5272 cardiac arrests between 2005 and 2009 were analyzed according to the type of CPR performed. During the study period, the number of bystanders performing any type of CPR increased from 28.2% in 2005 to 39.9% in 2009 ($P < .001$), while the proportion of bystanders performing COCPR increased from 19.6% to 75.9% during the same time period. The rate of survival to hospital discharge was 5.2% (95% confidence interval [CI], 4.4%-6.0%) for the no bystander CPR group, 7.8% (95% CI, 5.8-9.8%) for conventional CPR group, and 13.3% (95% CI, 11.0%-15.6%) for COCPR group. As shown in Table 3 in the original article, odds of survival were improved with COCPR compared with no bystander CPR (odds ratio, 1.59; 95% CI, 1.18-2.13) and conventional CPR (odds ratio, 1.60; 95% CI, 1.08-2.35). Overall survival increased from 3.7% (95% CI, 2.2%-5.2%) to 9.8% (95% CI, 9.0%-11.6%; $P < .001$).

There are several important findings in this study that have widespread implications for improvement in out-of-hospital cardiac arrest. First, it demonstrates the effectiveness of a public health campaign aimed at increasing awareness of the necessity for bystander CPR. Second, the results also suggest that COCPR is not only an alternative to traditional CPR but for the first time has been shown to be a superior method by increasing survival to hospital discharge and may be a preferable strategy for lay rescuers. Lastly, in addition to improved relative survival compared with conventional CPR, by increasing the number of bystanders performing CPR, this method also increases the absolute number of patients surviving out-of-hospital cardiac arrest. Despite these advances in provision and quality of bystander CPR, significant improvements are still required for patients with out-of-hospital cardiac arrest.

M. R. Gold, MD, PhD

41 Cardiac Surgery

Diabetic and Nondiabetic Patients With Left Main and/or 3-Vessel Coronary Artery Disease: Comparison of Outcomes With Cardiac Surgery and Paclitaxel-Eluting Stents

Banning AP, Westaby S, Morice M-C, et al (John Radcliffe Hosp, Oxford, UK; Institut Hospitalier Jacques Cartier, Massy, France; et al)

J Am Coll Cardiol 55:1067-1075, 2010

Objectives.—This study was designed to compare contemporary surgical revascularization (coronary artery bypass graft surgery [CABG]) versus TAXUS Express (Boston Scientific, Natick, Massachusetts) paclitaxel-eluting stents (PES) in diabetic and nondiabetic patients with left main and/or 3-vessel disease.

Background.—Although the prevalence of diabetes mellitus is increasing, the optimal coronary revascularization strategy in diabetic patients with complex multivessel disease remains controversial.

Methods.—The SYNTAX (SYNergy between percutaneous coronary intervention with TAXus and cardiac surgery) study randomly assigned 1,800 patients (452 with medically treated diabetes) to receive PES or CABG.

Results.—The overall 1-year major adverse cardiac and cerebrovascular event rate was higher among diabetic patients treated with PES compared with CABG, but the revascularization method did not impact the death/stroke/myocardial infarction rate for nondiabetic patients (6.8% CABG vs. 6.8% PES, $p = 0.97$) or for diabetic patients (10.3% CABG vs. 10.1% PES, $p = 0.96$). The presence of diabetes was associated with significantly increased mortality after either revascularization treatment. The incidence of stroke was higher among nondiabetic patients after CABG (2.2% vs. PES 0.5%, $p = 0.006$). Compared with CABG, mortality was higher after PES use for diabetic patients with highly complex lesions (4.1% vs. 13.5%, $p = 0.04$). Revascularization with PES resulted in higher repeat revascularization for nondiabetic patients (5.7% vs. 11.1%, $p < 0.001$) and diabetic patients (6.4% vs. 20.3%, $p < 0.001$).

Conclusions.—Subgroup analyses suggest that the 1-year major adverse cardiac and cerebrovascular event rate is higher among diabetic patients with left main and/or 3-vessel disease treated with PES compared with CABG, driven by an increase in repeat revascularization. However, the composite safety end point (death/stroke/myocardial infarction) is comparable between the 2 treatment options for diabetic and nondiabetic patients. Although further study is needed, these exploratory results may extend the evidence for PES use in selected patients with less complex left main and/or 3-vessel lesions. (SYNergy Between PCI With TAXus and Cardiac Surgery [SYNTAX]; NCT00114972).

▶ It is well known that diabetes increases the risk of developing cardiovascular disease and is a consistent predictor of mortality, myocardial infarction, and restenosis after percutaneous coronary intervention (PCI) and coronary artery bypass grafting (CABG). The SYNTAX (SYNergy between percutaneous coronary intervention with TAXus and cardiac surgery) study is the first to compare CABG with the TAXUS Express paclitaxel-eluting stent (PES) in nondiabetic and diabetic patients with complex left main and/or 3-vessel coronary disease. The 1-year SYNTAX results suggest that in patients with left main and/or 3-vessel disease, major adverse cardiac and cerebrovascular event is increased for PES-treated diabetic patients compared with CABG-treated patients, driven by an increase in repeat revascularization. Composite safety and mortality end points are comparable between the CABG and PES arms.

The SYNTAX study presents PCI as a viable general option with the following caveats: (1) multivessel PCI for diabetic patients performed without drug-eluting stents (DES) is likely associated with increased death and should not be done unless there is no reasonable surgical option and (2) diabetic patients undergoing PCI with DES remain at higher risk for repeat revascularization with PCI versus CABG. This is an excellent study performed by high-volume centers.

V. H. Thourani, MD

Should Patients With Severe Degenerative Mitral Regurgitation Delay Surgery Until Symptoms Develop?

Gillinov AM, Mihaljevic T, Blackstone EH, et al (Heart and Vascular Inst, Cleveland, OH; Cleveland Clinic, OH)
Ann Thorac Surg 90:481-488, 2010

Background.—The American College of Cardiology/American Heart Association practice guidelines recommending surgery for asymptomatic patients with severe mitral regurgitation caused by degenerative disease remain controversial. This study examined whether delaying surgery until symptoms occur causes adverse cardiac changes and jeopardizes outcome.

Methods.—From January 1985 to January 2008, 4,586 patients had primary isolated mitral valve surgery for degenerative mitral regurgitation; 4,253 (93%) underwent repair. Preoperatively, 30% were in New York Heart Association (NYHA) class I (asymptomatic), 56% in class II, 13% in class III, and 2% in class IV. Multivariable analysis and propensity matching were used to assess association of symptoms (NYHA class) with cardiac structure and function and postoperative outcomes.

Results.—Increasing NYHA class was associated with progressive reduction in left ventricular function, left atrial enlargement, and development of atrial fibrillation and tricuspid regurgitation. These findings were evident even in class II patients (mild symptoms). Repair was accomplished in 96% of asymptomatic patients, and in progressively fewer as NYHA class increased (93%, 86%, and 85% in classes II to IV, respectively; $p < 0.0001$). Hospital mortality was 0.37%, but was particularly high in class IV (0.29%, 0.20%, 0.67%, and 5.1% for classes I to IV, respectively; $p = 0.004$). Although long-term survival progressively diminished with increasing NHYA class, these differences were largely related to differences in left ventricular function and increased comorbidity.

Conclusions.—In patients with severe degenerative mitral regurgitation, the development of even mild symptoms by the time of surgical referral is associated with deleterious changes in cardiac structure and function. Therefore, particularly because successful repair is highly likely, early surgery is justified in asymptomatic patients with degenerative disease and severe mitral regurgitation.

▶ The American College of Cardiology/American Heart Association (ACC/AHA) practice guidelines recommending surgery for asymptomatic patients with severe mitral regurgitation caused by degenerative disease remain controversial. With this controversy in mind, researchers from the Cleveland Clinic shared their broad experience in mitral valve repair and documented results based on New York Heart Association (NYHA) classification. With increasing NYHA class, the likelihood of repair decreased significantly and the subsequent in-hospital mortality increased. Long-term survival was also decreased in patients with increased NYHA class, but this was likely related to decreases in left ventricular ejection fraction. This article stands as a seminal work to fortify the ACC/AHA guidelines for early surgical intervention in patients with severe asymptomatic mitral regurgitation.

V. H. Thourani, MD

42 Coronary Heart Disease

Early routine percutaneous coronary intervention after fibrinolysis vs. standard therapy in ST-segment elevation myocardial infarction: a meta-analysis
Borgia F, Goodman SG, Halvorsen S, et al (Royal Brompton Hosp and Imperial College, London, UK; Univ of Toronto, Canada; Oslo Univ Hosp, Ulleval, Norway; et al)
Eur Heart J 31:2156-2169, 2010

Aims.—Multiple trials in patients with ST-segment elevation myocardial infarction (STEMI) compared early routine percutaneous coronary intervention (PCI) after successful fibrinolysis vs. standard therapy limiting PCI only to patients without evidence of reperfusion (rescue PCI). These trials suggest that all patients receiving fibrinolysis should receive mechanical revascularization within 24 h from initial hospitalization. However, individual trials could not demonstrate a significant reduction in 'hard' endpoints such as death and reinfarction. We performed a meta-analysis of randomized controlled trials to define the benefits of early PCI after fibrinolysis over standard therapy on clinical and safety endpoints in STEMI.

Methods and Results.—We identified seven eligible trials, enrolling a total of 2961 patients. No difference was found in the incidence of death at 30 days between the two strategies. Early PCI after successful fibrinolysis reduced the rate of reinfarction (OR: 0.55, 95% CI: 0.36−0.82; $P = 0.003$), the combined endpoint death/reinfarction (OR: 0.65, 95% CI: 0.49−0.88; $P = 0.004$) and recurrent ischaemia (OR: 0.25, 95% CI: 0.13−0.49; $P < 0.001$) at 30-day follow-up. These advantages were achieved without a significant increase in major bleeding (OR: 0.93, 96% CI: 0.67−1.34; $P = 0.70$) or stroke (OR: 0.63, 95% CI: 0.31−1.26; $P = 0.21$). The benefits of a routine invasive strategy over standard therapy were maintained at 6−12 months, with persistent significant reduction in the endpoints reinfarction (OR: 0.64, 95% CI: 0.40−0.98; $P = 0.01$) and combined death/reinfarction (OR: 0.71, 95% CI: 0.52−0.97; $P = 0.03$).

Conclusion.—Early routine PCI after fibrinolysis in STEMI patients significantly reduced reinfarction and recurrent ischaemia at 1 month,

Death, 6-12 months

Study	Early PCI		Standard therapy			Odds ratio	Odds ratio
	Events	Total	Events	Total	Weight %	[M-H, Random, 95% CI]	[M-H, Random, 95% CI]
CARESS-IN-AMI	17	299	19	301	26.4	0.89 [0.46, 1.76]	
GRACIA-1	9	248	16	251	17.2	0.55 [0.24, 1.28]	
CAPITAL-AMI	3	86	3	84	4.5	0.98 [0.19, 4.98]	
SIAM-III	4	82	9	81	8.1	0.41 [0.12, 1.39]	
TRANSFER-AMI	30	537	23	522	38.7	1.28 [0.74, 2.24]	
NORDISTEMI	3	134	4	132	5.2	0.73 [0.16, 3.34]	
Total	66/1386		74/1371		100.0	0.88 [0.62, 1.25]	
	(4.8%)		(5.4%)				

Heterogeneity: $\tau^2 = 0.00$; $\chi^2 = 4.53$, df = 5 ($P = 0.48$); $I^2 = 0\%$
Test for overall effect: $Z = 0.70$ ($P = 0.48$)
Egger's regression test: P value 0.11

Favours early PCI   Favours standard therapy

Reinfarction, 6-12 months

Study	Early PCI		Standard therapy			Odds ratio	Odds ratio
	Events	Total	Events	Total	Weight %	[M-H, Random, 95% CI]	[M-H, Random, 95% CI]
CARESS-IN-AMI	13	299	9	301	18.2	1.47 [0.62, 3.50]	
GRACIA-1	9	248	15	251	19.6	0.59 [0.25, 1.38]	
CAPITAL-AMI	5	86	12	84	13.7	0.37 [0.12, 1.10]	
SIAM-III	2	82	2	81	5.0	0.99 [0.14, 7.18]	
TRANSFER-AMI	21	537	33	522	31.1	0.60 [0.34, 1.06]	
NORDISTEMI	4	134	12	132	12.5	0.31 [0.10, 0.98]	
Total	54/1386		83/1371		100.0	0.64 [0.40, 0.98]	
	(3.9%)		(6%)			NNT 46[26-187]	

Heterogeneity: $\tau^2 = 0.10$; $\chi^2 = 6.33$, df = 5 ($P = 0.28$); $I^2 = 21\%$
Test for overall effect: $Z = 2.12$ ($P = 0.03$)
Egger's regression test: P value 0.40

Favours early PCI   Favours standard therapy

Death-Reinfarction, 6-12 months

Study	Early PCI		Standard therapy			Odds ratio	Odds ratio
	Events	Total	Events	Total	Weight %	[M-H, Random, 95% CI]	[M-H, Random, 95% CI]
CARESS-IN-AMI	30	299	28	301	22.0	1.09 [0.63, 1.87]	
GRACIA-1	17	248	29	251	18.3	0.56 [0.30, 1.05]	
CAPITAL-AMI	8	86	15	84	10.1	0.47 [0.19, 1.18]	
SIAM-III	6	82	11	81	8.1	0.50 [0.18, 1.43]	
TRANSFER-AMI	51	537	56	522	31.5	0.87 [0.59, 1.30]	
NORDISTEMI	7	134	16	132	10.0	0.40 [0.16, 1.01]	
Total	119/1386		155/1371		100.0	0.71 [0.52, 0.97]	
	(8.6%)		(11.2%)			NNT 37[20-206]	

Heterogeneity: $\tau^2 = 0.04$; $\chi^2 = 6.49$, df = 5 ($P = 0.26$); $I^2 = 23\%$
Test for overall effect: $Z = 2.19$ ($P = 0.03$)
Egger's regression test: P value 0.03

Favours early PCI   Favours standard therapy

FIGURE 5.—Clinical endpoints at 6–12 months. Odds ratios and 95% confidence interval for death, reinfarction, and combined death/reinfarction between early PCI and standard therapy. Size of data markers indicates the weight of each trial. Benefits observed after early PCI on reduction of reinfarction and combined endpoint death/reinfarction are maintained in longer follow-up. (Reprinted from Borgia F, Goodman SG, Halvorsen S, et al. Early routine percutaneous coronary intervention after fibrinolysis vs. standard therapy in ST-segment elevation myocardial infarction: a meta-analysis. *Eur Heart J.* 2010;31:2156-2169, by permission of The European Society of Cardiology.)

with no significant increase in adverse bleeding events compared to standard therapy. Benefits of early PCI persist at 6–12 month follow-up (Fig 5).

▶ Many of the questions posed by the evolution of reperfusion therapy for ST-segment elevation myocardial infarction have been answered, but there remain areas of controversy. While it is widely accepted that primary percutaneous coronary intervention (PCI) is the best form of reperfusion therapy, an unanswered question is what degree of delay is acceptable in patients transferred directly to a PCI center.[1] Nonetheless, the geography of the United States and logistical constraints imposed by weather and long distances in rural areas will ensure a role for the initial administration of fibrinolytic drugs in many situations. The initial approach or reperfusion strategy will therefore vary markedly between regions and countries.

The optimal approach to the patient who has received fibrinolytic therapy in a community hospital has been a subject of some debate. The trials of facilitated PCI in which PCI is routinely performed as an emergency on arrival at the referral hospital fail to show a benefit, and there were some signals suggesting potential harm due to bleeding and perhaps balloon inflation in a thrombolytic milieu.

Subsequently, several trials strongly suggest that a routine invasive approach with angiography performed 3 to 24 hours following fibrinolytic drug administration is the preferred strategy in patients who are clinically stable with evidence of successful reperfusion therapy. This meta-analysis of 7 trials involving approximately 2900 patients strongly suggests that a routine invasive strategy performed early (3-24 hours), as opposed to immediate PCI, reduces reinfarction and recurrent ischemia with no significant increase in bleeding events. The umbrella term for this strategy is the pharmacoinvasive approach. A key component, however, of the pharmacoinvasive strategy is the ability to perform rescue PCI. The best approach, therefore, following lytic drugs administered in a non-PCI-capable hospital is immediate transfer if at all possible.

B. J. Gersh, MB, ChB, DPhil, FRCP

Reference

1. Gersh BJ, Stone GW, White HD, Holmes DR Jr. Pharmacological facilitation of primary percutaneous coronary intervention for acute myocardial infarction: is the slope of the curve the shape of the future? *JAMA.* 2005;293:979-986.

Comparative Effectiveness of ST-Segment–Elevation Myocardial Infarction Regionalization Strategies

Concannon TW, Kent DM, Normand S-L, et al (Tufts Med Ctr and Tufts Univ School of Medicine, Boston, MA; Harvard Med School, Boston, MA; et al)
Circ Cardiovasc Qual Outcomes 3:506-513, 2010

Background.—Primary percutaneous coronary intervention (PCI) is more effective on average than fibrinolytic therapy in the treatment of ST-segment–elevation myocardial infarction. Yet, most US hospitals are not equipped for PCI, and fibrinolytic therapy is still widely used. This study evaluated the comparative effectiveness of ST-segment–elevation myocardial infarction regionalization strategies to increase the use of PCI against standard emergency transport and care.

Methods and Results.—We estimated incremental treatment costs and quality-adjusted life expectancies of 2000 patients with ST-segment–elevation myocardial infarction who received PCI or fibrinolytic therapy in simulations of emergency care in a regional hospital system. To increase access to PCI across the system, we compared a base case strategy with 12 hospital-based strategies of building new PCI laboratories or extending the hours of existing laboratories and 1 emergency medical services–based strategy of transporting all patients with ST-segment–elevation myocardial infarction to existing PCI-capable hospitals. The base case resulted in 609 (95% CI, 569–647) patients getting PCI. Hospital-based strategies increased the number of patients receiving PCI, the costs of care, and quality-adjusted life years saved and were cost-effective under a variety of conditions. An emergency medical services–based strategy of transporting every patient to an existing PCI facility was less costly and more effective than all hospital expansion options.

Conclusion.—Our results suggest that new construction and staffing of PCI laboratories may not be warranted if an emergency medical services strategy is both available and feasible.

▶ This is an interesting cost-effectiveness analysis that has potentially major implications for the development of regional strategies for the delivery of reperfusion therapy.

It is increasingly accepted that if administered in a timely manner, primary percutaneous coronary intervention (PPCI) is the preferred form of reperfusion therapy. Nonetheless, since PPCI is not available in many hospitals, the key question is what degree of delay is acceptable during transfer to a PPCI facility as opposed to giving fibrinolytics at the primary presenting institution.[1] There is understandable interest, therefore, in increasing access to PPCI, and a number of regionalization strategies have been proposed.

This analysis using a recently developed triage and allocation model[2] compares the incremental benefits and costs of 2 approaches for increasing access to PPCI:

1. hospital-based in which new PPCI-capable facilities would be added;
2. emergency medical service (EMS)-based in which the key element is rapid transport to PCI-capable systems.

The bottom line is that providing additional catheterization laboratories does increase the number of patients receiving PPCI and could be cost effective in a variety of conditions. Nonetheless, the EMS-based strategy was less costly and more effective in all the scenarios that were tested.

What should be emphasized is that one size does not fit all, and the optimal strategy for a particular region will vary according to available resources, ambulance services, geographical constraints, including weather and distance. For many parts of the United States and other countries around the world, there will remain an important role for fibrinolytic therapy.[3]

B. J. Gersh, MB, ChB, DPhil, FRCP

References

1. Gersh BJ, Antman EM. Selection of the optimal reperfusion strategy for STEMI: does time matter? *Eur Heart J.* 2006;27:761-763.
2. Nallamothu BK, Bates ER, Wang Y, Bradley EH, Krumholz HM. Driving times and distances to hospitals with percutaneous coronary intervention in the United States: implications for prehospital triage of patients with ST-elevation myocardial infarction. *Circulation.* 2006;113:1189-1195.
3. Ting HH, Rihal CS, Gersh BJ, et al. Regional systems of care to optimize timeliness of reperfusion therapy for ST-elevation myocardial infarction: the Mayo Clinic STEMI Protocol. *Circulation.* 2007;116:729-736.

Primary angioplasty vs. fibrinolysis in very old patients with acute myocardial infarction: TRIANA (TRatamiento del Infarto Agudo de miocardio eN Ancianos) randomized trial and pooled analysis with previous studies
Bueno H, on behalf of the TRIANA Investigators (Hospital General Universitario Gregorio Marañón, Madrid, Spain; et al)
Eur Heart J 32:51-60, 2011

Aims.—To compare primary percutaneous coronary intervention (pPCI) and fibrinolysis in very old patients with ST-segment elevation myocardial infarction (STEMI), in whom head-to-head comparisons between both strategies are scarce.

Methods and Results.—Patients ≥75 years old with STEMI <6 h were randomized to pPCI or fibrinolysis. The primary endpoint was a composite of all-cause mortality, re-infarction, or disabling stroke at 30 days. The trial was prematurely stopped due to slow recruitment after enroling 266 patients (134 allocated to pPCI and 132 to fibrinolysis). Both groups were well balanced in baseline characteristics. Mean age was 81 years. The primary endpoint was reached in 25 patients in the pPCI group (18.9%) and 34 (25.4%) in the fibrinolysis arm [odds ratio (OR), 0.69; 95% confidence interval (CI) 0.38−1.23; $P = 0.21$]. Similarly, non-significant reductions were found in death (13.6 vs. 17.2%, $P = 0.43$), re-infarction (5.3 vs. 8.2%, $P = 0.35$), or disabling stroke (0.8 vs. 3.0%, $P = 0.18$). Recurrent ischaemia was less common in pPCI-treated patients (0.8 vs. 9.7%, $P < 0.001$). No differences were found in major bleeds. A pooled analysis with the two previous reperfusion trials performed in older patients showed an advantage of pPCI over fibrinolysis in reducing death, re-infarction, or stroke at 30 days (OR, 0.64; 95% CI 0.45−0.91).

Conclusion.—Primary PCI seems to be the best reperfusion therapy for STEMI even for the oldest patients. Early contemporary fibrinolytic therapy may be a safe alternative to pPCI in the elderly when this is not available.

▶ No one would dispute that primary percutaneous coronary intervention (pPCI) is the treatment of choice for patients presenting with ST-segment elevation myocardial infarction, providing the facilities and the expertise are available. Nonetheless, prior trials comparing pPCI with fibrinolysis either excluded or really enrolled patients in the elderly (age, ≥75 years) subgroup, and in fact, only 2 such trials have been performed and are with conflicting results.[1]

This trial from Spain was confined to patients age 75 years or older (mean age, 81 years) treated within 6 hours of symptoms. The trial was prematurely terminated because of slow recruitment, but in total, 266 patients were recruited. Patient's characteristics differ somewhat from those in the senior Primary Angioplasty in Myocardial Infarction trial in which the age cutoff was 70 years and above. The period of enrollment took 5 years, and the time limit was less than 12 hours in contrast to the enrollment period of 2 to 3 years in this trial.[2]

Although underpowered to provide definitive answers, the trends in regard to mortality, reinfarction, and stroke at 30 days (the primary end point) were in favor of pPCI as was recurrent ischemia. There was no difference in bleeding rates. A pooled analysis for the 2 other trials demonstrated statistical significance for the primary composite end point. Although a large community-based trial would be desirable, from a practical standpoint, this is unlikely to happen. Irrespective of the therapy, advanced stages are a powerful predictor of mortality and morbidity, but the risks of reperfusion therapy is more than outweighed from the potential for gain, as the elderly are a sicker group. Although the prompt early use of fibrinolytic therapy is a reasonable alternative to pPCI in the elderly in areas where the facilities for percutaneous coronary intervention are not available, it would appear that in the elderly and younger patients, pPCI remains the optimal therapeutic strategy.

B. J. Gersh, MB, ChB, DPhil, FRCP

References

1. Alexander KP, Newby LK, Armstrong PW, et al. American Heart Association Council on Clinical Cardiology, Society of Geriatric Cardiology. Acute coronary care in the elderly, part II: ST-segment-elevation myocardial infarction: a scientific statement for healthcare professionals from the American Heart Association Council on Clinical Cardiology: in collaboration with the Society of Geriatric Cardiology. *Circulation.* 2007;115:2570-2589.
2. Senior PAMI. Primary PCI not better than lytic therapy in elderly patients, http://www.theheart.org/article/581549.do. Accessed May 14, 2010.

Percutaneous Revascularization for Stable Coronary Artery Disease: Temporal Trends and Impact of Drug-Eluting Stents
Hilliard AA, From AM, Lennon RJ, et al (Mayo Clinic and Mayo Foundation, Rochester, MN)
J AM Coll Cardiol Intr 3:172-179, 2010

Objectives.—We sought to determine the characteristics, outcomes, and temporal trends among patients undergoing percutaneous coronary intervention (PCI) for stable coronary artery disease (CAD) from a single-center registry.

Background.—There is controversy regarding the generalizability of the findings from randomized trials of PCI for stable CAD to daily practice. An important perspective on the significance of the trial results can be achieved by clearly documenting past and present practice of PCI.

Methods.—This was a retrospective analysis of 8,912 consecutive patients undergoing elective PCI from 1979 through 2006 at a tertiary referral center. Clinical, angiographic, and procedural characteristics as well as in-hospital and long-term outcomes were measured in patients grouped into 4 eras depending on the dominant interventional strategy of that time: percutaneous transluminal coronary angioplasty, early stent, bare-metal stent, and drug-eluting stent.

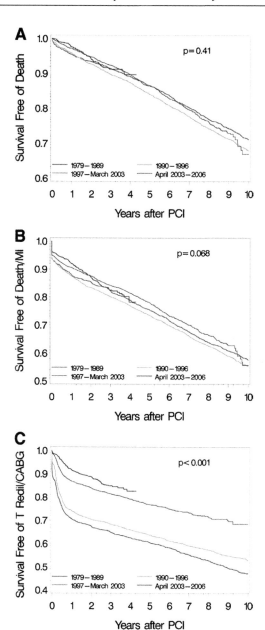

FIGURE 2.—Long-Term Mortality and Composite End Points of Death or MI and Repeat Target Lesion Redilation or CABG. Kaplan-Meier curves showing survival free of **(A)** death, **(B)** death/myocardial infarction (MI), and **(C)** target lesion redilation (T Redil)/coronary artery bypass grafting (CABG). PCI = percutaneous coronary intervention. (Reprinted from Hilliard AA, From AM, Lennon RJ, et al. Percutaneous revascularization for stable coronary artery disease: temporal trends and impact of drug-eluting stents. *JACC Cardiovasc Interv.* 2010;3:172-179, with permission The American College Of Cardiology Foundation.)

Results.—Procedural success rates have improved (81%, 92%, 96%, and 97%, respectively, p < 0.001), and in-hospital mortality has decreased significantly (1.0%, 0.8%, 0.1%, and 0.1%, respectively, p < 0.001) over time. Kaplan-Meier estimates of mortality at 4 years were 11%, 13%, 10%, and 10%, respectively (p = 0.4). The 1-year target lesion revascularization rates in the 4 groups were 29%, 26%, 13%, and 8%, respectively (p < 0.001).

Conclusions.—Procedural success rates in contemporary practice of PCI for stable CAD are excellent with very low in-hospital mortality. Introduction of drug-eluting stents has reduced target lesion revascularization but not mortality among all comers. Outcomes similar to that observed in recent clinical trials are being achieved in routine clinical practice (Fig 2).

▶ This study from the Mayo Clinic provides a sweeping perspective of the results of percutaneous coronary intervention in patients with stable coronary artery disease over almost 3 decades. Patients were divided into 4 groups that reflect the dominant interventional strategy at the time, beginning in 1976 through 2006. As shown in other studies, patients have been getting progressively older and sicker with an increased number of comorbid conditions, heavier, and the frequency of reduced ejection fraction and symptomatic heart failure has increased. Despite this, procedural success rates have steadily improved, in-hospital mortality has fallen from 1% to 0.1%, and the rate of repeat revascularization has declined following the introduction of stents, particularly drug-eluting stents. Nonetheless, Kaplan Meier estimates of mortality at 4 years were basically unchanged being 11%, 13%, 10%, and 10% in the 4 cohorts.

Of note, the composite end point of death and myocardial infarction at 4 years was almost identical to that reported in the Clinical Outcomes Utilizing Revascularization and Aggressive Drug Evaluation (COURAGE) trial.[1] This is interesting from a number of different perspectives. Firstly, these data suggest that the population enrolled in the COURAGE trial was probably very representative of patients seen in clinical practice. Secondly, the lack of any change in late death or myocardial infarction despite higher procedural success rates and the development of drug-eluting stents would suggest that late events are the consequence of disease progression and unrelated to the original target lesion.[2] Another factor underlying the lack of improvement in late mortality could be that the more recent cohort is a sicker subgroup and that late survival might have been increased in the event that the baseline characteristics were similar.

Irrespectively, these data provide a roadmap for the future. New developments in stent technology will probably improve success rates even further, particularly if innovative approaches to chronic total occlusions bear fruit. On the other hand, these developments need to go hand in hand with one other new technology in interventional cardiology, and that is secondary prevention and optimal medical therapy.

B. J. Gersh, MB, ChB, DPhil, FRCP

References

1. Boden WE, O'Rourke RA, Teo KK, et al. Optimal medical therapy with or without PCI for stable coronary artery disease. *N Engl J Med.* 2007;356:1503-1516.
2. Cutlip DE, Chhabra AG, Baim DS, et al. Beyond restenosis: five-year clinical outcomes from second-generation coronary stent trials. *Circulation.* 2004;110: 1226-1230.

Safety of Anacetrapib in Patients with or at High Risk for Coronary Heart Disease
Cannon CP, for the DEFINE Investigators (Brigham and Women's Hosp, Boston, MA; et al)
N Engl J Med 363:2406-2415, 2010

Background.—Anacetrapib is a cholesteryl ester transfer protein inhibitor that raises high-density lipoprotein (HDL) cholesterol and reduces low-density lipoprotein (LDL) cholesterol.

Methods.—We conducted a randomized, double-blind, placebo-controlled trial to assess the efficacy and safety profile of anacetrapib in patients with coronary heart disease or at high risk for coronary heart disease. Eligible patients who were taking a statin and who had an LDL cholesterol level that was consistent with that recommended in guidelines were assigned to receive 100 mg of anacetrapib or placebo daily for 18 months. The primary end points were the percent change from baseline in LDL cholesterol at 24 weeks (HDL cholesterol level was a secondary end point) and the safety and side-effect profile of anacetrapib through 76 weeks. Cardiovascular events and deaths were prospectively adjudicated.

Results.—A total of 1623 patients underwent randomization. By 24 weeks, the LDL cholesterol level had been reduced from 81 mg per deciliter (2.1 mmol per liter) to 45 mg per deciliter (1.2 mmol per liter) in the anacetrapib group, as compared with a reduction from 82 mg per deciliter (2.1 mmol per liter) to 77 mg per deciliter (2.0 mmol per liter) in the placebo group (P<0.001) — a 39.8% reduction with anacetrapib beyond that seen with placebo. In addition, the HDL cholesterol level increased from 41 mg per deciliter (1.0 mmol per liter) to 101 mg per deciliter (2.6 mmol per liter) in the anacetrapib group, as compared with an increase from 40 mg per deciliter (1.0 mmol per liter) to 46 mg per deciliter (1.2 mmol per liter) in the placebo group (P<0.001) — a 138.1% increase with anacetrapib beyond that seen with placebo. Through 76 weeks, no changes were noted in blood pressure or electrolyte or aldosterone levels with anacetrapib as compared with placebo. Prespecified adjudicated cardiovascular events occurred in 16 patients treated with anacetrapib (2.0%) and 21 patients receiving placebo (2.6%) (P=0.40). The prespecified Bayesian analysis indicated that this event distribution provided a predictive probability (confidence) of 94% that anacetrapib would not be associated with a 25% increase in cardiovascular events, as seen with torcetrapib.

Conclusions.—Treatment with anacetrapib had robust effects on LDL and HDL cholesterol, had an acceptable side-effect profile, and, within the limits of the power of this study, did not result in the adverse cardiovascular effects observed with torcetrapib. (Funded by Merck Research Laboratories; ClinicalTrials.gov number, NCT00685776.)

▶ Will the Details of the Determining the Efficacy and Tolerability of CETP Inhibition with Anacetrapib (DEFINE) trial be looked upon in the future as a defining moment in cardiology? We will all know in time, but for the present, this trial points us in the new clinical directions.

There is an abundant epidemiologic evidence to show that elevated low-density lipoprotein (LDL) cholesterol and reduced high-density lipoprotein (HDL) cholesterol levels are major risk factors for the development of cardiovascular disease. Despite the remarkable success of statins in reducing LDL cholesterol and cardiovascular events, in patients with and without coronary artery disease, it should be appreciated that a high residual risk of cardiovascular events persists even while on statins and particularly in the presence of other lipid abnormalities, that is, a low HDL cholesterol.[1]

One approach to raising HDL cholesterol is to inhibit the cholesteryl ester transfer protein (CETP), as this protein promotes the transfer of cholesteryl esters from HDL and other lipoprotein fractions. A previous trial with a CETP inhibitor or cetrapib was terminated because of an excess of deaths and cardiovascular events thought subsequently to be caused by drug-induced increases in aldosterone levels and blood pressure.[2] These adverse effects are thought, however, not to be related to CETP inhibition and as such are not necessarily shared by other members of the class of CETP inhibitors.

The DEFINE trial demonstrated quite emphatically a striking effect of anacetrapib on reducing LDL cholesterol and increasing HDL cholesterol (in patients already on statins) but without changes in blood pressure, aldosterone, or electrolyte levels.

This is a moderate sized safety study and demonstrates efficacy in regard to lipid levels, but this does not necessarily translate into a reduction in clinical events. A legitimate question is whether the HDL particles generated by inhibition of CETP are as protective functionally as naturally occurring HDL, which does appear to be atheroprotective. Preliminary in vitro studies in this respect are, however, encouraging.[3] It is interesting that in this study anacetrapib did not have any effect on C-reactive protein levels; what this means in terms of future clinical effectiveness is uncertain.

Whether elevating HDL cholesterol with CETP inhibitors would lead to a reduction in cardiovascular events awaits the results of large phase III studies. If these are positive, this will certainly usher in a new era in preventive cardiology, and it goes without saying that the results of these trials will be eagerly awaited.

B. J. Gersh, MB, ChB, DPhil, FRCP

References

1. LaRosa JC, Grundy SM, Waters DD, et al. Intensive lipid lowering with atorvastatin in patients with stable coronary disease. *N Engl J Med.* 2005;352:1425-1435.

2. Barter PJ, Caulfield M, Eriksson M, et al. Effects of torcetrapib in patients at high risk for coronary events. *N Engl J Med.* 2007;357:2109-2122.
3. Yvan-Charvet L, Kling J, Pagler T, et al. Cholesterol efflux potential and anti-inflammatory properties of high-density lipoprotein after treatment with niacin or anacetrapib. *Arterioscler Thromb Vasc Biol.* 2010;30:1430-1438.

Association of Marine Omega-3 Fatty Acid Levels With Telomeric Aging in Patients With Coronary Heart Disease

Farzaneh-Far R, Lin J, Epel ES, et al (San Francisco General Hosp, CA; Univ of California; et al)
JAMA 303:250-257, 2010

Context.—Increased dietary intake of marine omega-3 fatty acids is associated with prolonged survival in patients with coronary heart disease. However, the mechanisms underlying this protective effect are poorly understood.

Objective.—To investigate the association of omega-3 fatty acid blood levels with temporal changes in telomere length, an emerging marker of biological age.

Design, Setting, and Participants.—Prospective cohort study of 608 ambulatory outpatients in California with stable coronary artery disease recruited from the Heart and Soul Study between September 2000 and December 2002 and followed up to January 2009 (median, 6.0 years; range, 5.0-8.1 years).

Main Outcome Measures.—We measured leukocyte telomere length at baseline and again after 5 years of follow-up. Multivariable linear and logistic regression models were used to investigate the association of baseline levels of omega-3 fatty acids (docosahexaenoic acid [DHA] and eicosapentaenoic acid [EPA]) with subsequent change in telomere length.

Results.—Individuals in the lowest quartile of DHA + EPA experienced the fastest rate of telomere shortening (0.13 telomere-to-single-copy gene ratio [T/S] units over 5 years; 95% confidence interval [CI], 0.09-0.17), whereas those in the highest quartile experienced the slowest rate of telomere shortening (0.05 T/S units over 5 years; 95% CI, 0.02-0.08; $P < .001$ for linear trend across quartiles). Levels of DHA + EPA were associated with less telomere shortening before (unadjusted β coefficient $\times 10^{-3} = 0.06$; 95% CI, 0.02-0.10) and after (adjusted β coefficient $\times 10^{-3} = 0.05$; 95% CI, 0.01-0.08) sequential adjustment for established risk factors and potential confounders. Each 1-SD increase in DHA + EPA levels was associated with a 32% reduction in the odds of telomere shortening (adjusted odds ratio, 0.68; 95% CI, 0.47-0.98).

Conclusion.—Among this cohort of patients with coronary artery disease, there was an inverse relationship between baseline blood levels of marine omega-3 fatty acids and the rate of telomere shortening over 5 years.

▶ This is a fascinating study that attempts to link the benefits of omega-3 fatty acid levels with reduced aging of telomeres. A number of epidemiological studies and randomized trials have suggested that omega-3 fatty acids are associated with improved survival in patients with established cardiovascular disease.[1] These studies form the basis for the American Heart Association recommendations for the increased intake of oily fish and the use of omega-3 fatty acid supplements in the primary and secondary prevention of coronary heart disease.[2] The mechanisms underlying these apparently protective effects are, however, poorly understood and potentially include antiarrhythmic, anti-inflammatory, and antiplatelet effects among others.

Telomeres that form a protective cap at the ends of eukaryotic chromosomes may play a major role in cellular senescence or apoptosis. This has led to the concept that telomeric length is a novel marker of biological aging, and with respect to telomeric length, longer is better. Moreover, there is a strong association between reduced telomeric length and cardiovascular morbidity and mortality in some populations.[3]

In this prospective cohort study of 600 ambulatory patients with stable coronary artery disease in California, the authors correlated baseline levels of omega-3 fatty acids with leukocyte telomeric length at baseline and again after 5 years of follow-up. There was a strong inverse relationship suggesting that higher levels of omega-3 fatty acids were associated with reduced telomere shortening, which in a biological context is a favorable effect. Potential mechanisms are that the delayed telomere attrition is caused by a reduction in oxidative stress as reactive oxygen species significantly target telomeric DNA. Another possibility is that fish oils increase the activity of the enzyme telomerase, which may be beneficial in noncancerous lesions.

The findings in this study are purely observational and do not prove causality because it may well be that other favorable lifestyle behaviors are associated with a higher intake of omega-3 fatty acids, and no amount of statistical judgment can eliminate the potential bias. Nonetheless, the association is of great potential interest. It has been said that one is as old as the state of our arteries, but perhaps we need to add to this that we are as old as the length of our telomeres.

B. J. Gersh, MB, ChB, DPhil, FRCP

References

1. Lee JH, O'Keefe JH, Lavie CJ, Marchioli R, Harris WS. Omega-3 fatty acids for cardioprotection. *Mayo Clin Proc.* 2008;83:324-332.
2. Kris-Etherton PM, Harris WS, Appel LJ, American Heart Association Nutrition Committee. Fish consumption, fish oil, omega-3 fatty acids, and cardiovascular disease. *Circulation.* 2002;106:2747-2757.
3. Cawthon RM, Smith KR, O'Brien E, Sivatchenko A, Kerber RA. Association between telomere length in blood and mortality in people aged 60 years or older. *Lancet.* 2003;361:393-395.

Efficacy and safety of more intensive lowering of LDL cholesterol: a meta-analysis of data from 170 000 participants in 26 randomised trials

Cholesterol Treatment Trialists' (CTT) Collaboration (Clinical Trial Service Unit and Epidemiological Studies Unit (CTSU), Oxford, UK)
Lancet 376:1670-1681, 2010

Background.—Lowering of LDL cholesterol with standard statin regimens reduces the risk of occlusive vascular events in a wide range of individuals. We aimed to assess the safety and efficacy of more intensive lowering of LDL cholesterol with statin therapy.

Methods.—We undertook meta-analyses of individual participant data from randomised trials involving at least 1000 participants and at least 2 years' treatment duration of more versus less intensive statin regimens (five trials; 39 612 individuals; median follow-up 5·1 years) and of statin versus control (21 trials; 129 526 individuals; median follow-up 4·8 years). For each type of trial, we calculated not only the average risk reduction, but also the average risk reduction per 1·0 mmol/L LDL cholesterol reduction at 1 year after randomisation.

Findings.—In the trials of more versus less intensive statin therapy, the weighted mean further reduction in LDL cholesterol at 1 year was 0·51 mmol/L. Compared with less intensive regimens, more intensive regimens produced a highly significant 15% (95% CI 11–18; p<0·0001) further reduction in major vascular events, consisting of separately significant reductions in coronary death or non-fatal myocardial infarction of 13% (95% CI 7–19; p<0·0001), in coronary revascularisation of 19% (95% CI 15–24; p<0·0001), and in ischaemic stroke of 16% (95% CI 5–26; p=0·005). Per 1·0 mmol/L reduction in LDL cholesterol, these further reductions in risk were similar to the proportional reductions in the trials of statin versus control. When both types of trial were combined, similar proportional reductions in major vascular events per 1·0 mmol/L LDL cholesterol reduction were found in all types of patient studied (rate ratio [RR] 0·78, 95% CI 0·76–0·80; p<0·0001), including those with LDL cholesterol lower than 2 mmol/L on the less intensive or control regimen. Across all 26 trials, all-cause mortality was reduced by 10% per 1·0 mmol/L LDL reduction (RR 0·90, 95% CI 0·87–0·93; p<0·0001), largely reflecting significant reductions in deaths due to coronary heart disease (RR 0·80, 99% CI 0·74–0·87; p<0·0001) and other cardiac causes (RR 0·89, 99% CI 0·81–0·98; p=0·002), with no significant effect on deaths due to stroke (RR 0·96, 95% CI 0·84–1·09; p=0·5) or other vascular causes (RR 0·98, 99% CI 0·81–1·18; p=0·8). No significant effects were observed on deaths due to cancer or other non-vascular causes (RR 0·97, 95% CI 0·92–1·03; p=0·3) or on cancer incidence (RR 1·00, 95% CI 0·96–1·04; p=0·9), even at low LDL cholesterol concentrations.

Interpretation.—Further reductions in LDL cholesterol safely produce definite further reductions in the incidence of heart attack, of revascularisation, and of ischaemic stroke, with each 1·0 mmol/L reduction reducing the annual rate of these major vascular events by just over a fifth. There was no evidence of any threshold within the cholesterol range studied, suggesting that reduction of LDL cholesterol by 2–3 mmol/L would reduce risk by about 40–50%.

▶ Statins have been in clinical use for almost 2 decades and their efficacy in reducing vascular events in addition to their safety is not in doubt. What this meta-analysis from the Cholesterol Treatment Trialists' Collaboration using individual patient rather than summary data tells us is that reducing low-density lipoprotein (LDL) cholesterol below current targets is beneficial. This adds to current knowledge by showing that we can indeed go lower and that patients who started out at a target level of 70 mg/dL had a further reduction in vascular events when going from 70 mg/dL to 50 mg/dL. What is important is the absolute and not the relative risk reductions, and we need to emphasize that the data really only apply to patients at a high risk of cardiovascular events. Nonetheless, in patients with low baseline LDL levels, statins may still be indicated, and this would depend in part on the presence of other markers of cardiovascular risk, at least when primary prevention is the goal. The argument for a statin, however, is much less persuasive for people at low cardiovascular risk, such as young people with no other cardiovascular risk factors.

Another study in the same issue of the journal suggested that 80 mg of simvastatin was associated with a much higher incidence of myopathy so that the more potent statins, such as atorvastatin or rosuvastatin, may be a better approach because they have better safety profiles and greater efficacy.[1]

It is encouraging that the increase in hemorrhagic stroke was small and far outweighed by the reduction in ischemic stroke. An accompanying editorial, however, makes the point that perhaps we cannot extrapolate these data to other populations that have much higher rates of hemorrhagic stroke, such as patients from Japan and China.[2] In a 10-year population-based observational study from Japan, a low LDL cholesterol level was also an independent predictor of hemorrhagic stroke.[3]

In summary, at the population level, statins are underused, so an urgent priority is to identify those people who will benefit most from statin therapy and to lower their LDL cholesterol aggressively with higher doses and more potent statins, if necessary.

B. J. Gersh, MB, ChB, DPhil, FRCP

References

1. Study of the Effectiveness of Additional Reductions in Cholesterol and Homocysteine (SEARCH) Collaborative Group. Intensive lowering of LDL cholesterol with 80-mg versus 20-mg simvastatin daily in 12,064 survivors of myocardial infarction: a double-blind randomized trial. *Lancet.* 2010;376:1658-1669.
2. Cheung BNY, Lamb KSL. Is intensive LDL-cholesterol lowering beneficial and safe? *Lancet.* 2010;376:1622-1624.
3. Kumana CR, Cheung BM, Leuder IJ. Gauging the impact of statins using number needed to treat. *JAMA.* 1999;282:1899-1901.

Prospective Study of Obstructive Sleep Apnea and Incident Coronary Heart Disease and Heart Failure: The Sleep Heart Health Study
Gottlieb DJ, Yenokyan G, Newman AB, et al (VA Boston Healthcare System, MA; Johns Hopkins Univ, Baltimore, MD; Univ of Pittsburgh, PA; et al)
Circulation 122:352-360, 2010

Background.—Clinic-based observational studies in men have reported that obstructive sleep apnea is associated with an increased incidence of coronary heart disease. The objective of this study was to assess the relation of obstructive sleep apnea to incident coronary heart disease and heart failure in a general community sample of adult men and women.

Methods and Results.—A total of 1927 men and 2495 women ≥40 years of age and free of coronary heart disease and heart failure at the time of baseline polysomnography were followed up for a median of 8.7 years in this prospective longitudinal epidemiological study. After adjustment for multiple risk factors, obstructive sleep apnea was a significant predictor of incident coronary heart disease (myocardial infarction, revascularization procedure, or coronary heart disease death) only in men ≤70 years of age (adjusted hazard ratio 1.10 [95% confidence interval 1.00 to 1.21] per 10-unit increase in apnea-hypopnea index [AHI]) but not in older men or in women of any age. Among men 40 to 70 years old, those with AHI ≥30 were 68% more likely to develop coronary heart disease than those with AHI <5. Obstructive sleep apnea predicted incident heart failure in men but not in women (adjusted hazard ratio 1.13 [95% confidence interval 1.02 to 1.26] per 10-unit increase in AHI). Men with AHI ≥30 were 58% more likely to develop heart failure than those with AHI <5.

Conclusions.—Obstructive sleep apnea is associated with an increased risk of incident heart failure in community-dwelling middle-aged and older men; its association with incident coronary heart disease in this sample is equivocal.

▶ Sleep-disordered breathing is a major problem in the United States and presumably in other countries. It is estimated that approximately 40 million Americans have sleep disorders of whom approximately 25 million or more have sleep apnea (60%-80% of whom have not been diagnosed). The prevalence of sleep apnea as defined by an Apnea/Hypopnea Index of 5% or greater is estimated to be 9% in women and 24% in men.[1] The impact on mortality is unknown, but morbidity, including accidents, is considerable, as is the cost to society.

There are multiple pathophysiological interactions with sleep apnea that have potentially deleterious cardiovascular consequences. These have been the subject of several comprehensive reviews and include the direct contributions associated with apnea and arousal and their effect on intermediary mechanisms as well as the presence of comorbidities.[2] This makes it very difficult to tease out the effects of sleep apnea on cardiovascular morbidity and mortality as opposed to the impact of comorbid conditions. Moreover, clinical trials in symptomatic patients will be extremely difficult to perform given that we do have an effective form of therapy in continuous positive airway pressure.

The Wisconsin Sleep Heart Study has been an extremely valuable resource in the area of sleep-related research because it is a large prospective community study of patients aged 40 years or older followed for a median of 8.7 years. All patients were free of overt coronary heart disease and heart failure at the time of entry polysomnography. This analysis demonstrates a strong correlation with incident congestive heart failure after adjustment for traditional risk factors, but the association with incident coronary heart disease is equivocal. Other studies, however, do demonstrate a strong association between obstructive sleep apnea and cardiovascular conditions, such as atrial fibrillation and a temporal relationship to the timing of myocardial infarction and sudden cardiac death.[3]

Irrespective of whether cause or consequence has been unequivocally established, sleep apnea is not good for you. It should be diagnosed and treated, and elimination of the other underlying risk factors, that is, obesity, is a logical target.

B. J. Gersh, MB, ChB, DPhil, FRCP

References

1. Young T, Palta M, Dempsey J, Skatrud J, Weber S, Badr S. The occurrence of sleep-disordered breathing among middle-aged adults. *N Engl J Med.* 1993;328: 1230-1235.
2. Shamsuzzaman AS, Gersh BJ, Somers VK. Obstructive sleep apnea: implications for cardiac and vascular disease. *JAMA.* 2003;290:1906-1914.
3. Gami AS, Howard DE, Olson EJ, Somers VK. Day-night pattern of sudden death in obstructive sleep apnea. *N Engl J Med.* 2005;352:1206-1214.

Trends in Incidence, Severity, and Outcome of Hospitalized Myocardial Infarction
Roger VL, Weston SA, Gerber Y, et al (Mayo Clinic, Rochester, MN; et al)
Circulation 121:863-869, 2010

Background.—In 2000, the definition of myocardial infarction (MI) changed to rely on troponin rather than creatine kinase (CK) and its MB fraction (CK-MB). The implications of this change on trends in MI incidence and outcome are not defined.

Methods and Results.—This was a community study of 2816 patients hospitalized with incident MI from 1987 to 2006 in Olmsted County, Minnesota, with prospective measurements of troponin and CK-MB from August 2000 forward. Outcomes were MI incidence, severity, and survival. After troponin was introduced, 278 (25%) of 1127 incident MIs met only troponin-based criteria. When cases meeting only troponin criteria were included, incidence did not change between 1987 and 2006. When restricted to cases defined by CK/CK-MB, the incidence of MI declined by 20%. The incidence of non–ST-segment elevation MI increased markedly by relying on troponin, whereas that of ST-segment elevation MI declined regardless of troponin. The age- and sex-adjusted hazard ratio of death within 30 days for an infarction occurring in 2006 (compared with 1987) was 0.44 (95% confidence interval, 0.30 to 0.64). Among 30-day survivors, survival did not improve, but causes of death shifted from cardiovascular to noncardiovascular (P=0.001). Trends in long-term survival among 30-day survivors were similar regardless of troponin.

Conclusions.—Over the last 2 decades, a substantial change in the epidemiology of MI occurred that was only partially mediated by the introduction of troponin. Non—ST-segment elevation MIs now constitute the majority of MIs. Although the 30-day case fatality improved markedly, long-term survival did not change, and the cause of death shifted from cardiovascular to noncardiovascular.

▶ A problem in evaluating temporal trends in the incidence and prognosis of myocardial infarction (MI) is that the definition of MI is evolving. The adoption of the more sensitive troponins in the revised definition of MI in 2000 raised the possibility that this would lead to the increase in the incidence of MI and a lower mortality because of the inclusion of patients with smaller infarcts.[1] A previous study from Olmsted County demonstrated a large increase in the number of infarctions related to the identification of cases by troponin-based criteria,[2] but this article adds to the literature by analyzing trends over time in both incidence and severity. The ability to look at patients included on the basis of the troponins and on traditional creatine kinase (CK) and its MB fraction (CK-MB) measurements allows for a comparison of like versus like.

The results of this study are encouraging in that the incidence of MI (based upon CK-MB criteria) has declined substantially (20%), although if one includes patients with smaller infarcts based upon troponins, the MI incidence has remained the same. A striking reduction in the incidence of ST-segment elevation MI is noted, as is the case in the much developed world in contrast to countries like India in which ST-segment elevation MI dominates.[3] There has also been a marked decline in 30-day mortality between 1987 and 2000, but late survival has not changed much because of a shift from cardiovascular disease to noncardiovascular deaths, which is perhaps not surprising in a much older population. Nonetheless, the reduction in 30-day mortality is encouraging and suggests that there could be an improvement in long-term survival in those patients with MI unaccompanied by other comorbidities.

Explanations for the decline in the severity of MI over time are speculative, but the increasing use of aspirin and beta blockers may play a role, in addition to the aging of the population, because older patients have a higher incidence of multivessel disease with collaterals and non-ST-segment elevation acute coronary syndromes . Another potential factor might be the increasing population of patients who have undergone coronary revascularization, and this perhaps predisposes to smaller infarcts at a later time. A limitation of this study is that patients with silent MIs who may comprise a third of all infarcts were not captured nor were sudden cardiac deaths. Nonetheless, a previous study from the same group has shown that there has been a decline in sudden cardiac death comparable with the decline of infarctions meeting CK-MB criteria, so the lack of sudden cardiac death capture would not affect the validity of the results in this study.[4]

B. J. Gersh, MB, ChB, DPhil, FRCP

References

1. Alpert JS, Thygesen K, Antman E, Bassand JP. Myocardial infarction redefined—a consensus document of The Joint European Society of Cardiology/American College of Cardiology Committee for the redefinition of myocardial infarction. *J Am Coll Cardiol.* 2000;36:959-969.
2. Roger VL, Killian JM, Weston SA, et al. Redefinition of myocardial infarction: prospective evaluation in the community. *Circulation.* 2006;114:790-797.
3. Xavier D, Bais P, Devereaux PJ, et al. Treatment and outcomes of acute coronary syndromes in India (CREATE): a prospective analysis of registry data. *Lancet.* 2008;371:1435-1442.
4. Goraya TY, Jacobsen SJ, Kottke TE, Frye RL, Weston SA, Roger VL. Coronary heart disease death and sudden cardiac death: a 20-year population-based study. *Am J Epidemiol.* 2003;157:763-770.

HDL cholesterol and residual risk of first cardiovascular events after treatment with potent statin therapy: an analysis from the JUPITER trial

Ridker PM, for the JUPITER Trial Study Group (Harvard Med School, Boston, MA; et al)
Lancet 376:333-339, 2010

Background.—HDL-cholesterol concentrations are inversely associated with occurrence of cardiovascular events. We addressed, using the JUPITER trial cohort, whether this association remains when LDL-cholesterol concentrations are reduced to the very low ranges with high-dose statin treatment.

Methods.—Participants in the randomised placebo-controlled JUPITER trial were adults without diabetes or previous cardiovascular disease, and had baseline concentrations of LDL cholesterol of less than $3·37$ mmol/L and high-sensitivity C-reactive protein of 2 mg/L or more. Participants were randomly allocated by a computer-generated sequence to receive rosuvastatin 20 mg per day or placebo, with participants and adjudicators masked to treatment assignment. In the present analysis, we divided the participants into quartiles of HDL-cholesterol or apolipoprotein A1 and sought evidence of association between these quartiles and the JUPITER primary endpoint of first non-fatal myocardial infarction or stroke, hospitalisation for unstable angina, arterial revascularisation, or cardiovascular death. This trial is registered with ClinicalTrials.gov, number NCT00239681.

Findings.—For 17 802 patients in the JUPITER trial, rosuvastatin 20 mg per day reduced the incidence of the primary endpoint by 44% (p<0·0001). In 8901 (50%) patients given placebo (who had a median on-treatment LDL-cholesterol concentration of 2·80 mmol/L [IQR 2·43–3·24]), HDL-cholesterol concentrations were inversely related to vascular risk both at baseline (top quartile *vs* bottom quartile hazard ratio [HR] 0·54, 95% CI

0·35—0·83, p=0·0039) and on-treatment (0·55, 0·35—0·87, p=0·0047). By contrast, among the 8900 (50%) patients given rosuvastatin 20 mg (who had a median on-treatment LDL-cholesterol concentration of 1·42 mmol/L [IQR 1·14—1·86]), no significant relationships were noted between quartiles of HDL-cholesterol concentration and vascular risk either at baseline (1·12, 0·62—2·03, p=0·82) or on-treatment (1·03, 0·57—1·87, p= 0·97). Our analyses for apolipoprotein A1 showed an equivalent strong relation to frequency of primary outcomes in the placebo group but little association in the rosuvastatin group.

Interpretation.—Although measurement of HDL-cholesterol concentration is useful as part of initial cardiovascular risk assessment, HDL-cholesterol concentrations are not predictive of residual vascular risk among patients treated with potent statin therapy who attain very low concentrations of LDL cholesterol.

▶ Previous randomized trials of statin therapy have consistently reported large reductions in myocardial infarction, stroke, and vascular death in regard to both primary and secondary prevention. Nonetheless, significant vascular risk persists, and a legitimate question is whether this is related to low high-density lipoprotein (HDL) levels, which in themselves are a well-established baseline risk factor.

This intriguing substudy from the Justification for the Use of Statins in Primary Prevention: An Intervention Trial Evaluating Rosuvastatin (JUPITER) trial would suggest that the predictive value of HDL cholesterol is lost in patients given rosuvastatin who attain very low levels of low-density lipoprotein (LDL) cholesterol (in the range of 55 mg/dL). In contrast, another study demonstrated that the predictive value of HDL cholesterol was preserved even with LDL-cholesterol levels of less than 70 mg/dL.[1] Similarly, in the Framingham Offspring Study, the lower the pretreatment cholesterol, the greater the effect of increasing HDL cholesterol.[2] Moreover, in another study, HDL cholesterol remained a predictor of 1-year risk even when the LDL cholesterol was in the range of 62 mg/dL.[3]

An accompanying editorial speculates on why HDL-cholesterol concentrations did not predict cardiovascular risk in patients with low cardiovascular risk to begin with and who were then treated to very low concentrations of LDL cholesterol.[4] They do raise the question whether at very low LDL-cholesterol concentrations, other lipid measures, such as the apolipoprotein B to A1 ratio, would be of more benefit.

We also need to remember that this study does not mean that increasing HDL cholesterol levels in patients with low LDL levels will not be beneficial. This will require specifically designed randomized controlled trials. It should also be emphasized that the JUPITER trial was a trial of primary prevention in patients who did not have diabetes to begin with, and the study does not address the question of raising HDL cholesterol levels as part of a secondary prevention strategy. The findings should also not detract from the fact that raising HDL-cholesterol levels remains a major treatment strategy for the reduction of cardiovascular risks for most patients with elevated LDL-cholesterol concentrations, among whom many will not reach the concentrations obtained in this study. This remains a very interesting area, particularly given the ongoing development of HDL-elevating drugs that have the potential, but as yet unproven, to revolutionize the management of cardiovascular disease.[5]

B. J. Gersh, MB, ChB, DPhil, FRCP

References

1. Barter P, Gotto AM, LaRosa JC, et al. HDL cholesterol, very low levels of LDL cholesterol, and cardiovascular events. *N Engl J Med.* 2007;357:1301-1310.
2. Grover SA, Kaouache M, Joseph L, Barter P, Davignon J. Evaluating the incremental benefits of raising high-density lipoprotein cholesterol levels during lipid therapy after adjustment for the reductions in other blood lipid levels. *Arch Intern Med.* 2009;169:1775-1780.
3. deGoma EM, Leeper NJ, Heidenreich PA. Clinical significance of high-density lipoprotein cholesterol in patients with low low-density lipoprotein cholesterol. *J Am Coll Cardiol.* 2008;51:49-55.
4. Hausenloy DJ, Opie L, Yellon DM. Disassociating HDL cholesterol from cardiovascular risk. *Lancet.* 2010;376:305-306.
5. Natarajan P, Ray KK, Cannon CP. High-density lipoprotein in coronary heart disease: current and future therapies. *J Am Coll Cardiol.* 2010;55:1283-1299.

Relationship Between Cardiac Rehabilitation and Long-Term Risks of Death and Myocardial Infarction Among Elderly Medicare Beneficiaries

Hammill BG, Curtis LH, Schulman KA, et al (Duke Clinical Res Inst, Durham, NC)
Circulation 121:63-70, 2010

Background.—For patients with coronary heart disease, exercise-based cardiac rehabilitation improves survival rate and has beneficial effects on risk factors for coronary artery disease. The relationship between the number of sessions attended and long-term outcomes is unknown.

Methods and Results.—In a national 5% sample of Medicare beneficiaries, we identified 30 161 elderly patients who attended at least 1 cardiac rehabilitation session between January 1, 2000, and December 31, 2005. We used a Cox proportional hazards model to estimate the relationship between the number of sessions attended and death and myocardial infarction (MI) at 4 years. The cumulative number of sessions was a time-dependent covariate. After adjustment for demographic characteristics, comorbid conditions, and subsequent hospitalization, patients who attended 36 sessions had a 14% lower risk of death (hazard ratio [HR], 0.86; 95% confidence interval [CI], 0.77 to 0.97) and a 12% lower risk of MI (HR, 0.88; 95% CI, 0.83 to 0.93) than those who attended 24 sessions; a 22% lower risk of death (HR, 0.78; 95% CI, 0.71 to 0.87) and a 23% lower risk of MI (HR, 0.77; 95% CI, 0.69 to 0.87) than those who attended 12 sessions; and a 47% lower risk of death (HR, 0.53; 95% CI, 0.48 to 0.59) and a 31% lower risk of MI (HR, 0.69; 95% CI, 0.58 to 0.81) than those who attended 1 session.

Conclusions.—Among Medicare beneficiaries, a strong dose—response relationship existed between the number of cardiac rehabilitation sessions and long-term outcomes. Attending all 36 sessions reimbursed by Medicare was associated with lower risks of death and MI at 4 years compared with attending fewer sessions.

▶ It is well accepted that exercise-based cardiac rehabilitation has an important role to play in the management of patients with chronic stable angina, recent myocardial infarction, or prior bypass surgery among other conditions. Several trials and a meta-analysis have suggested that participation in a cardiac rehabilitation program improves survival and favorably modifies risk factors.[1] To what extent it is the exercise that is efficacious as opposed to the entire milieu of rehabilitation is uncertain, and there is also an obvious bias in favor of individuals who have both the time and the commitment to exercise and enter into a rehabilitation program.

One question addressed by this study is whether the optimal dose of cardiac rehabilitation and whether attending more cardiac rehabilitation sessions is better than attending fewer sessions and whether there is a specific threshold. This study on a national 5% sample of Medicare beneficiaries identified more than 30 000 elderly patients who had attended at least 1 cardiac rehabilitation session between 2000 and 2005. The qualifying indication for cardiac rehabilitation was coronary bypass surgery in the majority, recent myocardial infarction in 20.5%, stable angina in 14.9%, and unknown in 3.9%. Multivariant analysis using the number of sessions as a time-dependent covariant demonstrated that patients who attended all 36 sessions had a 14% lower incidence of death than those who attended 24 sessions, and there was also a lower risk of myocardial infarction. In summary, this study demonstrates at least on the surface a strong dose-response relationship and justifies the ongoing policy of Medicare reimbursement for cardiac rehabilitation.

An accompanying editorial appropriately emphasizes the potential for confounders in that sicker or severely disadvantaged patients were more likely to drop out of rehabilitation in addition to being at higher risk of events.[2] The conclusion is that the issue of causality remains uncertain and has not been proven by this study. This is certainly a subject for further investigation and perhaps a randomized trial. Nonetheless, for the present, cardiovascular rehabilitation should always be considered in the overall context of returning patients to a fully functional lifestyle, even though there is a need for more evidence-based medicine in this area.

B. J. Gersh, MB, ChB, DPhil, FRCP

References

1. Taylor RS, Brown A, Ebrahim S, et al. Exercise-based rehabilitation for patients with coronary heart disease: systematic review and meta-analysis of randomized controlled trials. *Am J Med.* 2004;116:682-692.
2. Weintraub WS. Do more cardiac rehabilitation visits reduce events compared with fewer visits? *Circulation.* 2010;121:8-9.

Statins and risk of incident diabetes: a collaborative meta-analysis of randomised statin trials

Sattar N, Preiss D, Murray HM, et al (Univ of Glasgow, UK; et al)
Lancet 375:735-742, 2010

Background.—Trials of statin therapy have had conflicting findings on the risk of development of diabetes mellitus in patients given statins. We aimed to establish by a meta-analysis of published and unpublished data whether any relation exists between statin use and development of diabetes.

Methods.—We searched Medline, Embase, and the Cochrane Central Register of Controlled Trials from 1994 to 2009, for randomised controlled endpoint trials of statins. We included only trials with more than 1000 patients, with identical follow-up in both groups and duration of more than 1 year. We excluded trials of patients with organ transplants or who needed haemodialysis. We used the I^2 statistic to measure heterogeneity between trials and calculated risk estimates for incident diabetes with random-effect meta-analysis.

Findings.—We identified 13 statin trials with 91 140 participants, of whom 4278 (2226 assigned statins and 2052 assigned control treatment) developed diabetes during a mean of 4 years. Statin therapy was associated with a 9% increased risk for incident diabetes (odds ratio [OR] 1·09; 95% CI 1·02—1·17), with little heterogeneity (I^2=11%) between trials. Meta-regression showed that risk of development of diabetes with statins was highest in trials with older participants, but neither baseline body-mass index nor change in LDL-cholesterol concentrations accounted for residual variation in risk. Treatment of 255 (95% CI 150—852) patients with statins for 4 years resulted in one extra case of diabetes.

Interpretation.—Statin therapy is associated with a slightly increased risk of development of diabetes, but the risk is low both in absolute terms and when compared with the reduction in coronary events. Clinical practice in patients with moderate or high cardiovascular risk or existing cardiovascular disease should not change (Fig 1).

▶ This meta-analysis is useful and timely given the findings of a recent randomized trial of rosuvastatin, which demonstrated an increased risk of developing diabetes.[1] This meta-analysis based on 13 large placebo-controlled trials involving 91 000 individuals demonstrated a 9% increase in risk (odds ratio 1.09 and 95% confidence interval is 1.02-1.17). This appears to be present mainly in older patients over the age of 60 years and is likely a class effect of all statins.

So statins join the list of other cardiovascular drugs associated with an increased risk of developing diabetes, including thiazide diuretics, β-blockers, and niacin. All drugs and interventions for that matter have side effects, and it is simply a question of striking a balance between risk and benefits.

In this respect an excellent accompanying editorial really places this issue in perspective.[2] The meta-analysis shows that for every 255 patients treated with

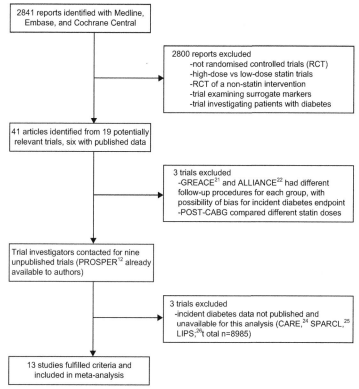

FIGURE 1.—Flow diagram of literature search to identify randomised placebo-controlled and standard care-controlled statin trials. (Reprinted from Sattar N, Preiss D, Murray HM, et al. Statins and risk of incident diabetes: a collaborative meta-analysis of randomised statin trials. *Lancet.* 2010;375:735-742, with permission from Elsevier.)

a statin for 4 years 1 additional patient would develop diabetes. In contrast the Cholesterol Treatment Trialist Collaboration estimated that over a 4-year period 5.4 deaths or myocardial infarctions would be avoided in addition to a similar number of strokes and coronary revascularization procedures .[3] Consequently, in the case of the statins, the benefits markedly outweigh the risks. Nonetheless, it is prudent to monitor patients and statins for the development of diabetes in addition to monitoring liver function and creatine kinase.

B. J. Gersh, MB, ChB, DPhil, FRCP

References

1. Ridker PM, Danielson E, Fonseca FA, et al. JUPITER Study Group. Rosuvastatin to prevent vascular events in men and women with elevated C-reactive protein. *N Engl J Med.* 2008;359:2195-2207.
2. Cannon CR. Balancing the benefits of statins versus a new risk-diabetes. *Lancet.* 2010;375:700-701.

3. Baigent C, Keech A, Kearney PM, et al. The Cholesterol Treatment Trialists' Collaborators. Efficacy and safety of cholesterol-lowering treatment: prospective meta-analysis of data from 90,056 participants in 14 randomized trials of statins. *Lancet.* 2005;366:1267-1278.

Projected Effect of Dietary Salt Reductions on Future Cardiovascular Disease

Bibbins-Domingo K, Chertow GM, Coxson PG, et al (Univ of California, San Francisco (UCSF); et al)
N Engl J Med 362:590-599, 2010

Background.—The U.S. diet is high in salt, with the majority coming from processed foods. Reducing dietary salt is a potentially important target for the improvement of public health.

Methods.—We used the Coronary Heart Disease (CHD) Policy Model to quantify the benefits of potentially achievable, population-wide reductions in dietary salt of up to 3 g per day (1200 mg of sodium per day). We estimated the rates and costs of cardiovascular disease in subgroups defined by age, sex, and race; compared the effects of salt reduction with those of other interventions intended to reduce the risk of cardiovascular disease; and determined the cost-effectiveness of salt reduction as compared with the treatment of hypertension with medications.

Results.—Reducing dietary salt by 3 g per day is projected to reduce the annual number of new cases of CHD by 60,000 to 120,000, stroke by 32,000 to 66,000, and myocardial infarction by 54,000 to 99,000 and to reduce the annual number of deaths from any cause by 44,000 to 92,000. All segments of the population would benefit, with blacks benefiting proportionately more, women benefiting particularly from stroke reduction, older adults from reductions in CHD events, and younger adults from lower mortality rates. The cardiovascular benefits of reduced salt intake are on par with the benefits of population-wide reductions in tobacco use, obesity, and cholesterol levels. A regulatory intervention designed to achieve a reduction in salt intake of 3 g per day would save 194,000 to 392,000 quality-adjusted life-years and $10 billion to $24 billion in health care costs annually. Such an intervention would be cost-saving even if only a modest reduction of 1 g per day were achieved gradually between 2010 and 2019 and would be more cost-effective than using medications to lower blood pressure in all persons with hypertension.

Conclusions.—Modest reductions in dietary salt could substantially reduce cardiovascular events and medical costs and should be a public health target.

▶ This complex study has huge potential ramifications for public health action by providing compelling evidence that reducing population-wide salt intake would markedly reduce the development of cardiovascular disease. The methodology is complicated and involves applying previously published data to a computer-simulation model. This model also involves a number of assumptions, namely that salt reduction lowers blood pressure and that this in turn reduces the incidence of stroke and cardiovascular disease. This is certainly a reasonable assumption, however, given much of the epidemiologic data and a few trials supporting this linkage.

The US diet is high in salt, and intake is much higher than the recommended target of 3.7 to 5.8 g of salt per day for individuals over the age of 40 years, those with hypertension, and in blacks.[1] The model suggests that a national effort to reduce salt intake by 3 g per day could translate into a massive impact upon the reduction of coronary heart disease, stroke, myocardial infarction, and all-cause mortality. These dramatic effects arising from an inexpensive intervention could be as beneficial as programs aimed at weight reduction, smoking cessation, and lipid lowering.

An accompanying editorial points out that even a reduction of 3 g per day would not achieve the desired targets for daily salt intake in many adults,[2] but the evidence to support a nationwide effort in the United States to reduce salt intake is nonetheless extremely strong. The same editorial, however, points out the magnitude of the problems involved in reducing salt intake. Given that the bulk of salt intake comes from processed foods, an individual approach would have relatively little impact. The level of salt in prepared and processed foods is excessively high, and this can only be changed by a national public health effort, which could be a relatively inexpensive but highly effective form of health care reform.

B. J. Gersh, MB, ChB, DPhil, FRCP

References

1. Centers for Disease Control and Prevention (CDC). Application of lower sodium intake recommendations to adults—United States, 1999–2006. *MMWR Morb Mortal Wkly Rep.* 2009;58:281-283.
2. Appel LJ, Anderson CAM. Compelling evidence for public health action to reduce salt intake. *N Engl J Med.* 2010;362:650-652.

43 Hypertension

Effect of self-measurement of blood pressure on adherence to treatment in patients with mild-to-moderate hypertension
van Onzenoort HAW, Verberk WJ, Kroon AA, et al (Univ Med Ctr St Radboud, Nijmegen, The Netherlands; Microlife Corporation, Taipei, Taiwan; Maastricht Univ, The Netherlands; et al)
J Hypertens 28:622-627, 2010

Background.—Poor adherence to treatment is one of the major problems in the treatment of hypertension. Self blood pressure measurement may help patients to improve their adherence to treatment.

Method.—In this prospective, randomized, controlled study coordinated by a university hospital, a total of 228 mild-to-moderate hypertensive patients were randomized to either a group that performed self-measurements at home in addition to office blood pressure measurements [the self-pressure group $(n = 114)$] or a group that only underwent office blood pressure measurement [the office pressure group $(n = 114)$]. Patients were followed for 1 year in which treatment was adjusted, if necessary, at each visit to the physician's office according to the achieved blood pressure. Adherence to treatment was assessed by means of medication event monitoring system TrackCaps.

Results.—Median adherence was slightly greater in patients from the self-pressure group than in those from the office pressure group (92.3 vs. 90.9%; $P = 0.043$). Although identical among both groups, in the week directly after each visit to the physician's office, adherence [71.4% (interquartile range $71-79\%$)] was significantly lower ($P<0.001$) than that at the last 7 days prior to each visit [100% (interquartile range $90-100\%$)]. On the remaining days between the visits, patients from the self-pressure group displayed a modestly better adherence than patients from the office pressure group (97.6 vs. 97.0%; $P = 0.024$).

Conclusion.—Although self-blood pressure measurement as an adjunct to office blood pressure measurement led to somewhat better adherence to treatment in this study, the difference was only small and not clinically significant. The time relative to a visit to the doctor seems to be a more important predictor of adherence.

▶ This article, derived from the randomized trial Home versus Office Measurements: Reduction of Unnecessary Treatment Study,[1] contradicts the conventional wisdom (now going back 35 years)[2] that self- (or home) monitoring of blood pressure is associated with better adherence to medication and thereafter to better blood pressure control.[3-5] The authors have a great deal of experience with the electronic medication monitoring system used in this study as the gold standard, and there is little reason to suspect that it didn't work as it usually does. A more likely explanation of why the extra home monitoring group did not have better adherence than the standard office blood pressure measurement group is that both groups were very well motivated to take their pills, being in a clinical trial that involved informed consent and a pill counter that tracked their adherence. This is most easily seen in the mean levels of adherence: 92.3% versus 90.9%, which is much higher than rates seen in routine clinical practice.

These authors have also redescribed in this article what is often called the toothbrush effect: adherence improves for the week or so prior to an office visit, as compared with the week afterward.[6] Dentists were among the first to show that the frequency of toothbrushing increases in the week or so prior to a dental appointment and that phenomenon has previously been seen in adherence with antihypertensive pills, especially when the electronic pill-cap monitoring system was used.

There are many reasons to recommend that many patients obtain home blood pressure readings, regardless of the conclusions of this work. The challenge for the health care system is how to have these readings interpreted and feedback given by the health care provider and paid for in the current reimbursement schemes.[7]

W. J. Elliott, MD, PhD

References

1. Verberk WJ, Kroon AA, Lenders JW, et al. for the Home Versus Office Measurement, Reduction of Unnecessary Treatment Study Investigators. Self-measurement of blood pressure at home reduces the need for antihypertensive drugs: a randomized, controlled trial. *Hypertension.* 2007;50:1019-1025.
2. Carnahan JE, Nugent CA. The effects of self-monitoring by patients on the control of hypertension. *Am J Med Sci.* 1975;269:69-73.
3. Vrijens B, Goetghebeur E. Comparing compliance patterns between randomized treatments. *Control Clin Trials.* 1997;18:187-203.
4. Márquez-Contreras E, Martell-Claros N, Gil-Guillén V, et al. Efficacy of a home blood pressure monitoring programme on therapeutic compliance in hypertension: The EAPACUM-HTA study. *J Hypertens.* 2006;24:169-175.
5. Ashida T, Sugiyama T, Okuno S, Ebihara A, Fujii J. Relationship between home blood pressure measurement and medication compliance and name recognition of antihypertensive drugs. *Hypertens Res.* 2000;23:21-24.
6. Waeber B, Burnier M, Brunner HR. How to improve adherence with prescribed treatment in hypertensive patients? *J Cardiovasc Pharmacol.* 2000;35:S23-S26.
7. Pickering TG, Miller NH, Ogedegbe G, Krakoff LR, Artinian NT, Goff D. Call to action on use and reimbursement for home blood pressure monitoring: executive summary: a joint scientific statement from the American Heart Association, American Society Of Hypertension, and Preventive Cardiovascular Nurses Association. *Hypertension.* 2008;52:1-9.

Prognostic significance of visit-to-visit variability, maximum systolic blood pressure, and episodic hypertension

Rothwell PM, Howard SC, Dolan E, et al (John Radcliffe Hosp, Headington, Oxford, UK; Connolly Hosp, Dublin, Ireland; et al)
Lancet 375:895-905, 2010

Background.—The mechanisms by which hypertension causes vascular events are unclear. Guidelines for diagnosis and treatment focus only on underlying mean blood pressure. We aimed to reliably establish the prognostic significance of visit-to-visit variability in blood pressure, maximum blood pressure reached, untreated episodic hypertension, and residual variability in treated patients.

Methods.—We determined the risk of stroke in relation to visit-to-visit variability in blood pressure (expressed as standard deviation [SD] and parameters independent of mean blood pressure) and maximum blood pressure in patients with previous transient ischaemic attack (TIA; UK-TIA trial and three validation cohorts) and in patients with treated hypertension (Anglo-Scandinavian Cardiac Outcomes Trial Blood Pressure Lowering Arm [ASCOT-BPLA]). In ASCOT-BPLA, 24-h ambulatory blood-pressure monitoring (ABPM) was also studied.

Findings.—In each TIA cohort, visit-to-visit variability in systolic blood pressure (SBP) was a strong predictor of subsequent stroke (eg, top-decile hazard ratio [HR] for SD SBP over seven visits in UK-TIA trial: $6\cdot22$, 95% CI $4\cdot16-9\cdot29$, p<$0\cdot0001$), independent of mean SBP, but dependent on precision of measurement (top-decile HR over ten visits: $12\cdot08$, $7\cdot40-19\cdot72$, p<$0\cdot0001$). Maximum SBP reached was also a strong predictor of stroke (HR for top-decile over seven visits: $15\cdot01$, $6\cdot56-34\cdot38$, p<$0\cdot0001$, after adjustment for mean SBP). In ASCOT-BPLA, residual visit-to-visit variability in SBP on treatment was also a strong predictor of stroke and coronary events (eg, top-decile HR for stroke: $3\cdot25$, $2\cdot32-4\cdot54$, p<$0\cdot0001$), independent of mean SBP in clinic or on ABPM. Variability on ABPM was a weaker predictor, but all measures of variability were most predictive in younger patients and at lower (<median) values of mean SBP in every cohort.

Interpretation.—Visit-to-visit variability in SBP and maximum SBP are strong predictors of stroke, independent of mean SBP. Increased residual variability in SBP in patients with treated hypertension is associated with a high risk of vascular events.

▶ This report, published in the same issue with 2 others[1,2] (an essentially unprecedented feat), with an accompanying editorial,[3] and simultaneously with another study on a similar topic in *Lancet Neurology*[4] (with its own editorial[5]) probably is the most important scientific contribution to hypertension in 2010, if not many years or even the new millennium. It should force us to rethink the usual blood pressure paradigm, which traditionally placed emphasis on the average level of blood pressure over a defined time period.

The use of sophisticated statistical analyses and the plethora of graphs from such analyses have probably deterred many from giving this article the study it deserves. Most practicing clinicians are aware of the greater risk of a high degree of within-individual variability in heart rate (eg, sick sinus syndrome) or plasma glucose levels (hypoglycemic coma vs hyperosmolar coma), but a similar degree of variability in blood pressure has not previously been cause for much concern. Professor Rothwell is trying to change that.

The efforts of the investigative team in this article are remarkable. They gathered patient-specific blood pressure from every visit and outcomes data from 5 clinical trials (data from the Anglo-Scandinavian Cardiac Outcomes Trial [ASCOT][5] included 1.12 million measurements), characterized their standard deviation and coefficient of variation (standard deviation/mean), and then, created a third statistical variable (variation independent of the mean, VID) related to the coefficient of variation, but dividing the standard deviation by the mean, raised to the x power, where x is derived from curve fitting of the standard deviation of systolic blood pressure (y-axis) versus mean systolic blood pressure (x-axis). This parameter has no significant correlation with mean blood pressure (as do both the standard deviation and the coefficient of variation). It turned out that all of these factors were more predictive of stroke than the mean level of blood pressure; the most predictive was visit-to-visit variability in blood pressure. They had consistent findings from each of the 4 trials that were used to develop the analytical techniques and discovered similar significant relationships in each randomized arm of the main ASCOT trial data.

They took their concept a giant step further by performing similar analyses on the 24-hour ambulatory blood pressure monitoring (ABPM) data from 1905 patients in ASCOT. Perhaps because of limited power (because of the smaller number of outcome events; the coefficients of variability were more precise because of the greater number of blood pressure measurements per session), the results were not quite as strong. However, the daytime coefficient of variation of systolic blood pressure on the ABPMs done during the 6th to 30th months of follow-up was still a significant predictor of cardiovascular events.

These results have important implications for clinical practice and future research. The first is that we need not "toss out the baby with the bathwater," and reject the importance of control of (mean) blood pressure. Recall that these analyses all adjust for mean blood pressure, so these are second-order effects, even if they account for a great deal of the residual variance of cardiovascular event prevention with drug therapy. The authors suggest that episodic hypertension is intrinsically risky and should not be an exclusion criterion for clinical trials. Similarly, stabilization of blood pressures may be a useful target for treatment and drug development. It is difficult to predict whether these concepts will be accepted by regulatory authorities, but the recent approval of single-pill combinations containing different agents with multiple dosing options is consistent with the authors' interpretations.[6]

W. J. Elliott, MD, PhD

References

1. Webb AJS, Fischer U, Mehta Z, Rothwell PM. Effects of antihypertensive-drug class on interindividual variation in blood pressure and risk of stroke: a systematic review and meta-analysis. *Lancet.* 2010;375:906-915.
2. Rothwell PM. Limitations of the usual blood-pressure hypothesis and importance of variability, instability, and episodic hypertension. *Lancet.* 2010;375:938-948.
3. Carlberg B, Lindholm LH. Stroke and blood-pressure variation: new permutations on an old theme. *Lancet.* 2010;375:867-869.
4. Rothwell PM, Howard SC, Dolan E, et al. Effects of beta blockers and calcium-channel blockers on within-individual variability in blood pressure and risk of stroke. *Lancet Neurol.* 2010;9:469-480.
5. Gorelick PB. Reducing blood pressure variability to prevent stroke? *Lancet Neurol.* 2010;9:448-449.
6. Donlan E, O'Brien E. Blood pressure variability: clarity for clinical practice. *Hypertension.* 2010;56:179-181.

Target Blood Pressure for Treatment of Isolated Systolic Hypertension in the Elderly: Valsartan in Elderly Isolated Systolic Hypertension Study

Ogihara T, for the Valsartan in Elderly Isolated Systolic Hypertension Study Group (Osaka Univ Graduate School of Medicine, Japan; et al)
Hypertension 56:196-202, 2010

In this prospective, randomized, open-label, blinded end point study, we aimed to establish whether strict blood pressure control (<140 mm Hg) is superior to moderate blood pressure control (≥140 mm Hg to <150 mm Hg) in reducing cardiovascular mortality and morbidity in elderly patients with isolated systolic hypertension. We divided 3260 patients aged 70 to 84 years with isolated systolic hypertension (sitting blood pressure 160 to 199 mm Hg) into 2 groups, according to strict or moderate blood pressure treatment. A composite of cardiovascular events was evaluated for ≥2 years. The strict control (1545 patients) and moderate control (1534 patients) groups were well matched (mean age: 76.1 years; mean blood pressure: 169.5/81.5 mm Hg). Median follow-up was 3.07 years. At 3 years, blood pressure reached 136.6/74.8 mm Hg and 142.0/76.5 mm Hg, respectively. The blood pressure difference between the 2 groups was 5.4/1.7 mm Hg. The overall rate of the primary composite end point was 10.6 per 1000 patient-years in the strict control group and 12.0 per 1000 patient-years in the moderate control group (hazard ratio: 0.89; [95% CI: 0.60 to 1.34]; $P=0.38$). In summary, blood pressure targets of <140 mm Hg are safely achievable in relatively healthy patients ≥70 years of age with isolated systolic hypertension, although our trial was underpowered to definitively determine whether strict control was superior to less stringent blood pressure targets.

▶ The optimal target blood pressure for older patients with isolated systolic hypertension is debatable. The landmark clinical trial, the Systolic Hypertension in the Elderly Program, found a highly significant benefit on stroke (and other cardiovascular end points, notably heart failure) with a chlorthalidone-based antihypertensive regimen, compared with placebo, but the target systolic blood pressure was < 160 mm Hg and/or a drop in systolic blood pressure by ≥20 mm Hg.[1] A post hoc analysis of the data showed significant benefits on stroke with achieved systolic blood pressures of < 160 mm Hg and < 150 mm Hg, but not < 140 mm Hg, presumably because so few patients achieved that level of systolic blood pressure with the antihypertensive drug regimens used in the late 1980s.[2] Similarly, the Systolic Hypertension in Europe and China trials showed significant prevention of stroke, but other end points were less impressive (perhaps again because the primary end point was so well prevented).[3,4] The most recent clinical trial, Hypertension in the Very Elderly Trial, had a target systolic blood pressure of < 150 mm Hg, but did not show a significant benefit on stroke, perhaps because the Data Safety and Monitoring Board recommended stopping the study early because of a significant mortality benefit of active treatment.[5] Disciples of evidence-based medicine thus assert that the clinical trial evidence favors a systolic blood pressure target of < 150 mm Hg, but not lower, in patients with isolated systolic hypertension. They discount the results of the Cardio-Sis trial because it included younger patients, without isolated systolic hypertension, and it was a secondary end point that showed a benefit of the lower target (< 130/80 mm Hg) on cardiovascular events.[6]

Unfortunately, the results of this Prospective, Randomized, Open-label Blinded Endpoints clinical trial failed to show a significant difference between blood pressure targets. One could argue that the trial itself was underpowered, should have used stroke as the primary end point (rather than a veritable hodge-podge of cardiovascular and renal events), might have done better with a diuretic as initial therapy,[1,5] or had many other potential criticisms. For reasons that are not clear, the trial's designers did not use the evidence-based target of < 150 mm Hg in their referent group, somewhat reminiscent of the Action to Control Cardiovascular Risk in Diabetes-Blood Pressure trial, which ignored the currently recommended target of < 130/80 mm Hg in patients with diabetes in favor of comparing the systolic targets of < 120 and < 140 mm Hg.[7]

These data add to the point of view espoused by recent Cochrane Collaboration meta-analysts, who claim that there are no good data to support any blood pressure targets < 140/90 mm Hg.[8] Whether guideline committees will agree with them remains to be seen.

W. J. Elliott, MD, PhD

References

1. Prevention of stroke by antihypertensive drug treatment in older persons with isolated systolic hypertension. Final results of the Systolic Hypertension in the Elderly Program (SHEP). SHEP Cooperative Study Group. *JAMA.* 1991;265:3255-3264.
2. Perry HM Jr, Davis BR, Price TR, et al. Effect of treating isolated systolic hypertension on the risk of developing various types and subtypes of stroke. the Systolic Hypertension in the Elderly Program (SHEP). *JAMA.* 2000;284:465-471.
3. Staessen JA, Fagard R, Thijs L, et al. for the Systolic Hypertension—Europe (Syst-EUR) Trial Investigators. Morbidity and mortality in the placebo-controlled European Trial on Isolated Systolic Hypertension in the Elderly. *Lancet.* 1997;350: 757-764.

4. Wang JG, Staessen JA, Gong L, Liu L. Chinese trial on isolated systolic hypertension in the elderly. Systolic Hypertension in China (Syst-China) Collaborative Group. *Arch Intern Med.* 2000;160:211-220.
5. Beckett NS, Peters R, Fletcher AE, et al. Treatment of hypertension in patients 80 years of age or older. *N Engl J Med.* 2008;358:1887-1898.
6. Verdecchia P, Staessen JA, Angeli F, et al. for the Cardio-Sis Investigators. Usual versus tight control of systolic blood pressure in non-diabetic patients with hypertension (Cardio-Sis): an open-label randomised trial. *Lancet.* 2009;374:525-533.
7. Cushman WC, Evans GW, Byington RP, et al. on behalf of The Action to Control Cardiovascular Risk in Diabetes (ACCORD) Study Group. Effects of intensive blood-pressure control in type 2 diabetes mellitus. *N Engl J Med.* 2010;362: 1575-1585.
8. Arguedas JA, Perez MI, Wright JM. Treatment blood pressure targets for hypertension. *Cochrane Database Syst Rev.* 2009;(4) 10.1002/14651858.CD004349.pub2, mrw. interscience.wiley.com/cochrane/clsysrev/articles/CD004349/frame.htm. Accessed October 10, 2010.

Continuous positive airway pressure treatment in sleep apnea patients with resistant hypertension: a randomized, controlled trial

Lozano L, Tovar JL, Sampol G, et al (Universitat Autònoma de Barcelona, Spain)
J Hypertens 28:2161-2168, 2010

Objectives.—This controlled trial assessed the effect of continuous positive airway pressure (CPAP) on blood pressure (BP) in patients with obstructive sleep apnea (OSA) and resistant hypertension (RH).

Methods.—We evaluated 96 patients with resistant hypertension, defined as clinic BP at least 140/90 mmHg despite treatment with at least three drugs at adequate doses, including a diuretic. Patients underwent a polysomnography and a 24-h ambulatory BP monitoring (ABPM). They were classified as consulting room or ABPM-confirmed resistant hypertension, according to 24-h BP lower or higher than 125/80 mmHg. Patients with an apnea-hypopnea index at least 15 events/h ($n = 75$) were randomized to receive either CPAP added to conventional treatment ($n = 38$) or conventional medical treatment alone ($n = 37$). ABPM was repeated at 3 months. The main outcome was the change in systolic and diastolic BP.

Results.—Sixty-four patients completed the follow-up. Patients with ABPM-confirmed resistant hypertension treated with CPAP ($n = 20$), unlike those treated with conventional treatment ($n = 21$), showed a decrease in 24-h diastolic BP (-4.9 ± 6.4 vs. 0.1 ± 7.3 mmHg, $P = 0.027$). Patients who used CPAP > 5.8 h showed a greater reduction in daytime diastolic BP $\{-6.12$ mmHg [confidence interval (CI) $-1.45; -10.82], P = 0.004\}$, 24-h diastolic BP ($-6.98$ mmHg [CI $-1.86; -12.1], P = 0.009$) and 24-h systolic BP (-9.71 mmHg [CI $-0.20; -19.22], P = 0.046$). The number of patients with a dipping pattern significantly increased in the CPAP group (51.7% vs. 24.1%, $P = 0.008$).

Conclusion.—In patients with resistant hypertension and OSA, CPAP treatment for 3 months achieves reductions in 24-h BP. This effect is seen in patients with ABPM-confirmed resistant hypertension who use CPAP more than 5.8 h.

▶ Most authorities agree that sleep apnea is an important cause of hypertension and appears to be even more common in patients with resistant hypertension.[1] Many previous observational studies have shown that patients with sleep apnea benefit from continuous positive airway pressure (CPAP), both in terms of blood pressure lowering[2] and in mortality,[3] but proper long-term randomized trials could typically not be done in this patient population because some would be randomized to not receive the standard-of-care therapy, CPAP.

These authors have now some short-term data from a randomized clinical trial (although only 64 of their 96 patients completed follow-up), showing a 3-month lowering in blood pressure (using the very sensitive technique of ambulatory blood pressure monitoring) as well as a restoration of the normal dipping pattern of blood pressure at night.

It now seems timely to organize the large clinical trial comparing CPAP and a selective aldosterone antagonist in a large number of hypertensive patients with obstructive sleep apnea, using both blood pressure and cardiovascular events as outcomes.[4,5] As both spironolactone and eplerenone are now generically available, such a study would likely require governmental funding and would require so many patients to be enrolled that its cost would likely be very high.

W. J. Elliott, MD, PhD

References

1. Calhoun DA, Jones D, Textor S, et al. Resistant hypertension: diagnosis, evaluation, and treatment. A scientific statement from the American Heart Association Professional Education Committee of the Council for High Blood Pressure Research. *Hypertension.* 2008;51:1403-1419.
2. Haentjens P, Van Meerhaeghe A, Moscariello A, et al. The impact of continuous positive airway pressure on blood pressure in patients with obstructive sleep apnea syndrome: evidence from a meta-analysis of placebo-controlled randomized trials. *Arch Intern Med.* 2007;167:757-764.
3. Marin JM, Carrizo SJ, Vicente E, Agusti AG. Long-term cardiovascular outcomes in men with obstructive sleep apnoea-hypopnoea with or without treatment with continuous positive airway pressure: an observational study. *Lancet.* 2005;365:1046-1053.
4. Nishizaka MK, Zaman MA, Calhoun DA. Efficacy of low-dose spironolactone in subjects with resistant hypertension. *Am J Hypertens.* 2003;16:925-930.
5. Ouzan J, Pérault C, Lincoff AM, Carré E, Mertes M. The role of spironolactone in the treatment of patients with refractory hypertension. *Am J Hypertens.* 2002;15:333-339.

Myocardial infarction and stroke associated with diuretic based two drug antihypertensive regimens: population based case-control study

Boger-Megiddo I, Heckbert SR, Weiss NS, et al (Univ of Washington, Seattle; et al)
BMJ 340:c103, 2010

Objective.—To examine the association of myocardial infarction and stroke incidence with several commonly used two drug antihypertensive treatment regimens.

Design.—Population based case-control study.

Setting.—Group Health Cooperative, Seattle, WA, USA.

Participants.—Cases (n=353) were aged 30-79 years, had pharmacologically treated hypertension, and were diagnosed with a first fatal or non-fatal myocardial infarction or stroke between 1989 and 2005. Controls (n=952) were a random sample of Group Health members who had pharmacologically treated hypertension. We excluded individuals with heart failure, evidence of coronary heart disease, diabetes, or chronic kidney disease.

Exposures.—One of three common two drug combinations: diuretics plus β blockers; diuretics plus calcium channel blockers; and diuretics plus angiotensin converting enzyme inhibitors or angiotensin receptor blockers.

Main Outcome Measures.—Myocardial infarction or stroke.

Results.—Compared with users of diuretics plus β blockers, users of diuretics plus calcium channel blockers had an increased risk of myocardial infarction (adjusted odds ratio (OR) 1.98, 95% confidence interval 1.37 to 2.87) but not of stroke (OR 1.02, 95% CI 0.63 to 1.64). The risks of myocardial infarction and stroke in users of diuretics plus angiotensin converting enzyme inhibitors or angiotensin receptor blockers were slightly but not significantly lower than in users of diuretics plus β blockers (myocardial infarction: OR 0.76, 95% CI 0.52 to 1.11; stroke: OR 0.71, 95% CI 0.46 to 1.10).

Conclusions.—In patients with hypertension, diuretics plus calcium channel blockers were associated with a higher risk of myocardial infarction than other common two drug treatment regimens. A large trial of second line antihypertensive treatments in patients already on low dose diuretics is required to provide a solid basis for treatment recommendations.

▶ This report is similar to 2 others: a prospective cohort study from the Women's Health Initiative (by many of the same authors)[1] and the infamous case-control study (by many of the same authors)[2] that launched the calcium channel blocker scare of 1995 and (many believe) may have been the impetus for National Institutes of Health to fund the Antihypertensive and Lipid-Lowering treatment to prevent Heart Attack Trial.[3] One of the major challenges to these case-control studies is the possibility of indication bias, which has been well described by one of this article's senior authors, who has suggested measures that make it less likely.[4] This type of bias is notoriously difficult to detect, either by the researchers or by readers of their reports.[5] Some have suggested that this was the major reason that these authors' 1995 study suggested a significant 60% increased risk of myocardial infarction with calcium antagonists (compared with a diuretic),[2] whereas the prospective, randomized, double-blinded, clinical trial showed a nonsignificant 2% reduction in said risk.[3] In the penultimate paragraph of the methods section, the authors discuss the steps they took to minimize indication bias in this report.

The authors interpret their findings of higher risk of diuretic + calcium antagonist to be consistent with the renin hypothesis[6] and the British National Institute for Health and Clinical Excellence guidelines.[7] In their discussion of trials of second-line antihypertensive therapy, they do not mention either the Study on Cognition and Prognosis in the Elderly (which added candesartan or other agents to hydrochlorothiazide 12.5 mg/d)[8] or the Felodipine Event Reduction trial, which showed significant benefit over placebo on stroke in Chinese patients whose blood pressures were not controlled with hydrochlorothiazide 12.5 mg/d.[9] They concluded by extolling the virtues of the recent National Institutes of Health (NIH) Consensus Conference,[10] which called for a large randomized trial of different second-line antihypertensive therapies and mentioned Systolic blood Pressure Intervention Trial (SPRINT) as a trial currently in planning that could address this important topic. An NIH meeting in 2007 concluded that the issue of the optimal second drug for hypertensive patients was not as important as determination of an optimal blood pressure target.[11] The current description of the SPRINT protocol on the ClinicalTrials.gov Web site makes no mention of a second randomization to different classes of antihypertensive agents but instead only to systolic blood pressure targets of <120 or <140 mm Hg.[12]

W. J. Elliott, MD, PhD

References

1. Wassertheil-Smoller S, Psaty BM, Greenland P, et al. Association between cardiovascular outcomes and antihypertensive drug treatment in older women. *JAMA*. 2004;292:2849-2859.
2. Psaty BM, Heckbert SR, Koepsell TD, et al. The risk of myocardial infarction associated with antihypertensive drug therapies. *JAMA*. 1995;274:620-625.
3. The ALLHAT Officers and Coordinators for the ALLHAT Collaborative Research Group. Major outcomes in high-risk hypertensive patients randomized to angiotensin-converting enzyme inhibitor or calcium channel blocker vs. diuretic: The Antihypertensive and Lipid-Lowering Treatment to Prevent Heart Attack Trial (ALLHAT). *JAMA*. 2002;288:2981-2997.
4. Psaty BM, Siscovick DS. Minimizing bias due to confounding by indication in comparative effectiveness research: the importance of restriction. *JAMA*. 2010; 304:897-898.
5. Joffe MM. Confounding by indication: the case of calcium channel blockers. *Pharmacoepidemiol Drug Saf*. 2000;9:37-41.
6. Laragh JH. Laragh's lessons in pathophysiology and clinical pearls for treating hypertension. Lesson XVI: how to choose the correct drug treatment for each hypertensive patient using a plasma renin-based method and the volume-vasoconstriction analysis. *Am J Hypertens*. 2001;14:491-503.
7. Littlejohns P, Ranson P, Sealey C, et al. for the National Collaborating Centre for Chronic Conditions. Hypertension: Management of hypertension in adults in primary care (partial update of NICE Clinical Guideline 18). National Institute

for Health and Clinical Excellence, http://www.nice.org.uk/page.aspx?o=278167. Accessed June 25, 2006.

8. Lithell H, Hansson L, Skoog I, et al. SCOPE Study Group. The Study on Cognition and Prognosis in the Elderly (SCOPE): principal results of a randomized double-blind intervention trial. *J Hypertens.* 2003;21:875-886.
9. Liu L, Zhang Y, Liu G, Li W, Zhang X, Zanchetti A, FEVER Study Group. The Felodipine Event Reduction (FEVER) study: a randomized long-term placebo-controlled trial in Chinese hypertensive patients. *J Hypertens.* 2005;23:2157-2172.
10. National Heart, Lung, and Blood Institute Working Group on Future Directions in Hypertension Treatment Trials. Major clinical trials of hypertension: what should be done next? *Hypertension.* 2005;46:1-6.
11. Working Group Report: Expert Panel on a Hypertension Treatment Trial Initiative Meeting Summary, http://www.nhlbi.nih.gov/meetings/workshops/hypertsnsion-full.pdf. Accessed November 01, 2010.
12. Systolic Blood Pressure Intervention Trial (SPRINT), http://www.clinicaltrials.gov/ct2/show/NCT01206062. Accessed November 01, 2010.

Angiotensin-Converting Enzyme Inhibitor Associated Cough: Deceptive Information from the *Physicians' Desk Reference*

Bangalore S, Kumar S, Messerli FH (Harvard Med School, Boston, MA; Columbia Univ College of Physicians & Surgeons, NY)
Am J Med 123:1016-1030, 2010

Background.—Dry cough is a common, annoying adverse effect of all angiotensin-converting enzyme (ACE) inhibitors. The present study was designed to compare the rate of coughs reported in the literature with reported rates in the *Physicians' Desk Reference (PDR)*/drug label.

Methods.—We searched MEDLINE/EMBASE/CENTRAL for articles published from 1990 to the present about randomized clinical trials (RCTs) of ACE inhibitors with a sample size of at least 100 patients in the ACE inhibitors arm with follow-up for at least 3 months and reporting the incidence or withdrawal rates due to cough. Baseline characteristics, cohort enrolled, metrics used to assess cough, incidence, and withdrawal rates due to cough were abstracted.

Results.—One hundred twenty-five studies that satisfied our inclusion criteria enrolled 198,130 patients. The pooled weighted incidence of cough for enalapril was 11.48% (95% confidence interval [CI], 9.54% to 13.41%), which was ninefold greater compared to the reported rate in the *PDR*/drug label (1.3%). The pooled weighted withdrawal rate due to cough for enalapril was 2.57% (95% CI, 2.40-2.74), which was 31-fold greater compared to the reported rate in the *PDR*/drug label (0.1%). The incidence of cough has increased progressively over the last 2 decades with accumulating data, but it has been reported consistently several-fold less in the *PDR* compared to the RCTs. The results were similar for most other ACE inhibitors.

Conclusion.—The incidence of ACE inhibitor-associated cough and the withdrawal rate (the more objective metric) due to cough is significantly greater in the literature than reported in the *PDR*/drug label and is likely to be even greater in the real world when compared with the data from

RCTs. There exists a gap between the data available from the literature and that which is presented to the consumers (prescribing physicians and patients).

▶ The authors' conclusion that the real incidence of cough associated with angiotensin-converting enzyme (ACE) inhibitor therapy is much higher than reported in the Food and Drug Administration (FDA)-approved package insert information is not a big surprise because the data that comprise the latter are typically drawn from the placebo-controlled randomized trials that supported the New Drug Application. In the case of the ACE inhibitors, it is not surprising that cough was not reported (either spontaneously or in response to the usual question, "Have you had any changes in your health status since your last visit?"), as there were no drugs that were recognized as causing cough at the time. Cough was first reported to be associated with ACE inhibitors in the English literature in 1985,[1] about 6 to 7 years after they were first given to hypertensive patients in clinical trials. It is a good reminder of the old saying, "You won't find a fever if you don't take a temperature."

The authors have compiled an impressive body of data from clinical trials in which cough was reported as a secondary (or lower) and/or safety end point and did not include some trials that compared an ACE inhibitor and an angiotensin receptor blocker for which cough was the prespecified primary end point.[2-9] They also excluded some studies that enrolled patients who had previously reported a cough with an ACE inhibitor, which is a very strong predictor of a second episode of coughing with another ACE inhibitor.[10]

The authors and editorialist[11] recommend that the FDA-approved prescription be updated periodically to reflect gathered information. The drug's registration trials would break new ground; however, updates would likely strain the already overburdened agency with contentious discussions with the drug's sponsors. These sponsors would wish to severely limit both the perception of hazards and the amount of printing required in order to disseminate the updated information.

W. J. Elliott, MD, PhD

References

1. Sesoko S, Kaneko Y. Cough associated with the use of captopril. *Arch Intern Med.* 1985;145:1524-1525.
2. Maillion JM, Goldberg AL. Global efficacy and tolerability of losartan, an angiotensin II subtype 1-receptor antagonist, in the treatment of hypertension. *Blood Press Suppl.* 1996;2:82-86.
3. Larochelle P, Flack JM, Marbury TC, Sareli P, Krieger EM, Reeves RA. Effects and tolerability of irbesartan versus enalapril in patients with severe hypertension. irbesartan Multicenter investigators. *Am J Cardiol.* 1997;80:1613-1615.
4. Malmqvist K, Kahan T, Dahl M. Angiotensin II type 1 (AT1) receptor blockade in hypertensive women: benefits of candesartan cilexetil versus enalapril or hydrochlorothiazide. *Am J Hypertens.* 2000;13:504-511.
5. McInnes GT, O'Kane KP, Istad H, Keinänen-Kiukaanniemi S, Van Mierlo HF. Comparison of the AT1-receptor blocker, candesartan cilexetil, and the ACE-inhibitor, lisinopril, in fixed combination with low dose hydrochlorothiazide in hypertensive patients. *J Hum Hypertens.* 2000;14:263-269.

6. Ogihara T, Arakawa K. Clinical efficacy and tolerability of candesartan cilexetil. Candesartan Study Groups in Japan. *J Hum Hypertens.* 1999;13:S27-S31.
7. Karlberg BE, Lins L-E, Hermansson K. Efficacy and safety of telmisartan, a selective AT1 receptor antagonist, compared with enalapril in elderly patients with primary hypertension. TEES Study Group. *J Hypertens.* 1999;17:293-302.
8. Lacourcière Y. A multicenter, randomized, double-blind study of the antihypertensive efficacy and tolerability of irbesartan in patients aged ≥ 65 years with mild-to-moderate hypertension. *Clin Ther.* 2000;22:1213-1224.
9. Ogihara T, Yoshinaga K. The clinical efficacy and tolerability of the angiotensin II-receptor antagonist losartan in Japanese patients with hypertension. *Blood Press Suppl.* 1996;2:78-81.
10. Elliott WJ. Cough with ACE-inhibitors or angiotensin II receptor blockers: Meta-analysis of randomized hypertension studies. *J Hypertens.* 2002;20:S161.
11. Serebruany VL. Realistic assessment of drug-induced adverse events: a double-edged sword. *Am J Med.* 2010;123:971.

Definition of ambulatory blood pressure targets for diagnosis and treatment of hypertension in relation to clinic blood pressure: prospective cohort study

Head GA, for the Ambulatory Blood Pressure Working Group of the High Blood Pressure Research Council of Australia (Baker IDI Heart and Diabetes Inst, Melbourne, Victoria, Australia; et al)
BMJ 340:c1104, 2010

Background.—Twenty-four hour ambulatory blood pressure thresholds have been defined for the diagnosis of mild hypertension but not for its treatment or for other blood pressure thresholds used in the diagnosis of moderate to severe hypertension. We aimed to derive age and sex related ambulatory blood pressure equivalents to clinic blood pressure thresholds for diagnosis and treatment of hypertension.

Methods.—We collated 24 hour ambulatory blood pressure data, recorded with validated devices, from 11 centres across six Australian states (n=8575). We used least product regression to assess the relation between these measurements and clinic blood pressure measured by trained staff and in a smaller cohort by doctors (n=1693).

Results.—Mean age of participants was 56 years (SD 15) with mean body mass index 28.9 (5.5) and mean clinic systolic/diastolic blood pressure 142/82 mm Hg (19/12); 4626 (54%) were women. Average clinic measurements by trained staff were 6/3 mm Hg higher than daytime ambulatory blood pressure and 10/5 mm Hg higher than 24 hour blood pressure, but 9/7 mm Hg lower than clinic values measured by doctors. Daytime ambulatory equivalents derived from trained staff clinic measurements were 4/3 mm Hg less than the 140/90 mm Hg clinic threshold (lower limit of grade 1 hypertension), 2/2 mm Hg less than the 130/80 mm Hg threshold (target upper limit for patients with associated conditions), and 1/1 mm Hg less than the 125/75 mm Hg threshold. Equivalents were 1/2 mm Hg lower for women and 3/1 mm Hg lower in older people compared with the combined group.

Conclusions.—Our study provides daytime ambulatory blood pressure thresholds that are slightly lower than equivalent clinic values. Clinic blood pressure measurements taken by doctors were considerably higher than those taken by trained staff and therefore gave inappropriate estimates of ambulatory thresholds. These results provide a framework for the diagnosis and management of hypertension using ambulatory blood pressure values.

▶ The results of this large Australian undertaking suggest 2 major conclusions. The first is that the daytime average of a 24-hour ambulatory blood pressure monitoring (ABPM) is lower than the corresponding office reading for important thresholds of blood pressure, with the difference mainly depending on the absolute level of blood pressure (eg, for clinic thresholds of 130/80 or 180/110 mm Hg, the corresponding daytime ABPM readings are 128/78 and 168/105 mm Hg, respectively). Second, like many other investigators, more than 25 years ago[1] and since,[2] they found that doctors' office blood pressures are higher than 24-hour ABPM daytime averages, whereas other trained health care providers' measurements are very similar to the ABPM daytime averages. The implication is that physicians ought not to be taking office readings to minimize the white-coat effect.

As might be expected, there was some inconsistency in the way the readings were obtained. Different ABPM machines were used at different sites, which probably is inconsequential. Doctors' readings were reported only for a small subset of the patients studied; those more than 2 weeks in time away from the ABPM session were excluded. The routine assignment of sleep and wake times for data analysis can be inaccurate for patients who do not work the usual 9AM to 5PM shift. The differences observed between genders are not well explained in the article but could result from differences in physical activity, which is known to influence daytime ABPM averages.

It is likely that these results are generalizable to non-Australian populations, as the overall averages for comparable situations are quite similar to those from other national and international databases.[3,4] Whether Australians have a larger white-coat effect than Americans is uncertain, but other studies have suggested that it is more common in Italians, Spaniards, and perhaps Mexicans. Because of the many problems inherent in office measurements of blood pressure, a prominent Canadian physician has recently recommended that automated sphygmomanometers can be used for all in-office readings, with the health care provider out of the examination room.[5]

W. J. Elliott, MD, PhD

References

1. Mancia G, Bertinieri G, Grassi G, et al. Effects of blood-pressure measurement by the doctor on patient's blood pressure and heart rate. *Lancet.* 1983;2:695-698.
2. Mancia G, Parati G, Pomidossi G, Grassi G, Casadei R, Zanchetti A. Alerting reaction and rise in blood pressure during measurement by physician and nurse. *Hypertension.* 1987;9:209-215.
3. Pickering TG, Hall JE, Appel LJ, et al. Recommendations for blood pressure measurement in humans and experimental animals: Part 1: blood pressure

measurement in humans: a statement for professionals from the Subcommittee of Professional and Public Education of the American Heart Association Council on High Blood Pressure Research. *Hypertension*. 2005;45:142-161.
4. Staessen JA, O'Brien ET, Atkins N, Amery AK. Short report: ambulatory blood pressure in normotensive compared with hypertensive subjects. The Ad-Hoc Working Group. *J Hypertension*. 1993;11:1289-1297.
5. Myers MG. A proposed algorithm for diagnosing hypertension using automated office blood pressure measurement. *J Hypertens*. 2010;28:703-708.

Screening renal artery angiography in hypertensive patients undergoing coronary angiography and 6-month follow-up after ad hoc percutaneous revascularization
Rimoldi SF, de Marchi SF, Windecker S, et al (Univ Hosp Bern, Switzerland)
J Hypertens 28:842-847, 2010

Objective.—To determine the prevalence and independent predictors of significant atherosclerotic renal artery stenosis (RAS) in unselected hypertensive patients undergoing coronary angiography and to assess the 6-month outcome of those patients with a significant RAS.

Methods.—One thousand, four hundred and three consecutive hypertensive patients undergoing drive-by renal arteriography were analyzed retrospectively. Univariate and multivariate logistic regression analyses were performed to identify independent predictors of RAS. In patients with significant RAS ($\geq 50\%$ luminal narrowing), 6-month follow-up was assessed and outcome was compared between patients with or without renal revascularization.

Results.—The prevalence of significant RAS was 8%. After multivariate analysis, coronary [odds ratio 5.3; 95% confidence interval (CI) 2.7—10.3; $P < 0.0001$], peripheral (odds ratio 3.3; 95% CI 2.0—5.5; $P < 0.0001$), and cerebral artery (odds ratio 2.8; 95% CI 1.5—5.3; $P = 0.001$) diseases, and impaired renal function (odds ratio 2.9; 95% CI 1.8—4.5; $P < 0.0001$) were found as independent predictors. At least one of these predictors was present in 96% of patients with RAS. In 74 patients (66%) with significant RAS, an ad hoc revascularization was performed. At follow-up, creatinine clearance was significantly higher in revascularized than in nonrevascularized patients (69.2 vs. 55.5 ml/min per 1.73 m, $P = 0.029$). By contrast, blood pressure was comparable between both groups, but nonrevascularized patients were taking significantly more antihypertensive drugs as compared with baseline (2.7 vs. 2.1, follow-up vs. baseline; $P = 0.0066$).

Conclusion.—The prevalence of atherosclerotic RAS in unselected hypertensive patients undergoing coronary angiography was low. Coronary, peripheral, and cerebral artery diseases, and impaired renal function were independent predictors of RAS. Ad hoc renal revascularization was associated with better renal function and fewer intake of antihypertensive drugs at follow-up.

▶ This article rather strongly contradicts much other information in the literature. Several series of American patients put the prevalence of significant renal artery stenosis at 11% to 39% among patients undergoing cardiac catheterization,[1] which would be a much larger clinical burden of disease than this group sees in Switzerland. The American Heart Association had to publish guidelines for appropriate investigation of renal artery stenosis during cardiac catheterization[2] because so many angiographers were performing drive-by renal angiograms. Because renal artery stenosis is more common in older patients, patients with obstructive atherosclerotic disease in other vascular beds, and patients with increasing degrees of renal impairment,[3] it would be interesting to know if the authors' cohort was much different than many American series with regard to these parameters; the descriptive data provided by the authors in Table 1 would suggest any such differences were minor.

The other area in which these authors' conclusions differ from those of other investigators is the improved outcomes in patients who received renal angioplasty. At least 3 large clinical trials have now shown no benefit of such therapy in intention-to-treat analyses, compared with maximal medical therapy alone.[4-6] One wonders about the possibility of indication bias that might account for the authors' observation that the patients they selected for angioplasty were different from those that they chose not to intervene. This may be another instance in which case series and cohort studies come to different conclusions than randomized clinical trials about the efficacy of a given therapy.

It is unlikely that angiographers in the United States will soon have a chance to repeat these findings because it took more than 3 years of work to accumulate 1043 subjects in Switzerland. Most health care financing authorities in the United States now routinely deny prior authorization requests for angiography and renal artery angioplasty, with or without stenting, unless very specific criteria are met and maximal medical therapy has been unsuccessful in lowering blood pressure over a defined (and relatively long) time period.

W. J. Elliott, MD, PhD

References

1. de Mast Q, Beutler JJ. The prevalence of atherosclerotic renal artery stenosis in risk groups: a systematic literature review. *J Hypertens.* 2009;27:1333-1340.
2. White CJ, Jaff MR, Haskal ZJ, et al. Indications for renal arteriography at the time of coronary arteriography: A science advisory from the American Heart Association Committee on Diagnostic and Interventional Cardiac Catheterization, Council on Clinical Cardiology, and the Councils on Cardiovascular Radiology and Intervention and on Kidney in Cardiovascular Disease. *Circulation.* 2006; 114:1892-1895.
3. Buller CE, Nogareda JG, Ramanathan K, et al. The profile of cardiac patients with renal artery stenosis. *J Am Coll Cardiol.* 2003;43:1606-1613.
4. van Jaarsveld BC, Krijnen P, Pieterman H, et al. The effect of balloon angioplasty on hypertension in atherosclerotic renal-artery stenosis. Dutch Renal Artery Stenosis Intervention Cooperative Study Group. *N Engl J Med.* 2000;342:1007-1014.
5. Bax L, Woittiez A-J, Kouwenberg HJ, et al. Stent placement in patients with atherosclerotic renal artery stenosis and impaired renal function: a randomized trial. *Ann Intern Med.* 2009;150:840-848.
6. Wheatley K, Ives N, Kalra PA, et al. on behalf of the Angioplasty and Stenting for Renal Artery Lesions (ASTRAL) Investigators. Revascularization versus medical therapy for renal-artery stenosis. *N Engl J Med.* 2009;361:1953-1962.

Tight Blood Pressure Control and Cardiovascular Outcomes Among Hypertensive Patients With Diabetes and Coronary Artery Disease
Cooper-DeHoff RM, Gong Y, Handberg EM, et al (Univ of Florida, Gainesville; et al)
JAMA 304:61-68, 2010

Context.—Hypertension guidelines advocate treating systolic blood pressure (BP) to less than 130 mm Hg for patients with diabetes mellitus; however, data are lacking for the growing population who also have coronary artery disease (CAD).

Objective.—To determine the association of systolic BP control achieved and adverse cardiovascular outcomes in a cohort of patients with diabetes and CAD.

Design, Setting, and Patients.—Observational subgroup analysis of 6400 of the 22 576 participants in the International Verapamil SR-Trandolapril Study (INVEST). For this analysis, participants were at least 50 years old and had diabetes and CAD. Participants were recruited between September 1997 and December 2000 from 862 sites in 14 countries and were followed up through March 2003 with an extended follow-up through August 2008 through the National Death Index for US participants.

Intervention.—Patients received first-line treatment of either a calcium antagonist or β-blocker followed by angiotensin-converting enzyme inhibitor, a diuretic, or both to achieve systolic BP of less than 130 and diastolic BP of less than 85 mm Hg. Patients were categorized as having tight control if they could maintain their systolic BP at less than 130 mm Hg; usual control if it ranged from 130 mm Hg to less than 140 mm Hg; and uncontrolled if it was 140 mm Hg or higher.

Main Outcome Measures.—Adverse cardiovascular outcomes, including the primary outcomes which was the first occurrence of all-cause death, nonfatal myocardial infarction, or nonfatal stroke.

Results.—During 16 893 patient-years of follow-up, 286 patients (12.7%) who maintained tight control, 249 (12.6%) who had usual control, and 431 (19.8%) who had uncontrolled systolic BP experienced a primary outcome event. Patients in the usual-control group had a cardiovascular event rate of 12.6% vs a 19.8% event rate for those in the uncontrolled group (adjusted hazard ratio [HR], 1.46; 95% confidence interval [CI], 1.25-1.71; $P<.001$). However, little difference existed between those with usual control and those with tight control. Their respective event rates were 12.6% vs 12.7% (adjusted HR, 1.11; 95% CI, 0.93-1.32; $P=.24$). The all-cause mortality rate was 11.0% in the tight-control group vs 10.2% in the usual-control group (adjusted HR, 1.20; 95% CI, 0.99-1.45; $P=.06$); however, when extended follow-up was included, risk of all-cause mortality was 22.8% in the tight control vs 21.8% in the usual control group (adjusted HR, 1.15; 95% CI, 1.01-1.32; $P=.04$).

Conclusion.—Tight control of systolic BP among patients with diabetes and CAD was not associated with improved cardiovascular outcomes compared with usual control.

Trial Registration.—clinicaltrials.gov Identifier: NCT00133692.

▶ Like a recent meta-analysis,[1] this report questions the long-held belief that patients with diabetes ought to have lower blood pressures than the nondiabetic hypertensive population. The authors point out that in previous clinical trials in hypertensive patients with diabetes, systolic blood pressure was seldom, if ever, reduced to < 130 mm Hg, as current guidelines recommend.[2,3] These data suggest that there is no benefit on cardiovascular end points associated with achieving systolic blood pressure < 130 mm Hg. The authors performed many sensitivity analyses to consider multiple variations on their data sets, including a 5-year extension of follow-up for mortality in patients enrolled at centers in the United States.

This report also addresses some of the controversy arising from the American Heart Association's Scientific Statement in 2007 that recommended a blood pressure target of < 130/80 mm Hg for hypertensive patients with established heart disease,[4] based primarily on a post hoc subgroup analysis of the intravascular ultrasound substudy of the Comparison of Amlodipine versus Enalapril to Limit Occurrences of Thrombosis trial,[5] and the general impression that high-risk patients should benefit from a lower blood pressure target.[2]

There are some challenges in accepting these conclusions as public health policy, however. These data are derived from a randomized clinical trial, but the analyses constituted a post hoc cohort study and performed many statistical adjustments for baseline variables, which may or may not lead to proper conclusions. For example, patients were trichotomized into those whose systolic blood pressures were, on average, < 130 mm Hg, between 130 and 139 mm Hg, or ≥140 mm Hg. This enriches the tight control group with those who were known to have an increased risk of myocardial infarction in the entire International Verapamil SR-Trandolapril Study data set.[6] Recent data have suggested that in addition to the average office blood pressure, its inter-visit variability may be an important determinant of cardiovascular outcomes.[7] There are also concerns about interpreting the results of this study too broadly, as it included subjects with both diabetes and coronary heart disease. Lastly, it may be dangerous to form policy based on potentially confounded observational studies; most would prefer clinical trials that randomized and successfully treated at-risk individuals to different blood pressure targets, as was recently done in the Avoiding Cardiovascular Complications in Diabetes trial.[8]

W. J. Elliott, MD, PhD

References

1. Arguedas JA, Perez MI, Wright JM. Treatment blood pressure targets for hypertension. *Cochrane Database Syst Rev.* 2009;(3):CD004349. 10.1002/14651858.CD004349. pub2, mrw.interscience.wiley.com/cochrane/clsysrev/articles/CD004349/frame.htm. Accessed July 10, 2009.
2. Chobanian AV, Bakris GL, Black HR, et al. National High Blood Pressure Education Program Coordinating Committee. Seventh report of the Joint National Committee on Prevention, Detection, Evaluation and Treatment of High Blood Pressure. *Hypertension.* 2003;42:1206-1252.
3. American Diabetes Association. Standards of medical care in diabetes—2010. *Diabetes Care.* 2010;33:S11-S61.

4. Rosendorff C, Black HR, Cannon CP, et al. Treatment of hypertension in the prevention and management of ischemic heart disease: a scientific statement from the American Heart Association Council for High Blood Pressure Research and the Councils on Clinical Cardiology and Epidemiology and Prevention. *Circulation.* 2007;115:2761-2788.
5. Sipahi I, Tuzcu EM, Schoenhagen P, et al. Effects of normal, pre-hypertensive, and hypertensive blood pressure levels on progression of coronary atherosclerosis. *J Am Coll Cardiol.* 2006;48:833-838.
6. Messerli FH, Mancia G, Conti CR, et al. for the International Verapamil-Trandolapril Study Investigators. Dogma disputed: can aggressively lowering blood pressure in hypertensive patients with coronary artery disease be dangerous? *Ann Intern Med.* 2006;144:884-893.
7. Rothwell PM. Limitations of the usual blood-pressure hypothesis and importance of variability, instability, and episodic hypertension. *Lancet.* 2010;375:938-948.
8. Cushman WC, Evans GW, Byington RP, et al. ACCORD Study Group. Effects of intensive blood-pressure control in type 2 diabetes mellitus. *N Engl J Med.* 2010; 362:1575-1585.

Coenzyme Q$_{10}$, Rosuvastatin, and Clinical Outcomes in Heart Failure: A Pre-Specified Substudy of CORONA (Controlled Rosuvastatin Multinational Study in Heart Failure)

McMurray JJV, on behalf of the CORONA Study Group (Univ of Glasgow, UK; et al)

J Am Coll Cardiol 56:1196-1204, 2010

Objectives.—The purpose of this study was to determine whether coenzyme Q$_{10}$ is an independent predictor of prognosis in heart failure.

Background.—Blood and tissue concentrations of the essential cofactor coenzyme Q$_{10}$ are decreased by statins, and this could be harmful in patients with heart failure.

Methods.—We measured serum coenzyme Q$_{10}$ in 1,191 patients with ischemic systolic heart failure enrolled in CORONA (Controlled Rosuvastatin Multinational Study in Heart Failure) and related this to clinical outcomes.

Results.—Patients with lower coenzyme Q$_{10}$ concentrations were older and had more advanced heart failure. Mortality was significantly higher among patients in the lowest compared to the highest coenzyme Q$_{10}$ tertile in a univariate analysis (hazard ratio: 1.50, 95% confidence interval: 1.04 to 2.6, p = 0.03) but not in a multivariable analysis. Coenzyme Q$_{10}$ was not an independent predictor of any other clinical outcome. Rosuvastatin reduced coenzyme Q$_{10}$ but there was no interaction between coenzyme Q$_{10}$ and the effect of rosuvastatin.

Conclusions.—Coenzyme Q$_{10}$ is not an independent prognostic variable in heart failure. Rosuvastatin reduced coenzyme Q$_{10}$, but even in patients with a low baseline coenzyme Q$_{10}$, rosuvastatin treatment was not associated with a significantly worse outcome. (Controlled Rosuvastatin Multinational Study in Heart Failure [CORONA]; NCT00206310).

▶ For years, there have been hundreds of articles examining the significance of low levels of coenzyme Q$_{10}$ (ubiquinone) in patients with heart failure (HF).

Q_{10} acts as an electron transporter and is a lipid-soluble essential cofactor in mitochondrial oxidative phosphorylation and generation of adenosine triphosphate.[1,2] Another possible action is as a lipophilic antioxidant protecting cell membranes and lipoproteins from oxidation.[1-3] Because the synthesis of Q_{10} is through the mevalonate pathway that is blocked by statins,[1-3] theoretically, Q_{10} depletion could lead to muscle dysfunction, both peripheral and myocardial, of especial concern in patients with HF. In an article by Molyneux and colleagues,[4] low Q_{10} serum levels were found to be an independent predictor of mortality in patients with HF. These facts have resulted in some physicians recommending Q_{10} supplements and avoiding indicated statins in patients with HF, causing the Food and Drug Administration to request that this study be done to examine the relationship of Q_{10} to adverse events in patients with HF. Compared with the previously mentioned study, this study is 5 times as large with 350 versus 76 deaths. Although this study also found that a low serum Q_{10} level was associated with worse outcomes in patients with HF, the low serum Q_{10} level served as a marker for advanced disease and was not independent of a low left ventricular ejection fraction, reduced glomerular filtration rate, higher New York Heart Association class, or increased N-terminal pro—B-type natriuretic peptide concentration as a predictor of mortality in patients with HF. Finally, in the study by Molyneux and colleagues, multivariable analysis adjusted for only 5 baseline variables in addition to Q_{10} levels, whereas in this study, 14 independent variables previously shown to be predictors of outcome were used. All these differences make this study more robust and its conclusions more likely to be correct. Additionally, there was evidence that statins increased muscle symptoms or creatine kinase in patients with low Q_{10} serum levels. Hopefully, this article will dampen the enthusiasm for prescribing Q_{10} to patients with HF and eliminate the hesitation for giving statins to patients where they are indicated.

M. D. Cheitlin, MD

References

1. Crane FL. Discovery of ubiquinone (coenzyme Q) and an overview of function. *Mitochondrion.* 2007;7:S2-S7.
2. Bentinger M, Brismar K, Dallner G. The antioxidant role of coenzyme Q. *Mitochondrion.* 2007;7:S41-S50.
3. Rustin P, Munnich A, Rötig A. Mitochondrial respiratory chain dysfunction caused by coenzyme Q deficiency. *Methods Enzymol.* 2004;382:81-88.
4. Molyneux SL, Florkowski CM, George PM, et al. Coenzyme Q10: an independent predictor of mortality in chronic heart failure. *J Am Coll Cardiol.* 2008;52:1435-1441.

44 Non-Coronary Heart Disease in Adults

Combination of Loop Diuretics With Thiazide-Type Diuretics in Heart Failure

Jentzer JC, DeWald TA, Hernandez AF (Duke Univ School of Medicine, Durham, NC)

J Am Coll Cardiol 56:1527-1534, 2010

Volume overload is an important clinical target in heart failure management, typically addressed using loop diuretics. An important and challenging subset of heart failure patients exhibit fluid overload despite significant doses of loop diuretics. One approach to overcome loop diuretic resistance is the addition of a thiazide-type diuretic to produce diuretic synergy via "sequential nephron blockade," first described more than 40 years ago. Although potentially able to induce diuresis in patients otherwise resistant to high doses of loop diuretics, this strategy has not been subjected to large-scale clinical trials to establish safety and clinical efficacy. We summarize the existing literature evaluating the combination of loop and thiazide diuretics in patients with heart failure in order to describe the possible benefits and hazards associated with this therapy. Combination diuretic therapy using any of several thiazide-type diuretics can more than double daily urine sodium excretion to induce weight loss and edema resolution, at the risk of inducing severe hypokalemia in addition to hyponatremia, hypotension, and worsening renal function. We provide considerations about prudent use of this therapy and review potential misconceptions about this long-used diuretic approach. Finally, we seek to highlight the need for pragmatic clinical trials for this commonly used therapy (Fig 1, Tables 3 and 4).

▶ Patients with severe heart failure frequently present with fluid overload and first-line therapy with diuretics results in marked symptom relief. With chronic diuretic use, diuretic resistance occurs from an interaction between the pathophysiology of sodium retention in heart failure and the renal response to diuretic therapy.[1] For 40 years, the use of a combination of a thiazide and a loop diuretic, each working at different levels of the nephron has increased diuresis in these diuretic-resistant patients. A review of the literature reveals the fact that most of the studies involving combined diuretic use are small and nonplacebo controlled. This article is a very good summary of the history of diuretic

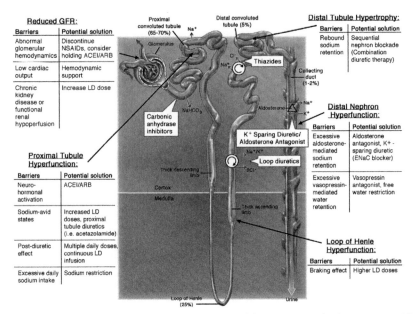

FIGURE 1.—Diuretic Resistance and the Nephron. Sites of diuretic action and sodium retention with suggested strategies to overcome diuretic resistance. Sodium delivery into tubular fluid is determined by glomerular filtration rate (GFR). Percentage of filtered sodium reabsorbed in each nephron segment is denoted in parentheses. Proximal convoluted tubule reabsorbs the majority of filtered sodium and proximal reabsorption is increased in sodium-retaining states under the control of neurohormones (alpha-1 adrenergic, angiotensin-II), producing the post-diuretic effect. Loop of Henle is the site of action of loop diuretics (LD) and absorbs most of the sodium that escapes the proximal tubule; braking effect appears to occur here due to up-regulation of the Na/K/Cl cotransporter after exposure to LD. Distal convoluted tubule reabsorbs a lesser amount of filtered sodium via NaCl cotransporter (inhibited by thiazide-type diuretics [TD]) but size and function may increase dramatically after chronic LD exposure, accounting for rebound sodium retention. Distal nephron collecting duct is the site of regulated sodium and water reabsorption under control of aldosterone and vasopressin via epithelial sodium channels (ENaC) and aquaporins, respectively. Multiple mechanisms of diuretic resistance may occur in a single patient, requiring a systematic approach to diuretic therapy. Figure illustration by Craig Skaggs based on the author's description and an example nephron from Ernst ME, Moser M. Use of diuretics in patients with hypertension. N Engl J Med 2009;36:2153−64. ACEI = angiotensin-converting enzyme inhibitor; ARB = angiotensin-receptor blocker. (Reprinted from Jentzer JC, DeWald TA, Hernandez AF. Combination of loop diuretics with thiazide-type diuretics in heart failure. *J Am Coll Cardiol.* 2010;56:1527-1534, copyright © 2010, with permission from the American College of Cardiology Foundation.)

TABLE 3.—Potential Benefits and Adverse Effects of CDT

Potential Benefits	Potential Adverse Effects
Overcoming diuretic resistance	Hypokalemia
Relief of fluid overload + edema	Worsening renal function/azotemia
Weight loss	Hyponatremia
Low drug cost	Hypochloremic metabolic alkalosis
Symptomatic improvement	Hypotension
Decrease in systemic congestion	Hypovolemia/dehydration
Diuresis in chronic renal failure	Worsening hepatic encephalopathy
Improved ventricular function	Cardiac arrhythmias/ectopy
Hospital discharge	Hypomagnesemia
Prevention of readmission	Hyperuricemia

CDT = combination diuretic therapy.

TABLE 4.—Important Considerations Regarding CDT

- Addition of thiazide-type diuretics can induce diuresis in patients refractory to massive loop diuretic doses
- Combination of loop + thiazide-type diuretics can be effective in patients with advanced chronic kidney disease
- Synergistic effects of thiazide-type diuretics on diuresis appear to be a class effect seen with all drugs studied
- Potentially dangerous hypokalemia can develop with CDT, warranting close laboratory monitoring
- Reversible increases in serum creatinine may be seen but are not the rule; reductions in creatinine can occur as well
- Safety and effects on morbidity and mortality with CDT are unknown

CDT = combination diuretic therapy.

resistance and the safety and effectiveness of combined diuretic therapy in patients with severe diuretic-resistant congestive heart failure.

M. D. Cheitlin, MD

Reference

1. Ellison DH. Diuretic therapy and resistance in congestive heart failure. *Cardiology*. 2001;96:132-143.

Improved Outcomes With Early Collaborative Care of Ambulatory Heart Failure Patients Discharged From the Emergency Department

Lee DS, Stukel TA, Austin PC, et al (Inst for Clinical Evaluative Sciences, Toronto, Ontario, Canada)
Circulation 122:1806-1814, 2010

Background.—The type of outpatient physician care after an emergency department visit for heart failure may affect patients' outcomes.

Methods and Results.—Using the National Ambulatory Care Reporting System, we examined the care and outcomes of heart failure patients who visited and were discharged from the emergency department in Ontario, Canada (April 2004 to March 2007). Early collaborative care by a cardiologist and primary care (PC) physician within 30 days after discharge was compared with PC alone. Care for 10 599 patients (age, 74.9 ± 11.9 years; 50.2% male) was provided by PC alone (n=6596), cardiologist alone (n=535), or concurrently by both cardiologist and PC (n=1478); 1990 did not visit a physician. Collaborative care patients were more likely to undergo assessment of left ventricular function (57.4% versus 28.7%), noninvasive stress testing (20.1% versus 7.8%), and cardiac catheterization (11.6% versus 2.7%) compared with PC. Drug prescriptions (patients ≥65 years of age) demonstrated higher use of angiotensin-converting enzyme inhibitors (58.8% versus 54.6%), angiotensin receptor blockers (22.7% versus 18.1%), β-adrenoceptor antagonists (63.4% versus 48.0%), loop diuretics (84.2% versus 79.6%), metolazone (4.8% versus

3.4%), and spironolactone (19.8% versus 12.7%) within 100 days after emergency department discharge for collaborative care compared with PC. In a propensity-matched model, mortality was lower with PC compared with no physician visit (hazard ratio, 0.75; 95% confidence interval, 0.64 to 0.87; $P<0.001$). Collaborative care reduced mortality compared with PC (hazard ratio, 0.79; 95% confidence interval, 0.63 to 1.00; $P=0.045$). Sole cardiology care conferred a trend to increased mortality (hazard ratio, 1.41 versus collaborative care; 95% confidence interval, 0.98 to 2.03; $P=0.067$).

Conclusions.—Early collaborative heart failure care was associated with increased use of drug therapies and cardiovascular diagnostic tests and better outcomes compared with PC alone.

▶ Heart failure (HF) is a major contributor to the rising cost of health care with most costs attributable to care in the emergency department (ED) and hospitalizations.[1] Patients with HF are frequently seen first in the ED. If they are hospitalized, they receive rapid treatment, and on discharge, arrangements are made for follow-up. If ambulatory patients are deemed low risk and discharged home from the ED, the care they receive as an outpatient is decided largely by the primary care physician (PCP), who is the gatekeeper of referral to specialists. Follow-up may be by a PCP, a cardiologist, or both concurrently. However, some receive no early physician follow-up at all. The impact of shared care in patients with HF is a source of debate, with some studies finding that patients receiving concurrent care by PCP and cardiologist after an acute myocardial infarction have lower mortality rates than those treated by either alone.[2] Others find that shared care in patients with HF involves a trade-off between lower mortality and higher hospitalization rates[3] or that there is no advantage to being followed by a cardiologist over a PCP.[4]

This study is a population-based study of patients with HF, who were seen in and discharged from the ED, examining the type of physician care received within a month after discharge. Those receiving collaborative care of a PCP and cardiologist within 30 days of discharge had a lower death rate, had lower repeat ED visits and rehospitalizations, were more likely to have important diagnostic tests (both for cardiac functional assessment and evaluation of the extent of myocardial ischemia), were more likely to have coronary revascularization, and received more evidence-based drugs than those followed by a PCP alone.

These improved outcomes are likely at least in part because of improved care resulting from knowledge of the importance of pathophysiology, targeted diagnostic tests, and pharmacotherapy for patients with HF among cardiologists.[5] Unfortunately, a large proportion of patients with HF discharged from the ED received no physician follow-up, and these patients had the greatest risk of death and adverse events. The study cohort by design had not been hospitalized, had survived the initial month(s) after discharge when the increased risk of adverse events occurs,[6,7] and therefore represented a milder spectrum of patients with HF.

The implications of the study are that patients with HF, considered to be low risk enough to be discharged from the ED, are at risk of death and serious morbidity and should require early follow-up. Furthermore, early collaborative physician involvement can lead to improved outcomes and a substantial decrease in morbidity and mortality.

M. D. Cheitlin, MD

References

1. Rydén-Bergsten T, Andersson F. The health care costs of heart failure in Sweden. *J Intern Med.* 1999;246:275-284.
2. Ayanian JZ, Landrum MB, Guadagnoli E, Gaccione P. Specialty of ambulatory care physicians and mortality among elderly patients after myocardial infarction. *N Engl J Med.* 2002;347:1678-1686.
3. Ezekowitz JA, van Walraven C, McAlister FA, Armstrong PW, Kaul P. Impact of specialist follow-up in outpatients with congestive heart failure. *CMAJ.* 2005; 172:189-194.
4. Franciosa JA, Massie BM, Lukas MA, et al. Beta-blocker therapy for heart failure outside the clinical trial setting: findings of a community-based registry. *Am Heart J.* 2004;148:718-726.
5. Baker DW, Hayes RP, Massie BM, Craig CA. Variations in family physicians' and cardiologists' care for patients with heart failure. *Am Heart J.* 1999;138:826-834.
6. Solomon SD, Dobson J, Pocock S, et al. Influence of nonfatal hospitalization for heart failure on subsequent mortality in patients with chronic heart failure. *Circulation.* 2007;116:1482-1487.
7. Lee DS, Schull MJ, Alter DA, et al. Early deaths in patients with heart failure discharged from the emergency department: a population-based analysis. *Circ Heart Fail.* 2010;3:228-235.

Ivabradine and outcomes in chronic heart failure (SHIFT): a randomised placebo-controlled study
Swedberg K, on behalf of the SHIFT Investigators (Univ of Gothenburg, Göteborg, Sweden; et al)
Lancet 376:875-885, 2010

Background.—Chronic heart failure is associated with high mortality and morbidity. Raised resting heart rate is a risk factor for adverse outcomes. We aimed to assess the effect of heart-rate reduction by the selective sinus-node inhibitor ivabradine on outcomes in heart failure.

Methods.—Patients were eligible for participation in this randomised, double-blind, placebo-controlled, parallel-group study if they had symptomatic heart failure and a left-ventricular ejection fraction of 35% or lower, were in sinus rhythm with heart rate 70 beats per min or higher, had been admitted to hospital for heart failure within the previous year, and were on stable background treatment including a β blocker if tolerated. Patients were randomly assigned by computer-generated allocation schedule to ivabradine titrated to a maximum of 7·5 mg twice daily or matching placebo. Patients and investigators were masked to treatment allocation. The primary endpoint was the composite of cardiovascular death or hospital admission for worsening heart failure. Analysis was by intention to treat. This trial is registered, number ISRCTN70429960.

Findings.—6558 patients were randomly assigned to treatment groups (3268 ivabradine, 3290 placebo). Data were available for analysis for 3241 patients in the ivabradine group and 3264 patients allocated placebo. Median follow-up was 22·9 (IQR 18—28) months. 793 (24%) patients in the ivabradine group and 937 (29%) of those taking placebo had a primary endpoint event (HR 0·82, 95% CI 0·75—0·90, p<0·0001). The effects were driven mainly by hospital admissions for worsening heart failure (672 [21%] placebo *vs* 514 [16%] ivabradine; HR 0·74, 0·66—0·83; p<0·0001) and deaths due to heart failure (151 [5%] *vs* 113 [3%]; HR 0·74, 0·58—0·94, p=0·014). Fewer serious adverse events occurred in the ivabradine group (3388 events) than in the placebo group (3847; p=0·025). 150 (5%) of ivabradine patients had symptomatic bradycardia compared with 32 (1%) of the placebo group (p<0·0001). Visual side-effects (phosphenes) were reported by 89 (3%) of patients on ivabradine and 17 (1%) on placebo (p<0·0001).

Interpretation.—Our results support the importance of heart-rate reduction with ivabradine for improvement of clinical outcomes in heart failure and confirm the important role of heart rate in the pathophysiology of this disorder.

▶ The treatment of heart failure (HF) has improved substantially over the last 20 years with the use of β-blockers and antagonists of the renin-angiotensin-aldosterone (RAAS) system. β-blockers reduce mortality and morbidity beyond that of RAAS blockade alone.[1] The effect of these drugs in improving left ventricular remodeling[2] and sudden death[3] may be in part associated with their effect on lowering the heart rate.[4,5] The heart rate—lowering effect of β-blockers attenuates the effect of energy depletion of the myocardium in HF[6] but has other undesirable effects such as a depressing effect on myocardial contractility. It is known that raised heart rate is a risk factor for mortality and cardiovascular outcomes in epidemiological and observational studies.[7,8] Patients with HF treated with β-blockers frequently still have an elevated heart rate,[9] so additional therapies to further reduce heart rate might be useful. This study is the first to specifically test the hypothesis that isolated heart rate reduction will decrease the incidence of adverse outcomes in a population of patients with HF. Ivabradine is a specific inhibitor of the I_f current in the sino-atrial node[10] and has no effect on myocardial contractility and intracardiac conduction. Patients with chronic systolic HF, an ejection fraction ≤35% on optimal medical management including β-blockers with a persistent heart rate ≥70 beats/min showed a significant decrease of 18% in the composite of cardiovascular deaths or hospital admissions for worsening HF in those taking ivabradine. Although there was no reduction in cardiovascular deaths or sudden deaths, there was a significant drop in deaths caused by HF and all-cause hospital admissions, all of which became apparent within 3 months of initiation of treatment. The effects were consistent across all prespecified subgroups, but were most striking in those with baseline higher heart rates. Before the authors concluded that ivabradine should be a part of optimal therapy for patients with HF with residual heart rate ≥70 beats/min, in this study, the minority of patients on β-blockers were at the recommended target dose, so the same result might have been found with higher doses of β-blockers. Also, the mechanism by which the reduction in the outcome end points was achieved by ivabradine is still unclear. However, any advance in therapy for patients with severe HF is important since the mortality and morbidity are still high.

M. D. Cheitlin, MD

References

1. Gheorghiade M, Colucci WS, Swedberg K. Beta-blockers in chronic heart failure. *Circulation.* 2003;107:1570-1575.
2. Udelson JE. Ventricular remodeling in heart failure and the effect of beta-blockade. *Am J Cardiol.* 2004;93:43B-48B.
3. MERIT-HF Study Group. Effect of metoprolol CR/XL in chronic heart failure: Metoprolol CR/XL Randomised Intervention Trial in Congestive Heart Failure (MERIT-HF). *Lancet.* 1999;353:2001-2007.
4. Lechat P, Hulot JS, Escolano S, et al. Heart rate and cardiac rhythm relationships with bisoprolol benefit in chronic heart failure in CIBIS II Trial. *Circulation.* 2001;103:1428-1433.
5. McAlister FA, Wiebe N, Ezekowitz JA, Leung AA, Armstrong PW. Meta-analysis: beta-blocker dose, heart rate reduction, and death in patients with heart failure. *Ann Intern Med.* 2009;150:784-794.
6. Katz AM. The myocardium in congestive heart failure. *Am J Cardiol.* 1989;63: 12A-16A.
7. Diaz A, Bourassa MG, Guertin MC, Tardif JC. Long-term prognostic value of resting heart rate in patients with suspected or proven coronary artery disease. *Eur Heart J.* 2005;26:967-974.
8. Wilhelmsen L, Berglund G, Elmfeldt D, et al. The multifactor primary prevention trial in Göteborg Sweden. *Eur Heart J.* 1986;7:279-288.
9. Komajda M, Follath F, Swedberg K, et al. The EuroHeart Failure Survey programme—a survey on the quality of care among patients with heart failure in Europe. Part 2: treatment. *Eur Heart J.* 2003;24:464-474.
10. DiFrancesco D. Funny channels in the control of cardiac rhythm and mode of action of selective blockers. *Pharmacol Res.* 2006;53:399-406.

Spironolactone use at discharge was associated with improved survival in hospitalized patients with systolic heart failure
Hamaguchi S, Kinugawa S, Tsuchihashi-Makaya M, et al (Hokkaido Univ Graduate School of Medicine, Sapporo, Japan)
Am Heart J 160:1156-1162, 2010

Background.—The RALES trial demonstrated that spironolactone improved the prognosis of patients with heart failure (HF). However, it is unknown whether the discharge use of spironolactone is associated with better long-term outcomes among hospitalized systolic HF patients in routine clinical practice. We examined the effects of spironolactone use at discharge on mortality and rehospitalization by comparing with outcomes in patients who did not receive spironolactone.

Methods.—The JCARE-CARD studied prospectively the characteristics and treatments in a broad sample of patients hospitalized with worsening

HF and the outcomes were followed with an average of 2.2 years of follow-up.

Results.—A total of 946 patients had HF with reduced left ventricular ejection fraction (LVEF) (<40%), among whom spironolactone was prescribed at discharge in 435 patients (46%), but not in 511 patients (54%). The mean age was 66.3 years and 72.2% were male. Etiology was ischemic in 39.7% and mean LVEF was 27.1%. After adjustment for covariates, discharge use of spironolactone was associated with a significant reduction in all-cause death (adjusted hazard ratio 0.612, $P = .020$) and cardiac death (adjusted hazard ratio 0.524, $P = .013$).

Conclusions.—Among patients with HF hospitalized for systolic dysfunction, spironolactone use at the time of discharge was associated with long-term survival benefit. These findings provide further support for the idea that spironolactone may be useful in patients hospitalized with HF and reduced LVEF (Fig 1).

▶ The treatment of patients with congestive heart failure (CHF) has markedly improved survival with the addition of β-blockers, angiotensin-converting enzyme inhibitors (ACEI), and angiotensin II receptor blockers and the addition of aldosterone blockade. Because aldosterone plays an important role in the progression of CHF by inducing vascular damage, myocardial hypertrophy, and fibrosis,[1-3] aldosterone antagonism by spironolactone and eplerenone, a selective aldosterone antagonist with fewer side effects than spironolactone, was an important advance in that both the Randomized Aldosterone Evaluation Study (RALES) and Eplerenone Post-Acute Myocardial Infarction Heart Failure Efficacy and Survival Study (EPHESUS) showed a significant decrease in mortality and morbidity in patients with systolic dysfunction CHF when added to β-blockers and ACEI.[4,5] Both the current American College of Cardiology/American Heart Association and European Society of Cardiology guidelines recommend spironolactone in patients with CHF, a reduced left ventricular ejection fraction (LVEF), and symptoms in spite of β-blockers, ACEI, and diuretics.[6,7] However, both these trials, like most randomized placebo-controlled trials, had a strictly limited inclusion population. The RALES trial included patients with New York Heart Association class III to IV symptoms with LVEF ≤ 35%. Further, they excluded patients with serum creatinine > 2.5 mg/dL and only 10% were taking a β-blocker. The CHF population taking aldosterone antagonists at present are older, are less symptomatic, and some have serum creatinine > 2.5 mg/dL. Therefore, it is not clear that spironolactone will have the same beneficial effect in these patients as in those in the controlled trials. The importance of this study is that unselected patients with CHF and an LVEF < 40% were divided into those taking and not taking spironolactone on hospital discharge, and it was found that spironolactone was associated with a 48% reduction in the risk for cardiac death when followed up for 2.2 years. There are a number of possible reasons that aldosterone antagonists could be beneficial. Spironolactone could induce reversed left ventricular (LV) remodeling,[8] improving LV function and exercise tolerance,[9] decrease cardiac fibrosis,[10] and improve endothelial function in asymptomatic

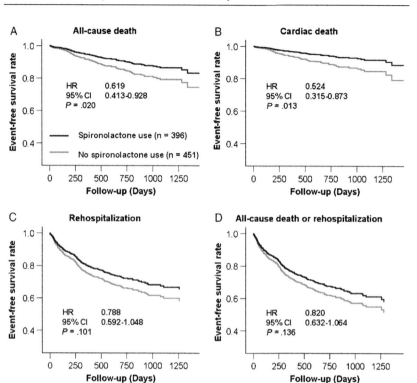

FIGURE 1.—Kaplan-Meier survival curves free from all-cause death (**A**), cardiac death (**B**), rehospitalization due to worsening HF (**C**), and all-cause death or rehospitalization (**D**) in hospitalized patients with spironolactone use (black lines, n = 396) versus no spironolactone use (red lines, n = 451) at discharge. For interpretation of the references to color in this figure legend, the reader is referred to web version of this article. (Reprinted from Hamaguchi S, Kinugawa S, Tsuchihashi-Makaya M, et al. Spironolactone use at discharge was associated with improved survival in hospitalized patients with systolic heart failure. *Am Heart J*. 2010;160:1156-1162, with permission from Mosby, Inc.)

or mildly symptomatic patients when added to optimal treatment including β-blockers.[11] This study therefore suggests that the beneficial effects of aldosterone antagonists seen in the RALES and EMPHSUS trials extend to a more unselected population of patients with systolic dysfunction CHF.

M. D. Cheitlin, MD

References

1. Rocha R, Rudolph AE, Frierdich GE, et al. Aldosterone induces a vascular inflammatory phenotype in the rat heart. *Am J Physiol Heart Circ Physiol*. 2002;283:H1802-H1810.
2. Schunkert H, Hense HW, Muscholl M, et al. Associations between circulating components of the renin-angiotensin-aldosterone system and left ventricular mass. *Heart*. 1997;77:24-31.
3. Weber KT, Brilla CG. Pathological hypertrophy and cardiac interstitium. Fibrosis and renin-angiotensin-aldosterone system. *Circulation*. 1991;83:1849-1865.

402 / Heart and Cardiovascular Disease

4. Pitt B, Zannad F, Remme WJ, et al. The effect of spironolactone on morbidity and mortality in patients with severe heart failure. Randomized Aldactone Evaluation Study Investigators. N Engl J Med. 1999;341:709-717.
5. Pitt B, Remme W, Zannad F, et al. Eplerenone, a selective aldosterone blocker, in patients with left ventricular dysfunction after myocardial infarction. N Engl J Med. 2003;348:1309-1321.
6. Hunt SA, Abraham WT, Chin MH, et al. ACC/AHA 2005 Guideline Update for the Diagnosis and Management of Chronic Heart Failure in the Adult: a report of the American College of Cardiology/American Heart Association Task Force on Practice Guidelines (Writing Committee to Update the 2001 Guidelines for the Evaluation and Management of Heart Failure): developed in collaboration with the American College of Chest Physicians and the International Society for Heart and Lung Transplantation: endorsed by the Heart Rhythm Society. Circulation. 2005;112:e154-235.
7. Dickstein K, Cohen-Solal A, Filippatos G, et al. ESC guidelines for the diagnosis and treatment of acute and chronic heart failure 2008: the Task Force for the Diagnosis and Treatment of Acute and Chronic Heart Failure 2008 of the European Society of Cardiology. Developed in collaboration with the Heart Failure Association of the ESC (HFA) and endorsed by the European Society of Intensive Care Medicine (ESICM). Eur Heart J. 2008;29:2388-2442.
8. Chan AK, Sanderson JE, Wang T, et al. Aldosterone receptor antagonism induces reverse remodeling when added to angiotensin receptor blockade in chronic heart failure. J Am Coll Cardiol. 2007;50:591-596.
9. Cicoira M, Zanolla L, Rossi A, et al. Long-term, dose-dependent effects of spironolactone on left ventricular function and exercise tolerance in patients with chronic heart failure. J Am Coll Cardiol. 2002;40:304-310.
10. Zannad F, Alla F, Dousset B, Perez A, Pitt B. Limitation of excessive extracellular matrix turnover may contribute to survival benefit of spironolactone therapy in patients with congestive heart failure: insights from the randomized aldactone evaluation study (RALES). Rales Investigators. Circulation. 2000;102:2700-2706.
11. Macdonald JE, Kennedy N, Struthers AD. Effects of spironolactone on endothelial function, vascular angiotensin converting enzyme activity, and other prognostic markers in patients with mild heart failure already taking optimal treatment. Heart. 2004;90:765-770.

Iron Overload Cardiomyopathy: Better Understanding of an Increasing Disorder

Gujja P, Rosing DR, Tripodi DJ, et al (Univ of Cincinnati, OH; Natl Insts of Health, Bethesda, MD)
J Am Coll Cardiol 56:1001-1012, 2010

The prevalence of iron overload cardiomyopathy (IOC) is increasing. The spectrum of symptoms of IOC is varied. Early in the disease process, patients may be asymptomatic, whereas severely overloaded patients can have terminal heart failure complaints that are refractory to treatment. It has been shown that early recognition and intervention may alter outcomes. Biochemical markers and tissue biopsy, which have traditionally been used to diagnose and guide therapy, are not sensitive enough to detect early cardiac iron deposition. Newer diagnostic modalities such as magnetic resonance imaging are noninvasive and can assess quantitative cardiac iron load. Phlebotomy and chelating drugs are suboptimal means of treating IOC; hence, the roles of gene therapy, hepcidin, and calcium channel blockers are being actively investigated. There is a need for the development of clinical guidelines in order to improve the management of this emerging complex disease (Figs 1 and 3).

▶ Most patients with cardiomyopathy at the time of diagnosis cannot get it reversed and treatment is directed at the pathophysiology of heart failure, with drugs targeted to treat the fluid overload and block the excessive neuro-hormonal activation that results in symptoms and progressive left ventricular dysfunction and death. In those with alcoholic cardiomyopathy, if patients stop drinking alcohol, a large number of these patients will recover ventricular function. Iron overload cardiomyopathy is one of the other few treatable cardiomyopathies that, if discovered early, can be stopped in its progression. The key to early treatment is early recognition of the disease. Excess iron accumulates in the body as a result of increased gastrointestinal absorption (hemochromatosis), excess administration of exogenous iron by dietary sources, or, more

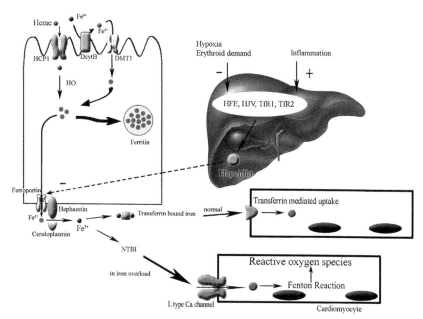

FIGURE 1.—Iron Kinetics. Heme is absorbed by Heme carrier protein (HCP)-1 and released from iron by hemoxygenase (HO)-1, but heme uptake overall still remains controversial. Non-heme iron is reduced by duodenal cytochrome b at the apical membrane of intestinal enterocytes (21), which is taken up by intestinal epithelium by the divalent metal transporter (DMT)-1 (22,23). Ferrous iron is then transported to the basolateral portion of the cell by iron carriers and later transported into the circulation by the duodenal iron exporter Ferroportin (regulated by hepcidin) when there is a need for iron. Ferrous iron is oxidized by ceruloplasmin in non-intestinal cells and also by a homolog of ceruloplasmin, Hephaestin, in intestinal cells to ferric iron and loaded on to transferrin. With the increase in intracellular concentrations of iron, ferritin synthesis also increases. Once the storage capacity is exceeded, metabolically active iron is released intracellularly in the form of hemosiderin and toxic nontransferrin-bound forms of iron (NTBI). *Editor's Note*: Please refer to original journal article for full references. (Reprinted from the Journal of the American College of Cardiology, Gujja P, Rosing DR, Tripodi DJ, et al. Iron overload cardiomyopathy: Better understanding of an increasing disorder. *J Am Coll Cardiol.* 2010;56:1001-1012. Copyright 2010, with permission from the American College of Cardiology Foundation.)

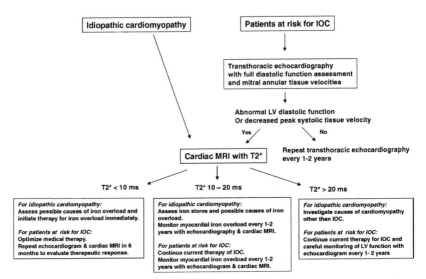

FIGURE 3.—Our Proposed Clinical Pathway to Evaluate Patients with Idiopathic Cardiomyopathy or Those at Risk for Iron Overload. IOC = iron overload cardiomyopathy; LV = left ventricle; MRI = magnetic resonance imaging. (Reprinted from the Journal of the American College of Cardiology, Gujja P, Rosing DR, Tripodi DJ, et al. Iron overload cardiomyopathy: Better understanding of an increasing disorder. *J Am Coll Cardiol.* 2010;56:1001-1012. Copyright 2010, with permission from the American College of Cardiology Foundation.)

commonly, red blood cell transfusions (hemosiderosis), the cornerstone of treatment for hereditary anemias such as thalassemia and sickle cell disease. The present paper is a very extensive review of the pathophysiology, diagnosis, and management of this disease. Described are the newer insights into iron homeostasis and a better understanding of how iron enters the body. Newer diagnostic techniques, including magnetic resonance imaging and diastolic function by tissue Doppler, are being developed to improve early diagnosis of iron overload, essential in treating early enough to halt progression to irreversible cardiomyopathy. To this end, a proposed clinical pathway algorithm is given to evaluate patients with idiopathic cardiomyopathy or those at risk of iron overload. New therapeutic options, other than repeated phlebotomy, include better chelating agents with fewer side effects, better efficacy, and absorption; calcium channel blocking agents; hepcidin, an amino acid that plays a major role in regulating iron homeostasis; genetic and stem cell therapy are being investigated. The incidence of iron overload cardiomyopathy is increasing worldwide, with patients with thalassemia and sickle cell disease living longer, and in individuals with hematologic malignancies and increased treatment, especially with bone marrow transplants and stem cell therapy. Because cardiologists take care of most of these patients, an excellent review paper on this subject is a valuable resource.

M. D. Cheitlin, MD

Risk of heart failure relapse in subsequent pregnancy among peripartum cardiomyopathy mothers

Fett JD, Fristoe KL, Welsh SN (Hôpital Albert Schweitzer, Deschapelles, Haiti; Peripartum Cardiomyopathy Support Network, Deschapelles, Haiti)
Int J Gynaecol Obstet 109:34-36, 2010

Objective.—To quantify the level of risk for heart failure relapse in a subsequent pregnancy in women who have had peripartum cardiomyopathy (PPCM), and to test the hypothesis that meeting additional criteria may help lower the risk.

Methods.—Prospectively-identified PPCM patients volunteering between 2003 and 2009 were identified from the PPCM Registry of Hôpital Albert Schweitzer, Deschapelles, Haiti, and an internet support group. Data were assessed for full adherence to monitoring and diagnostic criteria, clinical data, statistical analysis, and reporting.

Results.—Of 61 post-PPCM pregnancies identified, there were 18 relapses (29.5%) of heart failure. Of 26 pregnancies with a left ventricular ejection fraction (LVEF) of less than 0.55 prior to the pregnancy, relapse occurred in 12 (46.2%) pregnancies. Of 35 pregnancies with an LVEF of 0.55 or greater prior to the pregnancy, relapse occurred in 6 (17.1%) ($P < 0.01$). No relapses occurred in 9 women who also demonstrated adequate contractile reserve.

Conclusion.—The most important criterion associated with reduced risk for heart failure relapse in a post-PPCM pregnancy is recovery defined by an LVEF 0.55 or greater before the subsequent pregnancy. Exercise stress echocardiography showing adequate contractile reserve may help to identify women at an even lower risk of relapse (Figs 1 and 2, Table 1).

▶ Women with postpartum cardiomyopathy (PPCM) are at significant risk of relapsing heart failure during a subsequent pregnancy. To date, data support the concept that the risk of relapse in a subsequent pregnancy depends on the degree of left ventricular (LV) systolic functional recovery before becoming pregnant again. However, the degree of such risk is not well defined in these limited studies,[1-4] and there are no factors identified that are associated with the lowest risk. This study is the largest prospectively identified group of patients with PPCM with subsequent pregnancies, 61 post-PPCM pregnancies in 56 women, who were assessed for relapse of heart failure. In subsequent pregnancy, 18 relapses (29.5%) of heart failure occurred and the chance of recurrence was inversely related to the LV ejection fraction (LVEF) before the subsequent pregnancy. One of the important findings by these authors is that when a subsequent pregnancy occurred before the patient had fully recovered a LVEF > 50%, relapse of heart failure in the subsequent pregnancy occurred about 50% of the time.[1] Another unique observation in this study is that in patients with adequate contractile reserve before subsequent pregnancy, as defined by an increase of LVEF on exercise echocardiography at target exercise over resting heart rate ≥15%, there were no relapses of heart failure. Although the number of patients with exercise echocardiography was too small to reach

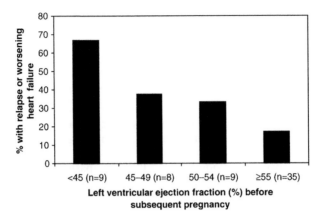

FIGURE 1.—Rate of relapse/worsening heart failure among 61 post-PPCM pregnancies, 2003–2009. (Reprinted from Fett JD, Fristoe KL, Welsh SN. Risk of heart failure relapse in subsequent pregnancy among peripartum cardiomyopathy mothers. *Int J Gynaecol Obstet.* 2010;109:34-36, with permission from Elsevier Ireland.)

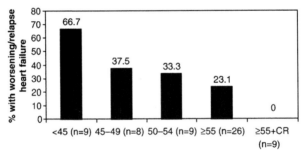

FIGURE 2.—Relapse or worsening of heart failure in 61 post-PPCM pregnancies, 2003–2009. (Reprinted from Fett JD, Fristoe KL, Welsh SN. Risk of heart failure relapse in subsequent pregnancy among peripartum cardiomyopathy mothers. *Int J Gynaecol Obstet.* 2010;109:34-36, with permission from Elsevier Ireland.)

TABLE 1.—Rate of Heart Failure Relapse Among 35 Post-PPCM Pregnancies in 30 Recovered (LVEF≥0.55) Patients From the USA, 2003–2009[a]

Criteria Met[b]	1 Only	1 and 2	1, 2, and 3	Total Relapses
Relapse of heart failure	3/11 (27.3)	3/15 (20.0)	0/9 (0)	6/35 (17.1)

[a]Values are given as number (percentage).
[b]Criterion 1: Recovered systolic heart function, with an LVEF of 0.55 or greater; Criterion 2: Maintained an LVEF of 0.55 or greater after phase-out of heart failure medications ("proof of recovery"); Criterion 3: Adequate contractile reserve demonstrated on exercise stress echocardiography (increase of LVEF at target exercise heart rate over resting heart rate by relative amount of at least 15%).

significance, it is probable that this exercise test provides evidence that the heart can respond adequately to the stress of pregnancy, labor, and delivery.[5-7] It is never possible to say that in a patient who had PPCM, a subsequent pregnancy will not precipitate relapse of heart failure. However, it is true that a subsequent pregnancy in such a patient is at high risk of relapse until the patient's LV systolic function, as represented by LVEF, has returned to ≥50% or better ≥55%. If the patient has adequate contractile reserve on exercise echocardiography, the risk of relapse is even lower.

M. D. Cheitlin, MD

References

1. Fett JD, Christie LG, Murphy JG. Brief communication: Outcomes of subsequent pregnancy after peripartum cardiomyopathy: a case series from Haiti. *Ann Intern Med.* 2006;145:30-34.
2. Fett JD, Christie LG, Carraway RD, Murphy JG. Five-year prospective study of the incidence and prognosis of peripartum cardiomyopathy at a single institution. *Mayo Clin Proc.* 2005;80:1602-1606.
3. Elkayam U, Tummala PP, Rao K, et al. Maternal and fetal outcomes of subsequent pregnancies in women with peripartum cardiomyopathy. *N Engl J Med.* 2001;344: 1567-1571.
4. Habli M, O'Brien T, Nowack E, Khoury S, Barton JR, Sibai B. Peripartum cardiomyopathy: prognostic factors for long-term maternal outcome. *Am J Obstet Gynecol.* 2008;199:415.e1-415.e5.
5. Lampert MB, Weinert L, Hibbard J, Korcarz C, Lindheimer M, Lang RM. Contractile reserve in patients with peripartum cardiomyopathy and recovered left ventricular function. *Am J Obstet Gynecol.* 1997;176:189-195.
6. Moonen M, Senechal M, Cosyns B, et al. Impact of contractile reserve on acute response to cardiac resynchronization therapy. *Cardiovasc Ultrasound.* 2008;6:65.
7. Sicari R, Nihoyannopoulos P, Evangelista A, et al. Stress echocardiography expert consensus statement: European Association of Echocardiography (EAE) (a registered branch of the ESC). *Eur J Echocardiogr.* 2008;9:415-437.

Comparison Between Transcatheter and Surgical Prosthetic Valve Implantation in Patients With Severe Aortic Stenosis and Reduced Left Ventricular Ejection Fraction

Clavel MA, Webb JG, Rodés-Cabau J, et al (Laval Univ, Québec, Canada; Univ of British Columbia, Vancouver; et al)
Circulation 122:1928-1936, 2010

Background.—Patients with severe aortic stenosis and reduced left ventricular ejection fraction (LVEF) have a poor prognosis with conservative therapy but a high operative mortality when treated surgically. Recently, transcatheter aortic valve implantation (TAVI) has emerged as an alternative to surgical aortic valve replacement (SAVR) for patients considered at high or prohibitive operative risk. The objective of this study was to compare TAVI and SAVR with respect to postoperative recovery of LVEF in patients with severe aortic stenosis and reduced LV systolic function.

Methods and Results.—Echocardiographic data were prospectively collected before and after the procedure in 200 patients undergoing

SAVR and 83 patients undergoing TAVI for severe aortic stenosis (aortic valve area $\leq 1 \text{ cm}^2$) with reduced LV systolic function (LVEF $\leq 50\%$). TAVI patients were significantly older (81 ± 8 versus 70 ± 10 years; $P<0.0001$) and had more comorbidities compared with SAVR patients. Despite similar baseline LVEF ($34 \pm 11\%$ versus $34 \pm 10\%$), TAVI patients had better recovery of LVEF compared with SAVR patients (ΔLVEF, $14 \pm 15\%$ versus $7 \pm 11\%$; $P=0.005$). At the 1-year follow-up, 58% of TAVI patients had a normalization of LVEF ($>50\%$) as opposed to 20% in the SAVR group. On multivariable analysis, female gender ($P=0.004$), lower LVEF at baseline ($P=0.005$), absence of atrial fibrillation ($P=0.01$), TAVI ($P=0.007$), and larger increase in aortic valve area after the procedure ($P=0.01$) were independently associated with better recovery of LVEF.

Conclusion.—In patients with severe aortic stenosis and depressed LV systolic function, TAVI is associated with better LVEF recovery compared with SAVR. TAVI may provide an interesting alternative to SAVR in patients with depressed LV systolic function considered at high surgical risk.

▶ Patients with severe aortic stenosis (AS) and reduced left ventricular ejection fraction (LVEF) have a poor prognosis without valve replacement and an increased perioperative mortality compared with those with a normal LVEF.[1,2] In such patients, improvement after surgical prosthetic valve change in LVEF is variable, with improvement occurring because of a decrease in a pressure afterload and worsening because of ischemia, cardioplegia, oxidative stress, and inflammation-causing myocardial damage.[3,4] After prosthetic valve replacement, studies have shown that patients with depressed LVEF are very sensitive to the residual pressure afterload imposed by prosthesis-patient mismatch.[5] With the development of transcatheter aortic valve implantation (TAVI), there is now an alternative to surgical prosthetic valve replacement that avoids some of the serious negative consequences of bypass surgery and is being considered for patients at high or prohibitive surgical risk.[6,7] This retrospective observational study compared outcomes in patients with severe AS and reduced LVEF after surgical prosthetic valve replacement with those with TAVI and showed at 1 year postprocedure that the number of patients improving to an LVEF $>50\%$ was significantly higher in the patients with thrombotic associated myocardial infarction. In another study by the same group, they reported that TAVI is associated with better hemodynamic performance and less incidence of prosthesis-patient mismatch compared with surgical valve replacement with either stented or stentless bioprostheses.[8] The duration of follow-up was short; the study was not a randomized study comparing surgical valve replacement with TAVI, but the results are extremely supportive in patients with severe AS and reduced LVEF or those considered inoperable of TAVI as an alternative therapy.

M. D. Cheitlin, MD

References

1. Powell DE, Tunick PA, Rosenzweig BP, et al. Aortic valve replacement in patients with aortic stenosis and severe left ventricular dysfunction. *Arch Intern Med.* 2000;160:1337-1341.
2. Pereira JJ, Lauer MS, Bashir M, et al. Survival after aortic valve replacement for severe aortic stenosis with low transvalvular gradients and severe left ventricular dysfunction. *J Am Coll Cardiol.* 2002;39:1356-1363.
3. Anselmi A, Abbate A, Girola F, et al. Myocardial ischemia, stunning, inflammation, and apoptosis during cardiac surgery: a review of evidence. *Eur J Cardiothorac Surg.* 2004;25:304-311.
4. Vähäsilta T, Saraste A, Kitö V, et al. Cardiomyocyte apoptosis after antegrade and retrograde cardioplegia. *Ann Thorac Surg.* 2005;80:2229-2234.
5. Ruel M, Al-Faleh H, Kulik A, Chan KL, Mesana TG, Burwash IG. Prosthesis-patient mismatch after aortic valve replacement predominantly affects patients with pre-existing left ventricular dysfunction: effect on survival, freedom from heart failure, and left ventricular mass regression. *J Thorac Cardiovasc Surg.* 2006;131:1036-1044.
6. Webb JG, Pasupati S, Humphries K, et al. Percutaneous transarterial aortic valve replacement in selected high-risk patients with aortic stenosis. *Circulation.* 2007; 116:755-763.
7. Rodés-Cabau J, Webb JG, Cheung A, et al. Transcatheter aortic valve implantation for the treatment of severe symptomatic aortic stenosis in patients at very high or prohibitive surgical risk: acute and late outcomes of the multicenter Canadian experience. *J Am Coll Cardiol.* 2010;55:1080-1090.
8. Clavel MA, Webb JG, Pibarot P, et al. Comparison of the hemodynamic performance of percutaneous and surgical bioprostheses for the treatment of severe aortic stenosis. *J Am Coll Cardiol.* 2009;53:1883-1891.

Comprehensive Diagnostic Strategy for Blood Culture–Negative Endocarditis: A Prospective Study of 819 New Cases

Fournier P-E, Thuny F, Richet H, et al (Université de la Méditerranée, France; Centre Hospitalo-Universitaire de Grenoble, France; et al)
Clin Infect Dis 51:131-140, 2010

Background.—Blood culture–negative endocarditis (BCNE) may account for up to 31% of all cases of endocarditis.

Methods.—We used a prospective, multimodal strategy incorporating serological, molecular, and histopathological assays to investigate specimens from 819 patients suspected of having BCNE.

Results.—Diagnosis of endocarditis was first ruled out for 60 patients. Among 759 patients with BCNE, a causative microorganism was identified in 62.7%, and a noninfective etiology in 2.5%. Blood was the most useful specimen, providing a diagnosis for 47.7% of patients by serological analysis (mainly Q fever and *Bartonella* infections). Broad-range polymerase chain reaction (PCR) of blood and *Bartonella*–specific Western blot methods diagnosed 7 additional cases. PCR of valvular biopsies identified 109 more etiologies, mostly streptococci, *Tropheryma whipplei*, *Bartonella* species, and fungi. Primer extension enrichment reaction and autoimmunohistochemistry identified a microorganism in 5 additional patients. No virus or *Chlamydia* species were detected. A noninfective cause of endocarditis, particularly neoplasic or autoimmune disease, was determined by histological analysis or by searching for antinuclear antibodies in 19 (2.5%) of the patients. Our diagnostic strategy proved useful and sensitive for BCNE workup.

Conclusions.—We highlight the major role of zoonotic agents and the underestimated role of noninfective diseases in BCNE. We propose serological analysis for *Coxiella burnetii* and *Bartonella* species, detection of antinuclear antibodies and rheumatoid factor as first-line tests, followed by specific PCR assays for *T. whipplei*, *Bartonella* species, and fungi in blood. Broad-spectrum 16S and 18S ribosomal RNA PCR may be performed on valvular biopsies, when available (Figs 1 and 2, Table 5).

▶ Blood culture-negative endocarditis (BCNE), where no microorganism can be grown using the usual blood culture methods, occurs in 2.5% to 31% of

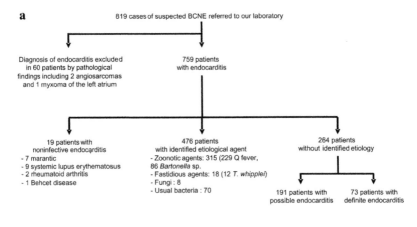

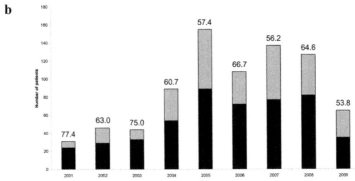

FIGURE 1.—Distribution of the 819 patients with suspected blood culture–negative endocarditis (BCNE) studied from 1 June 2001 to 1 September 2009, according to the etiological diagnosis *(a)* and the year *(b)*. *Black columns,* Number of patients per year for whom we obtained an etiological diagnosis (infectious or not). *Gray columns,* Number of patients without any etiological diagnosis. Values above each column represent percentages of etiological diagnoses obtained each year. Agents include *Tropheryma whipplei.* (Reprinted from Fournier P-E, Thuny F, Richet H, et al. Comprehensive diagnostic strategy for blood culture–negative endocarditis: a prospective study of 819 new cases. *Clin Infect Dis.* 2010;51:131-140, with permission from the Infectious Diseases Society of America and the University of Chicago.)

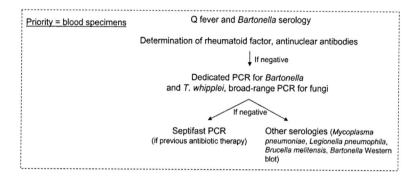

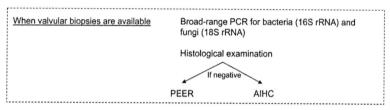

FIGURE 2.—Diagnostic tests applied to clinical specimens for identification of causative agents of blood culture–negative endocarditis. Agents include *Tropheryma whipplei*. AIHC, autoimmunohistochemistry; PCR, polymerase chain reaction; PEER, primer extension enrichment reaction; rRNA, ribosomal RNA. (Reprinted from Fournier P-E, Thuny F, Richet H, et al. Comprehensive diagnostic strategy for blood culture–negative endocarditis: a prospective study of 819 new cases. *Clin Infect Dis.* 2010;51:131-140, with permission from the Infectious Diseases Society of America and the University of Chicago.)

TABLE 5.—Comparison of Microorganisms Identified in Published Series of Blood Culture–Negative Endocarditis

Microorganism	Present Study[a] (n = 740)	France [3] (n = 348)	Study by Location [Reference] France [29] (n = 88)	Great Britain [30] (n = 63)	Algeria [31] (n = 62)
Bartonella species	12.4	28.4	0	9.5	22.6
Brucella melitensis	0	0	0	0	1.6
Chlamydia species	0	0	2.2	1.6	0
Corynebacterium species	0.5	0	1.1	0	1.6
Coxiella burnetii	37.0	48	7.9	12.7	3.2
Enterobacteriaceae	0.5	0	0	0	0
HACEK bacteria	0.5	0	0	0	3.2
Staphylococcus species	2.0	0	3.4	11.1	6.4
Streptococcus species	4.4	0	1.1	6.3	3.2
Tropheryma whipplei	2.6	0.3	0	0	0
Other bacteria	3.0	1.1	1.1	1.6	1.6
Fungi	1.0	0	0	6.3	1.6
No etiology	36.5	22.1	82.9	50.8	54.8

Note. Data are percentages. HACEK, Haemophilus, Actinobacillus, Cardiobacterium, Eikenella, Kingella.
Editor's Note: Please refer to original journal article for full references.
[a]Patients classified as excluded were not included in this analysis.

infective endocarditis cases.[1] The reasons for the variation in the incidence of negative blood cultures in different series may be differences in diagnostic criteria used, fastidious zoonotic agents, early use of antibiotics prior to drawing blood cultures, differences in timing of serologic testing,[2] or involvement of unknown organisms. This study is from an institution to which cases of BCNE are referred. The authors demonstrate the value of systematic serologic testing for not only various fastidious organisms such as *Coxiella burnetii* and *Bartonella* species but also *Brucella* species, *Legionella pneumophila*, and *Mycoplasma* species. Other methods that proved of value were histologic examination and molecular detection methods such as broad-range polymerase chain reaction, particularly when applied to excised valve tissue. Another useful tool in identifying the noninfectious cause of endocarditis was the detection of autoantibodies including rheumatoid factor, where 2.5% of the patients with BCNE were found to have marantic endocarditis, Libman-Sacks endocarditis, rheumatoid arthritis, and Behçet disease. Using this multimodal diagnostic strategy, they identified a causative microbial agent in 62.7% of 759 patients with BCNE and noninfective endocarditis in 2.5%. In hospitals where infective endocarditis is a relatively frequent problem, the physicians managing these patients should consult with their laboratory microbiologists whenever they have a case of BCNE and make certain that the patient has had the benefit of these latest techniques to make an etiologic diagnosis.

M. D. Cheitlin, MD

References

1. Brouqui P, Raoult D. Endocarditis due to rare and fastidious bacteria. *Clin Microbiol Rev.* 2001;14:177-207.
2. Raoult D, Casalta JP, Richet H, et al. Contribution of systematic serological testing in diagnosis of infective endocarditis. *J Clin Microbiol.* 2005;43:5238-5242.

45 Esophagus

Adherence and Adequacy of Therapy for Esophageal Varices Prophylaxis
Maddur H, Naik S, Siddiqui AA, et al (Univ of Texas Southwestern Med Ctr, Dallas)
Dig Dis Sci 2011 [Epub ahead of print]

Aims.—Esophageal varices (EVs) are prevalent among cirrhotics and their bleeding leads to substantial morbidity and mortality. Management guidelines available during this study recommended beta-blocker therapy for primary prophylaxis and beta-blocker or band ligation (EVL) for secondary prophylaxis. We evaluated prophylaxis practice patterns.

Methods.—We performed a retrospective cohort study of in and outpatient cirrhotics with known EVs at two University of Texas Southwestern teaching institutions. Use of prophylactic therapy and its adequacy (defined using published guidelines) was measured.

Results.—A total of 419 patients with cirrhosis and EVs warranting prophylaxis were identified, including 276 inpatients and 143 outpatients. Of those admitted with a first bleed (i.e. eligible for primary prophylactic therapy), 30/104 (29%) were on beta blocker. In this group, only 3/104 (3%) received optimal therapy (heart rate <55). Among inpatients with a previous EV bleed, 120/172 (70%) were on a beta blocker or had undergone EVL, although only 66/172 (38%) received optimal therapy. In the inpatient cohort, ten patients died of gastrointestinal hemorrhage, three of whom were receiving optimal therapy. Among outpatients, 94/121 (78%) without previous bleeding received primary prophylaxis and 20/22 (91%) of those with previous bleeding received some form of secondary prophylaxis. However, only 11 (9%) received adequate primary prophylaxis therapy, while 9 (41%) received appropriate secondary prophylaxis.

Conclusions.—Prophylaxis intent appears to be greatly improved compared to previous reports. However, implementation of optimal therapy appeared to be suboptimal. We conclude that efforts need to be made to ensure optimal treatment.

▶ Esophageal variceal hemorrhage remains a substantial cause of morbidity and mortality in patients with chronic liver disease. Current guidelines support the use of β-blockers to prevent bleeding. Although not addressed by this article and not part of current guidelines, there is also a growing body of evidence to support primary prophylaxis using esophageal variceal banding. Once a patient has bled, it has also been suggested that the majority of eligible patients get either no or insufficient prophylaxis (secondary). This study examined a large cohort of patients at a major teaching institution and found that there has been improvement in the proportion of patients getting primary or secondary prophylaxis (when compared with historical controls), but that the majority were not being optimally treated.

The authors suggest that the dissemination of treatment guidelines has resulted in the improvement seen in this study, although one cannot discount the fact that these data come from a major teaching institution and that internal education may be the real factor. While any treatment is superior to no treatment, very few of their patients were optimally treated. The most common issues were lack of follow-up after variceal banding and inadequate β-blocker therapy. Additional data should be obtained from community practices, and, if those results are similar or inferior to these, then additional education efforts are appropriate. The target is to obtain sufficient heart rate reduction (< 55) in all patients who tolerate β-blockers and to make sure that all patients who bled have at least 2 sessions of variceal banding (ideally banding continues until the varices are obliterated). It is likely that adherence to these guidelines will improve outcomes in this difficult-to-manage population.

K. R. DeVault, MD

ACCF/ACG/AHA 2010 Expert Consensus Document on the Concomitant Use of Proton Pump Inhibitors and Thienopyridines: A Focused Update of the ACCF/ACG/AHA 2008 Expert Consensus Document on Reducing the Gastrointestinal Risks of Antiplatelet Therapy and NSAID Use

Abraham NS, American College of Gastroenterology Representative, American College of Cardiology Foundation Representative, American Heart Association Representative (American College of Gastroenterology Representative, Bethesda, MD; et al)

Am J Gastroenterol 105:2533-2549, 2010

Background.—Expert consensus documents inform practitioners, payers, and other parties about changing areas of clinical practice or technological advances. Often the evidence base, experience with technology, or clinical practice has not yet developed to the point that a formal American College of Cardiology Foundation (ACCF) and American Heart Association (AHA) practice guideline can be formulated. These documents seek to inform clinical practice in the absence of rigorous evidence. The ACCF, AHA, and American College of Gastroenterology (ACG) issued an expert consensus document concerning the use of a proton pump inhibitor (PPI) in patients with risk factors for upper gastrointestinal (GI) bleeding who are receiving dual antiplatelet therapy, specifically thienopyridines and aspirin.

Major Findings and Recommendations.—Dual antiplatelet therapy with clopidogrel and aspirin reduces the number of major cardiovascular (CV) events compared to placebo or aspirin alone in patients who have established ischemic heart disease. This therapy also reduces coronary stent thrombosis. However, it is not recommended routinely for patients who have had an ischemic stroke because of the increased bleeding risk.

Clopidogrel, aspirin, and the combination of the two are all associated with an increased risk of GI bleeding. Patients who have had GI bleeding previously and are taking antiplatelet therapy are at the highest risk for recurrent bleeding. Higher risk is also associated with advanced age; concurrent use of anticoagulants, steroids, or nonsteroidal anti-inflammatory drugs (NSAIDs), including aspirin; and infection with *Helicobacter pylori.*

As the number of risk factors increases, so does the risk of GI bleeding. The risk of upper GI bleeding can be lowered by adding a PPI or a histamine H_2 receptor antagonist (H2RA). A comparison of PPIs and H2RAs shows that PPIs reduce upper GI bleeding more than H2RAs. PPIs are recommended for patients who have a history of upper GI bleeding and appropriate for those with multiple risk factors for GI bleeding who are taking antiplatelet therapy. The risk of complications must be weighed against the overall benefits of the PPI or H2RA treatment. Patients at lower risk for upper GI bleeding should not routinely receive a PPI or an H2RA because the potential for benefit is greatly reduced. The potential for both CV and GI complications must be considered. In addition, pharmacokinetic and pharmacodynamics studies using platelet assays as surrogate endpoints indicate that using clopidogrel and a PPI reduces the effectiveness of clopidogrel as an antiplatelet agent. Omeprazole and clopidogrel demonstrated the strongest interaction. The effect of using different surrogate endpoints is unknown. In addition, the effects on CV outcomes of concomitant use of thienopyridines and PPIs have been inconsistent in the available observational studies and single randomized clinical trial. Data are insufficient to rule out a clinically important interaction, especially in certain subgroups. Basing management decisions on either pharmacogenomic testing or platelet function testing is not currently feasible.

Conclusions.—PPIs and antiplatelet drugs are used together to reduce the higher risk of GI complications caused by the antiplatelet agents. GI protection is especially needed as the number of risk factors increases. Many gaps exist in the current knowledge about these agents and their interactions, so further research is needed.

▶ A potential negative interaction between proton pump inhibitors (PPIs) and activation of the antiplatelet agent clopidogrel has recently been reported and has led to a Food and Drug Administration black box warning on clopidogrel packaging. This is felt to be because of competitive inhibition of cytochrome CYP2C19, which is responsible for the metabolism of some PPIs and also for the activation of clopidogrel. This field is rapidly evolving, but the summary recommendations of this article are important for all physicians using these agents.

Summary of findings and consensus recommendations:

1. Clopidogrel reduces major cardiovascular (CV) events compared with placebo or aspirin.

2. Dual antiplatelet therapy with clopidogrel and aspirin, compared with aspirin alone, reduces major CV events in patients with established

ischemic heart disease, and it reduces coronary stent thrombosis but is not routinely recommended for patients with prior ischemic stroke because of the risk of bleeding.

3. Clopidogrel alone, aspirin alone, and their combination are all associated with increased risk of gastrointestinal (GI) bleeding.

4. Patients with prior GI bleeding are at highest risk for recurrent bleeding on antiplatelet therapy. Other clinical characteristics that increase the risk of GI bleeding include advanced age, concurrent use of anticoagulants, steroids, or nonsteroidal anti-inflammatory drugs, including aspirin, and *Helicobacter pylori* infection. The risk of GI bleeding increases as the number of risk factors increases.

5. Use of a PPI or histamine H_2 receptor antagonist (H2RA) reduces the risk of upper GI bleeding compared with no therapy. PPIs reduce upper GI bleeding to a greater degree than do H2RAs.

6. PPIs are recommended to reduce GI bleeding among patients with a history of upper GI bleeding. PPIs are appropriate in patients with multiple risk factors for GI bleeding who require antiplatelet therapy.

7. Routine use of either a PPI or an H2RA is not recommended for patients at lower risk of upper GI bleeding, who have much less potential to benefit from prophylactic therapy.

8. Clinical decisions regarding concomitant use of PPIs and thienopyridines must balance overall risks and benefits, considering both CV and GI complications.

9. Pharmacokinetic and pharmacodynamic studies, using platelet assays as surrogate end points, suggest that concomitant use of clopidogrel and a PPI reduces the antiplatelet effects of clopidogrel. The strongest evidence for an interaction is between omeprazole and clopidogrel. It is not established that changes in these surrogate end points translate into clinically meaningful differences.

10. Observational studies and a single randomized clinical trial have shown inconsistent effects on CV outcomes of concomitant use of thienopyridines and PPIs. A clinically important interaction cannot be excluded, particularly in certain subgroups, such as poor metabolizers of clopidogrel.

11. The role of either pharmacogenomic testing or platelet function testing in managing therapy with thienopyridines and PPIs has not yet been established.

Based on this article and others, the prudent approach is to avoid PPIs in patients who really do not need them and use PPIs carefully in those who require them for symptomatic control after an open discussion of the risks and benefits with the patient involved.

K. R. DeVault, MD

American Gastroenterological Association Medical Position Statement on the Management of Barrett's Esophagus

American Gastroenterological Association
Gastroenterology 140:1084-1091, 2011

Background.—A medical position statement issued by the American Gastroenterological Association Institute addresses the major clinical issues of treating patients with Barrett's esophagus. The condition was defined and recommendations for diagnosis and treatment offered.

Definition.—Barrett's esophagus is a condition in which any extent of metaplastic columnar epithelium that predisposes to the development of cancer replaces the stratified squamous epithelium naturally found lining the distal esophagus. Intestinal metaplasia is included in the definition, but cardia-type epithelium in the esophagus, while abnormal, is not because the degree of risk for malignancy with this type of epithelium is unknown. The traditional and still accepted endoscopic landmark that best identifies the level at which the esophagus ends and the stomach begins is the proximal extent of the gastric folds. Measuring and recording the extent of Barrett's metaplasia seen endoscopically is recommended and has clinical value. A diagnosis of Barrett's esophagus has marked influences on individual patients. The annual incidence of esophageal cancer is about 0.5%, but cardiovascular associations increase mortality, poor quality of life is common, and patients often suffer psychological stress and higher life and health insurance costs.

Recommendations.—Screening for Barrett's esophagus is recommended for patients with multiple risk factors related to esophageal adenocarcinoma but not for the general population with gastroesophageal reflux disease (GERD). Such factors include age 50 years or older, male gender, white race, chronic GERD, hiatal hernia, elevated body mass index, and intra-abdominal distribution of body fat. The diagnosis of dysplasia in Barrett's esophagus should be confirmed by two pathologists, at least one of whom is an expert in esophageal histopathology. For patients diagnosed with Barrett's esophagus, endoscopic surveillance is recommended every 3 to 5 years if there is no dysplasia, every 6 to 12 months if there is low-grade dysplasia, and every 3 months if there is high-grade dysplasia and no eradication therapy is performed. No molecular biomarkers provide sufficient predictive value to justify their use to either confirm the histologic diagnosis of dysplasia or contribute to risk stratification.

The biopsy protocol recommended for endoscopic surveillance of Barrett's esophagus should employ white light endoscopy and obtain four-quadrant biopsy specimens every 2 cm, except for patients with known or suspected dysplasia, whose specimens should be taken every 1 cm. Specific biopsy specimens of any mucosal irregularities should be submitted separately to the pathologist. Chromoendoscopy and advanced imaging techniques are not required for routine surveillance.

Measures not recommended for cancer prevention include eliminating esophageal acid exposure using proton pump inhibitors (PPIs) in doses exceeding once daily, esophageal pH monitoring to titrate PPI dosing, and antireflux surgery. Patients should be screened for cardiovascular risk factors treatable by aspirin therapy, but the use of aspirin solely to prevent esophageal adenocarcinoma with no other indications is not recommended. Endoscopic eradication therapy with radiofrequency ablation (RFA), photodynamic therapy (PDT), or endoscopic mucosal resection (EMR) is preferred to surveillance in patients with confirmed high-grade dysplasia in Barrett's esophagus. To determine the T stage of the neoplasia in patients with dysplasia in Barrett's esophagus and a visible mucosal irregularity, EMR is recommended, proving valuable as a diagnostic/staging procedure and a potentially therapeutic procedure.

Evidence indicates that complete eradication of all Barrett's epithelium is more effective therapeutically than removal of a localized area of dysplasia only. RFA and PDT achieve comparable efficacy, but RFA has fewer serious adverse effects. Treatment with eradication therapy is designed to achieve reversion to normal-appearing squamous epithelium throughout the length of the esophagus with no islands of buried intestinal metaplasia. RFA can produce this reversion in a high proportion of subjects at any stage of disease; the reversion lasts for up to 5 years. RFA therapy also reduces the progression to esophageal cancer in patients with high-grade dysplasia. If the patient has no dysplasia, endoscopic eradication therapy may be no more effective at reducing cancer risk and no more cost-effective than long-term endoscopic surveillance.

Conclusions.—The recommendations for clinical management of Barrett's esophagus are founded on the assumption that the diagnosis and the absence of low-grade and high-grade dysplasia are accurate to the highest degree possible according to the best current standards of practice. Over 90% of patients with low-grade dysplasia and 70% to 80% of patients who have high-grade dysplasia are successfully managed with endoscopic eradication therapy. Esophagectomy is another option, but should only be done at surgical centers that specialize in treating foregut cancers and high-grade dysplasia.

▶ A great deal of effort goes into the prevention of adenocarcinoma of the esophagus through the identification and surveillance of Barrett's esophagus (BE). The American Gastroenterological Association recently published these guidelines and a technical review article.[1] There were many consistencies and a few changes in the suggested approach to this condition compared with other recent statements. Endoscopic screening was suggested for gastroesophageal reflux disease (GERD) populations at increased risk for BE (particularly older white males with long-term GERD) but not the general population with GERD (other risk factors include elevated body mass index/abdominal obesity and hiatal hernia). Confirmation of dysplasia by expert pathologists was a recommendation. Suggested surveillance intervals for nondysplastic BE were expanded to 3 to 5 years, and low-grade intervals remained at 6 to 12 months. If surveillance was elected for high-grade dysplasia, it was suggested to be repeated on a 3-month interval. The standard 4-quadrant biopsy protocol obtained every 2 cm was advocated for nondysplastic BE with an increase to every 1 cm for dysplastic BE. In addition, any mucosal irregularity should be sampled separately. The Association did not feel that the data were strong enough to recommend routine high-dose proton pump inhibitor therapy or aspirin as chemopreventatives. Endoscopic mucosal resection was advocated for dysplastic lesions associated with a visible abnormality in a segment of BE. They suggested endoscopic ablation as the treatment of choice for high-grade dysplasia and a preferred approach compared with watchful waiting and esophagectomy.

K. R. DeVault, MD

Reference

1. Spechler SJ, Sharma P, Souza RF, Inadomi JM, Shaheen NJ. American Gastroenterological Association technical review on the management of Barrett's esophagus. *Gastroenterology.* 2011;140:e18-e52.

Acute development of gastroesophageal reflux after radiofrequency catheter ablation of atrial fibrillation
Martinek M, Hassanein S, Bencsik G, et al (Elisabethinen Univ Teaching Hosp, Linz, Austria; Univ of Szeged, Hungary)
Heart Rhythm 6:1457-1462, 2009

Background.—Induction of gastroesophageal reflux after radiofrequency catheter ablation (RFCA) of atrial fibrillation (AF) may have an impact on the progression of esophageal injury.

Objective.—The purpose of this study was to assess the acute effect of RFCA on distal esophageal acidity using leadless pH-metry capsules.

Methods.—A total of 31 patients (27 male and 4 female; 25 with paroxysmal AF) who underwent RFCA and esophagoscopy 24 hours before and after ablation were assessed for reflux and esophageal lesions. A leadless pH-metry capsule was inserted into the lower esophagus to screen for pH changes, number and duration of refluxes, and the DeMeester score (a standardized measure of acidity and reflux). No patient had a history of reflux or was taking proton pump inhibitors within 4 weeks before and 24 hours after ablation.

Results.—Five patients (16.1%) who presented with asymptomatic reflux prior to ablation were excluded from further examination. Of the remaining 26 patients, 5 (19.2%) demonstrated a significant pathologic increase in DeMeester score after ablation. No statistical differences in baseline parameters, method of sedation, ablation approach, and total energy delivered on the posterior wall were observed between patients with and those without a pathologic DeMeester score. One patient with asymptomatic reflux prior to ablation developed esophageal ulceration.

Conclusion.—A significant number of patients undergoing RFCA of AF develop pathologic acid reflux after ablation. In addition, a subgroup of patients has a preexisting condition of asymptomatic reflux prior to ablation. This finding may explain a potential mechanism for progression of esophageal injury to atrio-esophageal fistulas in patients undergoing RFCA.

▶ This small study performed ambulatory pH testing before and after radiofrequency ablation of atrial fibrillation. Approximately 20% of the patients demonstrated a significant increase in reflux as measured by the DeMeester score.

The esophagus and the heart are anatomically and embryologically connected. It is clear that chest pain may be produced by both organs and that stimulation of the organs produces similar symptoms. Catheter-based radiofrequency ablation of aberrant cardiac pathways has become commonly used. There have been reported gastrointestinal (GI) complications, including atrioesophageal fistulae and esophageal ulceration. These effects are local and likely related to direct trauma. Another possible mechanism of GI injury is inadvertent damage to esophageal nerves, either intramural or via vagal pathways. Gastroesophageal reflux (GER) is one possible complication of this therapy. While this study suggests a worsening in GER disease measurements after therapy in a small number of patients, one needs to consider the possibility that these changes are related to poor day-to-day reproducibility of pH monitoring, although if that were the case, then one would expect to see some patients actually get better on the second test. It would seem reasonable to consider proton pump inhibitor therapy after ablation and to be watchful for any new or worsened GI symptoms that may develop.

K. R. DeVault, MD

Gastroesophageal Reflux Symptoms in Patients With Celiac Disease and the Effects of a Gluten-Free Diet

Nachman F, Vázquez H, González A, et al (Dr C. Bonorino Udaondo Gastroenterology Hosp, Buenos Aires, Argentina)
Clin Gastroenterol Hepatol 9:214-219, 2011

Background & Aims.—Celiac disease (CD) patients often complain of symptoms consistent with gastroesophageal reflux disease (GERD). We aimed to assess the prevalence of GERD symptoms at diagnosis and to determine the impact of the gluten-free diet (GFD).

Methods.—We evaluated 133 adult CD patients at diagnosis and 70 healthy controls. Fifty three patients completed questionnaires every 3 months during the first year and more than 4 years after diagnosis. GERD symptoms were evaluated using a subdimension of the Gastrointestinal Symptoms Rating Scale for heartburn and regurgitation domains.

Results.—At diagnosis, celiac patients had a significantly higher reflux symptom mean score than healthy controls ($P < .001$). At baseline, 30.1% of CD patients had moderate to severe GERD (score >3) compared with 5.7% of controls ($P < .01$). Moderate to severe symptoms were significantly associated with the classical clinical presentation of CD (35.0%) compared with atypical/silent cases (15.2%; $P < .03$). A rapid improvement was evidenced at 3 months after initial treatment with a GFD ($P < .0001$) with reflux scores comparable to healthy controls from this time point onward.

Conclusions.—GERD symptoms are common in classically symptomatic untreated CD patients. The GFD is associated with a rapid and persistent improvement in reflux symptoms that resembles the healthy population.

► Symptoms from the upper gastrointestinal tract are often nonspecific. Gastroesophageal reflux disease (GERD), dyspepsia, gall bladder disease, and other disorders may present with similar and often overlapping presentations. This article provides further evidence for symptom overlap, this time between GERD and celiac disease (CD). They were able to demonstrate an increased prevalence of GERD symptoms in patients with CD compared with the control and, most importantly, demonstrated an impressive improvement in GERD symptoms once the patient was placed on a gluten-free diet.

How should we use these data? The data confirm that all heartburn is not caused by GERD. I suspect many of these patients could have been labeled refractory GERD and perhaps undergone additional tests and procedures had their CD not been diagnosed and treated. The mechanism of this association is not clear. It is possible that the GERD symptoms are nonspecific, but it is also possible that something related to the CD treatment is resulting in an actual decrease in gastroesophageal reflux. CD could adversely affect motility of the upper gastrointestinal tract either directly or perhaps because of some neurohumoral feedback mechanism. It is important to remember that these patients all had established CD and not to extrapolate into a routine search for CD in patients with reflux symptoms, although selective testing is certainly reasonable.

K. R. DeVault, MD

Laparoscopic Antireflux Surgery vs Esomeprazole Treatment for Chronic GERD: The LOTUS Randomized Clinical Trial
Galmiche J-P, for the LOTUS Trial Collaborators (Nantes Univ, France; et al)
JAMA 305:1969-1977, 2011

Context.—Gastroesophageal reflux disease (GERD) is a chronic, relapsing disease with symptoms that have negative effects on daily life. Two treatment options are long-term medication or surgery.

Objective.—To evaluate optimized esomeprazole therapy vs standardized laparoscopic antireflux surgery (LARS) in patients with GERD.

Design, Setting, and Participants.—The LOTUS trial, a 5-year exploratory randomized, open, parallel-group trial conducted in academic hospitals in 11 European countries between October 2001 and April 2009 among 554 patients with well-established chronic GERD who initially responded to acid suppression. A total of 372 patients (esomeprazole, n=192; LARS, n=180) completed 5-year follow-up.

Interventions.—Two hundred sixty-six patients were randomly assigned to receive esomeprazole, 20 to 40 mg/d, allowing for dose adjustments;

288 were randomly assigned to undergo LARS, of whom 248 actually underwent the operation.

Main Outcome Measure.—Time to treatment failure (for LARS, defined as need for acid suppressive therapy; for esomeprazole, inadequate symptom control after dose adjustment), expressed as estimated remission rates and analyzed using the Kaplan-Meier method.

Results.—Estimated remission rates at 5 years were 92% (95% confidence interval [CI], 89%-96%) in the esomeprazole group and 85% (95% CI, 81%-90%) in the LARS group (log-rank $P=.048$). The difference between groups was no longer statistically significant following best-case scenario modeling of the effects of study dropout. The prevalence and severity of symptoms at 5 years in the esomeprazole and LARS groups, respectively, were 16% and 8% for heartburn ($P=.14$), 13% and 2% for acid regurgitation ($P<.001$), 5% and 11% for dysphagia ($P<.001$), 28% and 40% for bloating ($P<.001$), and 40% and 57% for flatulence ($P<.001$). Mortality during the study was low (4 deaths in the esomeprazole group and 1 death in the LARS group) and not attributed to treatment, and the percentages of patients reporting serious adverse events were similar in the esomeprazole group (24.1%) and in the LARS group (28.6%).

Conclusion.—This multicenter clinical trial demonstrated that with contemporary antireflux therapy for GERD, either by drug-induced acid suppression with esomeprazole or by LARS, most patients achieve and remain in remission at 5 years.

Trial Registration.—clinicaltrials.gov Identifier: NCT00251927.

▶ When patients have well-documented chronic gastroesophageal reflux disease (GERD), management options include long-term proton pump inhibitor (PPI) therapy or surgical intervention. The advent of a laparoscopic approach to GERD has resulted in an increase in the use of this therapy. This article reports on more than 370 patients who were randomized to undergo laparoscopic anti-reflux surgery (LARS) or maintained on chronic esomeprazole (ESO) therapy. The remission rates between the groups were not statistically different (LARS 85%, ESO 92%), but there were other trends in the data. LARS was superior at controlling acid regurgitation at the cost of an increased rate of dyspahgia, bloating, and flatulence. Serious adverse events and mortality were no different.

How should we use these data? First, this study was actually not powered to find a difference and was labeled as "exploratory." That being said, the study does provide important, suggestive data. Second, these are clearly optimally treated patients. LARS was carried out by expert surgeons, and the medication was managed by study coordinators; both of these practices do not reflect the typical practice (at least in the United States), where the majority of surgeries are carried out by low-volume, less-experienced surgeons and it has been documented that a significant percentage of patients do not take their medications optimally. In any trial of this type, the end points for medical and surgical treatment are, by nature, different. Patients in the ESO group were started on 20 mg daily; but if they had breakthrough symptoms, they were escalated to 40 mg daily followed by 20 mg twice daily prior to being considered a failure.

To fail in the LARS group, you had to either be restarted on PPI therapy or have unacceptable side effects (none of the ESO patients failed because of side effects). Where do these data leave us? First, patients should understand that either treatment is generally effective. If acid regurgitation is the major symptom, then surgery may be superior. What is also clear from this study, and other studies, is that the side-effect profile of surgery is inferior to medical therapy, and patients must understand this going into this procedure or any other invasive procedure for which there is a similarly effective medical option.

K. R. DeVault, MD

Coffee intake and oral—oesophageal cancer: follow-up of 389 624 Norwegian men and women 40–45 years
Tverdal A, Hjellvik V, Selmer R (Norwegian Inst of Public Health, Nydalen, Oslo, Norway)
Br J Cancer 105:157-161, 2011

Background.—The evidence on the relationship between coffee intake and cancer of the oral cavity and oesophagus is conflicting and few follow-up studies have been done.

Methods.—A total of 389 624 men and women 40–45 years who participated in a national survey programme were followed with respect to cancer for an average of 14.4 years by linkage to the Cancer Registry of Norway. Coffee consumption at baseline was reported as a categorical variable (0 or <1 cup, 1–4, 5–8, 9+ cups per day).

Results.—Altogether 450 squamous oral or oesophageal cancers were registered during follow-up. The adjusted hazard ratios with 1–4 cups per day as reference were 1.01 (95% confidence interval: 0.70, 1.47), 1.16 (0.93, 1.45) and 0.96 (0.71, 1.14) for 0 or <1 cup, 5–8 and 9+ cups per day, respectively. Stratification by sex, type of coffee, smoking status and dividing the end point into oral and oesophageal cancers gave heterogeneous and non-significant estimates.

Conclusion.—This study does not support an inverse relationship between coffee intake and incidence of cancer in the mouth or oesophagus, but cannot exclude a weak inverse relationship.

▶ The affects of coffee consumption on the gastrointestinal tract have been long debated. Coffee and caffeine intake are thought to be risk factors for gastroesophageal reflux disease (GERD), and, therefore, one might assume that they would increase the risk of esophageal adenocarcinoma. In addition, some studies have suggested that high-temperature drinks may increase the risk of esophageal cancer. On the other hand, there are some data suggesting a protective effect against cancer of the esophagus and other organs in patients with moderate amounts of coffee intake. This large registry from Scandinavia was able to address this issue and found that coffee intake had no affect (positive or negative) on the risk of esophageal and oral carcinomas. There were some other interesting associations in the study. Heavy coffee users were more likely to be men, smokers, and heavier alcohol users, but they were less likely to be highly educated or physically active. Based on these data and others, we should continue to suggest moderation in coffee and caffeine intake in our patients with symptomatic GERD, but we should also counsel that there is little chance that this beverage changes the risk for esophageal cancer.

K. R. DeVault, MD

Esophageal Eosinophilic Infiltration Responds to Proton Pump Inhibition in Most Adults

Molina-Infante J, Ferrando-Lamana L, Ripoll C, et al (Hosp San Pedro de Alcantara, Caceres, Spain; Hosp Gregorio Marañon, Madrid, Spain)
Clin Gastroenterol Hepatol 9:110-117, 2011

Background & Aims.—Despite consensus recommendations, eosinophilic esophagitis (EoE) is commonly diagnosed upon esophageal eosinophilic infiltration (EEI; based on ≥15 eosinophils per high power field; eo/HPF). We evaluated the prevalence of EEI before and after proton pump inhibitor (PPI) therapy and assessed the accuracy of EEI and pH monitoring analyses.

Methods.—Biopsies were taken from the upper-middle esophagus of 712 adults with upper gastrointestinal symptoms who were referred for endoscopy due to upper gastrointestinal symptoms. Patients with EEI were treated with rabeprazole (20 mg, twice daily) for 2 months. EoE was defined by persistent symptoms and >15 eo/HPF following PPI therapy.

Results.—Thirty-five patients (4.9%) had EEI, of whom 55% had a history of allergies, and 70% had food impaction or dysphagia as their primary complaint. Twenty-six EEI patients (75%) achieved clinicopathological remission with PPI therapy; of these, 17 had GERD-like profile (EEI <35 eo/HPF and objective evidence of reflux, based on endoscopy or pH monitoring), and 9 had EoE-like profile (EEI 35−165 eo/HPF, typical EoE symptoms and endoscopic findings). The PPI response was 50% in the EoE-like profile patients. The PPI-response was 50% in EoE-like profile patients. Likewise, PPI-responsive EEI occurred with normal (33%) and pathologic (80%) pH monitoring. Higher histologic cut-off values improved specificity and positive predictive for EoE (35%−35% for >20 eo/HPF; 46%−39% for >24 eo/HPF; 65%−50% for 35 eo/HPF).

Conclusions.—In adults with EEI, 75% of unselected patients and 50% with an EoE phenotype respond to PPI therapy; pH monitoring is poorly predictive of response. Patients with PPI-responsive EEI >35 eo/HPF are phenotypically undistinguishable from EoE patients. EoE might be overestimated without clinical and pathologic follow-up of patient response to PPI.

▶ Eosinophilic esophagitis (EOE) is a commonly diagnosed condition in both children and adults, which is diagnosed based on eosinophilic infiltration (EEI) on examination of esophageal biopsies. There is considerable controversy about the best initial treatment of these patients; some experts suggest a trial of proton pump inhibitors (PPIs) and others suggest topical steroids. This study found that most patients with EOE respond to a course of PPIs. They also divided their patients into those whose symptoms and endoscopic findings were more GERD-like and those with a more typical EOE symptom (usually dysphagia) and endoscopic presentation. Both groups had at least a 50% response, but the response rate was higher in those who were more GERD-like. Interestingly, ambulatory pH testing did not predict whether the patients were going to respond to PPI treatment.

In this important study, the authors attempt to make a case that patients with EEI who respond to PPI do not have EOE. I do not think that can be clearly inferred from this study, and there are some emerging data that PPIs may actually downregulate some inflammatory markers seen in EOE independent of their affect on gastric acid.[1] The best we can say is that EOE symptoms (both typical and atypical) may respond to PPIs. The fact that pH results did not predict the response to PPIs is both surprising and troubling. It is possible that the pH test is not sufficiently sensitive in this population or that reflux amounts less than those usually considered abnormal might influence this particular population. Future studies are needed to confirm and expand these findings. The take-home message is a reinforcement of the concept that a trial of PPIs is an acceptable and perhaps preferred initial approach to most patients with EOE.

K. R. DeVault, MD

Reference

1. Cortes JR, Rivas MD, Molina-Infante J, et al. Omeprazole inhibits IL-4 and IL-13 signaling signal transducer and activator of transcription 6 activation and reduces lung inflammation in murine asthma. *J Allergy Clin Immunol.* 2009;124:607-610.

Budesonide Is Effective in Adolescent and Adult Patients With Active Eosinophilic Esophagitis

Straumann A, Conus S, Degen L, et al (Univ Hosp Basel, Switzerland; Univ of Bern, Switzerland; et al)
Gastroenterology 139:1526-1537, 2010

Background & Aims.—Eosinophilic esophagitis (EoE) is a chronic inflammatory disease of the esophagus characterized by dense tissue eosinophilia; it is refractory to proton pump inhibitor therapy. EoE affects all age groups but most frequently individuals between 20 and 50 years of age. Topical corticosteroids are effective in pediatric patients with EoE, but no controlled studies of corticosteroids have been reported in adult patients.

Methods.—We performed a randomized, double-blind, placebo-controlled trial to evaluate the effect of oral budesonide (1 mg twice daily for 15 days) in adolescent and adult patients with active EoE. Pretreatment and posttreatment disease activity was assessed clinically, endoscopically, and histologically. The primary end point was reduced mean numbers of eosinophils in the esophageal epithelium (number per highpower field

[hpf] = esophageal eosinophil load). Esophageal biopsy and blood samples were analyzed using immunofluorescence and immunoassays, respectively, for biomarkers of inflammation and treatment response.

Results.—A 15-day course of therapy significantly decreased the number of eosinophils in the esophageal epithelium in patients given budesonide (from 68.2 to 5.5 eosinophils/hpf; $P < .0001$) but not in the placebo group (from 62.3 to 56.5 eosinophils/hpf; $P = .48$). Dysphagia scores significantly improved among patients given budesonide compared with those given placebo (5.61 vs 2.22; $P < .0001$). White exudates and red furrows were reversed in patients given budesonide, based on endoscopy examination. Budesonide, but not placebo, also reduced apoptosis of epithelial cells and molecular remodeling events in the esophagus; no serious adverse events were observed.

Conclusions.—A 15-day course of treatment with budesonide is well tolerated and highly effective in inducing a histologic and clinical remission in adolescent and adult patients with active EoE.

▶ Eosinophilic esophagitis (EOE) is a commonly diagnosed condition in both children and adults. Treatment options include proton pump inhibitors (PPIs), topical steroids, and esophageal dilation (if dysphagia is the predominant symptom). Budesonide is a poorly absorbed steroid with limited side effects, which is readily available in a liquid formulation and would seem to be an ideal candidate for treating EOE topically. This agent produced both a decrease in esophageal eosinophils and an improvement in dysphagia when compared with placebo.[1]

If topical steroids are to be used in EOE, they could be used as a first-line therapy, as a second-line therapy for patients who fail a trial of PPIs, or either before or after the planned esophageal dilation. Unfortunately, both the exact role for topical steroids and the dosage and duration of EOE therapy are not clear. This study used 1 mg of budesonide twice daily for 15 days, whereas some others have used a lower dosage (500 μg) twice daily for 4 to 6 weeks. It is clear that the available data are not strong enough to make a strong recommendation either on dosage or duration. On the other hand, if topical steroids are to be used, budesonide seems to be a logical and reasonable agent for this indication. Although these authors used this agent in its liquid form, others have combined it with a sucralose-based product (Splenda in the United States) and have patients swallow this to possibly help with adherence to the esophageal mucosa.

K. R. DeVault, MD

Reference

1. Dohil R, Newbury R, Fox L, Bastian J, Aceves S. Oral viscous budesonide is effective in children with eosinophilic esophagitis in a randomized, placebo-controlled trial. *Gastroenterology.* 2010;139:418-429.

46 Gastrointestinal Cancers and Benign Polyps

Long-term effect of aspirin on colorectal cancer incidence and mortality: 20-year follow-up of five randomised trials
Rothwell PM, Wilson M, Elwin C-E, et al (Univ of Oxford, UK; Karolinska Institutet, Stockholm, Sweden; et al)
Lancet 376:1741-1750, 2010

Background.—High-dose aspirin (≥ 500 mg daily) reduces long-term incidence of colorectal cancer, but adverse effects might limit its potential for long-term prevention. The long-term effectiveness of lower doses (75—300 mg daily) is unknown. We assessed the effects of aspirin on incidence and mortality due to colorectal cancer in relation to dose, duration of treatment, and site of tumour.

Methods.—We followed up four randomised trials of aspirin versus control in primary (Thrombosis Prevention Trial, British Doctors Aspirin Trial) and secondary (Swedish Aspirin Low Dose Trial, UK-TIA Aspirin Trial) prevention of vascular events and one trial of different doses of aspirin (Dutch TIA Aspirin Trial) and established the effect of aspirin on risk of colorectal cancer over 20 years during and after the trials by analysis of pooled individual patient data.

Results.—In the four trials of aspirin versus control (mean duration of scheduled treatment 6·0 years), 391 (2·8%) of 14033 patients had colorectal cancer during a median follow-up of 18·3 years. Allocation to aspirin reduced the 20-year risk of colon cancer (incidence hazard ratio [HR] 0·76, 0·60—0·96, p=0·02; mortality HR 0·65, 0·48—0·88, p=0·005), but not rectal cancer (0·90, 0·63—1·30, p=0·58; 0·80, 0·50—1·28, p=0·35). Where subsite data were available, aspirin reduced risk of cancer of the proximal colon (0·45, 0·28—0·74, p=0·001; 0·34, 0·18—0·66, p=0·001), but not the distal colon (1·10, 0·73—1·64, p=0·66; 1·21, 0·66—2·24, p=0·54; for incidence difference p=0·04, for mortality difference p=0·01). However, benefit increased with scheduled duration of treatment, such that allocation to aspirin of 5 years or longer reduced risk of proximal colon cancer by about 70% (0·35, 0·20—0·63; 0·24, 0·11—0·52; both p<0·0001) and also reduced risk of

429

rectal cancer (0·58, 0·36—0·92, p=0·02; 0·47, 0·26—0·87, p=0·01). There was no increase in benefit at doses of aspirin greater than 75 mg daily, with an absolute reduction of 1·76% (0·61—2·91; p=0·001) in 20-year risk of any fatal colorectal cancer after 5-years scheduled treatment with 75—300 mg daily. However, risk of fatal colorectal cancer was higher on 30 mg versus 283 mg daily on long-term follow-up of the Dutch TIA trial (odds ratio 2·02, 0·70—6·05, p=0·15).

Interpretation.—Aspirin taken for several years at doses of at least 75 mg daily reduced long-term incidence and mortality due to colorectal cancer. Benefit was greatest for cancers of the proximal colon, which are not otherwise prevented effectively by screening with sigmoidoscopy or colonoscopy (Table 3).

▶ For decades, aspirin has been recognized as potential chemoprevention for colorectal cancer (CRC). In many respects it is an ideal agent because it is widely available, simple to administer (once-daily dosing), and inexpensive. Multiple lines of epidemiologic, cohort, and retrospective evidence support the concept that aspirin and related inhibitors of cyclo-oxygenase II reduce the rate and mortality of CRC. Because development of CRC is relatively uncommon and takes many years, trials in this field have used adenoma recurrence rates after colonoscopic polypectomy as a surrogate for cancer prevention. These studies have consistently demonstrated a reduction in recurrence of approximately 20%.

Multiple trials with placebo control in prevention of vascular disease have enrolled large numbers of patients on a variety of doses of aspirin. Long-term

TABLE 3.—Effect of Aspirin (75—1200 mg) Versus Control on Long-Term Risk of Colorectal Cancer

		All Patients Hazard Ratio			Scheduled Treatment Duration ≥5 Years Hazard Ratio		
	Events	(95% CI)	p		Events	(95% CI)	p
All cancers	397	0·76 (0·63-0·94)	0·01	316	0·68 (0·54-0·87)	0·002
Proximal colon	69	0·45 (0·28-0·74)	0·001	61	0·35 (0·20-0·63)	<0·0001
Distal colon	100	1·10 (0·73-1·64)	0·66	75	1·14 (0·69-1·86)	0·61
Colon (site unspecified)	109	0·74 (0·51-1·07)	0·11	93	0·81 (0·52-1·25)	0·34
All colon	278	0·76 (0·60-0·96)	0·02	229	0·75 (0·58-0·97)	0·03
Rectum	119	0·90 (0·63-1·30)	0·58	87	0·58 (0·36-0·92)	0·02
Fatal cancers	240	0·66 (0·52-0·86)	0·002	193	0·57 (0·42-0·78)	<0·0001
Proximal colon	41	0·34 (0·18-0·66)	0·001	37	0·24 (0·11-0·52)	<0·0001
Distal colon	44	1·21 (0·66-2·24)	0·54	30	1·24 (0·58-2·65)	0·58
Colon (site unspecified)	89	0·61 (0·40-0·94)	0·02	75	0·71 (0·44-1·17)	0·18
All colon	174	0·65 (0·48-0·88)	0·005	142	0·63 (0·45-0·87)	0·006
Rectum	70	0·80 (0·50—1·28)	0·35	54	0·47 (0·26-0·87)	0·01

Numbers differ slightly from those quoted for case-fatality in the main text because of inclusion of data from SALT. Stratified by site of tumour and by scheduled duration of treatment allocated in the initial randomised trial in a pooled analysis (Cox regression, stratified by trial) of the Thrombosis Prevention Trial, the Swedish Aspirin Low Dose Trial (SALT), the UK-TIA Aspirin Trial, and the British Doctors Aspirin Trial. The p values are taken from a Cox model stratified by study and the analysis of patients with longer scheduled trial treatments includes all events from the time of random assignment. The p values therefore differ slightly from those obtained from the log-rank test in analyses from different timepoints in figure 2. Two colorectal cancers at different sites are included in four patients in whom it was not possible to establish which cancer was responsible for death.

follow-up of 2 such studies showed a reduction in CRC risk, but the dose of aspirin was high (500 mg/d or higher). Bleeding complications associated with this dose of aspirin could negate the protective effect and limit the potential for chemoprevention. For example, the bleeding risk associated with daily aspirin use (including hemorrhagic stroke) makes the recommendation for daily acetylsalicylic acid prophylaxis against myocardial infarction, a much more common lethal condition than CRC, a controversial recommendation in average-risk subjects. Thus, although the complication rate of daily aspirin is definitely dose-dependent, the effect of dose on risk of CRC is unknown.

Indirect observational studies have suggested that higher doses of aspirin were necessary, and 2 large trials of low-dose alternate-day aspirin failed to show protection against CRC. However, the duration of the follow-up was 10 years, which may be insufficient to demonstrate a protective effect for cancer.

To try to address these deficiencies, these European authors examined the outcomes of 5 randomized trials of daily aspirin of various doses and obtained CRC rates after 20 years of follow-up. This important study made several key points highlighted in Table 3 from the article. Doses as low as 75 mg per day lowered the risk of CRC, which was almost exclusively due to reductions in right-sided colon cancer. The observation that mortality was reduced more than incidence suggests that aspirin might mitigate against the aggressiveness of CRC, perhaps especially proximal cancers that have a distinct pathobiology and are difficult to detect with colonoscopy.

Overall, the relative 70% and absolute 1.5% reduction in CRC mortality has implications for clinical practice. In patients with a secondary indication for antiplatelet treatment, aspirin should be favored over other drugs. Furthermore, reduced CRC mortality must be calculated in the finely balanced analysis of reduced cardiovascular mortality with major bleeding risk; this additional benefit of aspirin could tip the balance in favor of more patients qualifying for treatment. Finally, from an endoscopist's point of view, the importance of right-sided colon cancer prevention cannot be overemphasized. The failure of colonoscopy and polypectomy to reduce proximal colon cancer has been a consistent finding in recent large-scale observational studies. Daily aspirin combined with colonoscopy (possibly with less frequent surveillance intervals) could be synergistic and improve outcomes at reduced cost for CRC screening.

R. K. Pearson, MD

Feasibility and Yield of Screening in Relatives From Familial Pancreatic Cancer Families

Ludwig E, Olson SH, Bayuga S, et al (Memorial Sloan-Kettering Cancer Ctr, NY)
Am J Gastroenterol 106:946-954, 2011

Objectives.—Pancreatic adenocarcinoma is a lethal disease. Over 80% of patients are found to have metastatic disease at the time of diagnosis. Strategies to improve disease-specific outcome include identification and early detection of precursor lesions or early cancers in high-risk groups. In this study, we investigate whether screening at-risk relatives of familial pancreatic cancer (FPC) patients is safe and has significant yield.

Methods.—We enrolled 309 asymptomatic at-risk relatives into our Familial Pancreatic Tumor Registry (FPTR) and offered them screening with magnetic resonance cholangiopancreaticogram (MRCP) followed by endoscopic ultrasound (EUS) with fine needle aspiration if indicated. Relatives with findings were referred for surgical evaluation.

Results.—As of 1 August 2009, 109 relatives had completed at least one cycle of screening. Abnormal radiographic findings were present on initial screening in 18/109 patients (16.5%), 15 of whom underwent EUS. A significant abnormality was confirmed in 9 of 15 patients, 6 of whom ultimately had surgery for an overall diagnostic yield of 8.3% (9/109). Yield was greatest in relatives >65 years old (35%, 6/17) when compared with relatives 55–65 years (3%, 1/31) and relatives <55 years (3%, 2/61).

Conclusions.—Screening at-risk relatives from FPC families has a significant diagnostic yield, particularly in relatives >65 years of age, confirming prior studies. MRCP as initial screening modality is safe and effective.

▶ Pancreatic cancer (PC) is a devastating illness with a very poor prognosis. Established risk factors for the disease include advancing age, smoking, obesity, and a family history of pancreatic cancer. A positive family history is present in approximately 10% of patients with PC. None of these risk factors has an absolute risk high enough to warrant screening for the disease. Furthermore, there is no serologic test of sufficient accuracy to enrich a population for more expensive or invasive imaging tests, such as CT, MRI, or endoscopic ultrasound scan.

Familial PC is defined by multiple first-degree relatives (generally, 2 or more, or 1 under the age of 50) with PC and no known cancer syndrome. Because of their high absolute risk of PC, these kindreds have been studied in multiple centers in trials of screening. In this study from Memorial Sloan Kettering, 109 kindred members underwent screening initially with magnetic resonance cholangiopancreaticogram (MRCP), and if abnormal ductal changes were identified, endoscopic ultrasound scan (EUS) was performed. Patients with any suspicious lesions determined by cytology or carcinoembryonic antigen levels in aspirated cysts were seen in consultation by surgeons.

While the title of the article and conclusion suggest that the yield in these families is high, skeptics would counter with several cautions. First, only 1 invasive cancer was identified, and 5 other patients underwent resection for premalignant lesions, primarily dysplastic intraductal papillary mucinous neoplasia (IPMN) of the branch duct variety. These are quite common in the general population, and their management and risk are controversial subjects. Whether IPMN represents a higher risk for patients with a family history of PC remains to be established. Second, the false-positive rate for the MRCP screening was approximately 50%. Finally, all of the patients with significant findings on MRCP and EUS were identified on the initial screening round of testing. The role of surveillance in these kindreds remains completely unknown.

While it is tempting to offer screening for patients fearful of this disease because of a family history, this article should inspire caution. PC screening should not be undertaken outside of centers engaged in prospective clinical trials.

R. K. Pearson, MD

47 Gastrointestinal Motility Disorders/ Neurogastroenterology

Esomeprazole With Clopidogrel Reduces Peptic Ulcer Recurrence, Compared With Clopidogrel alone, in Patients With Atherosclerosis
Hsu P-I, Lai K-H, Liu C-P (Chia-Nan Univ of Pharmacy and Science, Tainan, Taiwan; Kaohsiung Veterans General Hosp and Natl Yang-Ming Univ, Taiwan)
Gastroenterology 140:791-798, 2011

Background & Aims.—We performed a prospective, randomized, controlled study to compare the combination of esomeprazole and clopidogrel vs clopidogrel alone in preventing recurrent peptic ulcers in patients with atherosclerosis and a history of peptic ulcers. We also investigated the effects of esomeprazole on the antiplatelet action of clopidogrel.

Methods.—From January 2008 to January 2010, long-term clopidogrel users with histories of peptic ulcers who did not have peptic ulcers at an initial endoscopy examination were assigned randomly to receive the combination of esomeprazole (20 mg/day, before breakfast) and clopidogrel (75 mg/day, at bedtime), or clopidogrel alone for 6 months. A follow-up endoscopy examination was performed at the end of the sixth month and whenever severe symptoms occurred. Platelet aggregation tests were performed on days 1 and 28 for 42 consecutive patients who participated in the pharmacodynamic study.

Results.—The cumulative incidence of recurrent peptic ulcer during the 6-month period was 1.2% among patients given the combination of esomeprazole and clopidogrel (n = 83) and 11.0% among patients given clopidogrel alone (n = 82) (difference, 9.8%; 95% confidence interval, 2.6%−17.0%; *P* =.009). In the group given the combination therapy, there were no differences in the percentages of aggregated platelets on days 1 and 28 (31.0% ± 20.5% vs 30.1% ± 16.5%).

Conclusions.—Among patients with atherosclerosis and a history of peptic ulcers, the combination of esomeprazole and clopidogrel reduced

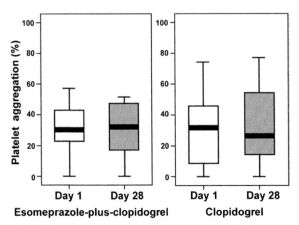

FIGURE 1.—Mean ADP-induced platelet aggregation on days 1 and 28. In the esomeprazole-plus-clopidogrel group, there were no differences between the PPAs on day 1 and day 28 (31.0% vs 30.1%; $P =.851$). In the clopidogrel group, the PPAs on days 1 and 28 also were similar (32.8% vs 35.0%; 95% confidence interval, -13.2 to 8.7; $P =.675$). In addition, there were no differences in the mean PPA between the 2 groups of patients on either day 1 or day 28. (Reprinted from Hsu P-I, Lai K-H, Liu C-P. Esomeprazole with clopidogrel reduces peptic ulcer recurrence, compared with clopidogrel alone, in patients with atherosclerosis. *Gastroenterology.* 2011;140:791-798, Copyright 2011, with permission from the AGA Institute.)

recurrence of peptic ulcers, compared with clopidogrel alone. Esomeprazole does not influence the action of clopidogrel on platelet aggregation (Fig 1).

▶ Clipodogrel may be slightly more effective than aspirin in the prevention of overall ischemic events, but what are the upper gastrointestinal (GI) risks, and how are these best prevented in clinical practice? Clopidogrel can induce upper GI bleeding, and this study suggests that 11% of patients with a peptic ulcer disease history may develop recurrent peptic ulceration from long-term use of clopidogrel. Prevention of peptic ulceration may be problematic because of concerns about an interaction between clopidogrel and proton pump inhibitors (PPIs) (omeprazole is both a substrate and an inhibitor of CYP2C19 and in vitro has been shown to decrease clopidogrel's inhibitory effect on platelets, leading to a potential loss of benefit of clopidogrel). In the current trial, ulcer disease was largely prevented by coadministration of a PPI (esomeprazole), and this was safe with no increase in ischemic events in the combination arm (although here the study was underpowered). Notably in this study, the patients were instructed to take esomeprazole before breakfast and clopidogrel at bedtime based on their half-lives, and no interaction was detected (Fig 1). A 14- to 16-hour separation may help minimize any theoretical interaction, although the jury is out whether this potential interaction is clinically relevant anyway, despite the current Food and Drug Administration warning. For example, a major trial failed to show any increase in cardiovascular events in the clopidogrel-omeprazole arm.[1] However, it seems reasonable not to prescribe a PPI to patients on clopidogrel who do not have any major indication for therapy, but in those at high risk of ulcer complications, PPI therapy should still be considered. Nonetheless, avoidance of omeprazole (and the isomer esomeprazole) and separating the dosing would be sensible based on current knowledge.

N. J. Talley, MD, PhD

Reference

1. Bhatt DL, Cryer BL, Contant CF, et al. Clopidogrel with or without omeprazole in coronary artery disease. *N Engl J Med.* 2010;363:1909-1917.

Prevention of peptic ulcers with esomeprazole in patients at risk of ulcer development treated with low-dose acetylsalicylic acid: A randomised, controlled trial (OBERON)
Scheiman JM, Devereaux PJ, Herlitz J, et al (Univ of Michigan Med Ctr, Ann Arbor; McMaster Univ, Hamilton, Ontario, Canada; Sahlgrenska Univ Hosp, Gothenburg, Sweden; et al)
Heart 97:797-802, 2011

Objective.—To determine whether once-daily esomeprazole 40 mg or 20 mg compared with placebo reduces the incidence of peptic ulcers over 26 weeks of treatment in patients taking low-dose acetylsalicylic acid (ASA) and who are at risk for ulcer development.

Design.—Multinational, randomised, blinded, parallel-group, placebo-controlled trial.

Setting.—Cardiology, primary care and gastroenterology centres (n=240).

Patients.—*Helicobacter pylori*-negative patients taking daily low-dose ASA (75—325 mg), who fulfilled one or more of the following criteria: age ≥18 years with history of uncomplicated peptic ulcer; age ≥60 years with either stable coronary artery disease, upper gastrointestinal symptoms and five or more gastric/duodenal erosions, or low-dose ASA treatment initiated within 1 month of randomisation; or age ≥65 years. All patients were ulcer-free at study entry.

Interventions.—Once-daily, blinded treatment with esomeprazole 40 mg, 20 mg or placebo for 26 weeks.

Main Outcome Measures.—The primary end point was the occurrence of endoscopy-confirmed peptic ulcer over 26 weeks.

Results.—A total of 2426 patients (52% men; mean age 68 years) were randomised. After 26 weeks, esomeprazole 40 mg and 20 mg significantly reduced the cumulative proportion of patients developing peptic ulcers; 1.5% of esomeprazole 40 mg and 1.1% of esomeprazole 20 mg recipients, compared with 7.4% of placebo recipients, developed peptic ulcers (both p<0.0001 vs placebo). Esomeprazole was generally well tolerated.

Conclusions.—Acid-suppressive treatment with once-daily esomeprazole 40 mg or 20 mg reduces the occurrence of peptic ulcers in patients at risk for ulcer development who are taking low-dose ASA (Fig 2).

▶ Low-dose aspirin is known to reduce cardiovascular risk, but there is a price: increased gastrointestinal (GI) toxicity—in particular, peptic ulcer disease and

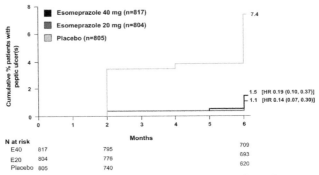

FIGURE 2.—Cumulative percentage of patients with peptic ulcer(s) by week 26 (intention-to-treat population, Kaplane–Meier curve). (Reprinted from Scheiman JM, Devereaux PJ, Herlitz J, et al. Prevention of peptic ulcers with esomeprazole in patients at risk of ulcer development treated with low-dose acetylsalicylic acid: a randomised, controlled trial (OBERON). *Heart.* 2011;97:797-802 Copyright 2011, with permission from the BMJ Publishing Group Ltd.)

upper GI bleeding. Enteric coating or buffering aspirin probably provides no additional protection. Concomitant *Helicobacter pylori* infection, advanced age, and a past history of peptic ulcer increase the risk of ulcer disease on aspirin, which is often silent in the elderly until bleeding occurs. In the present study, patients at increased risk of ulceration but who were serologically *H pylori* negative were randomized to the proton pump inhibitor (PPI) esomeprazole 40 mg and 20 mg once daily or placebo over 6 months. They observed that PPIs reduced the incidence of endoscopy-confirmed peptic ulcer disease versus placebo, but a higher dose added no benefit (Fig 2). These observations confirm other trial data,[1] and presumably the findings translate into lower ulcer complications on PPIs as well, although the study was not powered to detect such uncommon events. The PPIs produced similar protection in those taking higher doses (up to 325 mg) and lower doses (75–100 mg) of aspirin. About 20% of patients who were truly *H pylori* infected were accidentally included in the study (because they had false-negative *H pylori* serology results), but the PPI was equally protective in *H pylori*-positive and -negative cases. These results suggest that in patients at high risk of ulcer disease requiring low-dose aspirin for cardiovascular protection, coprescribing a PPI is reasonable to consider and is supported by expert opinion.[2]

N. J. Talley, MD, PhD

References

1. Yeomans N, Lanas A, Labenz J, et al. Efficacy of esomeprazole (20 mg once daily) for reducing the risk of gastroduodenal ulcers associated with continuous use of low-dose aspirin. *Am J Gastroenterol.* 2008;103:2465-2473.
2. Abraham NS, Hlatky MA, Antman EM, et al. ACCF/ACG/AHA 2010 expert consensus document on the concomitant use of proton pump inhibitors and thienopyridines: a focused update of the ACCF/ACG/AHA 2008 expert consensus document on reducing the gastrointestinal risks of antiplatelet therapy and NSAID use. *Am J Gastroenterol.* 2010;105:2533-2549.

Gluten Causes Gastrointestinal Symptoms in Subjects Without Celiac Disease: A Double-Blind Randomized Placebo-Controlled Trial

Biesiekierski JR, Newnham ED, Irving PM, et al (Monash Univ Dept of Medicine and Gastroenterology, Box Hill, Victoria, Australia; et al)
Am J Gastroenterol 106:508-514, 2011

Objectives.—Despite increased prescription of a gluten-free diet for gastrointestinal symptoms in individuals who do not have celiac disease, there is minimal evidence that suggests that gluten is a trigger. The aims of this study were to determine whether gluten ingestion can induce symptoms in non-celiac individuals and to examine the mechanism.

Methods.—A double-blind, randomized, placebo-controlled rechallenge trial was undertaken in patients with irritable bowel syndrome in whom celiac disease was excluded and who were symptomatically controlled on a gluten-free diet. Participants received either gluten or placebo in the form of two bread slices plus one muffin per day with a gluten-free diet for up to 6 weeks. Symptoms were evaluated using a visual analog scale and markers of intestinal inflammation, injury, and immune activation were monitored.

Results.—A total of 34 patients (aged 29–59 years, 4 men) completed the study as per protocol. Overall, 56 % had human leukocyte antigen (HLA)-DQ2 and/or HLA-DQ8. Adherence to diet and supplements was very high. Of 19 patients (68%) in the gluten group, 13 reported that symptoms were not adequately controlled compared with 6 of 15 (40%) on placebo ($P = 0.0001$; generalized estimating equation). On a visual analog scale, patients were significantly worse with gluten within 1 week for overall symptoms ($P = 0.047$), pain ($P = 0.016$), bloating ($P = 0.031$), satisfaction with stool consistency ($P = 0.024$), and tiredness ($P = 0.001$). Anti-gliadin antibodies were not induced. There were no significant changes in fecal lactoferrin, levels of celiac antibodies, highly sensitive C-reactive protein, or intestinal permeability. There were no differences in any end point in individuals with or without DQ2/DQ8.

Conclusions.—"Non-celiac gluten intolerance" may exist, but no clues to the mechanism were elucidated.

▶ Dietary manipulation appears to be of growing importance in the management of irritable bowel syndrome (IBS). There is limited evidence that fiber supplements (especially psyllium) can provide a benefit, although focusing on those with constipation and going slow is key to reducing bloating and noncompliance. More recent data suggest that removal of certain poorly absorbed short-chain carbohydrates (a low fermentable oligosaccharides, disaccharides, monosaccharides, and polyols diet) also appears to be useful based on evidence from Australia.[1] A second novel approach to dietary management in IBS is application of a gluten-free diet. Celiac disease is the great imitator in gastroenterology; patients with unrecognized celiac disease can present with classic IBS-like symptoms that appear to respond to gluten withdrawal. In this landmark Australian study, the authors assessed in a double-bind randomized trial the efficacy of a gluten-free diet in IBS where celiac disease was excluded (although half of them were HLA-DQ2 or DQ8 positive, indicating a potential genetic risk for celiac disease). They assessed treatment over only 6 weeks but observed that not only did gastrointestinal symptoms decrease on a gluten-free diet, but also fatigue improved. Other uncontrolled data suggest that 6 months of gluten withdrawal might be beneficial.[2] The findings support the concept that a subset of patients with IBS have gluten sensitivity that may in part explain their IBS symptoms, although the duration of needed dietary intervention and the durability of the response are unknown. Trialing a gluten-free diet now represents a reasonable strategy for patients with resistant IBS symptoms. The problem with a gluten-free diet is that it is restrictive, and compliance can be difficult. However, this is a safe strategy that accumulating evidence now supports; a translation into practice does not seem unreasonable in selected cases.

N. J. Talley, MD, PhD

References

1. Ong DK, Mitchell SB, Barrett JS, et al. Manipulation of dietary short chain carbohydrates alters the pattern of gas production and genesis of symptoms in irritable bowel syndrome. *J Gastroenterol Hepatol.* 2010;25:1366-1373.
2. Wahnschaffe U, Ullrich R, Riecken EO, Schulzke JD. Celiac disease-like abnormalities in a subgroup of patients with irritable bowel syndrome. *Gastroenterology.* 2001;121:1329-1338.

Survivors of Childhood Cancer Have Increased Risk of Gastrointestinal Complications Later in Life
Goldsby R, Chen Y, Raber S, et al (UCSF Benioff Children's Hosp; Univ of Alberta, Edmonton, Canada; et al)
Gastroenterology 140:1464-1471, 2011

Background & Aims.—Children who receive cancer therapy experience numerous acute gastrointestinal (GI) toxicities. However, the long-term GI consequences have not been extensively studied. We evaluated the incidence of long-term GI outcomes and identified treatment-related risk factors.

Methods.—Upper GI, hepatic, and lower GI adverse outcomes were assessed in cases from participants in the Childhood Cancer Survivor Study, a study of 14,358 survivors of childhood cancer who were diagnosed between 1970 and 1986; data were compared with those from randomly selected siblings. The median age at cancer diagnosis was 6.8 years (range, 0–21.0 years), and the median age at outcome assessment was 23.2 years (5.6–48.9 years) for survivors and 26.6 years (1.85–6.2 years) for siblings. Rates of self-reported late GI complications (occurred 5 or more years after cancer diagnosis) were determined and associated with patient characteristics and cancer treatments, adjusting for age, sex, and race.

Results.—Compared with siblings, survivors had increased risk of late-onset complications of the upper GI tract (rate ratio [RR], 1.8; 95% confidence interval [CI], 1.6–2.0), liver (RR, 2.1; 95% CI, 1.8–2.5), and lower GI tract (RR, 1.9; 95% CI, 1.7–2.2). The RRs for requiring colostomy/ileostomy, liver biopsy, or developing cirrhosis were 5.6 (95% CI, 2.4−13.1), 24.1 (95% CI, 7.5−77.8), and 8.9 (95% CI, 2.04−0.0), respectively. Older age at diagnosis, intensified therapy, abdominal radiation, and abdominal surgery increased the risk of certain GI complications.

Conclusions.—Individuals who received therapy for cancer during childhood have an increased risk of developing GI complications later in life (Fig 1).

► This is a fascinating study that suggests certain functional gastrointestinal (GI) disorders in addition to organic disease may develop up to 20 or more years after treatment for childhood cancer (Fig 1). In particular, dyspepsia, constipation, and diarrhea were associated with surviving childhood cancer. The comparison with sibling controls was reasonable, although how representative they are of the general population is unclear. It is well recognized that cancer therapy induces significant and unpleasant GI toxicity, including mucositis, nausea and vomiting, esophagitis, and enteritis. The present study raises the hypothesis that acute inflammation (or possibly severe symptoms alone) from

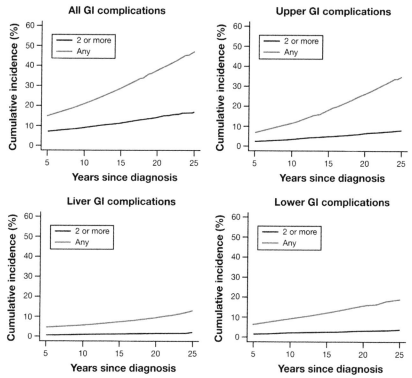

FIGURE 1.—Cumulative incidence of GI conditions (any, red; 2 or more, black) among 5-year survivors. For interpretation of the references to color in this figure legend, the reader is referred to web version of this article.(Reprinted from Goldsby R, Chen Y, Raber S, et al. Survivors of childhood cancer have increased risk of gastrointestinal complications later in life. *Gastroenterology.* 2011;140:1464-1471, Copyright 2011, with permission from the AGA Institute.)

chemoradiation can "wind up" the enteric or central nervous system (or both), and after a long latent period, unexplained GI symptoms may develop. Bias is possible in this study (how many cancer survivors had recent symptoms because of cancer recurrence is, for example, uncertain), but overall the research suggests more vigilance by clinicians who follow such patients in adult practice.

N. J. Talley, MD, PhD

Organic colonic lesions in 3,332 patients with suspected irritable bowel syndrome and lacking warning signs, a retrospective case–control study
Gu H-X, Zhang Y-L, Zhi F-C, et al (Southern Med Univ, Guangzhou, China)
Int J Colorectal Dis 26:935-940, 2011

Purpose.—The diagnosis of irritable bowel syndrome is symptom based, and colonoscopy is the most direct way to rule out organic colonic diseases. It is controversial on the necessity of colonoscopy for patients with suspected irritable bowel syndrome and lacking alarm features. This study was designed to verify the organic lesions and discuss the value of colonoscopy in this type of patients.

Methods.—Colonoscopy of 3,332 patients with suspected irritable bowel syndrome and lacking warning signs from 2000 to 2009 were reviewed. One thousand five hundred eighty-eight patients under 50 years of age who underwent colonoscopy screening for health care in the same period were used as controls. The prevalence of different colonic organic lesions was compared between two groups.

Results.—Organic colonic lesions were found in 30.3% of the patients with suspected irritable bowel syndrome (1,010/3,332) and 39.0% of the controls (619/1,588). Compared with controls, patients with suspected irritable bowel syndrome had higher prevalence of noninflammatory bowel disease and noninfectious colitis and terminal ileitis; however, they had lower prevalence of diverticular disease, adenomatous polyps, and non-adenomatous polyps (all $P<0.001$).

Conclusions.—The diagnostic sensitivity of symptom criteria on irritable bowel syndrome without colonoscopy is not more than 69.7% in patients with suspected irritable bowel syndrome lacking warning signs. Though the method of colonoscopy is hard to screen tumor in this type of patients, it is beneficial to uncover some other relevant organic lesions such as terminal ileitis. Colonoscopy should not be refused to suspected irritable bowel syndrome patients without warning signs.

▶ Many patients who present with irritable bowel syndrome (IBS)-like symptoms end up undergoing a colonoscopy despite the absence of alarm features. Gastroenterologists are trained to do procedures, and with referral filtering, they are more likely to encounter rare events (eg, colon cancer in a 20-year-old); therefore, they naturally have a low threshold for doing the test. However, there remains controversy about the potential risks (which are real) versus benefits of colonoscopy in IBS. Current American College of Gastroenterology guidelines do not recommend a colonoscopy for patients under the age of 50 without warning signs or symptoms. In this Chinese study, it is particularly interesting to note that IBS appeared to be protective in terms of finding polyps, both adenomatous and nonadenomatous. The reasons why IBS may be protective are unknown, but other evidence supports these observations. As expected, patients with IBS were more likely to be found to have evidence of inflammation in the colon. Others have reported that patients with microscopic colitis were more likely to present with IBS-like symptoms. Overall, the data from this study are reassuring and support current guidelines; colonoscopy is not usually indicated for those with typical IBS symptoms unless the patient is older (50 years and more) or there are alarm features, such as rectal bleeding, unexplained weight loss, or a strong family history of colon cancer.

N. J. Talley, MD, PhD

Irritable bowel syndrome and risk of colorectal cancer: a Danish nationwide cohort study
Nørgaard M, Farkas DK, Pedersen L, et al (Aarhus Univ Hosp, Aalborg, Denmark)
Br J Cancer 104:1202-1206, 2011

Background.—Little is known about the risk of colorectal cancer among patients with irritable bowel syndrome (IBS).

Methods.—We conducted a nationwide cohort study using data from the Danish National Registry of Patients and the Danish Cancer Registry from 1977 to 2008. We included patients with a first-time hospital contact for IBS and followed them for colorectal cancer. We estimated the expected number of cancers by applying national rates and we computed standardised incidence ratios (SIRs) by comparing the observed number of colorectal cancers with the expected number. We stratified the SIRs according to age, gender, and time of follow-up.

Results.—Among 57 851 IBS patients, we identified 407 cases of colon cancer during a combined follow-up of 506 930 years (SIR, 1.14 (95% confidence interval (CI): 1.03−1.25) and 115 cases of rectal cancer, corresponding to a SIR of 0.67 (95% CI: 0.52−0.85). In the first 3 months after an IBS diagnosis, the SIR was 8.42 (95% CI: 6.48−10.75) for colon cancer and 4.81 (95% CI: 2.85−7.60) for rectal cancer. Thereafter, the SIRs declined and 4−10 years after an IBS diagnosis, the SIRs for both colon and rectal cancer remained below 0.95.

Conclusion.—We found a decreased risk of colorectal cancer in the period 1−10 years after an IBS diagnosis. However, in the first 3 months after an IBS diagnosis, the risk of colon cancer was more than eight-fold increased and the risk of rectal cancer was five-fold increased. These increased risks are likely to be explained by diagnostic confusion because of overlapping symptomatology.

▶ The relationship between colorectal cancer and irritable bowel syndrome (IBS) has not been carefully investigated, but this is remedied by this large high-quality epidemiological study. At first glance, the results seem to suggest that patients who have IBS-like symptoms in the population are 8-fold more likely to have colorectal cancer, a frightening observation. However, when this was looked into more carefully, it becomes clear that this apparent increased risk is all because of detection bias. Overall, the risk of colon cancer is actually decreased in patients with long-standing IBS symptoms. The conclusions seem clear; colon cancer can present with IBS-like symptoms, but those with a firm diagnosis of IBS have a lower risk than normal for colon cancer (see also the Chinese study documenting a lower risk of adenomatous polyps in IBS in this volume). Why the risk of colon cancer is decreased in IBS is unknown. The data indicate that there is no requirement to change the current American College of Gastroenterology guidelines for diagnosis of IBS that recommend colonoscopy only in patients older than 50 years with IBS-like symptoms or those who have alarm features (eg, rectal bleeding, unexplained weight loss, or a strong family history of colon cancer).

N. J. Talley, MD, PhD

Domperidone Treatment for Gastroparesis: Demographic and Pharmacogenetic Characterization of Clinical Efficacy and Side-Effects
Parkman HP, Jacobs MR, Mishra A, et al (Temple Univ School of Medicine, Philadelphia, PA; Temple Univ School of Pharmacy, Philadelphia, PA)
Dig Dis Sci 56:115-124, 2011

Background.—Domperidone is a useful alternative to metoclopramide for treatment of gastroparesis due to better tolerability. Effectiveness and side-effects from domperidone may be influenced by patient-related factors including polymorphisms in genes encoding drug-metabolizing enzymes, drug transporters, and domperidone targets.

Aims.—The aim of this study was to determine if demographic and pharmacogenetic parameters of patients receiving domperidone are associated with response to treatment or side-effects.

Methods.—Patients treated with domperidone for gastroparesis provided saliva samples from which DNA was extracted. Fourteen single-nucleotide polymorphisms (SNPs) in seven candidate genes (*ABCB1, CYP2D6, DRD2, KCNE1, KCNE2, KCNH2, KCNQ1*) were used for genotyping. SNP microarrays were used to assess single-nucleotide polymorphisms in the *ADRA1A, ADRA1B,* and *ADRA1D* loci.

Results.—Forty-eight patients treated with domperidone participated in the study. DNA was successfully obtained from each patient. Age was associated with effectiveness of domperidone ($p = 0.0088$). Genetic polymorphism in KCNH2 was associated with effectiveness of domperidone ($p = 0.041$). The efficacious dose was associated with polymorphism in ABCB1 gene ($p = 0.0277$). The side-effects of domperidone were significantly associated with the SNPs in the promoter region of *ADRA1D* gene.

Conclusions.—Genetic characteristics associated with response to domperidone therapy included polymorphisms in the drug transporter gene

ABCB1, the potassium channel *KCNH2* gene, and α_{1D}—adrenoceptor *ADRA1D* gene. Age was associated with a beneficial response to domperidone. If verified in a larger population, this information might be used to help determine which patients with gastroparesis might respond to domperidone and avoid treatment in those who might develop side-effects (Fig 1).

▶ Domperidone is an old drug but remains widely used as a prokinetic (in part because there are relatively few alternatives). It is a dopamine receptor antagonist; dopamine inhibits gut motility. Although not approved in the United States by the Food and Drug Administration, under an Investigational New Drug program, the drug can be prescribed through compounding pharmacies. Some patients obtain the drug from Canada and Mexico. However, domperidone has potential side effects such as increased prolactin secretion (causing galactorrhea), and it may rarely prolong the QT interval causing serious arrhythmias. Interestingly, in this study older age was significantly associated with a better treatment response, which the authors speculate might be explained by dopamine receptors decreasing with age, so domperidone may be more efficient in the elderly. A goal of personalized medicine is to improve the benefit-to-risk ratio with drug therapy, and for this reason this study is worth reading.

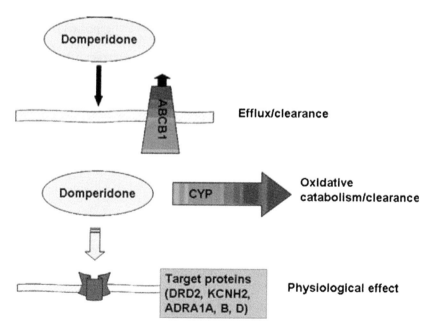

FIGURE 1.—Modulators of domperidone physiological activity. Modulators of domperidone physiological activity include the drug transporter ABCB1, the drug-metabolizing enzyme CYP2D6, and targets of domperidone (dopamine receptor D2, DRD2, α1-adrenergic receptors ADRA1A-D, and myocardial ion channels KCNE1/2, KCNH2, and KCNQ1). (Reprinted from Parkman HP, Jacobs MR, Mishra A, et al. Domperidone treatment for gastroparesis: demographic and pharmacogenetic characterization of clinical efficacy and side-effects. *Dig Dis Sci.* 2011;56:115-124, with permission from Springer Science+Business Media, LLC.)

While it represents a proof of concept study and the sample size was small, the results suggest that gene testing (Fig 1) will have a role in prescribing prokinetic treatments in the near future.

N. J. Talley, MD, PhD

Rifaximin Therapy for Patients with Irritable Bowel Syndrome without Constipation

Pimentel M, for the TARGET Study Group (Cedars–Sinai Med Ctr, Los Angeles, CA; et al)

N Engl J Med 364:22-32, 2011

Background.—Evidence suggests that gut flora may play an important role in the pathophysiology of the irritable bowel syndrome (IBS). We evaluated rifaximin, a minimally absorbed antibiotic, as treatment for IBS.

Methods.—In two identically designed, phase 3, double-blind, placebo-controlled trials (TARGET 1 and TARGET 2), patients who had IBS without constipation were randomly assigned to either rifaximin at a dose of 550 mg or placebo, three times daily for 2 weeks, and were followed for an additional 10 weeks. The primary end point, the proportion of patients who had adequate relief of global IBS symptoms, and the key secondary end point, the proportion of patients who had adequate relief of IBS-related bloating, were assessed weekly. Adequate relief was defined as self-reported relief of symptoms for at least 2 of the first 4 weeks after treatment. Other secondary end points included the percentage of patients who had a response to treatment as assessed by daily self-ratings of global IBS symptoms and individual symptoms of bloating, abdominal pain, and stool consistency during the 4 weeks after treatment and during the entire 3 months of the study.

Results.—Significantly more patients in the rifaximin group than in the placebo group had adequate relief of global IBS symptoms during the first 4 weeks after treatment (40.8% vs. 31.2%, P = 0.01, in TARGET 1; 40.6% vs. 32.2%, P = 0.03, in TARGET 2; 40.7% vs. 31.7%, P<0.001, in the two studies combined). Similarly, more patients in the rifaximin group than in the placebo group had adequate relief of bloating (39.5% vs. 28.7%, P = 0.005, in TARGET 1; 41.0% vs. 31.9%, P = 0.02, in TARGET 2; 40.2% vs. 30.3%, P<0.001, in the two studies combined). In addition, significantly more patients in the rifaximin group had a response to treatment as assessed by daily ratings of IBS symptoms, bloating, abdominal pain, and stool consistency. The incidence of adverse events was similar in the two groups.

Conclusions.—Among patients who had IBS without constipation, treatment with rifaximin for 2 weeks provided significant relief of IBS symptoms, bloating, abdominal pain, and loose or watery stools. (Funded by Salix Pharmaceuticals; ClinicalTrials.gov numbers, NCT00731679 and NCT00724126.) (Fig 4).

▶ There is accumulating evidence that antibiotic therapy temporarily improves irritable bowel syndrome (IBS) symptoms. In a previous randomized controlled

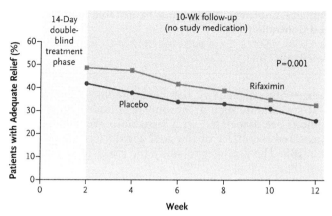

FIGURE 4.—Percentage of Patients with Adequate Relief of Global IBS Symptoms in the TARGET 1 and TARGET 2 Studies Combined. Adequate relief was defined as self-reported relief from symptoms for at least 1 week of every 2-week period. The P value was calculated on the basis of a longitudinal data analysis with the use of a generalized-estimating equation model, with fixed effects of treatment, analysis center, and week. Similar figures for the individual TARGET 1 and TARGET 2 trials are shown in the Supplementary Appendix. (Reprinted from Pimentel M, for the TARGET Study Group. Rifaximin therapy for patients with irritable bowel syndrome without constipation. *N Engl J Med.* 2011;364:22-32, Copyright 2011, Massachusetts Medical Society. All rights reserved.)

trial, 87 IBS patients who met Rome I criteria received 400 mg of rifaximin 3 times daily for 10 days or placebo; rifaximin resulted in greater improvement in global IBS symptoms and a lower bloating score over 10 weeks of follow-up.[1] These previous data suggested that a nonabsorbable antibiotic altered the natural history of IBS symptoms (the first treatment to be shown to alter the natural history of IBS at least over the short term). These results have been confirmed in the TARGET 1 and 2 Phase III trials. Although a higher dose was used and the new study excluded constipation-predominant IBS applying Rome III criteria, similar results were obtained (see Fig 4, with a number needed to treat of approximately 10). However, many questions remain. How durable is the effect (as the figure indicates, the effect wears off, and clinical experience suggests all patients relapse within several months)? Strategies to maintain response and the effect of retreatment are also uncertain (some respond to retreatment, others do not). We do not know whether breath testing to identify possible small bowel bacterial overgrowth predicts response (it may not). Furthermore, we do not know how this drug works and why only a minority of patients respond to it. Therefore, a conservative approach to the use of off-label rifaximin for IBS seems appropriate until more data emerge.

N. J. Talley, MD, PhD

Reference

1. Pimentel M, Park S, Mirocha J, Kane SV, Kong Y. The effect of a nonabsorbed oral antibiotic (rifaximin) on the symptoms of the irritable bowel syndrome: a randomized trial. *Ann Intern Med.* 2006;145:557-563.

Physical Activity Improves Symptoms in Irritable Bowel Syndrome: A Randomized Controlled Trial

Johannesson E, Simrén M, Strid H, et al (Univ of Gothenburg, Sweden)
Am J Gastroenterol 106:915-922, 2011

Objectives.—Physical activity has been shown to be effective in the treatment of conditions, such as fibromyalgia and depression. Although these conditions are associated with irritable bowel syndrome (IBS), no study has assessed the effect of physical activity on gastrointestinal (GI) symptoms in IBS. The aim was to study the effect of physical activity on symptoms in IBS.

Methods.—We randomized 102 patients to a physical activity group and a control group. Patients of the physical activity group were instructed by a physiotherapist to increase their physical activity, and those of the control group were instructed to maintain their lifestyle. The primary end point was to assess the change in the IBS Severity Scoring System (IBS-SSS).

Results.—A total of 38 (73.7 % women, median age 38.5 (19−65) years) patients in the control group and 37 (75.7 % women, median age 36 (18−65) years) patients in the physical activity group completed the study. There was a significant difference in the improvement in the IBS-SSS score between the physical activity group and the control group (−51 (−130 and 49) vs. −5 (−101 and 118), $P = 0.003$). The proportion of patients with increased IBS symptom severity during the study was significantly larger in the control group than in the physical activity group.

Conclusions.—Increased physical activity improves GI symptoms in IBS. Physically active patients with IBS will face less symptom deterioration compared with physically inactive patients. Physical activity should be used as a primary treatment modality in IBS.

▶ The initial management of irritable bowel syndrome (IBS) typically includes dietary manipulation (classically with the slow introduction of increased fiber or a fiber supplement), reassurance, and stress reduction. However, many patients fail this approach and require medical therapy, although most drugs prescribed target individual symptoms rather than altering the natural history of the disorder. Uncontrolled data indicate that patients who attend a formal IBS class do better than control subjects; in these classes, instructions regarding stress reduction and diet are provided, and patients may be asked to increase their physical activity.[1] This is the first randomized controlled trial to test the efficacy of physical activity in IBS. The results are interesting because increased physical activity did appear to improve gastrointestinal symptoms, rather than simply improving sense of well-being (which exercise is known to do in many settings). Further work is necessary to confirm that physical activity is efficacious in IBS, but on the basis of the available evidence, clinicians should consider counseling their patients to increase their activity and providing encouragement and assistance for those who can do so.

N. J. Talley, MD, PhD

Reference

1. Saito YA, Prather CM, Van Dyke CT, Fett S, Zinsmeister AR, Locke GR 3rd. Effects of multidisciplinary education on outcomes in patients with irritable bowel syndrome. *Clin Gastroenterol Hepatol.* 2004;2:576-584.

Vitamin D and Pelvic Floor Disorders in Women: Results From the National Health and Nutrition Examination Survey
Badalian SS, Rosenbaum PF (SUNY Upstate Med Univ, Syracuse, NY)
Obstet Gynecol 115:795-803, 2010

Objective.—To estimate the prevalence of vitamin D deficiency in women with pelvic floor disorders and to evaluate possible associations between vitamin D levels and pelvic floor disorders.

Methods.—Using 2005–2006 National Health and Nutrition Examination Survey data, we performed a cross-sectional analysis of nonpregnant women older than 20 years of age with data on both pelvic floor disorders and vitamin D measurements (n = 1,881). Vitamin D levels lower than 30 ng/mL were considered insufficient. The prevalence of demographic factors, pelvic floor disorders, and vitamin D levels were determined, accounting for the multi-stage sampling design; odds ratios (OR) and 95% confidence intervals (CI) were calculated to evaluate associations between vitamin D levels and pelvic floor disorders with control for known risk factors.

Results.—One or more pelvic floor disorders were reported by 23% of women. Mean vitamin D levels were significantly lower for women reporting at least one pelvic floor disorder and for those with urinary incontinence, irrespective of age. In adjusted logistic regression models, we observed significantly decreased risks of one or more pelvic floor disorders with increasing vitamin D levels in all women aged 20 or older (OR, 0.94; 95% CI, 0.88–0.99) and in the subset of women 50 years and older (OR, 0.92; 95% CI, 0.85–0.99). Additionally, the likelihood of urinary incontinence was significantly reduced in women 50 and older with vitamin D levels 30 ng/mL or higher (OR, 0.55; 95% CI, 0.34–0.91).

Conclusion.—Higher vitamin D levels are associated with a decreased risk of pelvic floor disorders in women.

▶ Pelvic floor disorders have been associated with osteoporosis. Vitamin D has been associated with severe osteoporosis but also muscle weakness. The study used data from the NHANES survey of Americans to show that lower vitamin D levels might predict pelvic floor disorders, especially pelvic organ prolapse and urinary and fecal incontinence. It appeared that lower levels of vitamin stores were associated with risk of pelvic floor disorders at all ages in adult women. Women older than 50 who had vitamin D levels higher than 30 had significantly fewer pelvic floor disorders than those with low levels. These symptoms were primarily urinary. The proposed mechanisms are related to the role of vitamin D in detrusor muscle function. Although one could conclude that vitamin D supplementation may be helpful, the possibility of a confounding explanation is possible. For example, vitamin D levels might be associated with sun exposure as a result of outdoor exercise; however, vitamin D deficiency can also occur in those exposed to sunlight. Nonetheless, this study will prompt more studies to understand the link between vitamin D stores and pelvic floor disorders and indeed other functional complaints.

J. A. Murray, MD

48 Inflammatory Bowel Disease

Dietary Intake and Risk of Developing Inflammatory Bowel Disease: A Systematic Review of the Literature
Hou JK, Abraham B, El-Serag H (Baylor College of Med, Houston, TX)
Am J Gastroenterol 106:563-573, 2011

Objectives.—The incidence of inflammatory bowel disease (IBD) is increasing. Dietary factors such as the spread of the "Western" diet, high in fat and protein but low in fruits and vegetables, may be associated with the increase. Although many studies have evaluated the association between diet and IBD risk, there has been no systematic review.

Methods.—We performed a systematic review using guideline-recommended methodology to evaluate the association between pre-illness intake of nutrients (fats, carbohydrates, protein) and food groups (fruits, vegetables, meats) and the risk of subsequent IBD diagnosis. Eligible studies were identified via structured keyword searches in PubMed and Google Scholar and manual searches.

Results.—Nineteen studies were included, encompassing 2,609 IBD patients (1,269 Crohn's disease (CD) and 1,340 ulcerative colitis (UC) patients) and over 4,000 controls. Studies reported a positive association between high intake of saturated fats, monounsaturated fatty acids, total polyunsaturated fatty acids (PUFAs), total omega-3 fatty acids, omega-6 fatty acids, mono- and disaccharides, and meat and increased subsequent CD risk. Studies reported a negative association between dietary fiber and fruits and subsequent CD risk. High intakes of total fats, total PUFAs, omega-6 fatty acids, and meat were associated with an increased risk of UC. High vegetable intake was associated with a decreased risk of UC.

Conclusions.—High dietary intakes of total fats, PUFAs, omega-6 fatty acids, and meat were associated with an increased risk of CD and UC. High fiber and fruit intakes were associated with decreased CD risk, and high vegetable intake was associated with decreased UC risk.

▶ Diet has often been suggested as contributing to the development of inflammatory bowel disease (IBD). Proof of causality is extremely difficult because of problems in obtaining accurate dietary histories, the potential for recall bias, and the difficulties in conducting prospective studies. Histories are typically reported among those already affected with IBD because true population-based studies with prospective longitudinal follow-up are not feasible. In this article, the authors review 19 (18 case-control and 1 cohort) studies. The conclusions, while interesting, are open to the same criticism as the articles that they have reviewed. Five of the studies reported dietary intake in the year prior to the IBD diagnosis. While the authors show that the conclusions of these studies are similar to other studies, basing diet history on the year prior to diagnosis is a potential problem. Patients with early symptoms of IBD may have adjusted their diet away from fruits and vegetables in favor of protein and fat because of worsening bloating or diarrhea. It's not surprising that high intake of fat and meat was associated with development of IBD because they increase the risk of many diseases. This is widely known in most Western populations, but do they really increase the risk of IBD? The fact that most of the studies say so is not enough to demonstrate causality. The authors, unfortunately, provide little critical appraisal of the literature. They declare that pooling studies (meta-analysis) is not possible because of the heterogeneity of the studies presented. While this may be true, they should provide more of a discussion outlining the strengths and weaknesses of the individual studies that suggest dietary associations. The quality of the studies is most important. Just because it makes sense that high fat and meat intake increase the risk of IBD does not necessarily mean this is true.

M. F. Picco, MD, PhD

Randomised clinical trial: early assessment after 2 weeks of high-dose mesalazine for moderately active ulcerative colitis - new light on a familiar question

Orchard TR, van der Geest SAP, Travis SPL (St Mary's Hosp, London, UK; Warner Chilcott UK Ltd, Larne; John Radcliffe Hosp, Oxford, UK)
Aliment Pharmacol Ther 33:1028-1035, 2011

Background.—Rapid resolution of rectal bleeding and stool frequency are important goals for ulcerative colitis therapy and may help guide therapeutic decisions.

Aim.—To explore patient diary data from ASCEND I and II for their relevance to clinical decision making.

Methods.—Data from two randomised, double-blind, Phase III studies were combined. Patients received mesalazine (mesalamine) 4.8 g/day (Asacol 800 mg MR) or 2.4 g/day (Asacol 400 mg MR). Time to improvement or resolution of rectal bleeding and stool frequency was assessed and the proportion of patients experiencing symptom improvement or resolution at day 14 evaluated using survival analysis. Symptoms after 14 days were compared to week 6. A combination of prespecified and *post hoc* analyses were used.

Results.—Median times to resolution and improvement of both rectal bleeding and stool frequency were shorter with 4.8 g/day than 2.4 g/day (resolution, 19 vs. 29 days, $P = 0.020$; improvement, 7 vs. 9 days, $P = 0.024$). In total, 73% of patients experienced improvement in both rectal bleeding and stool frequency by day 14 with 4.8 g/day, compared to 61%

with 2.4 g/day. More patients achieved symptom resolution by day 14 with 4.8 g/day than 2.4 g/day (43% vs. 30%; $P = 0.035$). Symptom relief after 14 days was associated with a high rate of symptom relief after 6 weeks.

Conclusions.—High-dose mesalazine 4.8 g/day provides rapid relief of the cardinal symptoms of moderately active ulcerative colitis. Symptom relief within 14 days was associated with symptom relief at 6 weeks in the majority of patients. Day 14 is a practical timepoint at which response to treatment may be assessed and decisions regarding therapy escalation made (Clinicaltrials.gov: NCT00577473, NCT00073021).

▶ The results of this study are not surprising, but they are reassuring. The finding of mesalamine treatment response at 14 days predicting response at 6 weeks confirms the validity of accepted clinical practice. The finding that 4.8 g/d is better than 2.4 g/d also fits with practice in that more mesalamine is better to treat mild to moderate ulcerative colitis (UC). Should we use the lack of response at 14 days to decide whether to escalate therapy? Although rates of response at 6 weeks were highest for those with response at 14 days, nearly half of those without symptom improvement in rectal bleeding at 14 days had symptom improvement at 6 weeks. Rates were lower for those without improvement in stool frequency at 14 days (25%). Should we abandon high-dose mesalamine for nonresponders at 14 days? The answer, not surprisingly, depends on the individual patient's clinical history and severity of symptoms. Patients who were receiving greater than 1.6 g/d of mesalamine were excluded from the study. This may have selected out a population more likely to respond and limited the applicability of the findings. Because most patients with UC are taking maintenance mesalamine at the time of a flare, this is an important exclusion. At best, assessment at 14 days of therapy provides a rough guide. Among patients with more severe symptoms or who worsen on treatment, changing therapy would be reasonable. It may be as simple as adding topical mesalamine or possibly topical or oral corticosteroids. For patients with mild symptoms who have an equivocal response or no response, adding topical mesalamine therapy or watchful waiting may be reasonable because many may respond and not require corticosteroids. Clinical judgment remains most important.

M. F. Picco, MD, PhD

Managing symptoms of irritable bowel syndrome in patients with inflammatory bowel disease
Camilleri M (Mayo Clinic, Rochester, MN)
Gut 60:425-428, 2011

Background.—Symptoms common to irritable bowel syndrome (IBS) may occur in patients who have inflammatory bowel disease (IBD) that appears stable or in remission. They experience abdominal pain, bloating, diarrhea, and urgency but have no significant inflammation, constitutional symptoms, or rectal bleeding. Another disease may be present.

Initial Screening.—Symptom management requires, first, that the absence of infection be confirmed, then screening tests are done to discriminate between IBD and IBS. This includes tests of fecal calprotectin, lactoferrin and S100A12, which is a calcium-binding proinflammatory protein secreted by granulocytes. Magnetic resonance (MR) and computed tomography (CT) enterography are equally sensitive for detecting active small bowel inflammation, but MR enteroclysis involves no radiation exposure and better characterizes stenotic lesions. CT provides better temporal resolution, mesenteric imaging, and a shorter examination time. Bile acid malabsorption (BAM) may also cause steatorrhea. Its diagnosis is confirmed through tests of serum 7α-hydroxy-4-cholesten-3-one, 48-hr fecal bile acid excretion, or 23-selena-25-homotaurocholate retention on scintigraphy. A surrogate test of fasting serum fibroblast growth factor 19 or therapeutic trials of cholestyramine (4 g three times a day) or oral colesevelam (625 mg tablets with up to two tablets three times a day) can also be used to detect BAM.

Conditions To Exclude.—Symptomatic patients with IBD but no overt inflammation are further screened to detect other conditions that may be causing symptoms. Small bowel bacterial overgrowth (SBO) may be suspected if there are anatomical aberrations that result from Crohn's disease or bypass surgery. No sensitive, specific, and easily performed test is available for SBO, so a therapeutic trial using a poorly absorbed antibiotic such as neomycin, metronidazole, quinolone, or rifaximin is the most practical approach.

Chronic pancreatic insufficiency is rare in these patients. Little evidence indicates that visceral hypersensitivity occurs in patients with IBD, but further studies of afferent and pelvic floor function associated with IBD are needed.

IBS with IBD.—Some patients whose IBD is in remission but who have persistent abdominal discomfort and diarrhea may also have IBS. IBS-like symptoms impair the patient's quality of life and global well-being. Patients with IBD who have IBS-like symptoms tend to have higher levels of anxiety and depression, and studies have linked anxiety and duration of disease as significantly predictive of developing IBS-like symptoms. The IBS can be managed symptomatically, observing caution with anti-motility agents to avoid complications related to the IBD.

Conclusions.—Patients with IBD can also have IBS. Treatment of IBS is tailored to the symptoms, with measurements of gastrointestinal and colonic transit used to guide therapy for patients whose transit values are significantly accelerated.

▶ Clinicians are often faced with the problem of determining whether a patient with inflammatory bowel disease (IBD) presenting with gastrointestinal symptoms has active disease. Testing for active disease typically relies on invasive and potentially dangerous procedures. Invasive testing may not confirm disease activity, and an alternative diagnosis should be considered. In this article, Camilleri provides a comprehensive review of these mimickers of IBD, including common organic conditions of enteric infection, bacterial overgrowth, bile salt malabsorption, and short bowel syndrome along with the more rare conditions of celiac disease and pancreatic insufficiency. Irritable bowel syndrome is a very important functional cause along with pelvic floor dysfunction. The first step to diagnosing these conditions is awareness, and the majority can be diagnosed without the need for invasive testing. Among patients with IBD, recognition of typical symptoms of these common conditions along with a clinical judgment that an individual's IBD is in remission may avoid invasive testing. Stool marker studies such as calprotectin and lactoferrin, while advocated by the author as a noninvasive method of documenting disease activity, lack acceptable sensitivity and specificity to recommend as part of routine practice. It all comes down to clinical judgment and assessment of symptom severity. For patients without overt symptoms or signs of severe IBD but with findings of an associated condition, directed treatment can avoid needless invasive testing.

M. F. Picco, MD, PhD

Prevalence of Colorectal Cancer Surveillance for Ulcerative Colitis in an Integrated Health Care Delivery System
Velayos FS, Liu L, Lewis JD, et al (Univ of California, San Francisco; Kaiser Permanente Northern California, Oakland, CA; Univ of Pennsylvania, Philadelphia; et al)
Gastroenterology 139:1511-1518, 2010

Background & Aims.—The absence of grade A supporting evidence for surveillance colonoscopy in patients with ulcerative colitis (UC) has led to controversy regarding its benefit, yet it is routinely recommended in practice guidelines. Limited data are available on rates of colonoscopy surveillance and factors associated with surveillance.

Methods.—A retrospective study of UC patients receiving care between 2006 and 2007 with ≥8 years history of UC was conducted. Primary outcome was the proportion of patients who underwent surveillance during this 2-year study period. Sociodemographic and disease factors were identified a priori from variables recorded electronically in the medical record; multivariable associations with surveillance were estimated using logistic regression.

Results.—Of 771 patients with ≥8 years history of UC, 24.6% of patients underwent at least 1 surveillance colonoscopy within the 2-year study period, with a maximum of 38.5% observed among patients with primary sclerosing cholangitis. In a multivariable analysis, gender, age, race, and education were not associated with surveillance. Factors associated with increasing surveillance included lack of significant comorbidity (Charlson-Deyo index 0 vs 1+: odds ratio [OR], 1.7; 95% confidence interval: 1.1−2.5), >3 inflammatory bowel disease-related outpatient visits (OR, 2.0; 95% CI: 1.4−3.0), and use of mesalamine (OR, 2.8; 95% CI: 1.7−4.4).

Conclusions.—Utilization of surveillance colonoscopy in a 2-year period was low, even among high-risk patients. Although specific factors recorded in computerized data were identified to be associated with surveillance, a greater understanding of how patients and physicians decide on surveillance is needed.

▶ The findings of this article are quite surprising. Rates of surveillance colonoscopy among a population derived from Kaiser Permanente Northern California with long-standing ulcerative colitis (UC) were very low. One would expect that the best rates of surveillance would come from such an integrated health system where patients receive all their health care within the plan and information on health care utilization would be complete. However, data acquisition was retrospective, and methods of identification of patients eligible for surveillance may have led to flawed estimates of surveillance rates. The first problem was that there is no code to identify surveillance procedures in UC. The authors relied on a computerized surveillance algorithm that identified surveillance colonoscopies. This resulted in a 20% false-negative level, suggesting that 20% of procedures classified as not for surveillance were in fact surveillance procedures. This may have contributed to a somewhat lower estimate of surveillance rates. In addition, the authors could not definitively separate patients based on extent of disease. The criteria used for identification and exclusion of proctitis patients was reasonable but the authors could not separate left-sided colitis from pancolitis. Patients with left-sided colitis may undergo surveillance later than 8 years of disease, which may have led to a lower overall estimate of surveillance rates because they admit that 59% of their population had left-side disease from a previous study. Despite these limitations, the findings are important. Even if case ascertainment was complete, surveillance rates would probably still be well below 100%. More work is needed to determine true patterns of surveillance across clinicians and reasons for disparities and barriers that interfere with compliance with current guidelines.

M. F. Picco, MD, PhD

A Multicenter Experience With Infliximab for Ulcerative Colitis: Outcomes and Predictors of Response, Optimization, Colectomy, and Hospitalization
Oussalah A, Evesque L, Laharie D, et al (Univ Hosp of Nancy, France; Univ of Nice Sophia Antipolis, France; Haut-Lévêque Hosp, Pessac, France; et al)
Am J Gastroenterol 105:2617-2625, 2010

Objectives.—The objective of this study was to evaluate short- and long-term outcomes of infliximab in ulcerative colitis (UC), including infliximab optimization, colectomy, and hospitalization.

Methods.—This was a retrospective multicenter study. All adult patients who received at least one infliximab infusion for UC were included. Cumulative probabilities of event-free survival were estimated by the Kaplan–Meier method. Independent predictors were identified using binary logistic regression or Cox proportionalhazards regression, and results were expressed as odds ratios or hazard ratios (HRs), respectively.

Results.—Between January 2000 and August 2009, 191 UC patients received infliximab therapy. Median follow-up per patient was 18 months (interquartile range = 25–75th, 8–32 months). Primary nonresponse was noted in 42 patients (22.0%). "Hemoglobin at infliximab initiation ≤ 9.4 g/dl" (odds ratio = 4.35; 95% confidence interval (CI) = 1.81–10.42) was a positive predictor of non-response to infliximab. Infliximab optimization was required in 36 (45.0%) of 80 patients on scheduled infliximab therapy. The only predictor of infliximab optimization was "infliximab indication for acute severe colitis" (HR = 2.75; 95% CI = 1.23–6.12). Thirty-six patients (18.8%) underwent colectomy. Predictors of colectomy were: "no clinical response after infliximab induction" (HR = 7.06; 95% CI = 3.36–14.83), "C-reactive protein at infliximab initiation > 10 mg/l" (HR = 5.11; 95% CI = 1.77–14.76), "infliximab indication for acute severe colitis" (HR = 3.40; 95% CI = 1.48–7.81), and "previous treatment with cyclosporine" (HR = 2.53; 95% CI = 1.22–5.28). Sixty-nine patients (36.1%) were hospitalized at least one time and UC-related hospitalizations rate was 29 per 100 patient-years (95% CI = 24–35 per 100 patient-years). Predictors of first hospitalization were: "no clinical response after infliximab induction" (HR = 3.87; 95% CI = 2.29–6.53), "infliximab indication for acute severe colitis" (HR = 3.13, 95% CI = 1.65–5.94), "disease duration at infliximab initiation ≤ 50 months" (HR = 2.14, 95% CI = 1.25–3.66), "hemoglobin at infliximab initiation ≤ 11.8 g/dl" (HR = 1.77; 95% CI = 1.03–3.04), and "previous treatment with methotrexate" (HR = 0.30; 95% CI = 0.09–0.97).

Conclusions.—Primary non-response to infliximab was noted in one fifth of patients and increased by seven and four the risks of colectomy and hospitalization, respectively. Infliximab optimization, colectomy, and hospitalization were required in half, one fifth, and one third of patients, respectively. Infliximab indication for acute severe colitis increased by three the risks of infliximab optimization, colectomy, and UC-related hospitalization.

▶ This is a large real-world experience on the use of infliximab in ulcerative colitis. Patient outcomes are measured from how infliximab is typically used in practice outside clinical trials. Unfortunately, the trial was retrospective, and there were no objective criteria to measure clinical response or maintenance of clinical benefit. These outcomes were measured by physician judgment with only limited objective data on individual patients. While physician judgment is typically how treatment decisions are based in practice, practices may vary, especially with regard to assessment for treatment response.

Despite these limitations, the conclusions are important. Median follow-up of 18 months was adequate. The mix of patients included both hospitalized patients and outpatients. Nearly 20% were cyclosporine failures. The predictors of response, optimization, and colectomy made sense and fit with most clinicians' experience with the drug. Of particularly importance is that severe colitis (where infliximab is typically used in practice) resulted in a 3-fold risk of infliximab failure. The finding that concomitant use of immunomodulators did not affect infliximab optimization was surprising, especially in light of Crohn's disease favoring combined usage in treatment-naive patients and the reported risk of malignancy and infection with combined immunosuppression. It is not clear whether these patients were immunodulator failures or had these medications started at the time of first infliximab.

Ultimately, a randomized clinical trial is the only way to understand what are the true predictors of treatment response or failure. Unfortunately, such a trial is unlikely. This study validates what many clinicians have learned from experience. It does also raise important questions about the use of concomitant immunosuppression, which need to be answered.

M. F. Picco, MD, PhD

Pregnancy outcome in patients with inflammatory bowel disease treated with thiopurines: cohort from the CESAME Study
Coelho J, for the CESAME pregancy study group (France) (Paris 7 Univ, France; et al)
Gut 60:198-203, 2011

Background and Aims.—Few studies have been conducted addressing the safety of thiopurine treatment in pregnant women with inflammatory bowel disease (IBD). The aim of this study was to evaluate the pregnancy outcome of women with IBD who have been exposed to thiopurines.

Methods.—215 pregnancies in 204 women were registered and documented in the CESAME cohort between May 2004 and October 2007. Physicians documented the following information from the women: last menstrual date, delivery term, details of pregnancy outcome, prematurity, birth weight and height, congenital abnormalities, medication history during each trimester, smoking history and alcohol ingestion. Data were compared between three groups: women exposed to thiopurines (group A), women receiving a drug other than thiopurines (group B) and women not receiving any medication (group C).

Results.—Mean age at pregnancy was 28.3 years. 75.7% of the women had Crohn's disease and 21.8% had ulcerative colitis, with a mean disease duration of 6.8 years at inclusion. Of the 215 pregnancies, there were 138 births (142 newborns), and the mean birth weight was 3135 g. There were 86 pregnancies in group A, 84 in group B and 45 in group C. Interrupted pregnancies occurred in 36% of patients enrolled in group A, 33% of patients enrolled in group B, and 40% of patients enrolled in group C; congenital abnormalities arose in 3.6% of group A cases and 7.1% of group B cases. No significant differences were found between the three groups in overall pregnancy outcome.

Conclusions.—The results obtained from this cohort indicate that thiopurine use during pregnancy is not associated with increased risks, including congenital abnormalities.

▶ Women with inflammatory bowel disease (IBD) are often diagnosed during or prior to their childbearing years. A woman's decision to become pregnant needs to be made with an understanding of the impact of IBD on pregnancy and the potential adverse effects of medications on fetal outcomes. Pregnancy outcomes are best among women in remission, but the decision on whether to continue medications that led to that remission may be difficult. The results of this article with regard to thiopurine use are encouraging. The CESAME cohort represents nearly 20 000 IBD patients followed in France over 3 years for cancer risk. Members of the cohort were invited to report pregnancies, and outcomes were followed. While 215 pregnancies in 204 women (86 had received thiopurines) do not seem like many, this represents one of the largest reported cohorts to date and demonstrates no increase in congenital anomalies. The first obvious criticism of this article is that the patient numbers are too small, and it does lack statistical power. This is true, as the authors concede, so that with number of pregnancies followed, only a 5-fold difference in anomalies from baseline 4% to 20% among those taking thiopurines could be detected. Furthermore, outcomes were patient reported and not verified by physicians. Overall, the conclusions from this study are severely limited. They are reassuring when taken along with the growing body of literature suggesting that thiopurines may be safe during pregnancy in doses used in IBD. The emphasis is on the "may," and a careful discussion should take place between patients and their physicians based on existing evidence well before pregnancy is contemplated. More information is needed in the form of more larger studies or a meta-analysis. Many clinicians will continue these medications among their patients with IBD, but this must be an individual decision.

M. F. Picco, MD, PhD

5-Aminosalicylates Prevent Relapse of Crohn's Disease After Surgically Induced Remission: Systematic Review and Meta-Analysis

Ford AC, Khan KJ, Talley NJ, et al (Leeds General Infirmary, UK; McMaster Univ, Hamilton, Ontario, Canada; Univ of Newcastle, New South Wales, Australia)

Am J Gastroenterol 106:413-420, 2011

Objectives.—Evidence from randomized controlled trials (RCTs) for the use of 5-aminosalicylic acid (5-ASA) drugs in Crohn's disease (CD) in remission after a surgical resection is conflicting. We conducted a systematic review and meta-analysis of RCTs to examine this issue.

Methods.—MEDLINE, EMBASE, and the Cochrane central register of controlled trials were searched (through April 2010). Eligible trials recruited adults with luminal CD in remission after a surgical resection and compared 5-ASAs with placebo, or no treatment. Dichotomous data were pooled to obtain relative risk (RR) of relapse of disease activity, with a 95% confidence interval (CI). The number needed to treat (NNT) was calculated from the reciprocal of the risk difference.

Results.—The search strategy identified 3,061 citations. Eleven RCTs were eligible for inclusion containing 1,282 patients. The RR of relapse of CD in remission after surgery with 5-ASA vs. placebo or no therapy was 0.86 (95% CI = 0.74–0.99) (NNT13). Sulfasalazine was of no benefit in preventing relapse in 448 patients (RR0.97; 95% CI = 0.72–1.31), but mesalamine was more effective than placebo or no therapy (RR = 0.80; 95% CI0.70–0.92) in 834 patients, with an NNT of 10.

Conclusions.—Mesalamine is of modest benefit in preventing relapse of CD in remission after surgery. Its use should be considered in those in whom immunosuppressive therapy is either not warranted or contraindicated.

▶ Currently, there is little enthusiasm for the use of mesalamine for Crohn's disease (CD). This conclusion is based on many studies that, while in some cases are conflicting, show little benefit. In this meta-analysis, the authors concluded that mesalamine is beneficial in prophylaxis after surgically induced remission. Mesalamine did show a "modest" benefit, but sulfasalazine did not. While the authors do conduct a careful meta-analysis to allow for bias and study heterogeneity, questions still remain as to the appropriate use of mesalamine among patients with a surgically induced remission. The first concern is the heterogeneity of the patients studied. The authors could not adjust for the location of CD or type of resection. Furthermore, we have no information regarding disease behavior. Both these factors may influence response to mesalamine. Behavior is particularly important. Patients included had "luminal disease," which does not distinguish disease confined to the lumen from penetrating or fibrostenotic disease. Each of these behaviors has its own postoperative prognosis. These factors, along with other patient-specific factors, such as smoking, may have influenced relapse rates. The authors suggest that treatment of 10 patients would result in prevention of one relapse. This may very well be the best possible treatment effect that can be expected in a group of low-risk patients in whom immunomodulator or biologic therapy would not be considered. As treatment of CD has become more aggressive, this represents very few patients. Other patients in whom immunosuppressive therapy is warranted but contraindicated are much less likely to respond to mesalamine. If there is no other choice, this meta-analysis suggests that there may be some benefit despite the high costs of these medications. Postoperative prophylaxis with mesalamine is marginally better than nothing and may be considered in select patients.

M. F. Picco, MD, PhD

Treatment of Relapsing Mild-to-Moderate Ulcerative Colitis with the Probiotic VSL#3 as Adjunctive to a Standard Pharmaceutical Treatment: A Double-Blind, Randomized, Placebo-Controlled Study

Tursi A, Brandimarte G, Papa A, et al ("Lorenzo Bonomo" Hosp, Andria, Italy; "Cristo Re" Hosp, Roma, Italy; Catholic Univ, Roma, Italy; et al)

Am J Gastroenterol 105:2218-2227, 2010

Objectives.—VSL#3 is a high-potency probiotic mixture that has been used successfully in the treatment of pouchitis. The primary end point of the study was to assess the effects of supplementation with VSL#3 in patients affected by relapsing ulcerative colitis (UC) who are already under treatment with 5-aminosalicylic acid (ASA) and/or immunosuppressants at stable doses.

Methods.—A total of 144 consecutive patients were randomly treated for 8 weeks with VSL#3 at a dose of 3,600 billion CFU/day (71 patients) or with placebo (73 patients).

Results.—In all, 65 patients in the VSL#3 group and 66 patients in the placebo group completed the study. The decrease in ulcerative colitis disease activity index (UCDAI) scores of 50% or more was higher in the VSL#3 group than in the placebo group (63.1 vs. 40.8; per protocol (PP) $P = 0.010$, confidence interval $CI_{95\%}$ 0.51–0.74; intention to treat (ITT) $P = 0.031$, $CI_{95\%}$ 0.47–0.69). Significant results with VSL#3 were recorded in an improvement of three points or more in the UCDAI score (60.5% vs. 41.4%; PP $P = 0.017$, $CI_{95\%}$ 0.51–0.74; ITT $P = 0.046$, $CI_{95\%}$ 0.47–0.69) and in rectal bleeding (PP $P = 0.014$, $CI_{95\%}$ 0.46–0.70; ITT $P = 0.036$, $CI_{95\%}$ 0.41–0.65), whereas stool frequency (PP $P = 0.202$, $CI_{95\%}$ 0.39–0.63; ITT $P = 0.229$, $CI_{95\%}$ 0.35–0.57), physician's rate of disease activity (PP $P = 0.088$, $CI_{95\%}$ 0.34–0.58; ITT $P = 0.168$, $CI_{95\%}$ 0.31–0.53), and endoscopic scores (PP $P = 0.086$, $CI_{95\%}$ 0.74–0.92; ITT $P = 0.366$, $CI_{95\%}$ 0.66–0.86) did not show statistical differences. Remission was higher in the VSL#3 group than in the placebo group (47.7% vs. 32.4%; PP $P = 0.069$, $CI_{95\%}$ 0.36–0.60; ITT $P = 0.132$, $CI_{95\%}$ 0.33–0.56). Eight patients on VSL#3 (11.2%) and nine patients on placebo (12.3%) reported mild side effects.

Conclusions.—VSL#3 supplementation is safe and able to reduce UCDAI scores in patients affected by relapsing mild-to-moderate UC who are under treatment with 5-ASA and/or immunosuppressants. Moreover, VSL#3 improves rectal bleeding and seems to reinduce remission in relapsing UC patients after 8 weeks of treatment, although these parameters do not reach statistical significance.

▶ Probiotics have been touted as beneficial treatments in numerous digestive diseases and are readily available at health food stores and on the Internet. Despite claims of efficacy, definitive evidence is lacking, and use remains controversial. It is important to understand that all probiotics are not created equal and may not be effective despite claims from their manufacturers. VSL#3 is the most tested of the probiotics for the treatment of inflammatory bowel disease and has an established place in the prevention of recurrent pouchitis among patients who have an ileal pouch construction following colectomy for ulcerative colitis. In this study, the authors claim that VSL#3 is beneficial as an adjunctive treatment among patients with active mild to moderate ulcerative colitis (UC) on maintenance therapy. While this conclusion does have some merit, it must be interpreted in the context of the patients studied. While the authors claim that VSL#3 is effective for mild to moderate UC, the majority of the patients studied had mild disease as evident from their activity index. This may have been the reason that the outcome of a 50% drop in index score was met but a decrease in stool frequency or improvement in physician-rated disease activity could not be shown. Most were only taking low-dose mesalamine with only few receiving immunomodulator therapy, again suggesting that their disease was probably milder and would have responded to increasing the dose of mesalamine. Finally, there was no difference in the endoscopic improvement between the 2 groups, although this may have been because of the short duration of the trial. Remission rates between VSL#3 and placebo were not different, although there was a trend toward a benefit of the probiotic. Overall, while these results are encouraging, much more evidence is needed before VSL#3 should be adopted into routine clinical practice. The correct patient population for these agents needs to be defined, and a clear benefit over existing therapies must be proven.

M. F. Picco, MD, PhD

49 Liver Disease

Noninvasive Tests for Fibrosis and Liver Stiffness Predict 5-Year Outcomes of Patients With Chronic Hepatitis C
Vergniol J, Foucher J, Terrebonne E, et al (Hôpital Haut-Lévêque, Pessac, France; et al)
Gastroenterology 140:1970-1979, 2011

Background & Aims.—Liver stiffness can be measured noninvasively to assess liver fibrosis in patients with chronic hepatitis C. In patients with chronic liver diseases, level of fibrosis predicts liver-related complications and survival. We evaluated the abilities of liver stiffness, results from noninvasive tests for fibrosis, and liver biopsy analyses to predict overall survival or survival without liver-related death with a 5-year period.

Methods.—In a consecutive cohort of 1457 patients with chronic hepatitis C, we assessed fibrosis and, on the same day, liver stiffness, performed noninvasive tests of fibrosis (FibroTest, the aspartate aminotransferase to platelet ratio index, FIB-4), and analyzed liver biopsy samples. We analyzed data on death, liver-related death, and liver transplantation collected during a 5-year follow-up period.

Results.—At 5 years, 77 patients had died (39 liver-related deaths) and 16 patients had undergone liver transplantation. Overall survival was 91.7% and survival without liver-related death was 94.4%. Survival was significantly decreased among patients diagnosed with severe fibrosis, regardless of the noninvasive method of analysis. All methods were able to predict shorter survival times in this large population; liver stiffness and results of FibroTest had higher predictive values. Patient outcomes worsened as liver stiffness and FibroTest values increased. Prognostic values of stiffness ($P < .0001$) and FibroTest results ($P < .0001$) remained after they were adjusted for treatment response, patient age, and estimates of necroinflammatory grade.

Conclusions.—Noninvasive tests for liver fibrosis (measurement of liver stiffness or FibroTest) can predict 5-year survival of patients with chronic hepatitis C. These tools might help physicians determine prognosis at earlier stages and discuss specific treatments, such as liver transplantation.

▶ The evaluation of extent of liver fibrosis is important in the management of patients with chronic liver disease. It is a deciding factor in consideration of the need to screen patients for complications of significant fibrosis, such as hepatocellular cancer and complications of portal hypertension, such as varices. Until recently, the only measure of liver fibrosis was liver biopsy. Liver biopsy is invasive and carries significant risk of complications. In addition, there can be bias in sampling variability. For these reasons, a noninvasive measure of liver fibrosis would be beneficial in patient management.

Liver stiffness measurement using a FibroScan probe has been shown to have a high degree of accuracy and reproducibility in predicting significant fibrosis in patients with chronic liver disease. Noninvasive markers, such as FibroTest, have been shown to be a surrogate marker of fibrosis and show a correlation with survival in patients with chronic liver disease. The aim of this study was to evaluate the 5-year prognostic value of noninvasive markers of liver fibrosis for predicting survival and liver-related death in patients with chronic hepatitis C virus (HCV) infection.

The results of this study independently validated the prognostic value of FibroTest and showed that markers of liver stiffness and FibroTest both predicted survival in patients with chronic HCV infection.

D. M. Harnois, DO

The natural history of nonalcoholic fatty liver disease with advanced fibrosis or cirrhosis: An international collaborative study

Bhala N, Angulo P, van der Poorten D, et al (Univ of Oxford, UK; Univ of Kentucky Med Ctr, Lexington; Univ of Sydney, Westmead, New South Wales, Australia; et al)
Hepatology 2011 [Epub ahead of print]

Information on the long-term prognosis of nonalcoholic fatty liver disease (NAFLD) is limited. We sought to describe the long-term morbidity and mortality of patients with NAFLD with advanced fibrosis or cirrhosis.

We conducted this prospective cohort study including 247 patients with NAFLD and 264 patients with HCV infection that were either naïve or non-responders to treatment. Both cohorts were Child-Pugh class A and had advanced (stage 3) fibrosis or cirrhosis (stage 4) confirmed by liver biopsy at enrolment.

In the NAFLD cohort, followed-up for 85.6 months mean (range 6-297), there were 48 (19.4%) liver-related complications and 33 (13.4%) deaths or liver transplants. In the HCV cohort, followed-up for 74.9 months mean (range 6-238), there were 47 (16.7%) liver-related complications and 25 (9.4%) deaths or liver transplants. When adjusting for baseline differences in age and gender, the cumulative incidence of liver-related complications was lower in the NAFLD than the HCV cohort (p=0.03), including incident hepatocellular cancer (6 vs 18; p=0.03), but that of cardiovascular events (p=0.17) and overall mortality (p=0.6) was similar in both groups. In the NAFLD cohort, platelet count, stage 4 fibrosis, and serum levels of cholesterol and ALT were associated with liver-related complications; an AST/ALT ratio <1 and older age were associated with overall mortality; and higher serum bilirubin levels and stage 4 fibrosis were associated with liver-related mortality.

Conclusions.—Patients with NAFLD with advanced fibrosis or cirrhosis have lower rates of liver-related complications and hepatocellular cancer than corresponding patients with HCV infection, but similar overall mortality. Some clinical and laboratory features predict outcomes in patients with NAFLD.

▶ Nonalcoholic fatty liver disease (NAFLD) has become the most prevalent cause of chronic liver disease worldwide. Regarded as the hepatic manifestation of the metabolic syndrome, NAFLD represents a histological spectrum of disease that extends from simple steatosis to steatohepatitis. NAFLD may be associated with advanced fibrosis or cirrhosis that can result in complications and mortality. Despite its prevalence, the prognosis of NAFLD with advanced fibrosis or cirrhosis remains poorly studied, and important aspects of the prognosis of patients with NAFLD still remain unclear. Finally, it is unclear which, if any, risk factors can independently predict liver, vascular, and overall morbidity and mortality.

To answer these questions, the investigators carried out an international, multicenter prospective study to assess the natural history and outcomes of liver biopsy—confirmed NAFLD with advanced fibrosis or cirrhosis. In this study from 4 countries, the investigators report the natural history of the biopsy-proven NAFLD with advanced fibrosis or cirrhosis. The NAFLD patients had well-compensated liver disease and no overt hepatic synthetic dysfunction at presentation. When they were compared with patients with liver disease secondary to chronic hepatitis C virus (HCV) infection with advanced fibrosis or cirrhosis of the same functional status, there were long-term differences, notably less liver-related complications and less hepatocellular carcinoma risk in patients with NAFLD as compared with patients with HCV infection. Interestingly, however, there were also remarkable long-term similarities for vascular disease and overall mortality in both groups. Larger prospective studies will be necessary to shed further understanding on the impact of NAFLD on liver- and vascular-related morbidity and mortality.

D. M. Harnois, DO

Prevalence of Nonalcoholic Fatty Liver Disease and Nonalcoholic Steatohepatitis Among a Largely Middle-Aged Population Utilizing Ultrasound and Liver Biopsy: A Prospective Study

Williams CD, Stengel J, Asike MI, et al (Brooke Army Med Ctr, Fort Sam Houston, TX)
Gastroenterology 140:124-131, 2011

Background & Aims.—Prevalence of nonalcoholic fatty liver disease (NAFLD) has not been well established. The purpose of this study was to prospectively define the prevalence of both NAFLD and nonalcoholic steatohepatitis (NASH).

Methods.—Outpatients 18 to 70 years old were recruited from Brooke Army Medical Center. All patients completed a baseline questionnaire and ultrasound. If fatty liver was identified, then laboratory data and a liver biopsy were obtained.

Results.—Four hundred patients were enrolled. Three hundred and twenty-eight patients completed the questionnaire and ultrasound. Mean age (range, 28–70 years) was 54.6 years (7.35); 62.5% Caucasian, 22% Hispanic, and 11.3% African American; 50.9% female; mean body mass index (BMI) (calculated as kg/m2) was 29.8 (5.64); and diabetes and hypertension prevalence 16.5% and 49.7%, respectively. Prevalence of NAFLD was 46%. NASH was confirmed in 40 patients (12.2% of total cohort, 29.9% of ultrasound positive patients). Hispanics had the highest prevalence of NAFLD (58.3%), then Caucasians (44.4%) and African Americans (35.1%). NAFLD patients were more likely to be male (58.9%), older ($P = .004$), hypertensive ($P < .00005$), and diabetic ($P < .00005$). They had a higher BMI ($P < .0005$), ate fast food more often ($P = .049$), and exercised less ($P = 0.02$) than their non-NAFLD counterparts. Hispanics had a higher prevalence of NASH compared with Caucasians (19.4% vs 9.8%; $P = .03$). Alanine aminotransferase, aspartate aminotransferase, BMI, insulin, Quantitative Insulin-Sensitivity Check Index, and cytokeratin-18 correlated with NASH. Among the 54 diabetic patients, NAFLD was found in 74% and NASH in 22.2%.

Conclusion.—Prevalence of NAFLD and NASH is higher than estimated previously. Hispanics and patients with diabetes are at greatest risk for both NAFLD and NASH.

▶ The health implications of the current epidemic of obesity are not fully understood. As the article points out, recent estimates suggest that obesity in adults has increased to 33.8%, and the prevalence of diabetes in adults ages 45 to 64 years has increased to 10.6% in the United States. One of the health consequences of obesity is metabolic syndrome and nonalcoholic fatty liver disease. Nonalcoholic fatty liver disease (NAFLD) encompasses a spectrum of liver disease ranging from simple noninflammatory steatosis to nonalcoholic steatohepatitis (NASH) and cirrhosis.

In this prospective study of outpatients 18 to 70 years of age recruited from Brooke Army Medical Center, the overall prevalence of NAFLD was 46%, and NASH was 12.2%. Hispanics had the highest prevalence followed by Caucasians and then African Americans. There was a prevalence, of NAFLD and NASH in diabetic patients. In this study, the prevalence of NASH in an asymptomatic adult population enrolled without regard to liver enzyme abnormalities was higher than previously estimated. In addition, 2.7% of patients had significant fibrosis (stage 2-4) secondary to NASH, many of these asymptomatic.

This study provides additional evidence with regard to the health implications of the current trend of obesity in the United States and the importance of health screening in these patients.

D. M. Harnois, DO

Rifaximin Improves Driving Simulator Performance in a Randomized Trial of Patients With Minimal Hepatic Encephalopathy

Bajaj JS, Heuman DM, Wade JB, et al (Virginia Commonwealth Univ and McGuire VA Med Ctr, Richmond; et al)
Gastroenterology 140:478-487, 2011

Background & Aims.—Patients with cirrhosis and minimal hepatic encephalopathy (MHE) have driving difficulties but the effects of therapy on driving performance is unclear. We evaluated whether performance on a driving simulator improves in patients with MHE after treatment with rifaximin.

Methods.—Patients with MHE who were current drivers were randomly assigned to placebo or rifaximin groups and followed up for 8 weeks (n = 42). Patients underwent driving simulation (driving and navigation tasks) at the start (baseline) and end of the study. We evaluated patients' cognitive abilities, quality of life (using the Sickness Impact Profile), serum levels of ammonia, levels of inflammatory cytokines, and model for end-stage-liver disease scores. The primary outcome was the percentage of patients who improved in driving performance, calculated as follows: total driving errors = speeding + illegal turns + collisions.

Results.—Over the 8-week study period, patients given rifaximin made significantly greater improvements than those given placebo in avoiding total driving errors (76% vs 31%; $P = .013$), speeding (81% vs 33%; $P = .005$), and illegal turns (62% vs 19%; $P = .01$). Of patients given rifaximin, 91% improved their cognitive performance, compared with 61% of patients given placebo ($P = .01$); they also made improvements in the psychosocial dimension of the Sickness Impact Profile compared with the placebo group ($P = .04$). Adherence to the assigned drug averaged 92%. Neither group had changes in ammonia levels or model for end-stage-liver disease scores, but patients in the rifaximin group had increased levels of the anti-inflammatory cytokine interleukin-10.

Conclusions.—Patients with MHE significantly improve driving simulator performance after treatment with rifaximin, compared with placebo.

▶ Patients with cirrhosis often have an underrecognized impairment in cognitive dysfunction known as minimal hepatic encephalopathy (MHE). These symptoms can significantly impact quality of life and ability to maintain job performance or life activities. Skills required to drive include balance, attention, and integration of various cognitive inputs. These are areas affected by MHE.

In this study, patients with cirrhosis who were not on treatment for encephalopathy and with no history of overt symptoms of encephalopathy were identified on testing as having MHE. These patients were randomized to treatment with rifaximin 550 mg twice daily versus placebo. Their driving skills were then tested. Patients treated with rifaximin had significant improvement in driving-simulator performance versus placebo.

Many patients with cirrhosis have unidentified symptoms of MHE that may significantly impact their life. It is important to diagnose these patients and consider therapy with lactulose and/or rifaximin.

D. M. Harnois, DO

Excess Mortality in Patients with Advanced Chronic Hepatitis C Treated with Long-Term Peginterferon
Di Bisceglie AM, for the HALT-C Trial Group (Saint Louis Univ School of Medicine, MO; et al)
Hepatology 53:1100-1108, 2011

Chronic hepatitis C virus infection can cause chronic liver disease, cirrhosis and liver cancer. The Hepatitis C Antiviral Long-term Treatment against Cirrhosis (HALT-C) Trial was a prospective, randomized controlled study of long-term, low-dose peginterferon therapy in patients with advanced chronic hepatitis C who failed to respond to a previous course of optimal antiviral therapy. The aim of this follow-up analysis is to describe the frequency and causes of death among this cohort of patients. Deaths occurring during and after the HALT-C Trial were reviewed by a committee of investigators to determine the cause of death and to categorize each death as liver- or nonliver-related and as related or not to complications of peginterferon. Rates of liver transplantation were also assessed. Over a median of 5.7 years, 122 deaths occurred among 1,050 randomized patients (12%), of which 76 were considered liver-related (62%) and 46 nonliver-related (38%); 74 patients (7%) underwent liver transplantation. At 7 years the cumulative mortality rate was higher in the treatment compared to the control group (20% versus 15%, $P = 0.049$); the primary difference in mortality was in patients in the fibrosis compared to the cirrhosis stratum (14% versus 7%, $P = 0.01$); comparable differences were observed when liver transplantation was included. Excess mortality, emerging after 3 years of treatment, was related largely to nonliver-related death; liver-related mortality was similar in the treatment and control groups. No specific cause of death accounted for the excess mortality and only one death was suspected to be a direct complication of peginterferon.

Conclusion.—Long-term maintenance peginterferon in patients with advanced chronic hepatitis C is associated with an excess overall mortality, which was primarily due to nonliver-related causes among patients with bridging fibrosis.

▶ Hepatitis C virus infection is an important cause of chronic liver disease. Beginning in 2000, the Hepatitis C Antiviral Long-term Treatment against Cirrhosis trial sought to answer the question of the benefit of low-dose maintenance therapy with peginterferon compared with no therapy in slowing progression of liver disease and preventing complications of end-stage liver disease. The trial ended in 2007 and failed to show a benefit of long-term interferon on clinical outcomes. In fact, an increase in mortality was seen in the group treated with interferon with advanced fibrosis but not cirrhosis. This study sought to more completely understand the explanation for that increased mortality rate.

The finding of higher mortality rates observed in the patients treated with pegylated interferon persisted when analyzed with a longer follow-up. The excess mortality did not begin to rise until after 3 years into the treatment and continued for several years after treatment was stopped. Nonetheless, a thorough review of the causes of death in these patients failed to identify a direct relationship as we currently understand it between the death rate and pegylated interferon therapy.

This study provides additional evidence that the use of long-term pegylated interferon therapy should be avoided or, at a minimum, be used cautiously.

D. M. Harnois, DO

Outcomes of Treatment for Hepatitis C Virus Infection by Primary Care Providers

Arora S, Thornton K, Murata G, et al (Univ of New Mexico, Albuquerque; et al)
N Engl J Med 364:2199-2207, 2011

Background.—The Extension for Community Healthcare Outcomes (ECHO) model was developed to improve access to care for underserved populations with complex health problems such as hepatitis C virus (HCV) infection. With the use of video-conferencing technology, the ECHO program trains primary care providers to treat complex diseases.

Methods.—We conducted a prospective cohort study comparing treatment for HCV infection at the University of New Mexico (UNM) HCV clinic with treatment by primary care clinicians at 21 ECHO sites in rural areas and prisons in New Mexico. A total of 407 patients with chronic HCV infection who had received no previous treatment for the infection were enrolled. The primary end point was a sustained virologic response.

Results.—A total of 57.5% of the patients treated at the UNM HCV clinic (84 of 146 patients) and 58.2% of those treated at ECHO sites (152 of 261 patients) had a sustained viral response (difference in rates between sites, 0.7 percentage points; 95% confidence interval, −9.2 to 10.7; $P = 0.89$). Among patients with HCV genotype 1 infection, the rate of sustained viral response was 45.8% (38 of 83 patients) at the UNM HCV clinic and 49.7% (73 of 147 patients) at ECHO sites ($P = 0.57$). Serious adverse events occurred in 13.7% of the patients at the UNM HCV clinic and in 6.9% of the patients at ECHO sites.

Conclusions.—The results of this study show that the ECHO model is an effective way to treat HCV infection in underserved communities. Implementation of this model would allow other states and nations to treat a greater number of patients infected with HCV than they are currently able to treat. (Funded by the Agency for Healthcare Research and Quality and others.)

▶ There is no question that, in the future, the structure of the medical system will look very different than it does today. Technology will provide a framework for greater data acquisition and potentially for sharing of information and expertise in ways never dreamed possible.

In the United States, there have been many articles written regarding the discrepancies in health care delivery among various populations. In particular, those people in underserved areas do not have access to many of the same treatments that are available in cities or in academic medical centers. Occasionally, this is an issue of technology, but sometimes it is simply a limitation of expertise and support for otherwise affordable treatments.

In the United States, it is estimated that a minimum of 3.2 million individuals are infected with the hepatitis C virus (HCV). Chronic hepatitis C accounts for 10 000 deaths per year in the United States and is the leading reason for liver transplantation. It is also clear that many patients who qualify for HCV treatment do not receive that treatment. There are many reasons why that is true, but in underserved areas, it is, in part, related to lack of specialty-care physicians in these communities.

In this article from *The New England Journal of Medicine*, a new model for health care delivery is reported. The ECHO model (Extension for Community Healthcare Outcomes) was developed to link the expertise of physicians at the University of New Mexico with patients at primary care clinics in rural areas and prisons in New Mexico. The target of treatment in this article was HCV infection. The results of this study show that the ECHO model was an effective way to treat HCV infection in underserved communities and may serve as a model to other states wishing to set up similar networks of care.

D. M. Harnois, DO

Association of caffeine intake and histological features of chronic hepatitis C
Costentin CE, Roudot-Thoraval F, Zafrani E-S, et al (Groupe Hospitalier Henri Mondor-Albert Chenevier, Créteil, France; INSERM, Créteil, France; et al)
J Hepatol 54:1123-1129, 2011

Background & Aims.—The severity of chronic hepatitis C (CHC) is modulated by host and environmental factors. Several reports suggest that caffeine intake exerts hepatoprotective effects in patients with chronic liver disease. The aim of this study was to evaluate the impact of caffeine consumption on activity grade and fibrosis stage in patients with CHC.

Methods.—A total of 238 treatment-naïve patients with histologically-proven CHC were included in the study. Demographic, epidemiological, environmental, virological, and metabolic data were collected, including daily consumption of alcohol, cannabis, tobacco, and caffeine during the six months preceding liver biopsy. Daily caffeine consumption was estimated as the sum of mean intakes of caffeinated coffee, tea, and caffeine-containing sodas. Histological activity grade and fibrosis stage were scored according to Metavir. Patients (154 men, 84 women, mean age: 45 ± 11 years) were categorized according to caffeine consumption quartiles: group 1 (<225 mg/day, $n = 59$), group 2 (225–407 mg/day, $n = 57$), group 3 (408–678 mg/day, $n = 62$), and group 4 (>678 mg/day, $n = 60$).

Results.—There was a significant inverse relationship between activity grade and daily caffeine consumption: activity grade >A2 was present in 78%, 61%, 52%, and 48% of patients in group 1, 2, 3, and 4, respectively ($p < 0.001$). By multivariate analysis, daily caffeine consumption greater than 408 mg/day was associated with a lesser risk of activity grade >A2 (OR = 0.32 (0.12–0.85). Caffeine intake showed no relation with fibrosis stage.

Conclusions.—Caffeine consumption greater than 408 mg/day (3 cups or more) is associated with reduced histological activity in patients with CHC. These findings support potential hepatoprotective properties of caffeine in chronic liver diseases.

▶ Many environmental factors may affect the degree of inflammation present in chronic hepatitis C. Caffeine and, in particular, coffee may have anti-inflammatory or antioxidant effects. Caffeine intake may reduce or protect against liver injury in patients with chronic liver diseases. High coffee consumption has been associated with a reduced risk of hepatocellular carcinoma in patients with chronic liver disease.[1] This study examined caffeine consumption in the 6 months before untreated patients with chronic hepatitis C underwent a liver biopsy.

Patients with high intakes (> 3 cups) of coffee had significantly less inflammation but no difference in fibrosis score, which suggests that coffee ingestion is not of any harm in patients with chronic hepatitis C. The other factors, such as degree of steatosis and age, were associated with increased degree of inflammation. Some unrecognized association with high caffeine consumption may confound these results and prior studies in chronic liver diseases; however, caffeine appears to be somewhat protective in 2 such confounders, age and alcohol consumption, which are associated with high coffee consumption. Although this study estimated caffeine consumption, it may be some other component of the primary source of caffeine, coffee, that is the source of benefit. Further study is needed to identify how the apparent benefit occurs. In the meantime, at the very least heavy coffee drinkers with hepatitis C should be encouraged to continue drinking their brew.

J. A. Murray, MD

Reference

1. Gelatti U, Covolo L, Franceschini M, et al. Coffee consumption reduces the risk of hepatocellular carcinoma independently of its aetiology: a case-control study. *J Hepatol.* 2005;42:528-534.

50 Nutrition and Celiac Disease

Morbidity and Mortality Among Older Individuals With Undiagnosed Celiac Disease
Godfrey JD, Brantner TL, Brinjikji W, et al (Mayo Clinic, Rochester, MN)
Gastroenterology 139:763-769, 2010

Background & Aims.—Outcomes of undiagnosed celiac disease (CD) are unclear. We evaluated the morbidity and mortality of undiagnosed CD in a population-based sample of individuals 50 years of age and older.

Methods.—Stored sera from a population-based sample of 16,886 Olmsted County, Minnesota, residents 50 years of age and older were tested for CD based on analysis of tissue transglutaminase and endomysial antibodies. A nested case-control study compared serologically defined subjects with CD with age- and sex-matched, seronegative controls. Medical records were reviewed for comorbid conditions.

Results.—We identified 129 (0.8%) subjects with undiagnosed CD in a cohort of 16,847 older adults. A total of 127 undiagnosed cases (49% men; median age, 63.0 y) and 254 matched controls were included in a systematic evaluation for more than 100 potentially coexisting conditions. Subjects with undiagnosed CD had increased rates of osteoporosis and hypothyroidism, as well as lower body mass index and levels of cholesterol and ferritin. Overall survival was not associated with CD status. During a median follow-up period of 10.3 years after serum samples were collected, 20 cases but no controls were diagnosed with CD (15.2% Kaplan–Meier estimate at 10 years).

Conclusions.—With the exception of reduced bone health, older adults with undiagnosed CD had limited comorbidity and no increase in mortality compared with controls. Some subjects were diagnosed with CD within a decade of serum collection, indicating that although most cases of undiagnosed CD are clinically silent, some result in symptoms. Undiagnosed CD can confer benefits and liabilities to older individuals.

▶ It is well known that there is increased morbidity and moderately increased mortality among patients with diagnosed celiac disease. The level of excess mortality varies depending on the studies. With regard to undiagnosed celiac disease, there have now been a number of studies that have suggested there may be increased mortality in individuals who have undiagnosed celiac disease[1,2]; however, not all studies suggest that there is increased mortality. A Finnish study showed no increase in mortality of these individuals. The study by Godfrey et al is important in that it studies a cohort of patients with undiagnosed celiac disease where serum had been saved in patients whose median age was 63 and whose follow-up was approximately 10 years. This study showed no excess mortality during this period of follow-up. There was some subtle morbidity in lower bone density and an increased propensity to hypothyroidism; however, there was no significant excess of gastrointestinal diagnoses or gastrointestinal procedures in this cohort. There was a trend toward lower body mass index and lower cholesterol in this cohort, suggesting some moderate nutritional impact of undiagnosed celiac disease. The conclusion of this study is that unrecognized celiac disease in patients first tested in their mid 60s followed for 10 years does not result in increased mortality. Interestingly, 16% of individuals were clinically recognized to have celiac disease by the end of the 10-year follow-up, suggesting that 1% of undiagnosed celiac disease will become symptomatic and will be diagnosed per year on average. What does this mean for practice? Routine screening of healthy people at an advanced age for celiac disease is probably not indicated; however, physicians should be aware that celiac disease seems to be quite common in people of this age group and may become symptomatic even at advanced ages. If there is no increased mortality over longer follow-ups than 10 years, then it is likely that patients who are found serendipitously without any symptoms may not necessarily vary greatly in terms of improved survival; however, it may prevent some morbidity.

J. A. Murray, MD

References

1. Rubio-Tapia A, Kyle RA, Kaplan EL, et al. Increased prevalence and mortality in undiagnosed celiac disease. *Gastroenterology.* 2009;137:88-93.
2. Metzger MH, Heier M, Mäki M, et al. Mortality excess in individuals with elevated IgA anti-transglutaminase antibodies: the KORA/MONICA Augsburg cohort study 1989-1998. *Eur J Epidemiol.* 2006;21:359-365.

A Biopsy Is Not Always Necessary to Diagnose Celiac Disease

Mubarak A, Wolters VM, Gerritsen SAM, et al (Univ Med Ctr Utrecht, The Netherlands)
J Pediatr Gastroenterol Nutr 52:554-557, 2011

Objectives.—Small intestinal histology is the criterion standard for the diagnosis of celiac disease (CD). However, results of serological tests such as anti-endomysium antibodies and anti-tissue transglutaminase antibodies (tTGA) are becoming increasingly reliable. This raises the question of whether a small intestinal biopsy is always necessary. The aim of the present study was, therefore, to investigate whether a small intestinal biopsy can be avoided in a selected group of patients.

Patients and Methods.—Serology and histological slides obtained from 283 pediatric patients suspected of having CD were examined retrospectively. The response to a gluten-free diet (GFD) in patients with a tTGA level ≥100 U/mL was investigated.

Results.—A tTGA level ≥100 U/mL was found in 128 of the 283 patients. Upon microscopic examination of the small intestinal epithelium, villous atrophy was found in 124 of these patients, confirming the presence of CD. Three patients had crypt hyperplasia or an increased number of intraepithelial lymphocytes. In 1 patient no histological abnormalities were found. This patient did not respond to a GFD.

Conclusions.—Pediatric patients with a tTGA level ≥100 U/mL in whom symptoms improve upon consuming a GFD may not need a small intestinal biopsy to confirm CD.

▶ The diagnosis of celiac disease currently requires duodenal biopsies for confirmation. Mubarak et al have studied the necessity for biopsies in patients with high positive tissue transglutaminase antibodies. They performed a retrospective analysis of consecutive patients referred to the pediatric gastrointestinal department for endoscopy. They had 301 patients in whom both serologic testing and biopsies were available. They excluded patients with giardiasis and immunoglobulin A (IgA) deficiency. A total of 57.6% of patients ultimately had a biopsy-proven diagnosis of celiac disease. They demonstrated that the overall specificity for celiac disease using the tissue transglutaminase IgA test was 83% with a sensitivity of 96%. Interestingly, they found the sensitivity of the endomysial antibody IgA was 96%; the specificity was only 66%. They demonstrated that in those patients in whom the tissue transglutaminase antibody levels were very high (> 100), the specificity went up to 97% and indeed showed that just 1 subject had a completely normal biopsy result. In this setting, they make the case that extremely high positive tissue transglutaminase antibodies, in this case > 100, were highly predictive of celiac disease, and in the 1 patient, who was truly a false-positive, no response to diet occurred. This study demonstrates that extremely positive serology for celiac disease using the specific test of tissue transglutaminase IgA is highly predictive of celiac disease and may, in certain circumstances, permit the avoidance of biopsy in children. One cause for concern is the low specificity of endomysial antibodies, suggesting that perhaps endomysial antibody is such a specialized test that it should only be performed in high volume, which could help maintain the expertise and consistency of reporting. The other potential weakness is that major criteria for undertaking biopsies are positive serologic test results, leading to a common weakness in many such retrospective studies, that is, positive selection bias for serologically positive individuals undergoing biopsies. This phenomenon would lead to the overestimation of the accuracy of the tests. Nonetheless, when faced with a patient with very positive serology, the chance of celiac disease is extremely high with a positive predictive value in patients with suspicious symptoms for celiac disease of 97%. Lower positive predictive values may occur when populations with a lower pretest prevalence are studied. However, not all authors agree; Freeman reported a significant minority of patients with strongly positive tissue transglutaminase antibodies who have normal biopsy results.[1]

J. A. Murray, MD

Reference

1. Freeman HJ. Strongly positive tissue transglutaminase antibody assays without celiac disease. *Can J Gastroenterol.* 2004;18:25-28.

51 Pancreaticobiliary Disease

A 6-month, open-label clinical trial of pancrelipase delayed-release capsules (Creon) in patients with exocrine pancreatic insufficiency due to chronic pancreatitis or pancreatic surgery

Gubergrits N, Malecka-Panas E, Lehman GA, et al (Donetsk Natl Med Univ, Ukraine; Med Univ of Lodz, Poland; Indiana Univ Med Ctr, Indianapolis; et al)

Aliment Pharmacol Ther 33:1152-1161, 2011

Background.—Pancreatic enzyme replacement therapy (PERT) is necessary to prevent severe maldigestion and unwanted weight loss associated with exocrine pancreatic insufficiency (EPI) due to chronic pancreatitis (CP) or pancreatic surgery (PS).

Aim.—To assess the long-term safety and efficacy of pancrelipase (pancreatin) delayed-release capsules (Creon) in this population.

Methods.—This was a 6-month, open-label extension of a 7-day, double-blind, placebo-controlled study enrolling patients ≥18 years old with confirmed EPI due to CP or PS who were previously receiving PERT. Patients received individualised pancrelipase doses as directed by investigators (administered as Creon 24 000-lipase unit capsules).

Results.—Overall, 48 of 51 patients completed the open-label phase; one withdrew due to the unrelated treatment-emergent adverse event (TEAE) of cutaneous burns and two were lost to follow-up. The mean age was 50.9 years, 70.6% of patients were male, 76.5% had CP and 23.5% had undergone PS. The mean ± s.d. pancrelipase dose was 186 960 ± 74 640 lipase units/day. TEAEs were reported by 22 patients (43.1%) overall. Only four patients (7.8%) had TEAEs that were considered treatment related. From double-blind phase baseline to end of the open-label period, subjects achieved a mean ± s.d. body weight increase of 2.7 ± 3.4 kg ($P < 0.0001$) and change in daily stool frequency of −1.0 ± 1.3 ($P < 0.001$). Improvements in abdominal pain, flatulence and stool consistency were observed.

Conclusions.—Pancrelipase was well tolerated over 6 months and resulted in statistically significant weight gain and reduced stool frequency in patients with EPI due to CP or PS previously managed with standard PERT.

▶ Exocrine pancreatic insufficiency leads to malabsorption and is often associated with weight loss and malnutrition. Pancreatic enzyme supplementation has been a well-accepted part of the management of these patients for many years; however, this is the first study to demonstrate meaningful increases in body weight and reduction in stool frequency over 6 months of treatment with an acceptable side-effect profile. The mean weight gain was 2.7 ± 3.4 kg, and there was a significant decrease in daily stool frequency from 2.8 to 1.8. The doses of enzyme replacement were higher than reported previously with a mean daily dosage of 186 960 ± 74 640 units of lipase, although the response was not dose dependent. No change was demonstrated in symptoms, such as abdominal pain, stool consistency or flatulence, clinical global improvement scores, or quality-of-life measures. Treatment-related adverse events occurred in 7.8% of patients and included mild abdominal pain, flatulence, diarrhea, and weight gain in a patient with a body mass index of 35.

Although healthy skepticism should be applied to any nonrandomized and company-funded research, this study does suggest enzyme supplementation has potential value in those patients with confirmed pancreatic insufficiency caused by chronic pancreatitis or pancreatic surgery, at least in terms of weight gain. The doses used in this study are higher than previously reported, and further study on optimal dosing schedules should be performed.

S. M. Philcox, MD

Outcome of Patients With Type 1 or 2 Autoimmune Pancreatitis
Maire F, Le Baleur Y, Rebours V, et al (Diderot-Paris VII Univ, Clichy, France; et al)
Am J Gastroenterol 106:151-156, 2011

Objectives.—Autoimmune pancreatitis (AIP) is better described than before, but there is still no international consensus for definition, diagnosis, and treatment. Our aims were to analyze the short- and long-term outcome of patients with focus on pancreatic endocrine and exocrine functions, to search for predictive factors of relapse and pancreatic insufficiency, and to compare patients with type 1 and type 2 AIP.

Methods.—All consecutive patients followed up for AIP in our center between 1999 and 2008 were included. Two groups were defined: (a) patients with type 1 AIP meeting HISORt (Histology, Imaging, Serology, Other organ involvement, and Response to steroids) criteria; (b) patients with definitive/probable type 2 AIP including those with histologically confirmed idiopathic duct-centric pancreatitis (definitive) or suggestive imaging, normal serum IgG4, and response to steroids (probable). AIP-related events and pancreatic exocrine/endocrine insufficiency were looked for during follow-up. Predictive factors of relapse and pancreatic insufficiency were analyzed.

Results.—A total of 44 patients (22 males), median age 37.5 (19–73) years, were included: 28 patients (64%) with type 1 AIP and 16 patients (36%) with type 2 AIP. First-line treatment consisted of steroids or pancreatic resection in 59 and 27% of the patients, respectively. Median follow-up was 41 (5–130) months. Steroids were effective in all treated patients.

Relapse was observed in 12 patients (27%), after a median delay of 6 months (1—70). Four patients received azathioprine because of steroid resistance/dependence. High serum IgG4 level, pain at time of diagnosis, and other organ involvement were associated with relapse (*P*<0.05). At the end point, pancreatic atrophy was observed in 35% of patients. Exocrine and endocrine insufficiencies were present in 34 and 39% of the patients, respectively. At univariate analysis, no factor was associated with exocrine insufficiency, although female gender (*P*=0.04), increasing age (*P*=0.006), and type 1 AIP (*P*=0.001) were associated with the occurrence of diabetes. Steroid/azathioprine treatment did not prevent pancreatic insufficiency. Type 2 AIP was more frequently associated with inflammatory bowel disease than type 1 AIP (31 and 3%, respectively), but relapse rates were similar in both groups.

Conclusions.—Relapse occurs in 27% of AIP patients and is more frequent in patients with high serum IgG4 levels at the time of diagnosis. Pancreatic atrophy and functional insufficiency occur in more than one-third of the patients within 3 years of diagnosis. The outcome of patients with type 2 AIP, a condition often associated with inflammatory bowel disease, is not different from that of patients with type 1 AIP, except for diabetes.

▶ Autoimmune pancreatitis (AIP) is a rare condition that can be mistaken for pancreatic cancer[1] given its similar radiological appearance and clinical presentation, so it is an important differential to consider. This article is a retrospective review of patients in a single center in France who were diagnosed with either type 1 or type 2 AIP over a 9-year period. The aim of the review was to document outcomes regarding pancreatic endocrine and exocrine function, to identify predictors of relapse and pancreatic insufficiency, and to see if there were differences between each type of AIP.

The selection of patients included in the study was based both on the Mayo Histology, Imaging, Serology, Other organ involvement, and Response to steroids (HISORt) criteria[2] for type 1 patients and a reasonable, but not universally accepted, definition of type 2 patients; this is consistent with recently published international consensus guidelines.[3] There were 28 type 1 patients and 16 type 2 patients identified over the 9-year period of the study, demonstrating how uncommon the disease is. Twelve patients were initially thought to have pancreatic cancer (27%) and underwent surgery, with an additional 26 patients commenced on steroids, 4 of whom also required azathioprine. Six patients required no treatment. Twelve patients relapsed, with a median time to relapse of 6 months, and most were treated again with steroids, with a 90% response rate.

There were several differences between the 2 groups that were statistically significant: The patients with type 2 were younger (median age 27 vs 48 years) and were more likely to have inflammatory bowel disease (5 vs 1 patients). Patients with type 1 were more likely to have other organ involvement (5 vs 2 patients) and have an elevated serum immunoglobulin (Ig) G4; this was seen in 12 patients with type 1 (43%) and in none with type 2. Type 1 patients were also more likely to be diabetic (16 patients, ie, 57% vs 1 patient), with an increase from 3 patients at the start to 17 patients by the finish. These data are suggestive of an association between type 1 AIP and the development of diabetes, although other factors, such as pancreatic surgery, age, or steroid use, may also play a role in this finding. Thirty-five percent of patients developed exocrine insufficiency, with no significant difference between the 2 types. Factors predictive of relapse included high serum IgG4 levels (odds ratio 5.5), abdominal pain as a presenting symptom, and other organ involvement.

This study is naturally limited by the retrospective observational design but raises several interesting points. All patients in this study responded to treatment, with 1 in 4 patients relapsing; relapse was associated with elevated serum IgG4 levels. Azathioprine was shown to be effective in avoiding relapse despite steroid cessation, although follow-up was limited to 3 years in these patients. Diabetes, particularly insulin-requiring, commonly developed in patients with type 1 AIP, although this may reflect older age, higher exposure to pancreatic surgery, and steroid use in this group. There were no significant differences between the 2 groups regarding exocrine insufficiency.

There was not enough information provided to assess whether the diagnostic criteria were used in a prospective or retrospective fashion; with 1 in 4 patients in this cohort undergoing unnecessary surgery, it is hoped that future studies will report these data prospectively. Although we were told 35% of the cohort developed pancreatic changes on imaging throughout the study, no initial imaging data were presented. Endoscopic ultrasound was underused, with only 25% of the cohort undergoing this assessment; it appeared that only 1 in 3 patients was identified as having elevated tissue IgG4 at fine-needle aspiration (FNA). No information was provided as to whether this was a core biopsy, which has been shown to be superior to FNA. Future studies will hopefully provide guidance as to the prospective utility of the HISORt criteria and whether there is clinical benefit and cost-effectiveness to assess all pancreatic masses with these guidelines in mind.

S. M. Philcox, MD

References

1. Song Y, Liu QD, Zhou NX, Zhang WZ, Wang DJ. Diagnosis and management of autoimmune pancreatitis: experience from China. *World J Gastroenterol.* 2008; 14:601-606.
2. Chari ST. Diagnosis of autoimmune pancreatitis using its five cardinal features: introducing the Mayo Clinic's HISORt criteria. *J Gastroenterol.* 2007;42:39-41.
3. Shimosegawa T, Chari ST, Frulloni L, et al. International consensus diagnostic criteria for autoimmune pancreatitis: guidelines of the International Association of Pancreatology. *Pancreas.* 2011;40:352-358.

PART EIGHT

ENDOCRINOLOGY, DIABETES, AND METABOLISM

DEREK LEROITH, MD, PHD

52 Calcium and Bone Metabolism

Effect of calcium supplements on risk of myocardial infarction and cardiovascular events: meta-analysis
Bolland MJ, Avenell A, Baron JA, et al (Univ of Auckland, New Zealand; Univ of Aberdeen, UK; Dartmouth Med School, NH)
BMJ 341:c3691, 2010

Objective.—To investigate whether calcium supplements increase the risk of cardiovascular events.

Design.—Patient level and trial level meta-analyses.

Data Sources.—Medline, Embase, and Cochrane Central Register of Controlled Trials (1966-March 2010), reference lists of meta-analyses of calcium supplements, and two clinical trial registries. Initial searches were carried out in November 2007, with electronic database searches repeated in March 2010.

Study Selection.—Eligible studies were randomised, placebo controlled trials of calcium supplements ($\geq$500 mg/day), with 100 or more participants of mean age more than 40 years and study duration more than one year. The lead authors of eligible trials supplied data. Cardiovascular outcomes were obtained from self reports, hospital admissions, and death certificates.

Results.—15 trials were eligible for inclusion, five with patient level data (8151 participants, median follow-up 3.6 years, interquartile range 2.7-4.3 years) and 11 with trial level data (11 921 participants, mean duration 4.0 years). In the five studies contributing patient level data, 143 people allocated to calcium had a myocardial infarction compared with 111 allocated to placebo (hazard ratio 1.31, 95% confidence interval 1.02 to 1.67, P=0.035). Non-significant increases occurred in the incidence of stroke (1.20, 0.96 to 1.50, P=0.11), the composite end point of myocardial infarction, stroke, or sudden death (1.18, 1.00 to 1.39, P=0.057), and death (1.09, 0.96 to 1.23, P=0.18). The meta-analysis of trial level data showed similar results: 296 people had a myocardial infarction (166 allocated to calcium, 130 to placebo), with an increased incidence of myocardial infarction in those allocated to calcium (pooled relative risk 1.27, 95% confidence interval 1.01 to 1.59, P=0.038).

Conclusions.—Calcium supplements (without coadministered vitamin D) are associated with an increased risk of myocardial infarction. As calcium supplements are widely used these modest increases in risk of cardiovascular disease might translate into a large burden of disease in the population. A reassessment of the role of calcium supplements in the management of osteoporosis is warranted.

▶ Calcium supplementation to maintain adequate calcium intake is recommended for the prevention and treatment of osteoporosis by most clinical guidelines.[1,2] Clinical studies have shown that calcium supplementation alone marginally reduces the risk of fracture.[3,4] Many adults older than 50 years are taking calcium supplements in the belief that these will help reduce their risk of future fracture. Previous observational studies suggested that increased calcium intake may prevent vascular disease,[5-7] consistent with interventional studies that showed calcium supplementation reduced some vascular risk factors.[8-10] Other studies have shown that patients with renal failure, both before and after starting dialysis, have increased vascular calcification and mortality when supplemented with calcium,[11-13] and a recent 5-year randomized trial of calcium supplements in healthy older women showed that calcium supplements increased risk of myocardial infarction (MI) and cardiovascular events.[14,15] The conflicting evidence regarding benefits and risks of calcium supplementation from these studies led to the meta-analysis in this study.

This study evaluated 15 trials of calcium supplementation in around 12 000 adults older than 40 years. Five of the trials included patient-level data, and 11 included trial-level data. The 5 trials with patient-level data contained 143 adults on calcium supplementation with MI and 111 adults on placebo with MI, with a significant difference between the 2 groups. Nonsignificant differences in stroke, composite end point of MI, stroke, or sudden death, and death were seen between the 2 groups. The 11 trials with trial-level data contained 166 adults on calcium supplementation with MI and 130 adults on placebo with MI, again with a significant difference between the 2 groups. The study concluded that calcium supplements without vitamin D are associated with about a 30% increased risk of MI and recommended that the role of calcium supplementation in the management of osteoporosis be reassessed.

The findings of this study are important because they suggest that calcium supplementation in patients with normal renal function may accelerate cardiovascular disease. Closer evaluation of the meta-analysis, however, shows that none of the single studies included showed a significant difference in risk of MI between calcium and placebo. Increased risk of MI was seen mainly with calcium supplementation above the median intake. None of the studies included vitamin D supplementation, which may be protective against cardiovascular disease. None of the trials evaluated cardiovascular events as primary end points, and data on cardiovascular events were not gathered in a standardized manner. Only 2 of the studies had data adjudicated by blinded trial investigators. No cardiovascular outcome data were reported for 7 of the included trials, accounting for about 15% of the total trial participants. Despite these weaknesses, the study conclusions raise concerns regarding calcium supplementation in older adults with osteoporosis. Further studies are needed to evaluate the vascular effects of calcium supplementation without vitamin D.

B. L. Clarke, MD

References

1. American Association of Clinical Endocrinologists medical guidelines for clinical practice for the prevention and treatment of postmenopausal osteoporosis. *Endocrine Pract.* 2003;9:545-564.
2. National Osteoporosis Foundation. *Physician's guide to prevention and treatment of osteoporosis.* National Osteoporosis Foundation; 2008.
3. Bischoff-Ferrari HA, Dawson-Hughes B, Baron JA, et al. Calcium intake and hip fracture risk in men and women: a meta-analysis of prospective cohort studies and randomized controlled trials. *Am J Clin Nutr.* 2007;86:1780-1790.
4. Tang BMP, Eslick GD, Nowson C, Smith C, Bensoussan A. Use of calcium or calcium in combination with vitamin D supplementation to prevent fractures and bone loss in people aged 50 years and older: a meta-analysis. *Lancet.* 2007; 370:657-666.
5. Knox EG. Ischaemic-heart-disease mortality and dietary intake of calcium. *Lancet.* 1973;1:1465-1467.
6. Bostick RM, Kushi LH, Wu Y, et al. Relation of calcium, vitamin D, and dairy food intake to ischemic heart disease mortality among postmenopausal women. *Am J Epidemiol.* 1999;149:151-161.
7. Iso H, Stampfer MJ, Manson JE, et al. Prospective study of calcium, potassium, and magnesium intake and risk of stroke in women. *Stroke.* 1999;30:1772-1779.
8. Griffith LE, Guyatt GH, Cook RJ, Bucher HC, Cook DJ. The influence of dietary and nondietary calcium supplementation on blood pressure: an updated meta-analysis of randomized controlled trials. *Am J Hypertens.* 1999;12:84-92.
9. Reid IR, Mason B, Home A, et al. Effects of calcium supplementation on serum lipid concentrations in normal older women: a randomized controlled trial. *Am J Med.* 2002;112:343-347.
10. Reid IR, Home A, Mason B, Ames R, Bava U, Gamble GD. Effects of calcium supplementation on body weight and blood pressure in normal older women: a randomized controlled trial. *J Clin Endocrinol Metab.* 2005;90:3824-3829.
11. Goodman WG, Goldin J, Kuizon BD, et al. Coronary-artery calcification in young adults with end-stage renal disease who are undergoing dialysis. *N Engl J Med.* 2000;342:1478-1483.
12. Block GA, Raggi P, Bellasi A, Kooienga L, Spiegel DM. Mortality effect of coronary calcification and phosphate binder choice in incident hemodialysis patients. *Kidney Int.* 2007;71:438-441.
13. Russo D, Miranda I, Ruocco C, et al. The progression of coronary artery calcification in predialysis patients on calcium carbonate or sevelamer. *Kidney Int.* 2007;72:1255-1261.
14. Reid IR, Mason B, Horne A, et al. Randomized controlled trial of calcium in healthy older women. *Am J Med.* 2006;119:777-785.
15. Bolland MJ, Barber PA, Doughty RN, et al. Vascular events in healthy older women receiving calcium supplementation: randomised controlled trial. *BMJ.* 2008;336:262-266.

Effects of Intravenous Zoledronic Acid Plus Subcutaneous Teriparatide [rhPTH(1−34)] in Postmenopausal Osteoporosis
Cosman F, Eriksen EF, Recknor C, et al (Helen Hayes Hosp, West Haverstraw, NY; Aker Univ Hosp, Oslo, Norway; United Osteoporosis Ctrs, Gainesville, GA; et al)
J Bone Miner Res 26:503-511, 2011

Clinical data suggest concomitant therapy with bisphosphonates and parathyroid hormone (PTH) may blunt the anabolic effect of PTH; rodent models suggest that infrequently administered bisphosphonates may interact differently. To evaluate the effects of combination therapy with an intravenous infusion of zoledronic acid 5 mg and daily subcutaneous recombinant human (rh)PTH(1−34) (teriparatide) 20 μg versus either agent alone on bone mineral density (BMD) and bone turnover markers, we conducted a 1-year multicenter, multinational, randomized, partial double-blinded, controlled trial. 412 postmenopausal women with osteoporosis (mean age 65 ± 9 years) were randomized to a single infusion of zoledronic acid 5 mg plus daily subcutaneous teriparatide 20 μg ($n = 137$), zoledronic acid alone ($n = 137$), or teriparatide alone ($n = 138$). The primary endpoint was percentage increase in lumbar spine BMD (assessed by dual-energy X-ray absorptiometry [DXA]) at 52 weeks versus baseline. Secondary endpoints included change in BMD at the spine at earlier time points and at the total hip, trochanter, and femoral neck at all time points. At week 52, lumbar spine BMD had increased 7.5%, 7.0%, and 4.4% in the combination, teriparatide, and zoledronic acid groups, respectively ($p < .001$ for combination and teriparatide versus zoledronic acid). In the combination group, spine BMD increased more rapidly than with either agent alone ($p < .001$ versus both teriparatide and zoledronic acid at 13 and 26 weeks). Combination therapy increased total-hip BMD more than teriparatide alone at all times (all $p < .01$) and more than zoledronic acid at 13 weeks ($p < .05$), with final 52-week increments of 2.3%, 1.1%, and 2.2% in the combination, teriparatide, and zoledronic acid groups, respectively. With combination therapy, bone formation (assessed by serum N-terminal propeptide of type I collagen [PINP]) increased from 0 to 4 weeks, declined minimally from 4 to 8 weeks, and then rose throughout the trial, with levels above baseline from 6 to 12 months. Bone resorption (assessed by serum β-C-telopeptide of type I collagen [β-CTX]) was markedly reduced with combination therapy from 0 to 8 weeks (a reduction of similar magnitude to that seen with zoledronic acid alone), followed by a gradual increase after week 8, with levels remaining above baseline for the latter half of the year. Levels for both markers were significantly lower with combination therapy versus teriparatide alone ($p < .002$). Limitations of the study included its short duration, lack of endpoints beyond DXA-based BMD (e.g., quantitative computed tomography and finite-element modeling for bone strength), lack of teriparatide placebo, and insufficient power for fracture outcomes. We conclude that while teriparatide increases spine BMD more than zoledronic acid and zoledronic acid increases hip BMD more than teriparatide, combination therapy provides the largest, most rapid increments when both spine and hip sites are considered.

▶ It has been proposed that the use of combination antiresorptive and anabolic therapies for osteoporosis treatment might stimulate a greater increase in bone density than therapy with either type of therapy alone. Theoretically, simultaneous stimulation of new bone formation and suppression of bone resorption should lead to a marked increase in bone formation and consequent increase in bone mineral density. However, previous studies have reported that simultaneous combination therapy with a potent antiresorptive agent, such as alendronate, and an anabolic agent, such as teriparatide or parathyroid hormone (PTH) 1-84, blunted the anabolic effect of teriparatide.[1-3]

This study evaluated the effect of a single infusion of zoledronic acid, 5 mg, over 15 minutes plus teriparatide, 20 μg, by subcutaneous injection once daily over 1 year versus zoledronic acid alone or teriparatide alone in 412 treatment-naive postmenopausal osteoporotic women. The results showed that the combination therapy led to a more rapid and greater increase in bone mineral density than either therapy alone at the lumbar spine and total hip. Markers of bone formation increased with combination therapy throughout the study, whereas markers of bone resorption decreased rapidly with combination therapy and then increased to above baseline in the latter half of the trial. The authors concluded that while teriparatide increased lumbar spine BMD more than zoledronic acid and zoledronic acid increased total hip BMD more than teriparatide, combination therapy provided the largest and most rapid increases in both.

These findings suggest that combination therapy with teriparatide and zoledronic acid in treatment-naive postmenopausal osteoporotic women improves bone mineral density more rapidly and to a greater degree than either therapy alone. Previous studies of combination therapy with teriparatide or PTH 1-84 and antiresorptive agents have given variable results depending on the antiresorptive agent used,[4-6] whether patients were treatment naive or on previous therapy when combination therapy was started.[2,7] And for patients on previous antiresorptive therapies, whether the antiresorptive therapy was continued or stopped when teriparatide or PTH 1-84 was started.[3] One previous study[2] found that treatment-naive patients randomized to alendronate alone, PTH 1-84 alone, or combination therapy had no evidence of additive benefit from combination therapy at the spine, but that combination therapy increased dual-energy x-ray absorptiometry bone density at the hip to a greater degree than teriparatide. Evaluation of trabecular bone's volumetric bone density by quantitative CT and bone turnover markers in this study suggested that combination therapy with alendronate might reduce the anabolic effect of PTH 1-84. These studies indicate that the response to combination therapies with teriparatide or PTH 1-84 and antiresorptive therapies for osteoporosis depends on the specific clinical situation.

B. L. Clarke, MD

References

1. Keaveny TM, Donley DW, Hoffmann PF, Mitlak BH, Glass EV, San Martin JA. Effects of teriparatide and alendronate on vertebral strength as assessed by finite element modeling of QCT scans in women with osteoporosis. *J Bone Miner Res.* 2007;22:149-157.
2. Black DM, Greenspan SL, Ensrud KE, et al. PaTH Study investigators. The effects of parathyroid hormone and alendronate alone or in combination in postmenopausal osteoporosis. *N Engl J Med.* 2003;349:1207-1215.
3. Cosman F, Wermers RA, Recknor C, et al. Effects of teriparatide in postmenopausal women with osteoporosis on prior alendronate or raloxifene: differences

between stopping and continuing the antiresorptive agent. *J Clin Endocrinol Metab.* 2009;94:3772-3780.

4. Lindsay R, Nieves J, Formica C, et al. Randomised controlled study of effect of parathyroid hormone on vertebral-bone mass and fracture incidence among postmenopausal women on oestrogen with osteoporosis. *Lancet.* 1997;350:550-555.

5. Cosman F, Nieves J, Woelfert L, et al. Parathyroid hormone added to established hormone therapy: effects on vertebral fracture and maintenance of bone mass after parathyroid hormone withdrawal. *J Bone Miner Res.* 2001;16:925-931.

6. Ettinger B, San Martin J, Crans G, Pavo I. Differential effects of teriparatide on BMD after treatment with raloxifene or alendronate. *J Bone Miner Res.* 2004; 19:745-751.

7. Finkelstein JS, Hayes A, Hunzelman JL, Wyland JJ, Lee H, Neer RM. The effects of parathyroid hormone, alendronate, or both in men with osteoporosis. *N Engl J Med.* 2003;349:1216-1226.

Cumulative Alendronate Dose and the Long-Term Absolute Risk of Subtrochanteric and Diaphyseal Femur Fractures: A Register-Based National Cohort Analysis

Abrahamsen B, Eiken P, Eastell R (Univ of Southern Denmark, Odense, Denmark; Hillerød Hosp, Denmark; Univ of Sheffield, UK)
J Clin Endocrinol Metab 95:5258-5265, 2010

Context.—Bisphosphonates are the mainstay of anti-osteoporotic treatment and are commonly used for a longer duration than in the placebo-controlled trials. A link to development of atypical subtrochanteric or diaphyseal fragility fractures of the femur has been proposed, and these fractures are currently the subject of a U.S. Food and Drug Administration review.

Objective.—Our objective was to examine the risk of subtrochanteric/diaphyseal femur fractures in long term users of alendronate.

Design.—We conducted an age- and gender-matched cohort study using national healthcare data.

Patients.—Patients were alendronate users, without previous hip fracture, who began treatment between January 1, 1996, and December 31, 2005 (n = 39,567) and untreated controls, (n = 158,268).

Main Outcome Measures.—Subtrochanteric or diaphyseal femur fractures were evaluated.

Results.—Subtrochanteric and diaphyseal fractures occurred at a rate of 13 per 10,000 patient-years in untreated women and 31 per 10,000 patient-years in women receiving alendronate [adjusted hazard ratio (HR) = 1.88; 95% confidence interval (CI) = 1.62−2.17]. Rates for men were six and 31 per 10,000 patient-years, respectively (HR = 3.98; 95% CI = 2.62−6.05). The HR for hip fracture was 1.37 (95% CI = 1.30−1.46) in women and 2.47 (95% CI = 2.07−2.95) in men. Risks of subtrochanteric/diaphyseal fracture were similar in patients who had received 9 yr of treatment (highest quartile) and patients who had stopped therapy after the equivalent of 3 months of treatment (lowest quartile).

Conclusions.—Alendronate-treated patients are at higher risk of hip and subtrochanteric/diaphyseal fracture than matched control subjects.

However, large cumulative doses of alendronate were not associated with a greater absolute risk of subtrochanteric/diaphyseal fractures than small cumulative doses, suggesting that these fractures could be due to osteoporosis rather than to alendronate.

▶ Recent case series and case-control studies have described atypical subtrochanteric or diaphyseal femoral shaft fractures in postmenopausal women who take long-term bisphosphonate therapy.[1-3] Most patients reported with this type of fracture have taken alendronate continuously for at least 5 years, but occasional patients have taken alendronate for less than 5 years, and some have never taken alendronate but have taken other antiresorptive drugs.[4] Some reports indicate that some patients with this type of fracture have never taken a bisphosphonate, raising the possibility that other factors are involved.[5]

This article, as well as one by Black et al, are important contributions to the literature in this area.[6] Abrahamsen et al evaluated the risk of subtrochanteric/diaphyseal fractures in long-term alendronate users in Denmark. The authors compared 39 567 alendronate users without prior hip fracture who started therapy between 1996 and 2005 with 158 268 age- and sex-matched nonusers. The hazard ratio for hip fracture in women was 1.37 (95% confidence interval [CI], 1.30-1.46), whereas that for men was 2.47 (95% CI, 2.07-2.95). Risks of subtrochanteric/diaphyseal fracture were not different in patients receiving 9 years of treatment (highest quartile) and those who had stopped therapy after the equivalent of 3 months of treatment (lowest quartile). The study concluded that alendronate-treated patients are at a higher risk of hip and subtrochanteric/diaphyseal fracture than matched control subjects, but that large cumulative doses of alendronate were not associated with a greater absolute risk of subtrochanteric/diaphyseal fractures than small cumulative doses. In the final assessment, the authors stated that these fractures could be because of osteoporosis rather than directly because of alendronate. The article by Black et al performed secondary analyses of 3 large prospective randomized trials of bisphosphonate therapy to assess the relative risk of subtrochanteric fractures in users of alendronate or zoledronic acid. In a review of 284 hip or femur fractures among 14 195 women in these trials, a total of 12 fractures in 10 patients were classified as occurring in the subtrochanteric or diaphyseal femur for a combined rate of 2.3 per 10 000 patient-years. Compared with placebo, the relative hazard ratios were 1.03 (95% CI, 0.06-16.46) for alendronate use in the Fracture Intervention Trial, 1.50 (95% CI, 0.25-9.00) for zoledronic acid use in the Health Outcomes and Reduced Incidence With Zoledronic Acid Once Yearly—Pivotal Fracture Trial, and 1.33 (95% CI, 0.12-14.67) for continued alendronate use in the Fracture Intervention Trial Long-term Extension trial. The authors concluded that the occurrence of subtrochanteric or diaphyseal femoral fractures was very rare, even among women who had been treated with bisphosphonates for as long as 10 years, and that there was no significant increase in risk associated with bisphosphonate use, although the study was underpowered for definitive conclusions.

These articles were unable to show that long-term bisphosphonate use increased the risk of subtrochanteric or diaphyseal femoral fractures. Despite large number of subjects, and long-term follow-up, an obvious increase in risk of fracture was not demonstrated. Larger longer-term studies will be required to demonstrate whether alendronate or other bisphosphonates increase the risk of this rare type of fracture.

B. L. Clarke, MD

References

1. Lenart BA, Neviaser AS, Lyman S, et al. Association of low-energy femoral fractures with prolonged bisphosphonate use: a case control study. *Osteoporos Int.* 2009;20:1353-1362.
2. Neviaser AS, Lane JM, Lenart BA, Edobor-Osula F, Lorich DG. Low-energy femoral shaft fractures associated with alendronate use. *J Orthop Trauma.* 2008;22:346-350.
3. Park-Wyllie LY, Mamdani MM, Juurlink DN, et al. Bisphosphonate use and the risk of subtrochanteric or femoral shaft fractures in older women. *JAMA.* 2011; 305:783-789.
4. Shane E, Burr D, Ebeling PR, et al. Atypical subtrochanteric and diaphyseal femoral fractures: report of a task force of the American Society for Bone and Mineral Research. *J Bone Miner Res.* 2010;25:2267-2294.
5. Vestergaard P, Schwartz F, Rejnmark L, Mosekilde L. Risk of femoral shaft and subtrochanteric fractures among users of bisphosphonates and raloxifene. *Osteoporos Int.* 2011;22:993-1001.
6. Black DM, et al. Bisphosphonates and fractures of the subtrochanteric or diaphyseal femur. *N Engl J Med.* 2010;362:1761-1771.

Cinacalcet HCl Reduces Hypercalcemia in Primary Hyperparathyroidism across a Wide Spectrum of Disease Severity

Peacock M, Bilezikian JP, Bolognese MA, et al (Indiana Univ School of Medicine, Indianapolis; Columbia Univ, NY; Bethesda Health Res, MD; et al)
J Clin Endocrinol Metab 96:E9-E18, 2011

Context.—Primary hyperparathyroidism (PHPT) is characterized by elevated serum calcium (Ca) and increased PTH concentrations.

Objective.—The objective of the investigation was to establish the efficacy of cinacalcet in reducing serum Ca in patients with PHPT across a wide spectrum of disease severity.

Design and Setting.—The study was a pooled analysis of data from three multicenter clinical trials of cinacalcet in PHPT.

Patients.—Patients were grouped into three disease categories for analysis based on the following: 1) history of failed parathyroidectomy (n = 29); 2) meeting one or more criteria for parathyroidectomy but without prior surgery (n = 37); and 3) mild asymptomatic PHPT without meeting criteria for either above category (n = 15).

Intervention.—The intervention in this study was treatment with cinacalcet for up to 4.5 yr.

Outcomes.—Measurements in the study included serum Ca, PTH, phosphate, and bone-specific alkaline phosphatase, and areal bone mineral density (aBMD). Vital signs, safety biochemical and hematological indices, and adverse events were monitored throughout the study period.

Results.—The extent of cinacalcet-induced serum Ca reduction, proportion of patients achieving normal serum Ca (≤10.3 mg/dl), reduction in serum PTH, and increase in serum phosphate were similar across all three categories. Except for decreased aBMD at the total femur indicated for parathyroidectomy group at 1 yr, no significant changes in aBMD occurred. The efficacy of cinacalcet was maintained for up to 4.5 yr of follow-up. AEs were mild and similar across the three categories.

Conclusions.—Cinacalcet is equally effective in the medical management of PHPT patients across a broad spectrum of disease severity, and overall cinacalcet is well tolerated.

▶ This study demonstrates for the first time that cinacalcet is effective in normalizing serum calcium and reducing plasma parathyroid hormone (PTH) in a heterogeneous sample of patients with primary hyperparathyroidism, including patients with and without indication for parathyroidectomy and patients with a history of failed parathyroidectomy. No previous studies have addressed the comparative efficacy of cinacalcet across a range of disease severity. Cinacalcet is an allosteric calcimimetic compound targeted to the calcium-sensing receptor (CaSR), which increases the sensitivity of the CaSR on parathyroid cells to extracellular calcium concentration, thereby decreasing PTH secretion.[1-3] Cinacalcet has been shown to be effective in treatment of intractable primary hyperparathyroidism,[4] long-term treatment of primary hyperparathyroidism,[5] inoperable parathyroid carcinoma,[6] and secondary hyperparathyroidism because of renal failure.[7] Cinacalcet is approved in the United States for treatment of secondary hyperparathyroidism in patients with chronic kidney disease on dialysis or hypercalcemia because of parathyroid carcinoma. Cinacalcet is approved in Europe for treatment of intractable hypercalcemia in patients with primary hyperparathyroidism for whom parathyroidectomy is indicated, but surgery is clinically inappropriate or is contraindicated.

This article summarizes the results of 3 separate small multicenter clinical trials of cinacalcet in patients with primary hyperparathyroidism. The study cohort included patients who had failed parathyroidectomy and had more severe primary hyperparathyroidism, patients who had indications for parathyroidectomy but not had surgery and had less severe hyperparathyroidism, and patients with mild asymptomatic primary hyperparathyroidism. The findings indicate that cinacalcet was similarly efficacious in all 3 groups in terms of normalizing serum calcium, increasing serum phosphorus, and reducing plasma PTH. Plasma PTH decreased more slowly than serum calcium but never normalized. Bone mineral density (BMD) by dual-energy x-ray absorptiometry did not improve but remained stable, except for decreased hip BMD in the parathyroidectomy group at 1 year. Cinacalcet appeared to be effective over long-term follow-up of up to 4 years.

These findings suggest that cinacalcet may be useful in the medical management of patients with a wide range of severity of primary hyperparathyroidism. Because surgery is highly effective at curing primary hyperparathyroidism, cinacalcet will likely be useful mainly in patients with more severe forms of the disease who are not able to be cured by surgery. This includes patients who have failed surgery, patients not eligible for surgery because of comorbidities, or patients who refuse surgery for personal reasons. This study showed that cinacalcet has a favorable safety and efficacy profile for long-term use.

B. L. Clarke, MD

References

1. Brown EM, Gamba G, Riccardi D, et al. Cloning and characterization of an extracellular Ca(2+)-sensing receptor from bovine parathyroid. *Nature.* 1993;366:575-580.
2. Nemeth EF, Fox J. Calcimimetic compounds: a direct approach to controlling plasma levels of parathyroid hormone in hyperparathyroidism. *Trends Endocrinol Metab.* 1999;10:66-71.
3. Chang W, Tu C, Chen TH, et al. Expression and signal transduction of calcium-sensing receptors in cartilage and bone. *Endocrinology.* 1999;140:5883-5893.
4. Marcocci C, Chanson P, Shoback D, et al. Cinacalcet reduces serum calcium concentration in patients with intractable primary hyperparathyroidism. *J Clin Endocrinol Metab.* 2009;94:2766-2772.
5. Peacock M, Bolognese MA, Borofsky M, et al. Cinacalcet treatment of primary hyperparathyroidism: biochemical and bone densitometric outcomes in a five-year study. *J Clin Endocrinol Metab.* 2009;94:4860-4867.
6. Silverberg SJ, Rubin MR, Faiman C, et al. Cinacalcet hydrochloride reduces the serum calcium concentrations in inoperable parathyroid carcinoma. *J Clin Endocrinol Metab.* 2007;92:3803-3808.
7. Harris RZ, Padhi D, Marbury TC, Noveck RJ, Salfi M, Sullivan JT. Pharmacokinetics, pharmacodynamics, and safety of cinacalcet hydrochloride in hemodialysis patients at doses of up to 200 mg once daily. *Am J Kid Dis.* 2004;44:1070-1076.

Efficacy and Safety of a Once-Yearly i.v. Infusion of Zoledronic Acid 5 mg Versus a Once-Weekly 70-mg Oral Alendronate in the Treatment of Male Osteoporosis: A Randomized, Multicenter, Double-Blind, Active-Controlled Study

Orwoll ES, Miller PD, Adachi JD, et al (Oregon Health Sciences Univ, Portland; Colorado Ctr for Bone Res, Lakewood; McMaster Univ, Hamilton, Ontario, Canada; et al)

J Bone Miner Res 25:2239-2250, 2010

Zoledronic acid (ZOL) has shown beneficial effects on bone turnover and bone mineral density (BMD) in postmenopausal osteoporosis. This study compared the efficacy and safety of a once-yearly i.v. infusion of ZOL with weekly oral alendronate (ALN) in men with osteoporosis. In this multicenter, double-blind, active-controlled, parallel-group study, participants ($n = 302$) were randomized to receive either once-yearly ZOL 5 mg i.v. or weekly oral ALN 70 mg for 24 months. Changes in BMD and bone marker levels were assessed. ZOL increased BMD at the lumbar spine, total hip, femoral neck, and trochanter and was not inferior to ALN at 24 months [least squares mean estimates of the percentage increases in lumbar spine BMD of 6.1% and 6.2%; difference approximately 0.13; 95% confidence interval (CI) 1.12−0.85 in the ZOL and ALN groups, respectively]. At month 12, the median change from baseline of markers for bone resorption [serum β-C-terminal telopeptide of type I collagen (β-CTx) and urine N-terminal telopeptide of type I collagen (NTx)] and formation [serum N-terminal propeptide of type I collagen (P1NP) and serum bone-specific alkaline phosphatase (BSAP)] were comparable between ZOL and ALN groups. Most men preferred i.v. ZOL over oral ALN. The incidence of adverse events and serious adverse events was similar in the treatment groups. It is concluded that a once-yearly i.v. infusion of ZOL 5 mg increased bone density and decreased bone turnover markers similarly to once-weekly oral ALN 70 mg in men with low bone density.

▶ Very few head-to-head comparison trials have been performed in postmenopausal women with osteoporosis. The available studies have been done in different populations with different study supplements, making it very difficult to draw comparison between the different drugs. Such studies have not previously been done in men, and none of these studies have been powered to show fracture reduction. Epidemiological studies have shown that 25% to 33% of men will sustain osteoporotic fractures during their lifetime[1] and that morbidity and mortality associated with osteoporotic fractures are greater in men than women.[2,3]

This multicenter randomized study assessed the efficacy and safety of once-yearly intravenous zoledronic acid compared with weekly oral alendronate over 24 months in 302 men with osteoporosis. Intravenous zoledronic acid increased bone mineral density by 6.1% at the lumbar spine, 2.5% at the total hip, 3.2% at the femoral neck, and 3.3% at the greater trochanter, whereas oral alendronate increased bone density by 6.2% at the lumbar spine, 3.0% at the total hip, 3.0% at the femoral neck, and 3.7% at the greater trochanter. The changes in bone density caused by zoledronic acid were noninferior to alendronate. Markers of bone turnover at 12 months were no different between the 2 groups. The incidence of adverse events and serious adverse events was similar with zoledronic acid or alendronate. The study concluded that intravenous zoledronic acid and oral alendronate over 2 years increased bone density and reduced markers of bone turnover similarly in men with osteoporosis.

This is the first head-to-head comparison of 2 bisphosphonates in men with osteoporosis. The study suggests that intravenous zoledronic acid and alendronate are comparable in the way they increase bone mineral density and reduce markers of bone turnover. This study was not powered to show fracture reduction, so no conclusions can be drawn regarding relative effectiveness of these agents in reducing fractures in men. Hopefully, future studies will address the issue of fracture reduction in men.

B. L. Clarke, MD

References

1. Khosla S. Update in male osteoporosis. *J Clin Endocrinol Metab.* 2010;95:3-10.
2. Khosla S, Amin S, Orwoll E. Osteoporosis in men. *Endocr Rev.* 2008;29:441-464.
3. Kamel HK. Male osteoporosis: new trends in diagnosis and therapy. *Drugs Aging.* 2005;22:741-748.

The Superiority of Minimally Invasive Parathyroidectomy Based on 1650 Consecutive Patients With Primary Hyperparathyroidism

Udelsman R, Lin Z, Donovan P (Yale Univ School of Medicine, New Haven, CT; Yale-New Haven Hosp, CT)

Ann Surg 253:585-591, 2011

Objective.—To compare the results of minimally invasive parathyroidectomy (MIP) and conventional parathyroid surgery.

Background.—Primary hyperparathyroidism is a common endocrine disorder often treated by surgical intervention. Outpatient MIP, employing image-directed focused exploration under cervical block anesthesia, has replaced traditional surgical approaches for many patients with primary hyperparathyroidism. This retrospective review of a prospective database compared MIP with conventional parathyroid surgery.

Methods.—One thousand six hundred fifty consecutive patients underwent surgery for primary hyperparathyroidism by a single surgeon between 1990 and 2009 at 2 tertiary care academic hospitals. Conventional bilateral cervical exploration under general anesthesia was performed in 613 patients and MIP was performed in 1037 cases. Cure rates, complication rates, pathologic findings, length of hospital stay, and total hospital costs were compared.

Results.—Minimally invasive parathyroidectomy is associated with improvements in the cure rate (99.4%) and the complication rate (1.45%) compared to conventional exploration with a cure rate of 97.1% and a complication rate of 3.10%. In addition, the hospital length of stay and total hospital charges were also improved compared to conventional surgery.

Conclusions.—Minimally invasive parathyroidectomy is a superior technique and should be adopted for the majority of patients with sporadic primary hyperparathyroidism.

▶ This article suggests that minimally invasive parathyroidectomy is a better approach than full neck exploration in patients with sporadic primary hyperparathyroidism. The first successful parathyroidectomy was done in Vienna by Dr Felix Mandl in 1925 in a patient with severe osteitis fibrosa cystica using full neck exploration.[1] Three normal glands were identified without preoperative imaging, and a fourth enlarged parathyroid gland was removed, with dramatic cure of the patient's hypercalcemia. The patient unfortunately developed recurrent disease 6 years later and eventually died of the disease.[2] Since that time, full neck exploration was the standard recommendation for most patients with primary hyperparathyroidism because all 4 parathyroid glands could be visualized at surgery, it was less likely that an abnormal gland or glands would be missed, and all visually abnormal glands could be removed. With advances in sestamibi and ultrasound preoperative parathyroid gland imaging,[3] however, minimally invasive approaches became popular because single adenomas could be localized reliably before surgery. In addition, advances in local and regional anesthesia allowed limited exploration on an outpatient basis,[4] and rapid and accurate intraoperative parathyroid hormone assays allowed surgeons to determine the adequacy of parathyroid gland removal during surgery.[5] The minimally invasive approach to parathyroidectomy became very popular with patients and surgeons over the last 20 years.

This study reports the large experience of a single academic surgeon with full neck exploration and minimally invasive parathyroidectomy over almost 20 years. About two-thirds of cases were done using a minimally invasive approach and the rest with traditional full neck exploration surgery. Both the cure and complication rates were better using the minimally invasive approach, and length of hospital stay and total hospital charges were reduced compared with full neck surgery. The study concluded that minimally invasive surgery is a better approach for sporadic primary hyperparathyroidism than full neck exploration and advocates using the minimally invasive approach in most patients with this disorder.

The minimally invasive approach offers obvious advantages compared with full neck exploration. However, occasional abnormal glands can be missed without full neck exploration. Preoperative imaging with sestamibi—single-photon emission computed tomography scanning, sestamibi-^{123}I subtraction scanning, neck ultrasound, 4D-CT scanning, or other techniques is very helpful in localizing abnormal parathyroid glands, but these imaging studies occasionally do not localize an abnormal gland or detect multiglandular disease, and false-positive scans occasionally complicate surgical decisions. This study was not a randomized clinical trial, but the experience reported nevertheless mirrors the current experience at other major surgical centers in the United States.

B. L. Clarke, MD

References

1. Mandl F. Therapeutischer versuch bein falls von osteitis fibrosa generalisata mittles. Extirpation eines epithelkorperchen tumors. *Wien Klin Wochenschr Zentral.* 1926;143:245-284.
2. Carney JA. The glandulae parathyroideae of Ivar Sandström. Contributions from two continents. *Am J Surg Pathol.* 1996;20:1123-1144.
3. Irvin GL III, Sfakianakis G, Yeung L, et al. Ambulatory parathyroidectomy for primary hyperparathyroidism. *Arch Surg.* 1996;31:1074-1078.
4. Chen H, Sokoll LJ, Udelsman R. Outpatient minimally invasive parathyroidectomy: a combination of sestamibi-SPECT localization, cervical block anesthesia, and intraoperative parathyroid hormone assay. *Surgery.* 1999;126:1016-1022.
5. Udelsman R. Six hundred fifty-six consecutive explorations for primary hyperparathyroidism. *Ann Surg.* 2002;235:665-670.

Bisphosphonates and Fractures of the Subtrochanteric or Diaphyseal Femur
Black DM, for the Fracture Intervention Trial and HORIZON Pivotal Fracture Trial Steering Committees (Univ of California at San Francisco; et al)
N Engl J Med 362:1761-1771, 2010

Background.—A number of recent case reports and series have identified a subgroup of atypical fractures of the femoral shaft associated with bisphosphonate use. A population-based study did not support this association. Such a relationship has not been examined in randomized trials.

Methods.—We performed secondary analyses using the results of three large, randomized bisphosphonate trials: the Fracture Intervention Trial (FIT), the FIT Long-Term Extension (FLEX) trial, and the Health Outcomes and Reduced Incidence with Zoledronic Acid Once Yearly (HORIZON) Pivotal Fracture Trial (PFT). We reviewed fracture records and radiographs (when available) from all hip and femur fractures to identify those below the lesser trochanter and above the distal metaphyseal flare (subtrochanteric and diaphyseal femur fractures) and to assess atypical features. We calculated the relative hazards for subtrochanteric and diaphyseal fractures for each study.

Results.—We reviewed 284 records for hip or femur fractures among 14,195 women in these trials. A total of 12 fractures in 10 patients were classified as occurring in the subtrochanteric or diaphyseal femur, a combined rate of 2.3 per 10,000 patient-years. As compared with placebo, the relative hazard was 1.03 (95% confidence interval [CI], 0.06 to 16.46) for alendronate use in the FIT trial, 1.50 (95% CI, 0.25 to 9.00) for zoledronic acid use in the HORIZON-PFT trial, and 1.33 (95% CI, 0.12 to 14.67) for continued alendronate use in the FLEX trial. Although increases in risk were not significant, confidence intervals were wide.

Conclusions.—The occurrence of fracture of the subtrochanteric or diaphyseal femur was very rare, even among women who had been treated with bisphosphonates for as long as 10 years. There was no significant increase in risk associated with bisphosphonate use, but the study was underpowered for definitive conclusions.

▶ Recent case series and case-control studies have described atypical subtrochanteric or diaphyseal femoral shaft fractures in postmenopausal women who take long-term bisphosphonate therapy.[1-3] Most patients reported with this type of fracture have taken alendronate continuously for at least 5 years, but occasional patients have taken alendronate for less than 5 years, and some have never taken alendronate but have taken other antiresorptive drugs.[4] Some reports indicate that some patients with this type of fracture have never taken a bisphosphonate, raising the possibility that other factors are involved.[5]

This article, as well as one by Abrahamsen et al, are important contributions to the literature in this area.[6] The article by Abrahamsen et al evaluated the risk of subtrochanteric/diaphyseal fractures in long-term alendronate users in Denmark. The authors compared 39 567 alendronate users without prior hip fracture who started therapy between 1996 and 2005 with 158 268 age- and sex-matched nonusers. The hazard ratio for hip fracture in women was 1.37 (95% confidence interval [CI], 1.30-1.46), whereas that for men was 2.47 (95% CI, 2.07-2.95). Risks of subtrochanteric/diaphyseal fracture were not different in patients receiving 9 years of treatment (highest quartile) and those who had stopped therapy after the equivalent of 3 months of treatment (lowest quartile). The study concluded that alendronate-treated patients are at a higher risk of hip and subtrochanteric/diaphyseal fracture than matched control subjects, but that large cumulative doses of alendronate were not associated with a greater absolute risk of subtrochanteric/diaphyseal fractures than small cumulative doses. In the final assessment, the authors stated that these fractures could be because of osteoporosis rather than directly because of alendronate. This article by Black et al performed secondary analyses of 3 large prospective randomized trials of bisphosphonate therapy to assess the relative risk of subtrochanteric fractures in users of alendronate or zoledronic acid. In a review of 284 hip or femur fractures among 14 195 women in these trials, a total of 12 fractures in 10 patients were classified as occurring in the subtrochanteric or diaphyseal femur for a combined rate of 2.3 per 10 000 patient-years. Compared with placebo, the relative hazard ratios were 1.03 (95% CI, 0.06-16.46) for alendronate use in the Fracture Intervention Trial, 1.50 (95% CI, 0.25-9.00) for zoledronic acid use in the Health Outcomes and Reduced Incidence With Zoledronic Acid Once Yearly—Pivotal Fracture Trial, and 1.33 (95% CI, 0.12-14.67) for continued alendronate use in the Fracture Intervention Trial Long-term Extension trial. The authors concluded that the occurrence of subtrochanteric or diaphyseal femoral fractures was very rare, even among women who had been treated with bisphosphonates for as long as 10 years, and that there was no significant increase in risk associated with bisphosphonate use, although the study was underpowered for definitive conclusions.

These articles were unable to show that long-term bisphosphonate use increased the risk of subtrochanteric or diaphyseal femoral fractures. Despite large number of subjects, and long-term follow-up, an obvious increase in risk of fracture was not demonstrated. Larger longer-term studies will be required to demonstrate whether alendronate or other bisphosphonates increase the risk of this rare type of fracture.

B. L. Clarke, MD

References

1. Lenart BA, Neviaser AS, Lyman S, et al. Association of low-energy femoral fractures with prolonged bisphosphonate use: a case control study. *Osteoporos Int.* 2009;20:1353-1362.
2. Neviaser AS, Lane JM, Lenart BA, Edobor-Osula F, Lorich DG. Low-energy femoral shaft fractures associated with alendronate use. *J Orthop Trauma.* 2008;22:346-350.
3. Park-Wyllie LY, Mamdami MM, Juurlink DM, et al. Bisphosphonate use and the risk of subtrochanteric or femoral shaft fractures in older women. *JAMA.* 2011; 305:783-789.
4. Shane E, Burr D, Ebeling PR, et al. Atypical subtrochanteric and diaphyseal femoral fractures: report of a task force of the American Society for Bone and Mineral Research. *J Bone Miner Res.* 2010;25:2267-2294.
5. Vestergaard P, Schwartz F, Rejnmark L, Mosekilde L. Risk of femoral shaft and subtrochanteric fractures among users of bisphosphonates and raloxifene. *Osteoporos Int.* 2011;22:993-1001.
6. Abrahamsen B, Eiken P, Eastell R. Cumulative alendronate dose and the long-term absolute risk of subtrochanteric and diaphyseal femur fractures: a register-based national cohort analysis. *J Clin Endocrinol Metab.* 2010;95:5258-5265.

53 Neuroendocrinology

Prevalence of Metabolic Syndrome in Adult Hypopituitary Growth Hormone (GH)-Deficient Patients Before and After GH Replacement
Attanasio AF, on behalf of the International Hypopituitary Control and Complications Study Advisory Board (Cascina del Rosone, Agliano Terme, Italy; et al)
J Clin Endocrinol Metab 95:74-81, 2010

Context and Objective.—Metabolic and body compositional consequences of GH deficiency (GHD) in adults are associated with a phenotype similar to the metabolic syndrome (MetS).

Patients.—We assessed MetS prevalence in adult GHD patients (n = 2531) enrolled in the Hypopituitary Control and Complications Study. Prevalence was assessed at baseline and after 3 yr of GH replacement in a subset of 346 adult-onset patients.

Results.—Baseline MetS crude prevalence was 42.3%; age-adjusted prevalence in the United States and Europe was 51.8 and 28.6% ($P < 0.001$), respectively. In the United States, age-adjusted prevalence was significantly higher ($P < 0.001$) than in a general population survey. Increased MetS risk at baseline was observed for age 40 yr or older (adjusted relative risk 1.34, 95% confidence interval 1.17–1.53, $P < 0.001$), females (1.15, 1.05–1.25, $P = 0.002$), and adult onset (1.77, 1.44–2.18, $P < 0.001$). In GH-treated adult-onset patients, MetS prevalence was not changed after 3 yr (42.5–45.7%, $P = 0.172$), but significant changes were seen for waist circumference (62.1–56.9%, $P = 0.008$), fasting glucose (26.0–32.4%, $P < 0.001$), and blood pressure (59.8–69.7%, $P < 0.001$). Significantly increased risk of MetS at yr 3 was associated with baseline MetS (adjusted relative risk 4.09, 95% confidence interval 3.02–5.53, $P < 0.001$) and body mass index 30 kg/m^2 or greater (1.53, 1.17–1.99, $P = 0.002$) and increased risk (with a P value < 0.1) for GH dose 600 μg/d or greater (1.18, 95% confidence interval 0.98–1.44, $P = 0.088$).

Conclusion.—MetS prevalence in GHD patients was higher than in the general population in the United States and higher in the United States than Europe. Prevalence was unaffected by GH replacement, but baseline MetS status and obesity were strong predictors of MetS after GH treatment.

▶ Growth hormone deficiency (GHD) in adults leads to a constellation of effects, including central weight gain, fatigue, lack of vigor, memory deficits, bone loss, and lipid abnormalities. This constellation of symptomatic and physical complaints is often referred to as the adult GHD syndrome. Many of the consequences of GHD on body composition are similar to that seen in metabolic syndrome. These authors evaluated data for 2531 adults with GHD followed in the Hypopituitary Control and Complications Study and assessed parameters of metabolic syndrome in a subset of 346 of these patients who were treated with GH for 3 years. They found that the incidence of metabolic syndrome was higher in patients with GHD than in the general population and was higher in the United States than in Europe. They noted that the overall prevalence of metabolic syndrome was unaffected by GH replacement (some parameters such as central obesity significantly improved, while other parameters worsened). These authors conclude that the treatment of both GHD and non-GHD risk factors must be addressed for patients to have a significant reduction in the overall presentation of the metabolic syndrome.

W. H. Ludlam, MD, PhD

Gamma Knife surgery for pituitary adenomas: factors related to radiological and endocrine outcomes

Sheehan JP, Pouratian N, Steiner L, et al (Univ of Virginia Health System, Charlottesville; et al)
J Neurosurg 114:303-309, 2011

Object.—Gamma Knife surgery (GKS) is a common treatment for recurrent or residual pituitary adenomas. This study evaluates a large cohort of patients with a pituitary adenoma to characterize factors related to endocrine remission, control of tumor growth, and development of pituitary deficiency.

Methods.—A total of 418 patients who underwent GKS with a minimum follow-up of 6 months (median 31 months) and for whom there was complete follow-up were evaluated. Statistical analysis was performed to evaluate for significant factors (p < 0.05) related to treatment outcomes.

Results.—In patients with a secretory pituitary adenoma, the median time to endocrine remission was 48.9 months. The tumor margin radiation dose was inversely correlated with time to endocrine remission. Smaller adenoma volume correlated with improved endocrine remission in those with secretory adenomas. Cessation of pituitary suppressive medications at the time of GKS had a trend toward statistical significance in regard to influencing endocrine remission. In 90.3% of patients there was tumor control. A higher margin radiation dose significantly affected control of adenoma growth.

New onset of a pituitary hormone deficiency following GKS was seen in 24.4% of patients. Treatment with pituitary hormone suppressive medication at the time of GKS, a prior craniotomy, and larger adenoma volume at the time of radiosurgery were significantly related to loss of pituitary function.

Conclusions.—Smaller adenoma volume improves the probability of endocrine remission and lowers the risk of new pituitary hormone deficiency with GKS. A higher margin dose offers a greater chance of endocrine remission and control of tumor growth.

▶ Pituitary surgery is the treatment of choice for most clinically significant pituitary lesions (other than prolactinomas that are typically treated medically). However, when pituitary surgery is not successful or is contraindicated, adjunct therapy with various forms of radiation may be indicated. Although radiation therapy offers many positive consequences in terms of stopping tumor growth or reducing hormonal activity, it also has the potential of inducing negative sequelae such as pituitary damage, frontal lobe necrosis, and vision loss. These authors retrospectively review their own patients at a single institution to assess the positive and negative effects of one form of stereotactic radiosurgery, specifically gamma knife surgery (GKS). These authors reviewed records for 418 patients who underwent GKS with a minimum follow-up of 6 months. They note that the median time to endocrine remission was 48.9 months, that smaller tumors had a shorter time to endocrine remission, and that a higher margin dose led to greater endocrine remission. New endocrine deficiencies were noted in 24.4%. GKS is a safe and effective means of creating control of tumor growth as well as endocrine remission, and it has minimal side effects.

W. H. Ludlam, MD, PhD

Pituitary Incidentaloma: An Endocrine Society Clinical Practice Guideline
Freda PU, Beckers AM, Katznelson L, et al (Columbia College of Physicians & Surgeons, NY; University of Liége Domaine Universitaire du Sart-Tilman, Belgium; Stanford Univ, CA; et al)
J Clin Endocrinol Metab 96:894-904, 2011

Objective.—The aim was to formulate practice guidelines for endocrine evaluation and treatment of pituitary incidentalomas.

Consensus Process.—Consensus was guided by systematic reviews of evidence and discussions through a series of conference calls and e-mails and one in-person meeting.

Conclusions.—We recommend that patients with a pituitary incidentaloma undergo a complete history and physical examination, laboratory evaluations screening for hormone hypersecretion and for hypopituitarism, and a visual field examination if the lesion abuts the optic nerves or chiasm. We recommend that patients with incidentalomas not meeting criteria for surgical removal be followed with clinical assessments, neuroimaging (magnetic resonance imaging at 6 months for macroincidentalomas, 1 yr for a microincidentaloma, and thereafter progressively less frequently if unchanged in size), visual field examinations for incidentalomas that abut or compress the optic nerve and chiasm (6 months and yearly), and endocrine testing for macroincidentalomas (6 months and yearly) after the initial evaluations. We recommend that patients with a pituitary incidentaloma be referred for surgery if they have a visual field deficit; signs of compression by the tumor leading to other visual abnormalities, such as ophthalmoplegia, or neurological compromise due to compression by the lesion; a lesion abutting the optic nerves or chiasm; pituitary apoplexy with visual disturbance; or if the incidentaloma is a hypersecreting tumor other than a prolactinoma.

▶ Pituitary lesions are often discovered incidentally when head MRIs are performed for reasons unrelated to symptoms of pituitary pathology (ie, headaches, hearing loss, stroke, etc). Knowing how to appropriately manage these incidentally discovered masses can be perplexing to many clinicians. To address this knowledge gap, the Endocrine Society has prepared a clinical guideline with evidence-based recommendations to help in the management of pituitary incidentalomas. Their recommendations include (but are not limited to) that patients with an incidentally discovered pituitary lesion should undergo a complete history, physical, and neuroendocrine evaluation. Those patients meeting the criteria for resection of their pituitary tumor (ie, tumor causing impingement of the vision apparatus, apoplexy with vision disturbance, or hormonal hypersecretion [other than with hyperprolactinemia]) should be referred to an experienced pituitary surgeon. Those patients not meeting the criteria for resection of their pituitary lesion should have a repeat MRI at 6 months for macroadenomas and at 1 year for microadenomas. If the lesion is nongrowing, the interval for subsequent MRIs should be progressively increased. Visual field testing and neuroendocrine testing should be repeated at the 6-month interval for macroadenomas. The guideline will likely be very helpful to many clinicians so that they appropriately react to incidentally found pituitary masses.

W. H. Ludlam, MD, PhD

Diagnosis and Treatment of Hyperprolactinemia: An Endocrine Society Clinical Practice Guideline
Melmed S, Casanueva FF, Hoffman AR, et al (Cedars Sinai Med Ctr, Los Angeles, CA; Univ of Santiago de Compostela, Spain; VA Palo Alto Health Care System, CA; et al)
J Clin Endocrinol Metab 96:273-288, 2011

Objective.—The aim was to formulate practice guidelines for the diagnosis and treatment of hyperprolactinemia.

Participants.—The Task Force consisted of Endocrine Society-appointed experts, a methodologist, and a medical writer.

Evidence.—This evidence-based guideline was developed using the Grading of Recommendations, Assessment, Development, and Evaluation (GRADE) system to describe both the strength of recommendations and the quality of evidence.

Consensus Process.—One group meeting, several conference calls, and e-mail communications enabled consensus. Committees and members of The Endocrine Society, The European Society of Endocrinology, and

The Pituitary Society reviewed and commented on preliminary drafts of these guidelines.

Conclusions.—Practice guidelines are presented for diagnosis and treatment of patients with elevated prolactin levels. These include evidence-based approaches to assessing the cause of hyperprolactinemia, treating drug-induced hyperprolactinemia, and managing prolactinomas in nonpregnant and pregnant subjects. Indications and side effects of therapeutic agents for treating prolactinomas are also presented.

▶ Adult growth hormone deficiency (AGHD) syndrome is characterized by fatigue, loss of vigor, central weight gain, memory impairment, bone loss, and distortion of lipid profile. The insulin tolerance test (ITT) has historically been the gold standard for diagnosing AGHD, but the arginine/growth hormone-releasing hormone (GHRH) test became widely used when it was shown to have a similar sensitivity and specificity to the ITT. However, with the current unavailability of the GHRH in the United States, alternate testing methods for diagnosing AGHD are needed. To help characterize alternative testing methods to the ITT, these authors review existing published data discussing various growth hormone stimulation tests. Of all the tests that have been historically performed to assess for AGHD, they note that the glucagon stimulation test (GST) is an excellent test based on its accuracy and reliability, availability, reproducibility, safety, and lack of being influenced by body mass index, gender, or presence of hypothalamic causes of AGHD. They conclude that the GST is an excellent test for diagnosing AGHD as long as GHRH continues to not be available in the United States and when the ITT is contraindicated or not desirable.

W. H. Ludlam, MD, PhD

54 Thyroid

High Rate of Persistent Hypothyroidism in a Large-Scale Prospective Study of Postpartum Thyroiditis in Southern Italy
Stagnaro-Green A, Schwartz A, Gismondi R, et al (George Washington Univ School of Medicine and Health Sciences, DC; Univ of Illinois, Chicago; Casa di Cura "Salus", Brindisi, Italy; et al)
J Clin Endocrinol Metab 96:652-657, 2011

Context.—The incidence of postpartum thyroiditis (PPT) varies widely in the literature. Limited data exist concerning the hormonal status of women with PPT at the end of the first postpartum year.

Objective.—Our aim was to conduct a large prospective study of the incidence and clinical course of PPT.

Design.—A total of 4394 women were screened for thyroid function and thyroid autoantibodies at 6 and 12 months postpartum. Women were classified as being at high or low risk of having thyroid disease before any thyroid testing.

Setting.—The study was conducted at two ambulatory clinics in southern Italy, an area of mild iodine deficiency.

Patients.—A total of 4394 pregnant women were studied.

Intervention.—There was no intervention.

Main Outcome Measures.—We measured incidence, clinical presentation, and course of postpartum thyroiditis.

Results.—The incidence of postpartum thyroiditis was 3.9% (169 of 4384). Women classified as being at high risk for thyroid disease had a higher incidence of PPT than women classified as low risk (11.1 vs. 1.9%; odds ratio, 6.69; 95% confidence interval, 4.63, 9.68). Eighty-two percent of the 169 women with PPT had a hypothyroid phase during the first postpartum year. At the end of the first postpartum year, 54% of the 169 women had persistent hypothyroidism.

Conclusions.—One of every 25 women in southern Italy developed PPT. Women at high risk for thyroid disease have an increased rate of PPT. The high rate of permanent hypothyroidism at 1 yr should result in a reevaluation of the widely held belief that most women with PPT are euthyroid at the end of the first postpartum year (Table 2).

▶ Postpartum thyroiditis (PPT) is the occurrence of transient thyroid hormonal abnormalities in the first year after delivery in women who were euthyroid before pregnancy. In its classic form, hyperthyroidism occurs within the first 3 to 6 months, followed by hypothyroidism, with a return to the euthyroid state

TABLE 2.—Clinical Progressions of PPT and Associated Thyroid Function Test Values at 6 and 12 Months

	Euthyroid at 6 Months		Hyperthyroid at 6 Months		Hypothyroid at 6 Months	
	Hypothyroid at 12 Months	Hyperthyroid at 12 Months	Hypothyroid at 12 Months	Euthyroid at 12 Months	Hypothyroid at 12 Months	Euthyroid at 12 Months
TSH at 6 months (median, IQR)	2.15 (1.58)	1.35 (1.88)	0.02 (0.04)	0.03 (0.05)	6.7 (1.8)[a]	5.2 (0.77)[a]
TSH at 12 months (median, IQR)	7.25 (5.5)[a]	0.04 (0.10)[a]	7.4 (6.0)[a]	2.0 (1.3)[a]	7.9 (3.8)[a]	3.05 (1.2)[a]
FT4 at 6 months	11.5 (2.3)	13.0 (1.8)	27.3 (6.3)	23.7 (4.9)	8.3 (0.69)	9.1 (0.65)
FT4 at 12 months	8.4 (0.85)[a]	17.8 (10.2)[a]	8.0 (0.93)[a]	12.8 (1.4)[a]	8.2 (0.82)[a]	10.9 (1.7)[a]
No. (%) of women with PPT with this progression	38 (22.5%)	4 (2.4%)	23 (13.6%)	27 (16.0%)	31 (18.3%)	46 (27.2%)

Values of thyroid function tests are given as means (SD), except where noted. IQR, Interquartile range.

[a]Values significantly different in paired comparisons between clinical progressions with a common 6-month thyroid status, based on Scheffe tests (for FT4) or Mann-Whitney U tests (for TSH).

(in the majority of women) before the conclusion of the first postpartum year. The incidence of PPT (in retrospective analyses) varies between 1.1% and 16.7%, with a quantitative review estimating that the incidence of PPT is 1 in every 12 women worldwide. The aim of this (prospective) study was to measure the incidence, clinical presentation, and course of PPT. A total of 4394 pregnant women were studied. The incidence of PPT was 3.9% (169 of 4384). Women classified as being at high risk for thyroid disease had a higher incidence of PPT than women classified as low risk. Eighty-two percent of the 169 women with PPT had a hypothyroid phase during the first postpartum year. At the end of the first postpartum year, 54% of the 169 women had persistent hypothyroidism. Detailed data are given in Table 2.

This study supports the high incidence of a hypothyroid phase in the course of PPT. The most unexpected finding, as stated by the authors, is the high incidence of permanent hypothyroidism in over 50% of their patients. The literature mentioned an incidence of 5% to 20% of permanent hypothyroidism at 12 months postpartum and an incidence of 20% to 60% of permanent hypothyroidism after 5 to 10 years. The authors speculated that the low incidence of PPT in their study represents an underestimation because of limited sampling only at 6 and 12 months postpartum. In addition, the incidence of PPT in this study was lower than that in other reports. This could be attributable to several reasons, as indicated by the authors, including the selection of patients; all their patients were euthyroid in the first trimester of pregnancy, and the thyroid tests were done routinely at 6 and 12 months postpartum. In other studies, thyroid tests were performed every 3 months for 12 months, and this could have yielded a higher incidence of women with PPT.[1]

M. Schott, MD, PhD

Reference

1. Mestman J. Over half of women with postpartum thyroiditis remain hypothyroid one year later. *Clinical Thyroidology.* 2011;23:16-19.

The Thyroid Epidemiology, Audit, and Research Study (TEARS): The Natural History of Endogenous Subclinical Hyperthyroidism
Vadiveloo T, Donnan PT, Cochrane L, et al (Univ of Dundee, Scotland, UK)
J Clin Endocrinol Metab 96:E1-E8, 2011

Objective.—For patients with subclinical hyperthyroidism (SH), the objective of the study was to define the rates of progression to frank hyperthyroidism and normal thyroid function.

Design.—Record-linkage technology was used retrospectively to identify patients with SH in the general population of Tayside, Scotland, from January 1, 1993, to December 31, 2009.

Patients.—All Tayside residents with at least two measurements of TSH below the reference range for at least 4 months from baseline and normal free T_4/total T_4 and total T_3 concentrations at baseline were included as potential cases. Using a unique patient identifier, data linkage enabled a cohort of SH cases to be identified from prescription, admission, and radioactive iodine treatment records. Cases younger than 18 yr of age were also excluded from the study.

Outcome Measures.—The status of patients was investigated at 2, 5, and 7 yr after diagnosis.

Results.—We identified 2024 cases with SH, a prevalence of 0.63% and an incidence of 29 per 100,000 in 2008. Most SH cases without thyroid treatment remained as SH at 2 (81.8%), 5 (67.5%), and 7 yr (63.0%) after diagnosis. Few patients (0.5–0.7%) developed hyperthyroidism at 2, 5, and 7 yr. The percentage of SH cases reverting to normal increased with time: 17.2% (2 yr), 31.5% (5 yr), and 35.6% (7 yr), and this was more common in SH patients with baseline TSH between 0.1 and 0.4 mU/liter.

Conclusion.—Very few SH patients develop frank hyperthyroidism, whereas a much larger proportion revert to normal, and many remain with SH (Table 5).

▶ Patients with subclinical hyperthyroidism have few or no symptoms of thyroid dysfunction. In the general population, the prevalence of subclinical hyperthyroidism has been reported to range from 0.7% to 12.4%. Recently, it has been recognized that patients with a suppressed thyrotropin (TSH) may have more profound disease than those with a low but unsuppressed TSH.[1] Low TSH concentration is defined as TSH level between 0.1 and 0.4 mU/L, and suppressed TSH is defined as a TSH concentration less than 0.1 mU/L. Some studies have suggested that patients with subclinical hyperthyroidism may develop overt hyperthyroidism at a rate of 1% to 5% per year.[2] However, some other studies have suggested that patients with subclinical hyperthyroidism revert to normal after diagnosis.[3] It has previously been assumed that more patients with a low but unsuppressed TSH revert to normality, and more patients with a suppressed TSH develop overt hyperthyroidism.[1] The aim of the study by Vadiveloo et al was to define the rates of conversion to frank hyperthyroidism and rates in which patients' results normalize.

The study by Vadiveloo et al is the largest study published thus far on the natural history of subclinical hyperthyroidism. The study classifies these patients into 2 groups. The authors conclude that the rate of development of overt hyperthyroidism, 10%, is small in those with a TSH of <0.1 mU/L, but they ignore the even higher proportion in this category who were given therapy for hyperthyroidism (Table 5). They base the diagnosis of hyperthyroidism on

TABLE 5.—Clinical Outcomes and Transition of Subclinical Cases that were Excluded After 1 yr

n (%)	SH (TSH 0.1–0.4)	SH (TSH < 0.1)	Normal	Hyperthyroid
SH (TSH 0.1–0.4)	1929 (70.0)	536 (19.4)	105 (3.8)	130 (4.7)
SH (TSH < 0.1)	302 (15.9)	1261 (66.2)	89 (4.7)	194 (10.2)

SH, Subclinical hyperthyroidism.

raised free thyroxine and free triiodothyronine levels, but it is likely that the physicians caring for these patients decided that the TSH of < 0.1 mU/L together with whatever thyroid hormone levels the patients had was a sufficient basis for the initiation of therapy. When the authors ignored those under therapy, the progression to overt hyperthyroidism was 6.1% of all patients at 1 year. They consider these patients as having incipient hyperthyroidism and differentiate them from those with stable subclinical hyperthyroidism. The authors tend to emphasize that most patients remain subclinically hyperthyroid or revert to normal, but the take-home message is that in 10% hyperthyroidism will develop within 1 year and that clinical judgment will dictate an intervention in an even higher proportion of patients as they are followed. Clearly, most of those who have slightly subnormal serum TSH levels make up the 2.5% of subjects below the lower 95% confidence interval limit and will probably not require intervention, but this study provides good evidence that those with serum TSH < 0.1 mU/L must be followed carefully. The results support the recommendations of the task force on subclinical thyroid disease some years ago in the *Journal of the American Medical Association.*[4]

M. Schott, MD, PhD

References

1. Mitchell AL, Pearce SH. How should we treat patients with low serum thyrotropin concentrations? *Clin Endocrinol (Oxf).* 2010;72:292-296.
2. Sawin CT, Geller A, Wolf PA, et al. Low serum thyrotropin concentrations as a risk factor for atrial fibrillation in older persons. *N Engl J Med.* 1994;331: 1249-1252.
3. Parle JV, Franklyn JA, Cross KW, Jones SC, Sheppard MC. Prevalence and follow-up of abnormal thyrotrophin (TSH) concentrations in the elderly in the United Kingdom. *Clin Endocrinol (Oxf).* 1991;34:77-83.
4. Surks MI, Ortiz E, Daniels GH, et al. Subclinical thyroid disease: scientific review and guidelines for diagnosis and management. *JAMA.* 2004;291:228-238.

Maternal Thyroid Function during Early Pregnancy and Cognitive Functioning in Early Childhood: The Generation R Study

Henrichs J, Bongers-Schokking JJ, Schenk JJ, et al (Erasmus Med Univ Ctr, Rotterdam, The Netherlands; Erasmus Med Ctr—Sophia Children's Hosp, Rotterdam, The Netherlands; Erasmus Univ, Rotterdam, The Netherlands)
J Clin Endocrinol Metab 95:4227-4234, 2010

Context.—Thyroid hormones are essential for neurodevelopment from early pregnancy onward. Yet population-based data on the association between maternal thyroid function in early pregnancy and children's cognitive development are sparse.

Objective.—Our objective was to study associations of maternal hypothyroxinemia and of early pregnancy maternal TSH and free T_4 (FT_4) levels across the entire range with cognitive functioning in early childhood.

Design and Setting.—We conducted a population-based cohort in The Netherlands.

Participants.—Participants included 3659 children and their mothers.

Main Measures.—In pregnant women with normal TSH levels at 13 wk gestation (SD = 1.7), mild and severe maternal hypothyroxinemia were defined as FT_4 concentrations below the 10th and 5th percentile, respectively. Children's expressive vocabulary at 18 months was reported by mothers using the MacArthur Communicative Development Inventory. At 30 months, mothers completed the Language Development Survey and the Parent Report of Children's Abilities measuring verbal and nonverbal cognitive functioning.

Results.—Maternal TSH was not related to the cognitive outcomes. An increase in maternal FT_4 predicted a lower risk of expressive language delay at 30 months only. However, both mild and severe maternal hypothyroxinemia was associated with a higher risk of expressive language delay across all ages [odds ratio (OR) = 1.44; 95% confidence interval (CI) = 1.09–1.91; $P = 0.010$ and OR = 1.80; 95% CI = 1.24–2.61; $P = 0.002$, respectively]. Severe maternal hypothyroxinemia also predicted a higher risk of nonverbal cognitive delay (OR = 2.03; 95% CI = 1.22–3.39; $P = 0.007$).

Conclusions.—Maternal hypothyroxinemia is a risk factor for cognitive delay in early childhood (Table 3).

▶ Clinical hypothyroidism is associated with subfertility, and in those women who conceive, there is an increased risk of miscarriage, stillbirth, preeclampsia, and preterm delivery. There is also some evidence that subclinical hypothyroidism, defined by an increased serum concentration of thyrotropin (TSH) in the presence of normal levels of free thyroxine (FT_4), may be associated with an increased risk for miscarriage, stillbirth, and preeclampsia. Moreover, there is evidence that subclinical hypothyroidism may affect the brain development of the children. In this article, the authors performed a large population-based cohort study with verbal and nonverbal cognitive measures in early childhood. The aim was to investigate whether low FT_4 concentrations in pregnant women with normal TSH levels negatively affect offspring cognitive development. To

TABLE 3.—Maternal Thyroid Function in Early Pregnancy and Nonverbal Cognitive Delay at Age 30 Months

Maternal Thyroid Function Measure	n	Nonverbal Cognitive Delay,[a] OR (95% CI), P
TSH, per SD	2588	0.98 (0.88–1.10), 0.759
FT_4, per SD	2606	0.85 (0.72–1.01), 0.057
Mild hypothyroxinemia[b]	2086[d]	1.37 (0.90 –2.07), 0.139
Severe hypothyroxinemia[c]	2086[d]	2.03 (1.22–3.39), 0.007

Models were adjusted for maternal age, maternal educational level, maternal smoking during pregnancy, maternal prenatal distress, gestational age at blood sampling, birth weight, and child ethnicity. The sample size of the respective analysis is represented by n.
[a]Nonverbal cognitive delay was defined as a score below the 15th age- and gender-specific percentile.
[b]Mild maternal hypothyroxinemia was defined as normal TSH levels and FT_4 concentrations below the 10th percentile.
[c]Severe maternal hypothyroxinemia was defined as normal TSH levels and FT_4 concentrations below the 5th percentile.
[d]Mothers with abnormal TSH levels during early pregnancy were excluded.

this aim, the authors defined mild and severe hypothyroxinemia, representing FT_4 concentrations below the 10th and fifth percentile, respectively, in line with previous research. The authors also examined whether continuous measures of maternal TSH and FT_4 levels in early pregnancy predict verbal cognitive functioning at 18 and 30 months and nonverbal cognitive functioning at 30 months. This study shows that maternal hypothyroxinemia in early pregnancy is a determinant of verbal and nonverbal cognitive functioning in early childhood. The findings of this large population-based study suggest that even in pregnant women with normal TSH levels, low FT_4 concentrations affect fetal brain development and put children at risk for subsequent neurodevelopmental deficits (Table 3). It is tempting to recommend thyroid function screening, including FT_4 measures, of women in early pregnancy. Yet, first clinical trials addressing the potentially beneficial effects of iodine treatment or T_4 supplementation in early pregnancy are needed before the implementation of FT_4 screening programs can be justified.

M. Schott, MD, PhD

Thyroid Function within the Upper Normal Range Is Associated with Reduced Bone Mineral Density and an Increased Risk of Nonvertebral Fractures in Healthy Euthyroid Postmenopausal Women
Murphy E, Glüer CC, Reid DM, et al (Imperial College London, UK; Universitätsklinikum Schleswig-Holstein, Kiel, Germany; Univ of Aberdeen, UK; et al)
J Clin Endocrinol Metab 95:3173-3181, 2010

Context.—The relationship between thyroid function and bone mineral density (BMD) is controversial. Existing studies are conflicting and confounded by differences in study design, small patient numbers, and sparse prospective data.

Objective.—We hypothesized that variation across the normal range of thyroid status in healthy postmenopausal women is associated with differences in BMD and fracture susceptibility.

Design.—The Osteoporosis and Ultrasound Study (OPUS) is a 6-yr prospective study of fracture-related factors.

Setting.—We studied a population-based cohort from five European cities.

Participants.—A total of 2374 postmenopausal women participated. Subjects with thyroid disease and nonthyroidal illness and those receiving drugs affecting thyroid status or bone metabolism were excluded, leaving a study population of 1278 healthy euthyroid postmenopausal women.

Interventions.—There were no interventions.

Main Outcome Measures.—We measured free T_4 (fT4) (picomoles/liter), free T_3 (fT3) (picomoles/liter), TSH (milliunits/liter), bone turnover markers, BMD, and vertebral, hip, and nonvertebral fractures.

Results.—Higher fT4 ($\beta = -0.091$; $P = 0.004$) and fT3 ($\beta = -0.087$; $P = 0.005$) were associated with lower BMD at the hip, and higher fT4

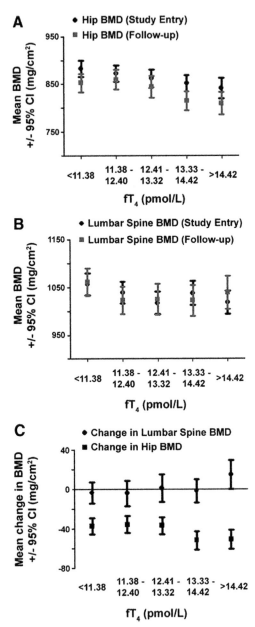

FIGURE 2.—Graphs showing hip (A) and lumbar spine (B) mean BMD ± 95% confidence interval (CI) at the time of entry into the study and after 6-yr follow-up in relation to quintiles of fT4 concentration. (C) Mean change in BMD ± 95% CI in relation to fT4. (Reprinted from Murphy E, Glüer CC, Reid DM, et al. Thyroid function within the upper normal range is associated with reduced bone mineral density and an increased risk of nonvertebral fractures in healthy euthyroid postmenopausal women. *J Clin Endocrinol Metab*. 2010;95:3173-3181, Copyright © 2010, with permission from The Endocrine Society.)

was associated with increasing bone loss at the hip ($\beta = -0.09; P = 0.015$). After adjustment for age, body mass index, and BMD, the risk of nonvertebral fracture was increased by 20% ($P = 0.002$) and 33%($P = 0.006$) in women with higher fT4 or fT3, respectively, whereas higher TSH was protective and the risk was reduced by 35% ($P = 0.028$). There were independent associations between fT3 and pulse rate ($\beta = 0.080; P = 0.006$), increased grip strength ($\beta = 0.171; P < 0.001$), and better balance ($\beta = 0.099; P < 0.001$), indicating that the relationship between thyroid status and fracture risk is complex.

Conclusions.—Physiological variation in normal thyroid status is related to BMD and nonvertebral fracture (Fig 2).

▶ Low bone mineral density (BMD), prior or parental history of fracture, low body mass index (BMI), use of glucocorticoids, smoking, excessive alcohol consumption, untreated thyrotoxicosis, and other factors increase susceptibility to osteoporosis. Even subclinical hyperthyroidism, defined by a suppressed thyrotropin (TSH) level in the presence of normal thyroid hormone concentrations, is associated with fracture, and treatment with T4 at doses that suppress TSH is associated with increased bone turnover and low BMD in postmenopausal women. The prevalence of thyroid disease increases with age: 3% of women older than 50 years receive T4, and more than 20% are overtreated. Subclinical hyperthyroidism affects a further 1.5% of women older than 60 years, and its prevalence increases with age. Nevertheless, the role of thyroid hormones in the pathogenesis of osteoporosis remains uncertain. The aim of this study by Murphy et al was to investigate the correlation between the thyroid status in healthy euthyroid postmenopausal women and differences in BMD and fracture susceptibility.

The authors enrolled 566 premenopausal and 2374 postmenopausal women. In 44 cases a spine fracture was detected. As shown in Fig 2, there was no correlation between thyroid function and fracture risk of the spine. In contrast, there was an increased risk in regard to hip fractures (+ 20% if free T4 (fT4) was within the upper quintile and + 33% if free T3 (fT3) was within the upper quintile). In contrast, a relatively high TSH level was somehow protective. These data clearly show that the effect of thyroid hormones on the bone is complex. Nonetheless, fT3 and fT4 levels within the upper normal range may already influence BMD.

M. Schott, MD, PhD

Outcome of Very Long-Term Treatment with Antithyroid Drugs in Graves' Hyperthyroidism Associated with Graves' Orbitopathy
Elbers L, Mourits M, Wiersinga W (Univ of Amsterdam, The Netherlands)
Thyroid 21:279-283, 2011

Background.—It is still debated which treatment modality for Graves' hyperthyroidism (GH) is most appropriate when Graves' orbitopathy (GO) is present. The preference in our center has been always to continue antithyroid drugs for GH (as the block-and-replace [B-R] regimen) until all medical and/or surgical treatments for GO are concluded and the eye disease does not require any further therapy (except prescription of lubricants). This usually takes more than 2 years. The aim of this study was to evaluate the outcome of long-term B-R regimen for GH in GO patients by assessment (after discontinuation of B-R) of (a) the recurrence rate of GH and (b) the relapse rate of GO and its association with recurrent GH and/or ^{131}I therapy.

Methods.—A retrospective follow-up study was done among all patients referred to the Academic Medical Center in Amsterdam between 1995 and 2005 for GO. The inclusion criteria for the study were a history of GH and GO and a history of treatment for GH with a B-R regimen for more than 2 years. The exclusion criteria were a history of ^{131}I therapy or thyroidectomy before the end of GO treatment. A questionnaire was sent to 255 patients and returned by 114. Of these patients, 73 qualified for the study. Recurrences of GH and/or GO as indicated by returned questionnaires were checked with treating physicians.

Results.—Patients were treated with B-R for a median of 41 months (range: 24−132). The median follow-up after discontinuation of the B-R regimen was 57 months (range: 12−170). Recurrent GH occurred in 27 of the 73 study patients (37%) at a median of 3 months (range: 1−65) after withdrawal of antithyroid drug therapy. Nineteen of the 27 patients with recurrent hyperthyroidism were treated with ^{131}I therapy. A relapse of GO was not encountered in any of the 73 patients.

Conclusion.—The study suggests that long-term B-R treatment of GH in GO patients is associated with a recurrence rate of hyperthyroidism of about 37%. With the regimen employed, recurrence of hyperthyroidism and recurrence of hyperthyroidism followed by treatment with ^{131}I appears not to be a likely cause of relapse of GO. The data suggest that B-R treatment of GH until GO has become inactive and does not require any further treatment is a feasible option and does not jeopardize the improvement that occurred in GO.

▶ There is much debate on the most appropriate way to treat Graves hyperthyroidism (GH) in the presence of moderate to severe Graves orbitopathy (GO). Each of the 3 available treatment modalities has its own advantages and disadvantages in this setting. Treatment with antithyroid drugs appears rather neutral with respect to the course of the eye changes, but its disadvantage is the risk of recurrent hyperthyroidism and an associated flare-up of the ophthalmopathy. [131]I therapy is associated with a small but definite risk of worsening of GO; the risk is greater when the eye disease is still active. The risk of developing or worsening of eye changes after ^{131}I therapy in patients with GH with no or mild GO can be greatly diminished by a course of prednisone (eg, 0.25 mg/kg per day for 12 weeks, or even lower doses for a shorter period of time) (3,5). There are, however, no good data on the effectiveness of these rather low doses of prednisone in preventing worsening of eye changes when ^{131}I therapy is given in patients with moderate to severe and active GO. Much higher doses are likely required, and one could opt for ^{131}I therapy immediately followed by weekly intravenous methylprednisolone pulses for 3 months. The aim of this study was to investigate the outcome of GO if patients receive a block-and-replace (B-R) regimen. The authors assessed the recurrence rate of GH after withdrawal of antithyroid drugs, the treatment of recurrences, and whether this affected the course of the ophthalmopathy. Within this study, none of the patients did, in fact, require further orbital therapy, which confirms the expertise of this group. Although patient questionnaires were initially used, the responses were confirmed by contacting the specialists treating the patients if the patients were no longer being followed at the Orbital Center. Nonetheless, only about one-third of patients invited to participate were finally included. Some were excluded because their thyroid disease had been prematurely treated with radioactive iodine or thyroidectomy; presumably, none of these cases was resistant to the antithyroid drug regimen. Despite these potential drawbacks to the study, several facts support the concept that prolonged antithyroid treatment can reduce recurrences: (1) Graves disease will eventually burn out in many patients, (2) thyroid-stimulating immunoglobulin levels do tend to drop following treatment with antithyroid drugs (or surgery), (3) certain thionamides appear to have immunosuppressive properties, and (4) some of the risk factors for a relapse of GH are also associated with increased risk of progression of Graves ophthalmopathy (eg, smoking and goiter size). If more specific thyrotropin receptor antibodies correlate consistently with the activity of orbitopathy, they could prove useful in determining when to perform reconstructive orbital surgery and/or discontinue antithyroid drug therapy.

M. Schott, MD, PhD

Maternal Thyroid Function during Early Pregnancy and Cognitive Functioning in Early Childhood: The Generation R Study

Henrichs J, Bongers-Schokking JJ, Schenk JJ, et al (Erasmus Med Univ Ctr, Rotterdam, The Netherlands; Erasmus Med Ctr—Sophia Children's Hosp, Rotterdam, the Netherlands; Erasmus Univ, Rotterdam, The Netherlands)

J Clin Endocrinol Metab 95:2010 [Epub ahead of print]

Context.—Thyroid hormones are essential for neurodevelopment from early pregnancy onward. Yet population-based data on the association between maternal thyroid function in early pregnancy and children's cognitive development are sparse.

Objective.—Our objective was to study associations of maternal hypothyroxinemia and of early pregnancy maternal TSH and free T_4 (FT_4) levels across the entire range with cognitive functioning in early childhood.

Design and Setting.—We conducted a population-based cohort in The Netherlands.

Participants.—Participants included 3659 children and their mothers.

Main Measures.—In pregnant women with normal TSH levels at 13 wk gestation (SD = 1.7), mild and severe maternal hypothyroxinemia were defined as FT_4 concentrations below the 10th and 5th percentile, respectively. Children's expressive vocabulary at 18 months was reported by mothers using the MacArthur Communicative Development Inventory. At 30 months, mothers completed the Language Development Survey and the Parent Report of Children's Abilities measuring verbal and nonverbal cognitive functioning.

Results.—Maternal TSH was not related to the cognitive outcomes. An increase in maternal FT$_4$ predicted a lower risk of expressive language delay at 30 months only. However, both mild and severe maternal hypothyroxinemia was associated with a higher risk of expressive language delay across all ages [odds ratio (OR) = 1.44; 95%confidence interval (CI) = 1.09−1.91; $P = 0.010$ and OR = 1.80; 95% CI = 1.24−2.61; $P = 0.002$, respectively]. Severe maternal hypothyroxinemia also predicted a higher risk of nonverbal cognitive delay (OR = 2.03; 95% CI = 1.22−3.39; $P = 0.007$).

Conclusions.—Maternal hypothyroxinemia is a risk factor for cognitive delay in early childhood.

▶ This study will undoubtedly add to the debate about whether routine prenatal screening of maternal thyroid function should be undertaken. Unlike a previous report of an adverse effect of mild maternal primary hypothyroidism on neuropsychological status in children at age 7 to 9,[1] this study included only mothers whose thyroid-stimulating hormone (TSH) was normal but whose free thyroxine (FT4) concentrations were low. The findings of an association between low FT4 and higher risk of expressive language delay (in both mild and severe hypothyroxinemia) and nonverbal cognitive delay (in severe maternal hypothyroxinemia) is troubling, especially as it is unclear whether these mothers had a true underlying thyroid condition and if so, what it was. Unfortunately, no information about prepregnancy thyroid levels or iodine status is provided. Additionally, the possibility that some of these women had central hypothyroidism is not discussed. However, the authors make the excellent point that association does not prove causality and that their findings could be the result of other variables linking thyroid function and early childhood cognitive development. Regardless, this is an important study to be aware of. Particular strengths include the large sample size, cognitive assessments at 2 critical time points, and inclusion of neonatal thyroid status in a subset of children. Randomized prospective studies to examine the effect of thyroxine supplementation on the offspring's cognitive function in maternal hypothyroxinemia are clearly needed.

E. Eugster, MD, PhD

Reference

1. Haddow JE, Palomaki GE, Allan WC, et al. Maternal thyroid deficiency during pregnancy and subsequent neuropsychological development of the child. *N Engl J Med.* 1999;341:549-555.

55 Lipoproteins and Atherosclerosis

Abdominal and gynoid adipose distribution and incident myocardial infarction in women and men
Wiklund P, Toss F, Jansson J-H, et al (Umeå Univ, Sweden; Skellefteå County Hosp, Sweden)
Int J Obes 34:1752-1758, 2010

Objective.—The relationships between objectively measured abdominal and gynoid adipose mass with the prospective risk of myocardial infarction (MI) has been scarcely investigated. We aimed to investigate the associations between fat distribution and the risk of MI.

Subjects.—Total and regional fat mass was measured using dual-energy X-ray absorptiometry (DEXA) in 2336 women and 922 men, of whom 104 subsequently experienced an MI during a mean follow-up time of 7.8 years.

Results.—In women, the strongest independent predictor of MI was the ratio of abdominal to gynoid adipose mass (hazard ratio (HR) = 2.44, 95% confidence interval (CI) 1.79−3.32 per s.d. increase in adipose mass), after adjustment for age and smoking. This ratio also showed a strong association with hypertension, impaired glucose tolerance and hypertriglyceridemia ($P < 0.01$ for all). In contrast, the ratio of gynoid to total adipose mass was associated with a reduced risk of MI (HR = 0.57, 95% CI 0.43−0.77), and reduced risk of hypertension, impaired glucose tolerance and hypertriglyceridemia ($P < 0.001$ for all). In men, gynoid fat mass was associated with a decreased risk of MI (HR = 0.69, 95% CI 0.48−0.98), and abdominal fat mass was associated with hypertriglyceridemia (P for trend 0.02).

Conclusion.—In summary, fat distribution was a strong predictor of the risk of MI in women, but not in men. These different results may be explained by the associations found between fat distribution and hypertension, impaired glucose tolerance and hypertriglyceridemia (Tables 1-3).

▶ Wiklund and coworkers provide important new insights into the impact of anatomical variation in adiposity and risk for myocardial infarction (MI) as well as for hypertension, impaired glucose tolerance, and hypertriglyceridemia. The study included 2280 women and 874 men from northern Sweden. Gynoid adipose tissue is defined as femorogluteal fat. Abdominal and gynoid fat estimates were

TABLE 1.—Physical Characteristics, Adipose Distribution and Background Data at Baseline in Relation to Whether the Female and Male Subjects Suffered an MI or Not During Follow-Up

Females	No MI During Follow-Up (N = 2280)	MI During Follow-Up (N = 56)
Age (years)	56.2 ± 13.2	57.9 ± 7.9
Weight (kg)	67.7 ± 12.9	68.3 ± 13.0
Height (m)	1.63 ± 0.07	1.61 ± 0.06**
BMI (kgm^{-2})	25.5 ± 4.5	26.4 ± 4.7
Total adipose mass (kg)	26.2 ± 9.7	27.5 ± 9.0
Abdominal adipose mass (g)	1510 ± 536	1726 ± 508**
Gynoid adipose mass (g)	2679 ± 841	2651 ± 770
Abdominal/gynoid adipose mass	0.56 ± 0.12	0.66 ± 0.14***
Gynoid/total adipose mass	0.11 ± 0.01	0.010 ± 0.01***
Diabetes (%)	4.6	30.4***
Hypertension (%)	27.4	65.5***
Hyperlipidemia (%)	9.0	24.0*
Current smoking (%)	20.4	22.2

Males	No MI during follow-up (N = 874)	MI during follow-up (N = 48)
Age (years)	51.8 ± 13.1	54.3 ± 8.6
Weight (kg)	81.6 ± 12.6	78.5 ± 12.5
Height (m)	1.77 ± 0.07	1.75 ± 0.05
BMI (kgm^{-2})	26.0 ± 3.6	25.5 ± 3.9
Total adipose mass (kg)	21.0 ± 7.7	20.3 ± 10.1
Abdominal adipose mass (g)	1484 ± 458	1473 ± 607
Gynoid adipose mass (g)	1856 ± 588	1754 ± 774
Abdominal/gynoid adipose mass	0.81 ± 0.15	0.85 ± 0.14*
Gynoid/total adipose mass	0.09 ± 0.01	0.09 ± 0.01
Diabetes (%)	9.8	35.4**
Hypertension (%)	30.4	48.9*
Hypertriglyceridemia (%)	15.6	30.8
Current smoking (%)	17.8	26.8

Abbreviations: BMI, body mass index; MI, myocardial infarction. Means and s.d. are presented.
*$P<0.05$.
**$P<0.01$.
***$P<0.001$.

performed using dual-energy x-ray absorptiometry. Over 7.8 years of follow-up, 104 subjects sustained an MI. Among women, short stature, abdominal adipose tissue mass, abdominal/gynoid adipose mass, gynoid/total adipose tissue mass, diabetes mellitus, hyperlipidemia, and hypertension all correlated with risk for MI (Table 1). Among men, abdominal/gynoid adipose mass, diabetes, and hypertension correlated with risk for MI (Table 1). In women, body mass index (BMI), total adipose mass, abdominal adipose mass, and abdominal/gynoid adipose mass all correlated positively with risk for hypertension, hypertriglyceridemia, and impaired glucose tolerance (Table 2). Gynoid adipose tissue mass was protective against each of these metabolic derangements. In men, BMI and adipose tissue mass correlated with hypertriglyceridemia, but none of the other adipose tissue measures achieved statistical significance for metabolic derangement. Adipose tissue distribution affected risk for MI. Among women, increased abdominal/gynoid adipose mass was associated with a 2.4-fold higher risk, while increased gynoid/total adipose tissue mass was protective against MI (hazard ratio [HR],

TABLE 2.—Associations Between Quartiles of the Different Adipose Mass Estimates and Hypertension or Treatment for Hypertension, Diabetes or Impaired Glucose Tolerance and Treatment for Hypertriglyceridemia or Hypertriglyceridemia After Adjustment for the Influence of Age and Smoking

Women	Hypertension OR	95% CI	P-Value	Impaired Glucose Tolerance OR	95% CI	P-Value	Hypertriglyceridemia OR	95% CI	P-Value
BMI	2.26	1.50–3.43	0.001	2.46	1.37–4.42	0.01	3.67	1.91–7.03	<0.001
Total adipose mass	2.62	1.70–4.03	<0.001	2.05	1.14–3.67	0.03	3.45	1.83–6.50	<0.001
Abdominal adipose mass	2.89	1.85–4.51	<0.001	2.93	1.59–5.38	0.001	8.39	3.48–20.20	<0.001
Gynoid adipose mass	1.89	1.26–2.86	0.02	1.55	0.89–2.71	0.37	1.69	0.95–3.01	0.07
Abdominal/gynoid adipose mass	2.54	1.63–3.97	<0.001	2.88	1.62–5.12	<0.001	8.48	3.50–20.57	<0.001
Gynoid/total adipose mass	0.40	0.26–0.61	<0.001	0.31	0.18–0.54	<0.001	0.10	0.04–0.24	<0.001

Men	Hypertension OR	95% CI	P for Trend	Impaired Glucose Tolerance OR	95% CI	P for Trend	Hypertriglyceridemia OR	95% CI	P for Trend
BMI	1.29	0.69–2.39	0.85	0.92	0.43–1.98	0.40	2.46	1.15–5.26	0.04
Total adipose mass	1.42	0.76–2.67	0.25	1.18	0.50–2.79	0.81	2.78	1.20–6.44	0.08
Abdominal adipose mass	1.59	0.84–3.01	0.49	0.98	0.42–2.30	0.61	3.01	1.29–7.05	0.02
Gynoid adipose mass	1.27	0.68–2.36	0.73	1.06	0.48–2.38	0.85	1.98	0.89–4.41	0.31
Abdominal/gynoid adipose mass	0.82	0.42–1.59	0.56	0.97	0.40–2.44	0.97	1.46	0.60–3.52	0.40
Gynoid/total adipose mass	0.53	0.27–1.06	0.22	0.95	0.38–2.35	0.83	0.37	0.16–0.86	0.12

Abbreviations: BMI, body mass index; CI, confidence interval; MI, myocardial infarction; OR, odds ratio. ORs and 95% CIs are presented for the fourth vs the first quartiles of the different fat estimates in 1040 women and 388 men. P-values are presented.

TABLE 3.—HRs for the Risk of MI per s.d. Increase in the Adipose Variables, Adjusted for Age and Smoking in 1439 Subjects Including 41 Males and 49 Females who Later Sustained an MI

	HR	Women 95% CI	P-Value	HR	Men 95% CI	P-Value
BMI	1.18	0.85–1.62	0.32	0.84	0.60–1.18	0.31
Total adipose mass	1.07	0.78–1.47	0.67	0.71	0.50–1.02	0.07
Abdominal adipose mass	1.53	1.10–2.12	0.01	0.80	0.55–1.17	0.25
Gynoid adipose mass	0.88	0.65–1.20	0.43	0.69	0.48–0.98	0.04
Abdominal/gynoid adipose mass	2.44	1.79–3.32	<0.01	1.29	0.89–1.85	0.18
Gynoid/total adipose mass	0.57	0.43–0.77	<0.01	1.05	0.75–1.48	0.78

Abbreviations: BMI, body mass index; CI, confidence interval; HR, hazard ratio; MI, myocardial infarction. The 95% CIs and P-values are presented.

0.57; Table 3). Among men, gynoid adipose tissue mass reduced risk for MI, with an HR of 0.69 ($P = .04$).

The relationship between adiposity and cardiovascular risk was stronger for women than men in this study. Moreover, none of the adiposity indices usually associated with increased risk for cardiovascular disease achieved statistical significance in men. Visceral adiposity did increase risk for MI in women. Gynoid adipose tissue was protective in both men and women. The lack of correlation between events and visceral adipose tissue in men may be attributable to the small sample size, although a correlation between these variables has not been consistently found. It is possible that the apparent protectiveness of gynoid adipose tissue is attributable to higher capacity for adiponectin production, better insulin sensitivity, and less responsiveness to circulating catecholamines, resulting in less release of free fatty acid mass and injurious adipocytokines. This study certainly suggests that region-specific fat depots affect risk for metabolic derangements and cardiovascular events in different and quantifiable ways. Much work remains to be done in this area before the relationships between the volume/mass of specific adipose tissue depots, insulin resistance, and risk for cardiovascular events can be quantified in a reliable and generalizable manner.

P. P. Toth, MD, PhD

Cardiovascular Event Reduction and Adverse Events Among Subjects Attaining Low-Density Lipoprotein Cholesterol <50 mg/dl With Rosuvastatin: The JUPITER Trial (Justification for the Use of Statins in Prevention: an Intervention Trial Evaluating Rosuvastatin)

Hsia J, MacFadyen JG, Monyak J, et al (AstraZeneca LP, Wilmington, DE; Harvard Med School, Boston, MA)

J Am Coll Cardiol 57:1666-1675, 2011

Objectives.—The purpose of this study was to assess the impact on cardiovascular and adverse events of attaining low-density lipoprotein cholesterol (LDL-C) levels <50 mg/dl with rosuvastatin in apparently healthy adults in the JUPITER (Justification for the Use of Statins in Prevention: an Intervention Trial Evaluating Rosuvastatin) trial.

Background.—The safety and magnitude of cardiovascular risk reduction conferred by treatment to LDL-C levels below current recommended targets remain uncertain.

Methods.—A cohort of 17,802 apparently healthy men and women with high-sensitivity C-reactive protein ≥2 mg/l and LDL-C <130 mg/dl were randomly allocated to rosuvastatin 20 mg daily or placebo, and followed up for all-cause mortality, major cardiovascular events, and adverse events. In a post-hoc analysis, participants allocated to rosuvastatin were categorized as to whether or not they had a follow-up LDL-C level <50 mg/dl.

Results.—During a median follow-up of 2 years (range up to 5 years), rates of the primary trial endpoint were 1.18, 0.86, and 0.44 per 100 person-years in the placebo group (n = 8,150) and rosuvastatin groups without LDL-C <50 mg/dl (n = 4,000) or with LDL-C <50 mg/dl (n = 4,154), respectively (fully-adjusted hazard ratio: 0.76; 95% confidence interval: 0.57 to 1.00 for subjects with no LDL-C <50 mg/dl vs. placebo and 0.35, 95% confidence interval: 0.25 to 0.49 for subjects attaining LDL-C <50 mg/dl; p for trend <0.0001). For all-cause mortality, corresponding event rates were 0.67, 0.65, and 0.39 (p for trend = 0.004). Rates of myalgia, muscle weakness, neuropsychiatric conditions, cancer, and diabetes mellitus were not significantly different among rosuvastatin-allocated participants with and without LDL-C <50 mg/dl.

Conclusions.—Among adults with LDL-C <130 mg/dl and high-sensitivity C-reactive protein ≥2 mg/l, rosuvastatin-allocated participants attaining LDL-C <50 mg/dl had a lower risk of cardiovascular events without a systematic increase in reported adverse events (Figs 2 and 3).

▶ There are lingering concerns over how low-density lipoprotein cholesterol (LDL-C) can be safely reduced. In addition, as LDL-C gets very low (< 70 mg/ dL), the relationship between LDL-C and risk for cardiovascular events becomes more curvilinear with potentially less and less risk reduction per milligram per deciliter decrease in this lipoprotein. In both the Pravastatin Or atorVastatin Evaluation and Infection Trial[1] and Treating to New Targets trial,[2] lower LDL-C level attainment correlated with improved risk reduction. In the Justification for the Use of Statins in Primary Prevention: An Intervention Trial Evaluating Rosuvastatin trial, a mean attained LDL-C of 55 mg/dL was found to be both safe and efficacious relative to placebo.[3] In this investigation by Hsia et al, a post hoc analysis of event rates was performed among subjects attaining an LDL-C < 50 mg/dL or LDL-C > 50 mg/dL with rosuvastatin compared with placebo. The patients who attained LDL-C < 50 mg/dL clearly had substantially lower risk for cardiovascular events and mortality compared with LDL > 50 mg/dL or placebo (Fig 2). Compared with placebo, LDL-C > 50 mg/dL and < 50 mg/dL were associated with statistically highly significant reductions in the primary composite end point of 24% and 65%, respectively. Compared with both placebo and attained LDL-C > 50 mg/dL, those patients achieving an LDL-C < 50 mg/dL

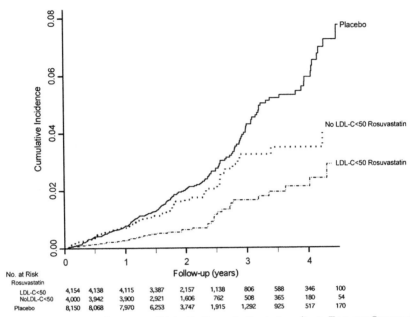

FIGURE 2.—Time to Occurrence of Major Cardiovascular Events According to Treatment Group and Achieved LDL-C Concentrations. Kaplan-Meier curves for the primary study endpoint, time to first occurrence of cardiovascular death, myocardial infarction, stroke, arterial revascularization, or hospitalized unstable angina for subjects allocated to placebo (**solid line**), rosuvastatin with no low-density lipoprotein cholesterol (LDL-C) <50 mg/dl (**dashed line**), and rosuvastatin with LDL-C <50 mg/dl (**dotted line**); p for trend <0.0001. (Reprinted from Hsia J, MacFadyen JG, Monyak J, et al. Cardiovascular event reduction and adverse events among subjects attaining low-density lipoprotein cholesterol <50 mg/dl with rosuvastatin: the JUPITER trial (Justification for the Use of Statins in Prevention: an Intervention Trial Evaluating Rosuvastatin). *J Am Coll Cardiol.* 2011;57:1666-1675, Copyright 2011, with permission from the American College of Cardiology.)

experienced superior benefit in the primary composite end point across all prespecified subgroups (Fig 3). In the group with LDL-C < 50 mg/dL, all-cause mortality was significantly reduced by 46% compared with placebo. When comparing subjects in the LDL-C < 50 mg/dL group with the placebo and LDL-C > 50 mg/dL groups, there was no significant increase in risk for adverse events, including hemorrhagic stroke, new onset diabetes mellitus, myalgia, myopathy, or liver toxicity.

While these analyses are post hoc and must be considered hypothesis generating, they are most certainly consistent with the conclusion that reducing LDL-C even beyond current recommendations for very high risk patients (ie, < 70 mg/dL)[4,5] is both efficacious and safe. These findings are consistent with another analysis of PROVE-IT, which showed that among patients who sustained an acute coronary syndrome, the patients with the lowest risk for recurrent events were those with an attained LDL-C of < 40 mg/dL on statin therapy.[6] It would be particularly important to investigate this issue further in a prospective randomized trial in patients at highest risk for recurrent events, such as those with a history of unstable angina pectoris

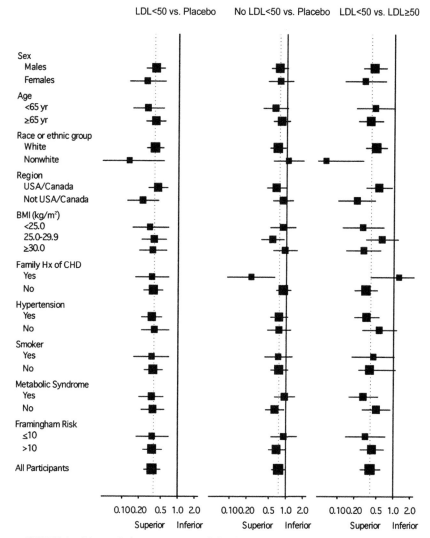

FIGURE 3.—Primary Endpoint in Pre-Specified Subgroups Within JUPITER Trial, Stratified by Achieved LDL-C. Hazard ratios and 95% confidence intervals for the primary endpoint are shown for patients without and with low-density lipoprotein cholesterol (LDL-C) <50 mg/dl compared with placebo and for rosuvastatin-allocated patients with versus without LDL-C <50 mg/dl. Among the 30 subgroups assessed, p values for interaction were all >0.05, except for family history (Hx) of premature coronary heart disease (CHD) in the rosuvastatin-allocated group without LDL <50 mg/dl versus placebo (p for interaction = 0.003) and white versus nonwhite ethnicity for rosuvastatin-allocated patients with versus without LDL-C <50 mg/dl (p for interaction = 0.03). BMI = body mass index. (Reprinted from Hsia J, MacFadyen JG, Monyak J, et al. Cardiovascular event reduction and adverse events among subjects attaining low-density lipoprotein cholesterol <50 mg/dl with rosuvastatin: the JUPITER trial (Justification for the Use of Statins in Prevention: an Intervention Trial Evaluating Rosuvastatin). *J Am Coll Cardiol.* 2011;57:1666-1675, Copyright 2011, with permission from the American College of Cardiology.)

and previous myocardial infarction and those who undergo frequent percutaneous coronary stenting despite comprehensive risk factor goal attainment.

P. P. Toth, MD, PhD

References

1. Cannon CP, Braunwald E, McCabe CH, et al. Intensive versus moderate lipid lowering with statins after acute coronary syndromes. *N Engl J Med.* 2004;350: 1495-1504.
2. LaRosa JC, Grundy SM, Waters DD, et al. Intensive lipid lowering with atorvastatin in patients with stable coronary disease. *N Engl J Med.* 2005;352:1425-1435.
3. Ridker PM. The JUPITER trial: results, controversies, and implications for prevention. *Circ Cardiovasc Qual Outcomes.* 2009;2:279-285.
4. Grundy SM, Cleeman JI, Merz CN, et al. Implications of recent clinical trials for the National Cholesterol Education Program Adult Treatment Panel III Guidelines. *Circulation.* 2004;110:227-239.
5. Smith SC Jr, Allen J, Blair SN, et al. AHA/ACC, National Heart, Lung, and Blood Institute. AHA/ACC guidelines for secondary prevention for patients with coronary and other atherosclerotic vascular disease: 2006 update: endorsed by the National Heart, Lung, and Blood Institute. *Circulation.* 2006;113:2363-2372.
6. Wiviott SD, Cannon CP, Morrow DA, Ray KK, Pfeffer MA, Braunwald E. Can low-density lipoprotein be too low? The safety and efficacy of achieving very low low-density lipoprotein with intensive statin therapy: a PROVE it-TIMI 22 substudy. *J Am Coll Cardiol.* 2005;46:1411-1416.

Dose-response effects of omega-3 fatty acids on triglycerides, inflammation, and endothelial function in healthy persons with moderate hypertriglyceridemia

Skulas-Ray AC, Kris-Etherton PM, Harris WS, et al (Pennsylvania State Univ, Univ Park; Univ of South Dakota, Vermillion; et al)
Am J Clin Nutr 93:243-252, 2011

Background.—Eicosapentaenoic acid (EPA) and docosahexaenoic acid (DHA) have been shown to reduce cardiovascular mortality at a dose of ≈ 1 g/d. Studies using higher doses have shown evidence of reduced inflammation and improved endothelial function. Few studies have compared these doses.

Objective.—The objective of this study was to compare the effects of a nutritional dose of EPA+DHA (0.85 g/d) with those of a pharmaceutical dose (3.4 g/d) on serum triglycerides, inflammatory markers, and endothelial function in healthy subjects with moderately elevated triglycerides.

Design.—This was a placebo-controlled, double-blind, randomized, 3-period crossover trial (8 wk of treatment, 6 wk of washout) that compared the effects of 0.85 and 3.4 g EPA+DHA/d in 23 men and 3 postmenopausal women with moderate hypertriglyceridemia (150–500 mg/dL).

Results.—The higher dose of EPA+DHA lowered triglycerides by 27% compared with placebo (mean ± SEM: 173 ± 17.5 compared with 237 ± 17.5 mg/dL; $P = 0.002$), whereas no effect of the lower dose was observed on lipids. No effects on cholesterol (total, LDL, and HDL), endothelial function [as assessed by flow-mediated dilation, peripheral arterial tonometry/EndoPAT (Itamar Medical Ltd, Caesarea, Israel), or Doppler measures of hyperemia], inflammatory markers (interleukin-1β, interleukin-6, tumor necrosis factor-α, and high-sensitivity C-reactive protein), or the expression of inflammatory cytokine genes in isolated lymphocytes were observed.

Conclusion.—The higher dose (3.4 g/d) of EPA+DHA significantly lowered triglycerides, but neither dose improved endothelial function or inflammatory status over 8 wk in healthy adults with moderate hypertriglyceridemia. The trial was registered at clinicaltrials.gov as NCT00504309 (Tables 3 and 4).

► The fish oils eicosapentaenoic acid (EPA) and docosahexaenoic acid (DHA) have been shown to reduce risk for acute cardiovascular events in secondary prevention trials and to provide incremental cardiovascular benefit when

TABLE 3.—Effects of Treatment on Plasma and Serum Measures $(n = 26)$[1]

		EPA+DHA		*P* value for
	0 g/d	0.85 g/d	3.4 g/d	Treatment Effect[2]
Lipids and lipoproteins				
TG (mg/dL)	237.3 ± 17.5[a]	215.3 ± 17.5[a]	173.7 ± 17.5[b]	0.002
TC (mg/dL)	209.0 ± 7.9	212.1 ± 7.9	207.9 ± 7.9	0.60
LDL-C (mg/dL)	123.3 ± 7.6	127.6 ± 7.6	130.3 ± 7.6	0.21
HDL-C (mg/dL)	42.6 ± 1.9	42.7 ± 1.9	43.2 ± 1.9	0.76
non-HDL-C (mg/dL)	166.4 ± 7.1	169.4 ± 7.1	164.7 ± 7.1	0.54
non-HDL-C:HDL-C	4.03 ± 0.2	4.04 ± 0.2	3.95 ± 0.2	0.74
LDL-C:HDL-C	2.94 ± 0.2	3.00 ± 0.2	3.11 ± 0.2	0.15
TC:HDL-C	5.03 ± 0.2	5.04 ± 0.2	4.95 ± 0.2	0.74
Glucose metabolism				
Glucose (mg/dL)	96.1 ± 2.0	98.0 ± 1.9	99.2 ± 1.9	0.14
Insulin (μIU/mL)	14.6 ± 1.4	15.5 ± 1.4	15.0 ± 1.4	0.31
HOMA-IR	3.55 ± 0.4	3.75 ± 0.4	3.64 ± 0.4	0.46
QUICKI	0.14 ± 0.002	0.14 ± 0.002	0.14 ± 0.002	0.36
Markers of inflammation (plasma protein concentrations)				
hs-CRP (mg/L)	1.45 ± 0.2	1.32 ± 0.2	1.29 ± 0.2	0.72
IL-1β (pg/mL)	0.15 ± 0.02	0.15 ± 0.02	0.14 ± 0.02	0.89
IL-6 (pg/mL)	0.87 ± 0.15	0.85 ± 0.15	0.87 ± 0.15	0.89
TNF-α (pg/mL)	1.16 ± 0.07	1.07 ± 0.07	1.10 ± 0.07	0.20
Markers of inflammation (normalized gene expression in isolated PBMCs)				
IL-1β expression	1.10 ± 0.09	1.06 ± 0.09	1.08 ± 0.09	0.92
IL-6 expression	0.73 ± 0.16	0.73 ± 0.16	0.69 ± 0.16	0.70
TNF-α expression	1.00 ± 0.07	0.94 ± 0.07	0.97 ± 0.07	0.82
Liver enzymes (IU/L)				
AST	20.3 ± 1.1	21.1 ± 1.1	21.9 ± 1.1	0.18
ALT	27.4 ± 3.1	30.4 ± 3.1	32.4 ± 3.1	0.11
Erythrocyte omega-3 fatty acid content (% by weight)				
EPA	0.57 ± 0.09[a]	1.15 ± 0.09[b]	2.30 ± 0.09[c]	< 0.0001
DPA	2.74 ± 0.08[a]	3.04 ± 0.08[b]	3.40 ± 0.08[c]	< 0.0001
DHA	4.39 ± 0.15[a]	5.34 ± 0.15[b]	6.49 ± 0.15[c]	< 0.0001
Omega-3 index	4.96 ± 0.21[a]	6.49 ± 0.21[b]	8.79 ± 0.21[c]	< 0.0001

[1]All values are as means ± SEMs. LDL-C, LDL cholesterol; HDL-C, HDL cholesterol; TG, triglycerides; TC, total cholesterol; hs-CRP, high-sensitivity C-reactive protein; IL, interleukin; TNF, tumor necrosis factor; AST, aspartate aminotransferase; ALT, alanine aminotransferase; HOMA-IR, homeostatic model of insulin resistance; QUICKI, quantitative insulin-sensitivity check index; EPA, eicosapentaenoic acid; DPA, docosapentaenoic acid (n−3); DHA, docosahexaenoic acid; PBMCs, peripheral blood mononuclear cells. Values with different superscript letters are significantly different, $P < 0.05$ (Tukey-adjusted values from post hoc tests).

[2]P values are for the main effect of treatment based on the MIXED procedure (version 9.2; SAS Institute Inc, Cary, NC). Lipids and lipoproteins are the average of 2 samples taken on 2 separate days.

TABLE 4.—Effects of Treatment on Measures of Endothelial Function (n = 26)[1]

	0 g/d	EPA+DHA 0.85 g/d	3.4 g/d	P value[2] For Treatment Effect	For Period Effect
Reactive hyperemia outcomes from FMD					
FMD (% change in artery diameter)	5.00 ± 0.48	4.03 ± 0.48	4.14 ± 0.48	0.11	0.73
ΔArtery diameter (mm, peak-base)	0.24 ± 0.02	0.19 ± 0.02	0.19 ± 0.02	0.07	0.80
Peak flow:resting flow[3]	6.28 ± 0.44	6.59 ± 0.45	6.84 ± 0.44	0.55	0.001
RHI from EndoPAT					
RHI	1.84 ± 0.10	1.82 ± 0.10	1.86 ± 0.10	0.86	0.02
Framingham RHI	0.28 ± 0.06	0.27 ± 0.07	0.33 ± 0.07	0.66	0.17
Pulse wave properties and HR from EndoPAT					
AI	−9.33 ± 1.6	−9.52 ± 1.6	−9.25 ± 1.6	0.97	0.56
AI standardized for HR of 75 bpm[4]	−16.9 ± 1.6	−17.5 ± 1.5	−18.1 ± 1.5	0.53	0.91
Heart rate (beats/min)[4]	62.9 ± 1.6	62.7 ± 1.6	61.0 ± 1.6	0.09	0.03
Resting artery diameter and blood flow values (Doppler ultrasound)					
Artery diameter (mm)[5]	4.83 ± 0.13	4.92 ± 0.13	4.87 ± 0.13	0.09	0.005
Velocity time integral (m)[5]	0.17 ± 0.01	0.17 ± 0.01	0.18 ± 0.01	0.88	0.003
Maximum velocity (m/s)	0.98 ± 0.06	0.95 ± 0.06	1.00 ± 0.06	0.49	0.10
Average flow velocity (m/s)[5]	0.19 ± 0.02	0.19 ± 0.02	0.20 ± 0.02	0.84	0.01
Flow (mL/min)[5]	201 ± 17.5	207 ± 17.7	206 ± 17.5	0.94	0.0007
Postocclusion artery diameter and blood flow values (Doppler ultrasound)					
Artery diameter (mm)[5]	5.07 ± 0.13	5.10 ± 0.13	5.06 ± 0.13	0.55	0.01
Velocity time integral (m)	0.97 ± 0.05	0.99 ± 0.05	1.02 ± 0.05	0.45	0.43
Maximum velocity (m/s)	1.76 ± 0.07	1.76 ± 0.07	1.78 ± 0.07	0.83	0.22
Average flow velocity (m/s)	1.02 ± 0.04	1.01 ± 0.04	1.02 ± 0.04	0.83	0.57
Flow (mL/min)	1193 ± 77	1219 ± 77	1238 ± 77	0.68	0.47

[1] Values are expressed as means ± SEMs. EndoPAT, Itamar Medical Ltd, Caesarea, Israel. RHI, Reactive Hyperemia Index; AI, Augmentation Index; HR, heart rate; FMD, flow-mediated dilation; EPA, eicosapentaenoic acid; DHA, docosahexaenoic acid.

[2] P values are for the main effect of treatment and period based on the MIXED procedure with both fixed effects in the model when period effects were significant (version 9.2; SAS Institute Inc, Cary, NC). When the period was nonsignificant, it was removed from the model to determine treatment effects. None of the Tukey-adjusted P values for pairwise comparisons for treatment effects were significant (P > .05).

[3] First-visit values were significantly greater than visit 2 and visit 3 values (P < 0.005, Tukey-adjusted).

[4] First-visit values were significantly lower than visit 3 values (P = 0.04, Tukey-adjusted).

[5] First-visit values were significantly lower than visit 2 and visit 3 values (P < 0.05, Tukey-adjusted).

given in addition to a statin.[1,2] In the Gruppo Italiano per lo Studio della Sopravvivenza nell'Infarto Miocardico 3 trial, fish oils had demonstrable capacity to significantly reduce risk for reinfarction and sudden cardiovascular death.[3] Fish oils have been ascribed roles in reducing inflammation, thrombosis, and arrhythmogenesis. The ω-3 fish oils are widely used to treat severe hypertriglyceridemia (triglycerides > 500 mg/dL) and are catabolized to form a variety of prostaglandins and leukotrienes. The ω-3 fish oils appear to reduce serum triglyceride levels by promoting intrahepatic mitochondrial β-oxidation, inhibiting triglyceride biosynthesis, and activating lipoprotein lipase.

The investigation by Skulas-Ray and coworkers was designed to evaluate the impact of high- (3.4 g/d) and low-dose (0.85 g/d) ω-3 fatty acids on measures of serum lipids and lipoproteins, markers of inflammation, and arterial vasoreactivity compared with placebo. Sample size was relatively small at 26 patients who were mildly hypertriglyceridemic with baseline triglycerides of 223 mg/dL. High-dose fish oils reduced serum triglycerides by 27%, but other components of the lipid profile were unchanged (Table 3). The low dose of fish oil had no impact of any component of the lipid profile. Serum glucose and insulin levels were not affected relative to placebo at either dose. Levels of inflammatory mediators (C-reactive protein, interleukins 1 and 6, and tumor necrosis factor α) were unchanged in plasma, and no changes were noted in rates of monocyte gene expression at either dose of fish oil, despite the fact that high levels of ω-3 fish oils were taken up by red cell membranes. No improvements in endothelial function or in vasoreactivity were noted (Table 4).

The reduction in serum triglycerides is expected at the high dose of fish oils given the fact that these agents are indicated in the management of sever hypertriglyceridemia. The findings do not support previous conclusions that the fish oils reduce systemic inflammatory tone and improve arterial vasoreactivity. The sample size was small and the severity of hypertriglyceridemia was mild. It is possible that to detect the types of alterations in inflammation and endothelial function these investigators were trying to assess, a larger sample size of patients with much more substantial elevations in serum triglycerides might constitute a more appropriate study population. Moreover, 8 weeks of treatment may not be enough to adequately correct endothelial dysfunction and heightened systemic inflammatory tone. This study does not negate the considerable benefit the ω-3 fish oils confer on patients with dyslipidemia in both the primary and secondary prevention settings.

P. P. Toth, MD, PhD

References

1. Burr ML, Fehily AM, Gilbert JF, et al. Effects of changes in fat, fish, and fibre intakes on death and myocardial reinfarction: diet and reinfarction trial (DART). *Lancet.* 1989;2:757-761.
2. Yokoyama M, Origasa H, Matsuzaki M, et al. Effects of eicosapentaenoic acid on major coronary events in hypercholesterolaemic patients (JELIS): A randomised open-label, blinded endpoint analysis. *Lancet.* 2007;369:1090-1098.
3. Marchioli R, Barzi F, Bomba E, et al. Early protection against sudden death by n-3 polyunsaturated fatty acids after myocardial infarction: time-course analysis of the results of the gruppo italiano per lo studio della sopravvivenza nell'infarto miocardico (gissi)-prevenzione. *Circulation.* 2002;105:1897-1903.

Relation of Albuminuria to Angiographically Determined Coronary Arterial Narrowing in Patients With and Without Type 2 Diabetes Mellitus and Stable or Suspected Coronary Artery Disease

Rein P, Vonbank A, Saely CH, et al (Vorarlberg Inst for Vascular Investigation and Treatment, Feldkirch, Austria; et al)
Am J Cardiol 107:1144-1148, 2011

Albuminuria is associated with atherothrombotic events and all-cause mortality in patients with and without diabetes. However, it is not known whether albuminuria is associated with atherosclerosis per se in the same manner. The present study included 914 consecutive white patients who had been referred for coronary angiography for the evaluation of established or suspected stable coronary artery disease (CAD). Albuminuria was defined as a urinary albumin/creatinine ratio ≥ 30 μg/mg. Microalbuminuria was defined as 30 to 300 μg albumin/mg creatinine, and macroalbuminuria as a urinary albumin/creatinine ratio of ≥ 300 μg/mg. The prevalence of stenoses of $\geq 50\%$ was significantly greater in patients with albuminuria than in those with normoalbuminuria (66% vs 51%; $p < 0.001$). Logistic regression analysis, adjusted for age, gender, diabetes, smoking, hypertension, low-density lipoprotein cholesterol, high-density lipoprotein cholesterol, C-reactive protein, body mass index, estimated glomerular filtration rate, and the use of angiotensin-converting enzyme inhibitors/angiotensin II antagonists, aspirin, and statins, confirmed that albuminuria was significantly associated with stenoses $\geq 50\%$ (standardized adjusted odds ratio [OR] 1.68, 95% confidence interval [CI] 1.15 to 2.44; $p = 0.007$). The adjusted OR was 1.54 (95% CI 1.03 to 2.30; $p = 0.034$) for microalbuminuria and 2.55 (95% CI 1.14 to 5.72; $p = 0.023$) for macroalbuminuria. This association was significant in the subgroup of patients with type 2 diabetes (OR 1.66, 95% CI 1.01 to 2.74; $p = 0.045$) and in those without diabetes (OR 1.42, 95% CI 1.05 to 1.92; $p = 0.023$). An interaction term urinary albumin/creatinine ratio*diabetes was not significant ($p = 0.579$). In conclusion, micro- and macroalbuminuria were strongly associated with angiographically determined coronary atherosclerosis in both patients with and those without type 2 diabetes mellitus, independent of conventional cardiovascular risk factors and the estimated glomerular filtration rate (Fig 1).

▶ Microalbuminuria is a widely acknowledged adverse prognostic indicator of increased risk for cardiovascular events in patients with and without diabetes mellitus.[1,2] Albuminuria is a manifestation of glomerular injury and systemic endothelial dysfunction. Endothelial dysfunction potentiates a large number of pathophysiologic changes within arterial walls, ultimately resulting in heightened intravascular inflammation and atherogenesis. In this study by Rein et al, the magnitude of albuminuria is correlated with risk of angiographically determined obstructive coronary artery disease (CAD) in 914 consecutive patients referred for coronary angiography. These investigators found a dose-response

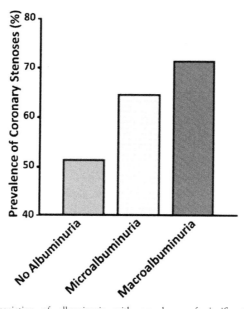

FIGURE 1.—Association of albuminuria with prevalence of significant coronary stenoses ($p_{trend} = 0.001$). (Reprinted from Rein P, Vonbank A, Saely CH, et al. Relation of albuminuria to angiographically determined coronary arterial narrowing in patients with and without type 2 diabetes mellitus and stable or suspected coronary artery disease. *Am J Cardiol*. 2011;107:1144-1148, Copyright 2011, with permission from Elsevier.)

relationship between severity of albuminuria and prevalence of coronary plaques that were ≥50% obstructive (normoalbuminuria, 51%; microalbuminuria, 65%; and macroalbuminuria, 71%) (Fig 1). Moreover, microalbuminuria was an independent risk factor for obstructive disease after adjusting for age, gender, diabetes status, smoking, hypertension, low-density lipoprotein cholesterol, high-density lipoprotein cholesterol, C-reactive protein, and body mass index. The relationship of microalbuminuria to risk of obstructive CAD remained significant after further adjusting for estimated glomerular filtration rate and use of angiotensin-converting enzyme inhibitors, angiotensin receptor blockers, statins, and aspirin. Compared with patients with normoalbuminuria, the presence of microalbuminuria and macroalbuminuria correlated with odds ratios for obstructive CAD of 1.54 ($P = .034$) and 2.55 ($P = .023$) compared with normoalbuminuria. These relationships held in patients who either had or did not have diabetes mellitus.

Microalbuminuria and its progression to macroalbuminuria/proteinuria are associated with increased risk for cardiovascular events as well as chronic kidney disease, end-stage renal disease, and need for dialysis/transplantation in diabetics and nondiabetics. This study shows that micro/macroalbuminuria also correlate with risk for obstructive CAD even after adjusting for all other established CAD risk factors and background medications. An important next step will be to determine in a prospective randomized manner whether or not albuminuria/proteinuria reduction either slows or halts the progression of angiographically identifiable CAD.

P. P. Toth, MD, PhD

References

1. Arnlöv J, Evans JC, Meigs JB, et al. Low-grade albuminuria and incidence of cardiovascular disease events in nonhypertensive and nondiabetic individuals: the Framingham Heart Study. *Circulation.* 2005;112:969-975.
2. Gerstein HC, Mann JF, Yi Q, et al. Albuminuria and risk of cardiovascular events, death, and heart failure in diabetic and nondiabetic individuals. *JAMA.* 2001;286: 421-426.

Early Signs of Atherosclerosis in Diabetic Children on Intensive Insulin Treatment: A population-based study
Margeirsdottir HD, Stensaeth KH, Larsen JR, et al (Oslo Univ Hosp, Norway; Oslo Diabetes Res Centre, Norway)
Diabetes Care 33:2043-2048, 2010

Objective.—To evaluate early stages of atherosclerosis and predisposing factors in type 1 diabetic children and adolescents compared with age- and sex-matched healthy control subjects.

Research Design and Methods.—All children and adolescents with type 1 diabetes, aged 8−18 years in Health Region South-East in Norway were invited to participate in the study ($n = 800$). A total of 40% ($n = 314$) agreed to participate and were compared with 118 age-matched healthy control subjects. Carotid artery intima-media thickness (cIMT) and elasticity were measured using standardized methods.

Results.—Mean age of the diabetic patients was 13.7 years, mean diabetes duration was 5.5 years, and mean A1C was 8.4%; 97% were using intensive insulin treatment, and 60% were using insulin pumps. Diabetic patients had more frequently elevated cIMT than healthy control subjects: 19.5% were above the 90th centile of healthy control subjects, and 13.1% were above the 95th centile ($P < 0.001$). Mean cIMT was higher in diabetic boys than in healthy control subjects (0.46 ± 0.06 vs. 0.44 ± 0.05 mm, $P = 0.04$) but not significantly so in girls. There was no significant difference between the groups regarding carotid distensibility, compliance, or wall stress. None of the subjects had atherosclerotic plaque formation. Although within the normal range, the mean values of systolic blood pressure, total cholesterol, LDL cholesterol, and apolipoprotein B were significantly higher in the diabetic patients than in the healthy control subjects.

Conclusions.—Despite short disease duration, intensive insulin treatment, fair glycemic control, and no signs of microvascular complications, children and adolescents with type 1 diabetes had slightly increased cIMT compared with healthy control subjects, and the differences were more prominent in boys (Tables 1 and 3).

▶ The hyperglycemic milieu characteristic of diabetes mellitus (DM) is injurious to arterial vessel walls and promotes atherogenesis. Agonizing receptors of advanced glycosylated end products promote intravascular inflammation and oxidation. In the Diabetes Control and Complications Trial/Epidemiology of Diabetes Interventions and Complications study, tight glycemic control was shown to reduce rates of carotid intima media thickness (CIMT) progression better than less tight control.[1] Atherosclerosis begins early in life, and multiple studies of unfortunate young (18-25 years) men killed in the Korean War and the Vietnam War demonstrated significant coronary atherosclerosis in almost half of the subjects autopsied. Tight glycemic control is well documented for reducing risk of microangiopathy. While we still lack definitive convincing evidence (trends are observed) for significant cardiovascular event reduction in response to intensive glycemic control, there is little question as to the significant long-term risk for cardiovascular disease in children who develop type 1 DM.

In this investigation by Margeirsdottir and coworkers, 314 children with a mean age of 13.7 years, mean A1c level of 8.4%, and mean duration of DM of 5.5 years underwent CIMT screening and were compared with nondiabetic control subjects. A significant percentage of these children (19.5%) were above the 90th percentile for age for CIMT. There was no difference in CIMT between diabetic and nondiabetic girls. The boys did manifest a statistically significant difference in CIMT. Consistent with the fact that at 0.46 mm there is very little lipid accumulation, there were no differences between groups for carotid distensibility, wall stress, or compliance. When comparing diabetic and nondiabetic subjects, diabetic ones had significantly higher total cholesterol and low-density lipoprotein cholesterol. There was also a mean 3/2 mm Hg difference in the systolic/diastolic blood pressure between groups, and diabetic children on average weighed 7 kg more than their nondiabetic counterparts.

For the boys in this study, intensive insulin therapy did not appear to offer adequate protection against the earliest changes underlying carotid atherosclerosis. With a 7-kg difference in weight between groups, over time and with continued weight gain in response to intensive insulin therapy, many of these children could also develop insulin resistance, which could antagonize glucose control and exacerbate blood pressure elevations and dyslipidemia. There is considerable uncertainty and caution about the use of statins in children. There are no long-term safety or outcome studies with statins in children. The role of statins in children with familial hypercholesterolemia is reasonably well defined, with multiple statins having an indication for use in these children from the age of 10 years. Children with type 1 DM pose significant challenges, but the use of statin therapy should be expanded to children with type 1 DM especially if there is evidence of CIMT thickening with or without concomitant dyslipidemia. Statins either alone[2] or in combination with niacin[3] or ezetimibe[4] have been shown to reduce rates of CIMT progression. It is critical that more be

TABLE 1.—Clinical Characteristics and Metabolic and Anthropometric Data of the Particpants

	Total			Male			Female		
	Diabetes	Control	P	Diabetes	Control	P	Diabetes	Control	P
n	314	118		155	53		159	65	
Age (years)	13.8±2.8	13.2±2.6	0.73	13.4±2.80	13.3±2.44	0.7	14.1±2.85	13.2±2.7	0.03
Duration of diabetes (years)	5.5±3.4			5.6±3.4	0		5.4±3.4		0
Pubertal stage (Tanner)	3.2±1.5	2.9±1.4	0.36	2.9±1.6	2.8±1.4	0.52	3.5±1.4	3.0±1.4	0.15
Height (cm)	160.4±14.4	156.8±13.6	0.02	160.6±14.7	157.6±16.2	0.24	160.3±12.3	156.2±12.6	0.02
Weight (kg)	54.9±16.7	47.9±13.4	<0.001	53.3±17.4	46.9±12.1	0.004	56.5±14.4	48.7±14.4	0.001
BMI (kg/m^2)	20.9±3.939	19.1±0.3	<0.001	20.1±3.6	18.6±2.3	0.001	21.6±4.1	19.5±3.6	0.001
Waist circumference (cm)	71.2±10.0	66.7±6.7	<0.001	70.3±10.0	65.9±6.5	0.001	72.1±9.9	67.4±6.8	<0.001
SBP (mmHg)	101.0±10.1	98.0±10.2	0.006	101.0±9.8	96.8±10.7	0.01	101.0±10.3	99.0±9.6	0.18
DBP (mmHg)	60.5±8.3	58.5±7.8	0.22	59.6±8.4	58.1±9.2	0.29	61.5±8.2	58.8±6.2	0.009
Smoking	11 (3.5)	2 (2)	0.53	2 (1.3)	0 (0)	1	9 (5.7)	2 (3.1)	0.52
Urinary albumin-tocreatinine ratio	1.4±3.7	1.3±1.9	0.72	1.8±4.9	1.1±1.7	0.32	1.0±1.1	1.5±2.0	0.11
S-creatinine (μmol/l)	53.1±10.3	54.5±10.1	0.23	53.7±10.8	55.5±10.2	0.3	52.5±9.7	53.6±9.9	0.43
Fasting blood glucose (mmol/l)	10.9±4.8	4.9±0.4	<0.001	10.1±5.1	4.9±0.4	<0.001	10.8±4.5	4.8±0.5	<0.001
A1C (%)	8.4±1.3	5.3±0.5	<0.001	8.3±1.2	5.3±0.6	<0.001	8.4±1.3	5.3±0.4	<0.001
Mean A1C (%)	8.2±1.0			8.1±1.0			8.2±1.0		
A1 months*	119±104.1			120.8±107.1			117.9±101.5		
Total cholesterol (mmol/l)	4.6±0.9	4.3±0.8	0.002	4.6±0.8	4.3±0.8	0.11	4.7±0.8	4.4±0.7	0.004
HDL cholesterol (mmol/l)	1.8±0.4	1.70±0.4	0.07	1.8±0.4	1.7±0.5	0.8	1.8±0.4	1.7±0.3	0.20
LDL cholesterol (mmol/l)	2.5±0.7	2.3±0.7	0.028	2.5±0.7	2.2±0.7	0.13	2.5±0.7	2.4±0.7	0.09
LDL-to-HDL cholesterol ratio	1.5±0.6	1.5±0.7	0.7	1.5±0.7	1.4±0.7	0.48	1.5±0.6	1.5±0.6	0.99
Total-to-LDL cholesterol ratio	2.7±0.8	2.7±0.8	0.7	2.7±0.8	2.6±0.8	0.48	2.7±0.7	2.7±0.7	0.89
Triglycerides (mmol/l)	0.8±0.4	0.7±0.4	0.32	0.8±0.4	0.7±04	0.35	0.8±0.4	0.8±0.4	0.51
ApoB (g/l)	0.7±0.2	0.7±0.2	<0.001	0.7±0.2	0.7±0.2	0.02	0.8±0.2	0.7±0.2	0.006
ApoA1 (g/l)	1.6±0.3	1.5±0.3	0.003	1.6±0.3	1.5±0.3	0.48	1.6±0.3	1.4±0.3	<0.001
ApoB-to-ApoA1 ratio	0.5±0.2	0.5±0.3	0.75	0.5±1.6	0.5±0.2	0.37	0.5±0.1	0.5±0.3	0.44
Insulin dose (U/kg/day)	0.9±0.4			0.9±0.3			0.9±0.4		
Injections per day									

1–2	1 (0.4)	0	1 (0.6)
3	6 (2.4)	3 (2.5)	3 (2.3)
≥4	95 (37.5)	45 (37.5)	50 (37.6)
Insulin pumps	151 (59.7)	72 (60)	79 (59.3)

Data are means ± SD and n (%).

*The number of months from the diagnosis until the first registered A1C value multiplied by A1C units above the upper normal reference value (6.4%) of the first registered value, plus the number of months from the first to second registration multiplied by A1C units above the upper normal reference value of the second registered value, and so on until the time of cIMT analysis.

TABLE 3.—CIMT and Vessel Elasticity

	Total			Male			Female		
	Diabetes	Control	P	Diabetes	Control	P	Diabetes	Control	P
cIMT (mm)	0.45 ± 0.054	0.44 ± 0.045	0.11	0.46 ± 0.057	0.44 ± 0.057	0.04	0.44 ± 0.050	0.44 ± 0.044	0.94
DC (kPa^{-1})	0.35 ± 0.026	0.36 ± 0.023	0.48	0.35 ± 0.025	0.35 ± 0.020	0.93	0.36 ± 0.027	0.36 ± 0.024	0.42
CC (m^2/kPa^{-1})	9.95 ± 0.657	9.90 ± 0.564	0.48	10.08 ± 0.680	10.06 ± 0.534	0.83	9.82 ± 0.610	9.78 ± 0.560	0.58
Young's modulus (kPa)	4.17 ± 1.438	4.30 ± 0.951	0.38	4.29 ± 1.075	4.37 ± 1.013	0.62	4.06 ± 1.718	4.24 ± 0.901	0.42

Data are means ± SD.

done therapeutically in the setting of primordial prevention to reduce risk of both macrovascular and microvascular events in children with type 1 DM.

P. P. Toth, MD, PhD

References

1. Nathan DM, Lachin J, Cleary P, et al. Intensive diabetes therapy and carotid intima-media thickness in type 1 diabetes mellitus. *N Engl J Med.* 2003;348:2294-2303.
2. Crouse JR 3rd, Raichlen JS, Riley WA, et al. Effect of rosuvastatin on progression of carotid intima-media thickness in low-risk individuals with subclinical atherosclerosis: the meteor trial. *JAMA.* 2007;297:1344-1353.
3. Taylor AJ, Lee HJ, Sullenberger LE. The effect of 24 months of combination statin and extended-release niacin on carotid intima-media thickness: ARBITER 3. *Curr Med Res Opin.* 2006;22:2243-2250.
4. Fleg JL, Mete M, Howard BV, et al. Effect of statins alone versus statins plus ezetimibe on carotid atherosclerosis in type 2 diabetes: The SANDS (Stop Atherosclerosis in Native Diabetics Study) trial. *J Am Coll Cardiol.* 2008;52:2198-2205.

56 Diabetes

Effects of Aerobic and Resistance Training on Hemoglobin A$_{1c}$ Levels in Patients With Type 2 Diabetes: A Randomized Controlled Trial
Church TS, Blair SN, Cocreham S, et al (Louisiana State Univ System, Baton Rouge; Univ of South Carolina, Columbia; et al)
JAMA 304:2253-2262, 2010

Context.—Exercise guidelines for individuals with diabetes include both aerobic and resistance training although few studies have directly examined this exercise combination.

Objective.—To examine the benefits of aerobic training alone, resistance training alone, and a combination of both on hemoglobin A$_{1c}$ (HbA$_{1c}$) in individuals with type 2 diabetes.

Design, Setting, and Participants.—A randomized controlled trial in which 262 sedentary men and women in Louisiana with type 2 diabetes and HbA$_{1c}$ levels of 6.5% or higher were enrolled in the 9-month exercise program between April 2007 and August 2009.

Intervention.—Forty-one participants were assigned to the nonexercise control group, 73 to resistance training 3 days a week, 72 to aerobic exercise in which they expended 12 kcal/kg per week; and 76 to combined aerobic and resistance training in which they expended 10 kcal/kg per week and engaged in resistance training twice a week.

Main Outcome.—Change in HbA$_{1c}$ level. Secondary outcomes included measures of anthropometry and fitness.

Results.—The study included 63.0% women and 47.3% nonwhite participants who were a mean (SD) age of 55.8 years (8.7 years) with a baseline HbA$_{1c}$ level of 7.7% (1.0%). Compared with the control group, the absolute mean change in HbA$_{1c}$ in the combination training exercise group was −0.34% (95% confidence interval [CI], −0.64% to −0.03%; $P=.03$). The mean changes in HbA$_{1c}$ were not statistically significant in either the resistance training (−0.16%; 95% CI, −0.46% to 0.15%; $P=.32$) or the aerobic (−0.24%; 95% CI, −0.55% to 0.07%; $P=.14$) groups compared with the control group. Only the combination exercise group improved maximum oxygen consumption (mean, 1.0 mL/kg per min; 95% CI, 0.5-1.5, $P<.05$) compared with the control group. All exercise groups reduced waist circumference from −1.9 to −2.8 cm compared with the control group. The resistance training group lost a mean of −1.4 kg fat mass (95% CI, −2.0 to −0.7 kg; $P<.05$) and combination training group lost a mean of −1.7 (−2.3 to −1.1 kg; $P<.05$) compared with the control group.

Conclusions.—Among patients with type 2 diabetes mellitus, a combination of aerobic and resistance training compared with the nonexercise control group improved HbA_{1c} levels. This was not achieved by aerobic or resistance training alone.

Trial Registration.—clinicaltrials.gov Identifier: NCT00458133.

▶ Sedentary lifestyle is one of the major problems in Western societies. Physical activity can prevent and cure metabolic disease. However, it is not clear how to motivate people to exercise and which type of exercise is most efficient. This study addressed the latter question. Patients with typical features of type 2 diabetes mellitus were included: The mean age was 55 years, hemoglobin A_{1c} (HbA_{1c}) level was 7.7%, and the body mass index (BMI) was 34.9 kg/m^2. These patients did not exercise regularly at study entry. Patients were enrolled to different exercise regimes: either aerobic or resistance training or a combination of both. The primary end point after 9 months was the change in HbA_{1c}. With every type of exercise, HbA_{1c} and related parameters (BMI, waist circumference, etc) were improved. However, only the combination of aerobic and resistance training reached statistical significance.

How were the exercise programs defined? Aerobic training aimed for consumption of 12 kcal/kg body weight per week. This was achieved after approximately 150 minutes of moderate training. Notably, the combined training group differed only slightly with respect to energy consumption (10 vs 12 kcal/kg body weight per week). Therefore, aerobic training was the major contribution for both treatment regimes. However, studies like this are important to translate findings from physiology and theoretical recommendations into clinical practice. Knowing an exact exercise plan might help to motivate patients to eventually take part in it. This study is very useful for clinicians, as it is one of the few publications in this field leading to clinical recommendations.

S. Schinner, MD, PhD

Long-Term Effects of Intensive Glucose Lowering on Cardiovascular Outcomes

The ACCORD Study Group (McMaster Univ and Hamilton Health Sciences, Ontario, Canada; Wake Forest Univ School of Medicine, Winston-Salem, NC; Case Western Reserve Univ, Cleveland, OH; et al)
N Engl J Med 364:818-828, 2011

Background.—Intensive glucose lowering has previously been shown to increase mortality among persons with advanced type 2 diabetes and a high risk of cardiovascular disease. This report describes the 5-year outcomes of a mean of 3.7 years of intensive glucose lowering on mortality and key cardiovascular events.

Methods.—We randomly assigned participants with type 2 diabetes and cardiovascular disease or additional cardiovascular risk factors to receive intensive therapy (targeting a glycated hemoglobin level below 6.0%) or standard therapy (targeting a level of 7 to 7.9%). After termination of the intensive therapy, due to higher mortality in the intensive-therapy group, the target glycated hemoglobin level was 7 to 7.9% for all participants, who were followed until the planned end of the trial.

Results.—Before the intensive therapy was terminated, the intensive-therapy group did not differ significantly from the standard-therapy group in the rate of the primary outcome (a composite of nonfatal myocardial infarction, nonfatal stroke, or death from cardiovascular causes) (P=0.13) but had more deaths from any cause (primarily cardiovascular) (hazard ratio, 1.21; 95% confidence interval [CI], 1.02 to 1.44) and fewer nonfatal myocardial infarctions (hazard ratio, 0.79; 95% CI, 0.66 to 0.95). These trends persisted during the entire follow-up period (hazard ratio for death, 1.19; 95% CI, 1.03 to 1.38; and hazard ratio for nonfatal myocardial infarction, 0.82; 95% CI, 0.70 to 0.96). After the intensive intervention was terminated, the median glycated hemoglobin level in the intensive-therapy group rose from 6.4% to 7.2%, and the use of glucose-lowering medications and rates of severe hypoglycemia and other adverse events were similar in the two groups.

Conclusions.—As compared with standard therapy, the use of intensive therapy for 3.7 years to target a glycated hemoglobin level below 6% reduced 5-year nonfatal myocardial infarctions but increased 5-year mortality. Such a strategy cannot be recommended for high-risk patients with advanced type 2 diabetes. (Funded by the National Heart, Lung and Blood Institute; ClinicalTrials.gov number, NCT00000620.)

▶ This study reports on the extension of the observation period of the initial Action to Control Cardiovascular Risk in Diabetes (ACCORD) study. As reported in 2008, the intensified treatment group of the initial ACCORD study was stopped after 3.7 years because of increased mortality in this group. The study compared cardiovascular outcomes in patients with long-standing type 2 diabetes mellitus and a high burden of preexisting cardiovascular disease under conventional (glycated hemoglobin A_{1c} [HbA_{1c}] goal 7.0%-7.9%) versus intensified (HbA_{1c} goal < 6.0%) therapy.[1-3]

This study reports a follow-up of the patients who were initially ascribed to the intensified group and subsequently switched to a conventional treatment regime aiming for an HbA_{1c} target of 7.0% to 7.9%. Consequently, the mean HbA_{1c} level in these patients rose from 6.4% to 7.2%.

The outcomes were now assessed after a total of 5 years, of which 3.7 years were under an intensified glucose-lowering regime. As in the initial observation, the risk of death by any cause was slightly higher in the former intensified group, whereas the risk for nonfatal myocardial infarction was lower. The incidence of severe hypoglycemia was equal in both groups after the intensified group was switched to conventional treatment.

What is new in this study?

As expected, HbA_{1c} and hypoglycemia risk were now equal in both groups. Still, the initial trend with a decreased risk for myocardial infarction but increased risk of death was maintained.

How come?

Apparently, 3.7 years of intensive treatment prolonged by a 1.3-year postinterventional follow-up does not significantly improve cardiovascular outcomes. This is not surprising and in line with the follow-up study of the United Kingdom Prospective Diabetes Study. In the latter study, cardiovascular risk after stricter glucose control was reduced 10 years after the intervention was stopped. One major point that we learned from this study was that benefits for cardiovascular end points need time to develop.[4] Therefore, it is not surprising that 1.3 additional years of postinterventional follow-up do not change the overall trend of the initial study with respect to cardiovascular end points.

Why is the mortality still increased, although hypoglycemia risk is comparable between the 2 groups?

This finding does indeed argue against hypoglycemia as the major cause for increased mortality in the intensified group. Although it is still not clear why patients initially under strict glucose control have still a higher mortality even after switching to standard therapy, drug interactions might be one possible explanation.

Taken together, these data further argue against an HbA$_{1c}$ target < 6% in patients with high cardiovascular risk and long-standing diabetes mellitus.

S. Schinner, MD, PhD

References

1. Gerstein HC, Miller ME, Byington RP, et al. Action to Control Cardiovascular Risk in Diabetes Study Group. Effects of intensive glucose lowering in type 2 diabetes. *N Engl J Med.* 2008;358:2545-2559.
2. Calles-Escandón J, Lovato LC, Simons-Morton DG, et al. Effect of intensive compared with standard glycemia treatment strategies on mortality by baseline subgroup characteristics: the Action to Control Cardiovascular Risk in Diabetes (ACCORD) trial. *Diabetes Care.* 2010;33:721-727.
3. Riddle MC, Ambrosius WT, Brillon DJ, et al. Epidemiologic relationships between A1C and all-cause mortality during a median 3.4-year follow-up of glycemic treatment in the ACCORD trial. *Diabetes Care.* 2010;33:983-990.
4. Holman RR, Paul SK, Bethel MA, Matthews DR, Neil HA. 10-Year follow-up of intensive glucose control in type 2 diabetes. *N Engl J Med.* 2008;359:1577-1589.

Diabetes Mellitus, Fasting Glucose, and Risk of Cause-Specific Death

The Emerging Risk Factors Collaboration (Univ of Cambridge, UK; et al)

N Engl J Med 364:829-841, 2011

Background.—The extent to which diabetes mellitus or hyperglycemia is related to risk of death from cancer or other nonvascular conditions is uncertain.

Methods.—We calculated hazard ratios for cause-specific death, according to baseline diabetes status or fasting glucose level, from individual-participant data on 123,205 deaths among 820,900 people in 97 prospective studies.

Results.—After adjustment for age, sex, smoking status, and body-mass index, hazard ratios among persons with diabetes as compared with persons without diabetes were as follows: 1.80 (95% confidence interval [CI], 1.71 to 1.90) for death from any cause, 1.25 (95% CI, 1.19 to 1.31) for death from cancer, 2.32 (95% CI, 2.11 to 2.56) for death from vascular causes, and 1.73 (95% CI, 1.62 to 1.85) for death from other causes. Diabetes (vs. no diabetes) was moderately associated with death from cancers of the liver, pancreas, ovary, colorectum, lung, bladder, and breast. Aside from cancer and vascular disease, diabetes (vs. no diabetes) was also associated with death from renal disease, liver disease, pneumonia and other infectious diseases, mental disorders, nonhepatic digestive diseases, external causes, intentional self-harm, nervous-system disorders, and chronic obstructive pulmonary disease. Hazard ratios were appreciably reduced after further adjustment for glycemia measures, but not after adjustment for systolic blood pressure, lipid levels, inflammation or renal markers. Fasting glucose levels exceeding 100 mg per deciliter (5.6 mmol per liter), but not levels of 70 to 100 mg per deciliter (3.9 to 5.6 mmol per liter), were associated with death. A 50-year-old with diabetes died, on average, 6 years earlier than a counterpart without diabetes, with about 40% of the difference in survival attributable to excess nonvascular deaths.

Conclusions.—In addition to vascular disease, diabetes is associated with substantial premature death from several cancers, infectious diseases, external causes, intentional self-harm, and degenerative disorders, independent of several major risk factors. (Funded by the British Heart Foundation and others.)

▶ The glucose thresholds to define the diagnosis of diabetes mellitus (DM) are based on the risk for retinopathy. However, it has been shown in numerous studies that DM is associated with increased macrovascular complication and cardiovascular death.[1,2] This study investigates not only the effects of DM on nonvascular death but also the relationship of fasting plasma glucose levels with the risk of death. Even after adjustment for body mass index and other risk factors, DM was associated with a strong increase in the risk for not only cardiovascular death but also death by cancer. The latter is of particular interest, as the relationship between glycemic control and the antihyperglycemic medication and cancer risk has been intensively discussed. In fact, DM appears as an independent risk factor for a number of cancer entities. These include cancers of the liver, pancreas, ovary, colorectum, lung, bladder, and breast. In principle, the nature of this study is correlative. However, it is highly plausible that DM plays a causative role for the excessive risk of death even from cancer. Of course, possible underlying mechanisms cannot be explained by this study. Reasonable explanations are based on the fact that glucose and insulin can both promote tumor growth. However, it cannot be ruled out that the underlying causes for diabetes (nutrition, lack of physical activity) are themselves causal cofactors for the excess death.

Another interesting aspect of this study is the definition of the cutoff for the fasting plasma glucose level, namely 100 mg/dL, for the risk of death. Of note, this is well below the current diabetes definition and underlines furthermore the fact that the current diabetes definitions derive from retinopathy risk assessments (and not from macrovascular risk or risk of death).

S. Schinner, MD, PhD

References

1. Sarwar N, Gao P, Seshasai SR. The Emerging Risk Factors Collaboration. Diabetes mellitus, fasting blood glucose concentration, and risk of vascular disease: a collaborative meta-analysis of 102 prospective studies. *Lancet.* 2010;375:2215-2222.
2. Coutinho M, Gerstein HC, Wang Y, Yusuf S. The relationship between glucose and incident cardiovascular events. A metaregression analysis of published data from 20 studies of 95,783 individuals followed for 12.4 years. *Diabetes Care.* 1999;22:233-240.

57 Adrenal Cortex

18F-FDG PET for the Identification of Adrenocortical Carcinomas among Indeterminate Adrenal Tumors at Computed Tomography Scanning
Nunes ML, Rault A, Teynie J, et al (Centre Hospitalier Universitaire de Bordeaux, Pessac, France)
World J Surg 34:1506-1510, 2010

Background.—18F-fluorodeoxyglucose positron emission tomography (18F-FDG PET) has been proposed for the evaluation of adrenal tumors. However, only scarce data are available to evaluate its usefulness for the identification of primary adrenal carcinomas in patients with no previous history of cancer and equivocal tumors on computed tomography (CT) scan. The objective of the present study was to evaluate the diagnostic performance of 18F-FDG-PET to predict malignancy in such patients.

Methods and Patients.—This was a retrospective study carried out from 2006 to 2009 in a single university hospital center. Twenty-three consecutive patients without previous history of cancer investigated for adrenal tumors without features of benign adrenocortical adenoma on CT scan but no obvious ACC underwent 18F-FDG PET. All patients underwent adrenalectomy because of CT scan characteristics regardless of the results of 18F-FDG PET. The ratio of maxSUV adrenal tumor on maxSUV liver (adrenal/liver maxSUV ratio) during 18F-FDG PET was compared to Weiss pathological criteria.

Results.—Seventeen patients had an adrenal adenoma, 2 had small size adrenal carcinomas (<5 cm), 1 had an angiosarcoma, and 3 had noncortical benign lesions. An adrenal/liver maxSUV ratio above 1.6 provided 100% sensitivity, 90% specificity, and 100% negative predictive value for the diagnosis of malignant tumor.

Conclusions.—Because of its excellent negative predictive value, 18F-FDG-PET may be of help in avoiding unnecessary surgery in patients with non-secreting equivocal tumors at CT scanning and low 18F-FGD uptake.

▶ Imaging criteria for identifying benign adrenal masses are a measurement of < 10 unenhanced density on unenhanced CT and contrast washout of > 60% at 15 minutes after contrast injection. Sensitivity of unenhanced CT is 98%, specificity 92%, and washout sensitivity and specificity almost 100%. Lipid-rich benign lesions can also be detected by their drop in signal with chemical shift MRI with comparable sensitivity and specificity. The problem is with indeterminate adrenal masses that do not reach the cutoff criteria. Nunes et al propose the use of 18F-fluorodeoxyglucose positron emission tomography (18F-FDG PET) as helpful in determining which of these lesions are likely to be malignant. An adrenal/liver max standardized uptake value ratio above 1.6 provided 100% sensitivity, 90% specificity, and 100% negative predictive value for diagnosing malignancy. The PET would also be helpful in detecting metastases and helping to stage the tumor. In a series of 23 patients, they discovered 2 adrenocortical carcinomas (ACCs) and 1 angiosarcoma, while the rest were benign adrenocortical adenomas. They conclude that 18F-FDG PET can be useful in patients with indeterminate adrenal masses. Of interest in this series is that the 2 patients with small ACCs were treated by laparoscopic surgery and developed local recurrence and peritoneal carcinomatosis. We have observed these complications frequently with laparoscopic resections and have strongly recommended open adrenalectomies in all cases of ACC regardless of tumor size or surgical skill.

D. E. Schteingart, MD

Reversible Sympathetic Overactivity in Hypertensive Patients with Primary Aldosteronism

Kontak AC, Wang Z, Arbique D, et al (Univ of Texas Southwestern Med Ctr, Dallas; et al)
J Clin Endocrinol Metab 95:4756-4761, 2010

Context.—Aldosterone has been shown to exert a central sympathoexcitatory action in multiple animal models, but evidence in humans is still lacking.

Objectives.—Our objective was to determine whether hyperaldosteronism causes reversible sympathetic activation in humans.

Methods.—We performed a cross-sectional comparison of muscle sympathetic nerve activity (SNA, intraneural microelectrodes) in 14 hypertensive patients with biochemically proven primary aldosteronism (PA) with 20 patients with essential hypertension (EH) and 18 age-matched normotensive (NT) controls. Seven patients with aldosterone-producing adenoma (APA) were restudied 1 month after unilateral adrenalectomy.

Results.—Mean blood pressure values in patients with PA and EH and NT controls was $145 \pm 4/88 \pm 2$, $150 \pm 4/90 \pm 2$, and $119 \pm 2/76 \pm 2$ mm Hg, respectively. The major new findings are 2-fold: 1) baseline SNA was significantly higher in the PA than the NT group (40 ± 3 vs. 30 ± 2 bursts/min, $P = 0.014$) but similar to the EH group (41 ± 3 bursts/min) and 2) after unilateral adrenalectomy for APA, SNA decreased significantly from 38 ± 5 to 27 ± 4 bursts/min ($P = 0.01$), plasma aldosterone levels fell from 72.4 ± 20.3 to 11.4 ± 2.3 ng/dl ($P < 0.01$), and blood pressure decreased from $155 \pm 8/94 \pm 3$ to $117 \pm 4/77 \pm 2$ mm Hg ($P < 0.01$).

Conclusion.—These data provide the first evidence in humans that APA is accompanied by reversible sympathetic overactivity, which may contribute to the accelerated hypertensive target organ disease in this condition.

▶ It is generally agreed that the mechanism of hypertension in patients with primary aldosteronism is mineralocorticoid-mediated sodium retention and volume expansion. Aldosterone also has direct effects on the heart and kidneys, inducing fibrosis. There may be other contributing factors in the pathogenesis of hypertension in primary aldosteronism, including a central sympathoexcitatory action of aldosterone. This putative effect had been shown in animal models but not in humans. Kontak et al compared muscle sympathetic nerve activity (SNA) in 14 patients with primary aldosteronism, 20 patients with essential hypertension, and 18 age-matched normotensive controls. Studies were repeated in some patients with primary aldosteronism after adrenalectomy. As shown in Fig 4 in the original article, SNA was significantly increased in primary aldosteronism and essential hypertension and was consistently reversed after adrenalectomy. These studies suggest a possible benefit of sympathetic blockers in treating patients with primary aldosteronism.

D. E. Schteingart, MD

Glucocorticoids in the prefrontal cortex enhance memory consolidation and impair working memory by a common neural mechanism
Barsegyan A, Mackenzie SM, Kurose BD, et al (Univ of Groningen, The Netherlands; Univ of California, Irvine)
Proc Natl Acad Sci U S A 107:16655-16660, 2010

It is well established that acute administration of adrenocortical hormones enhances the consolidation of memories of emotional experiences and, concurrently, impairs working memory. These different glucocorticoid effects on these two memory functions have generally been considered to be independently regulated processes. Here we report that a glucocorticoid receptor agonist administered into the medial prefrontal cortex (mPFC) of male Sprague-Dawley rats both enhances memory consolidation and impairs working memory. Both memory effects are mediated by activation of a membrane-bound steroid receptor and depend on noradrenergic activity within the mPFC to increase levels of cAMP-dependent protein kinase. These findings provide direct evidence that glucocorticoid effects on both memory consolidation and working memory share a common neural influence within the mPFC.

▶ Glucocorticoids (GCs) have direct brain effects and have been shown to induce hippocampal structure and function changes affecting memory in both experimental animals and people with corticosteroid therapy, endogenous Cushing syndrome, and depression. GCs can affect other brain areas such as the prefrontal cortex and cause alteration in different types of memory in a complex manner. For example, GCs impair working memory but enhance memory consolidation. Barsegyan et al dissected the mechanism of this effect of GCs on the prefrontal cortex in male rats and show that the changes in these 2 types of memory are linked by common nongenomic mechanisms involving activation of a noradrenergic and protein kinase A (PKA) signaling pathway. While these observations suggest that GC antagonists, β-adrenoceptor antagonists, and PKA inhibitors may be used to treat prefrontal cortex cognitive dysfunction during chronic stress, aging, or other pathological conditions, the fact the 2 types of memory are interdependent and in opposite directions could result in further impairment of cognitive function.

D. E. Schteingart, MD

Addison's Disease in Women Is a Risk Factor for an Adverse Pregnancy Outcome
Björnsdottir S, Cnattingius S, Brandt L, et al (Karolinska Institutet, Stockholm, Sweden; et al)
J Clin Endocrinol Metab 95:5249-5257, 2010

Context.—Autoimmune Addison's disease (AAD) tends to affect young and middle-aged women. It is not known whether the existence of undiagnosed or diagnosed AAD influences the outcome of pregnancy.

Objective.—The aim of the study was to compare the number of children and pregnancy outcomes in individuals with AAD and controls.

Design and Setting.—We conducted a population-based historical cohort study in Sweden.

Patients.—Through the Swedish National Patient Register and the Total Population Register, we identified 1,188 women with AAD and 11,879 age-matched controls who delivered infants between 1973 and 2006.

Main Outcome Measures.—We measured parity and pregnancy outcome.

Results.—Adjusted odds ratios (ORs) for infants born to mothers with deliveries 3 yr or less before the diagnosis of AAD were 2.40 [95% confidence interval (CI), 1.27−4.53] for preterm birth ($\leq$37 wk), 3.50 (95% CI, 1.83−6.67) for low birth weight (<2500 g), and 1.74 (95% CI, 1.02−2.96) for cesarean section. Compared to controls, women who gave birth after their AAD diagnosis were at increased risk of both cesarean delivery (adjusted OR, 2.35; 95% CI, 1.68−3.27) and preterm delivery (adjusted OR, 2.61; 95% CI, 1.69−4.05). Stratifying by isolated AAD and concomitant type 1 diabetes and/or autoimmune thyroid disease in the mother did not essentially influence these risks. There were no differences in risks of congenital malformations or infant death. Women with AAD had a reduced overall parity compared to controls ($P < 0.001$).

Conclusion.—Clinically undiagnosed and diagnosed AAD both entail increased risks of unfavorable pregnancy outcomes. AAD also influences the number of childbirths.

▶ Taking advantage of a comprehensive register, Björnsdottir et al examined all the patients in Sweden with autoimmune Addison disease (AAD) between 1973 and 2006 for evidence of adverse pregnancy outcomes. They identified 1188 women with AAD and compared them with 11 879 age-matched controls who delivered during that period. Adjusted odds ratios for women who delivered 3 or less years before diagnosis were 2.4 for preterm birth, 3.5 for low birth weight, and 1.7 for cesarean section, and for those who delivered after diagnosis, 2.6 for preterm birth and 2.3 for cesarean section. The data are impressive in terms of the number of patients examined but leave many questions the registry is unable to answer. The health status of women who became pregnant prior to diagnosis and the adequacy of treatment of those whose diagnosis had already been established. These are limitations of the registry. The management of patients with AAD has evolved over the 40 years the data was collected, and most pregnant women with those conditions are currently being followed up in high-risk pregnancy clinics where replacement is monitored and adjusted on an ongoing basis. Perhaps preterm birth and cesarean section can be avoided in these patients with better endocrine care.

D. E. Schteingart, MD

58 Obesity

Remission of Type 2 Diabetes After Gastric Bypass and Banding: Mechanisms and 2 Year Outcomes

Pournaras DJ, Osborne A, Hawkins SC, et al (Musgrove Park Hosp, Taunton, Somerset, UK; et al)

Ann Surg 252:966-971, 2010

Objective.—To investigate the rate of type 2 diabetes remission after gastric bypass and banding and establish the mechanism leading to remission of type 2 diabetes after bariatric surgery.

Summary Background Data.—Glycemic control in type 2 diabetic patients is improved after bariatric surgery.

Methods.—In study 1, 34 obese type 2 diabetic patients undergoing either gastric bypass or gastric banding were followed up for 36 months. Remission of diabetes was defined as patients not requiring hypoglycemic medication, fasting glucose below 7 mmol/L, 2 hour glucose after oral glucose tolerance test below 11.1 mmol/L, and glycated haemoglobin (HbA1c) <6%. In study 2, 41 obese type 2 diabetic patients undergoing either bypass, banding, or very low calorie diet were followed up for 42 days. Insulin resistance (HOMA-IR), insulin production, and glucagon-like peptide 1 (GLP-1) responses after a standard meal were measured.

Results.—In study 1, HbA1c as a marker of glycemic control improved by 2.9% after gastric bypass and 1.9% after gastric banding at latest follow-up ($P < 0.001$ for both groups). Despite similar weight loss, 72% (16/22) of bypass and 17% (2/12) of banding patients ($P = 0.001$) fulfilled the definition of remission at latest follow-up. In study 2, within days, only bypass patients had improved insulin resistance, insulin production, and GLP-1 responses (all $P < 0.05$).

Conclusions.—With gastric bypass, type 2 diabetes can be improved and even rapidly put into a state of remission irrespective of weight loss. Improved insulin resistance within the first week after surgery remains unexplained, but increased insulin production in the first week after surgery may be explained by the enhanced postprandial GLP-1 responses.

▶ Bariatric surgery is currently the most efficacious treatment option for sustained substantial weight loss in severely and morbidly obese individuals. Roux-en-Y gastric bypass (RYGB) is the most commonly performed bariatric surgery, followed by laparoscopic gastric banding. RYGB is increasingly recognized as a major treatment modality for morbidly obese individuals with diabetes. In fact, the 2010 Diabetes Surgery Summit consensus conference has considered the notion to designate weight loss surgery as a diabetes surgery.[1] The RYGB procedure creates a small gastric pouch that is anastomosed to the small intestine below the proximal jejunum, ultimately bypassing nutrient exposure of the duodenum and proximal jejunum.[2] Drastic immediate improvements in glucose metabolism are observed shortly after RYGB that cannot be explained entirely by caloric restriction and weight loss alone. Hence, studies have been initiated to understand the underlying mechanisms accounting for the rapid improvement in glycemic control following RYGB. It is hypothesized that rapid delivery of nutrients to the distal small bowel increases the secretion of gut hormones, including glucagon-like peptide 1 (GLP-1) and gastric inhibitory peptide. GLP-1 is secreted by the L cells of the distal small intestine, and increased plasma levels have been shown to improve glucose metabolism by increasing the secretion of insulin and reducing the secretion of glucagon.[2]

In this study under review, Pournaras et al attempted to determine the effects of RYGB and gastric banding on diabetes remission and glucose metabolism in obese patients with type 2 diabetes. The first study that was conducted determined glycemic control in bariatric surgery patients with type 2 diabetes. Similar improvements in glycated hemoglobin A_{1c} were reported between subjects with type 2 diabetes who had RYGB and gastric banding at 1-year follow-up. However, a greater proportion of RYGB patients (72%) achieved fasting glucose concentrations < 7 mmol/L compared with gastric banding patients (17%) with similar weight loss after 1 year. In addition, RYGB patients had greater and faster rates of remission of diabetes relative to gastric banding patients (Fig 2 in the original article). This provides persuasive evidence that weight loss alone does not account for the rapid improvement in glycemic control in obese patients with type 2 diabetes following RYGB.

Pournaras et al also examined the mechanisms of improved glycemic control following bariatric surgery compared with caloric restriction. One of the key strengths of this study is that the authors attempted to tease out the effects of caloric deprivation induced by surgery by including a nonsurgical caloric-restricted group. However, one criticism of this approach is that the caloric-restricted group was not exposed to a surgical procedure, which limits our interpretation of the findings. Nevertheless, significant improvements in insulin resistance as assessed by homeostatic model assessment of insulin resistance were observed in patients with type 2 diabetes within 7 days of RYGB, whereas no improvements were observed in this short time frame for patients without diabetes or those who underwent gastric banding or caloric restriction (1000 kcal/d). Moreover, increased postprandial GLP-1 secretion was observed as early as 2 days postoperatively in the RYGB group. It should be noted that the authors did not report changes in GLP-1 levels for the patients who underwent gastric banding or caloric restriction. Despite the relatively small sample size (n = 5-17/group), these results suggest that the early improvements in insulin secretion and resistance observed in RYGB patients with type 2 diabetes may be because of increased GLP-1 secretion that was induced by the anatomical rearrangements of the gut.

This study provides compelling evidence that the physical rearrangements of the gut during RYGB induce early (≤7 days postoperatively) improvements in insulin resistance, which may be mediated by increased secretion of postprandial

GLP-1. These findings not only improve our understanding of the importance of gut-derived hormones in early improvements in glucose homeostasis after bariatric surgery but also support potential pharmaceutical targets for the medical management of insulin resistance in obesity.

M. R. Ruth, PhD

References

1. Rubino F, Kaplan LM, Schauer PR, Cummings DE. The Diabetes Surgery Summit consensus conference: recommendations for the evaluation and use of gastrointestinal surgery to treat type 2 diabetes mellitus. *Ann Surg.* 2010;251:399-405.
2. Beckman LM, Beckman TR, Earthman CP. Changes in gastrointestinal hormones and leptin after Roux-en-Y gastric bypass procedure: a review. *J Am Diet Assoc.* 2010;110:571-584.

Sustained improvement in mild obstructive sleep apnea after a diet- and physical activity–based lifestyle intervention: postinterventional follow-up
Tuomilehto H, for the Kuopio Sleep Apnea Group (Univ of Eastern Finland, Kuopio, Finland; et al)
Am J Clin Nutr 92:688-696, 2010

Background.—Obesity is the most important risk factor for obstructive sleep apnea (OSA). Weight-reduction programs have been observed to represent effective treatment of overweight patients with OSA. However, it is not known whether beneficial changes remain after the end of the intervention.

Objective.—The aim of the study was to assess the long-term efficacy of a lifestyle intervention based on a healthy diet and physical activity in a randomized, controlled, 2-y postintervention follow-up in OSA patients.

Design.—Eighty-one consecutive overweight [body mass index (in kg/m^2): 28–40] adult patients with mild OSA were recruited. The intervention group completed a 1-y lifestyle modification regimen that included an early 12-wk weight-reduction program with a very-low-calorie diet. The control group received routine lifestyle counseling. During the second year, no dietary counseling was offered. Change in the apnea-hypopnea index (AHI) was the main objective outcome variable, and changes in symptoms were used as a subjective measurement.

Results.—A total of 71 patients completed the 2-y follow-up. The mean (± SD) changes in diet and lifestyle with simultaneous weight reduction (-7.3 ± 6.5 kg) in the intervention group reflected sustained improvements in findings and symptoms of OSA. After 2 y, the reduction in the AHI was significantly greater in the intervention group ($P = 0.049$). The intervention lowered the risk of OSA at follow-up; the adjusted odds ratio for OSA was 0.35 (95% CI: 0.12–0.97; $P = 0.045$).

Conclusion.—Favorable changes achieved by a 1-y lifestyle intervention aimed at weight reduction with a healthy diet and physical activity were sustained in overweight patients with mild OSA after the termination of supervised lifestyle counseling. This trial was registered at clinicaltrials. gov as NCT00486746.

▶ Obstructive sleep apnea (OSA) is characterized by repeated episodes of apnea and hypopnea during sleep. It is associated with insulin resistance, type 2 diabetes mellitus, and cardiovascular morbidity and mortality. Obesity is the most important risk factor predisposing for OSA. OSA perpetuates obesity possibly through hormonal changes because of stress caused by hypoxemia and inflammation.[1,2] Although the increased risk of cardiovascular disease is mainly encountered in patients with more severe OSA, patients with mild OSA (apnea-hypopnea index [AHI] between 5 and 15 events/h) are also at increased risk. Weight loss has been shown to improve OSA; therefore, lifestyle changes are an integral part of therapy in overweight/obese patients with OSA.[3]

Tuomilehto et al investigated whether the beneficial effect of weight loss on OSA persists 1 year after the end of a 1-year lifestyle intervention study. This study reports the 2-year follow-up study of overweight/obese patients with mild OSA initially randomized to 12-week very-low-calorie diet followed by intensive lifestyle changes for 1 year, while the control group received routine dietary counseling. After 1 year no dietary counseling was offered to either group, and the main outcome was change in AHI in both groups. After 2 years, the study group lost 7.3 ± 6.5 kg and the control group lost 2.4 ± 2.1 kg ($P = .09$). The change in body mass index and waist circumference was statistically significant in the intervention group. Although the intervention group gained some of the weight lost through the lifestyle intervention at the follow-up, they still had a 65% reduced risk of OSA and a 50% decrease in the progression of the disease compared with the control group. The beneficial effect of weight loss on OSA was also observed in patients of the control group that succeeded in losing weight.

This study was able to show a sustained beneficial effect of weight loss in patients with OSA 1 year after the cessation of the active intervention. Because obesity is a risk factor not only for OSA but also for type 2 diabetes and cardiovascular disease, weight loss has beneficial effects well beyond improvement in respiratory function. This study emphasizes the value of weight loss also as primary therapy for mild OSA.

R. Ness-Abramof, MD

References

1. Vgontzas AN. Does obesity play a major role in the pathogenesis of sleep apnoea and its associated manifestations via inflammation, visceral adiposity, and insulin resistance? *Arch Physiol Biochem.* 2008;114:211-223.
2. Trakada G, Chrousos G, Pejovic S, Vgontzas A. Sleep Apnea and its association with the Stress System, Inflammation, Insulin Resistance and Visceral Obesity. *Sleep Med Clin.* 2007;2:251-261.
3. Foster GD, Borradaile KE, Sanders MH, et al. Sleep AHEAD Research Group of Look AHEAD Research Group. A randomized study on the effect of weight loss on obstructive sleep apnea among obese patients with type 2 diabetes: the Sleep AHEAD study. *Arch Intern Med.* 2009;169:1619-1626.

Insufficient Sleep Undermines Dietary Efforts to Reduce Adiposity

Nedeltcheva AV, Kilkus JM, Imperial J, et al (The Univ of Chicago, IL; Univ of Wisconsin, Madison)
Ann Intern Med 153:435-441, 2010

Background.—Sleep loss can modify energy intake and expenditure.

Objective.—To determine whether sleep restriction attenuates the effect of a reduced-calorie diet on excess adiposity.

Design.—Randomized, 2-period, 2-condition crossover study.

Setting.—University clinical research center and sleep laboratory.

Patients.—10 overweight nonsmoking adults (3 women and 7 men) with a mean age of 41 years (SD, 5) and a mean body mass index of 27.4 kg/m^2 (SD, 2.0).

Intervention.—14 days of moderate caloric restriction with 8.5 or 5.5 hours of nighttime sleep opportunity.

Measurements.—The primary measure was loss of fat and fat-free body mass. Secondary measures were changes in substrate utilization, energy expenditure, hunger, and 24-hour metabolic hormone concentrations.

Results.—Sleep curtailment decreased the proportion of weight lost as fat by 55% (1.4 vs. 0.6 kg with 8.5 vs. 5.5 hours of sleep opportunity, respectively; $P = 0.043$) and increased the loss of fat-free body mass by 60% (1.5 vs. 2.4 kg; $P = 0.002$). This was accompanied by markers of enhanced neuroendocrine adaptation to caloric restriction, increased hunger, and a shift in relative substrate utilization toward oxidation of less fat.

Limitation.—The nature of the study limited its duration and sample size.

Conclusion.—The amount of human sleep contributes to the maintenance of fat-free body mass at times of decreased energy intake. Lack of sufficient sleep may compromise the efficacy of typical dietary interventions for weight loss and related metabolic risk reduction.

▶ Sleep restriction and obesity are both linked to the modern way of living. Epidemiological studies have shown that short sleep duration is associated with obesity in children and adults.[1] Possible mechanisms by which sleep deprivation may promote weight gain include increase in appetite because of changes in orexigenic hormones (increase in ghrelin and decrease of leptin levels)[2] and increased food intake to fight fatigue or cope with stress, among other possible mechanisms. The question remains whether short sleep is the cause or correlates with obesity. Short-term studies have shown an increase in hunger in adults deprived of sleep, but the effect of sleep deprivation on weight loss has not been well studied.

Nedeltcheva and colleagues investigated whether sleep restriction attenuates the effect of a reduced-calorie diet on adiposity. They recruited 10 overweight adults who had a normal sleep duration (slept between 6.5-8.5 hours per day). The patients were randomly assigned to sleep 5.5 hours or 8.5 hours and to caloric restriction (90% of the resting metabolic rate) during 14 days. Sleep deprivation decreased the proportion of weight loss as fat by 55% and increased the loss of fat-free mass by 60% (Fig 2 in the original article). Sleep-deprived patients were hungrier and had less fat oxidation. In this study, sleep restriction was not accompanied by an increase in cortisol, serum triiodothyronine, free thyroxine, and plasma catecholamines. Leptin levels were similar between groups.

The main limitation of the study is the small number of patients and the wide range of total body expenditure between the 2 sleep conditions. The main question is whether sleep-deprived obese subjects will improve fat loss by increasing sleep duration. This study suggests that recommendations for lifestyle changes to induce weight loss should include a good night's sleep.

R. Ness-Abramof, MD

References

1. Cappuccio FP, Taggart FM, Kandala NB, et al. Meta-analysis of short sleep duration and obesity in children and adults. *Sleep.* 2008;31:619-626.
2. Taheri S, Lin L, Austin D, Young T, Mignot E. Short sleep duration is associated with reduced leptin, elevated ghrelin, and increased body mass index. *PLoS Med.* 2004;1:e62.

Weight Loss, Exercise, or Both and Physical Function in Obese Older Adults
Villareal DT, Chode S, Parimi N, et al (Washington Univ School of Medicine, St Louis; et al)
N Engl J Med 364:1218-1229, 2011

Background.—Obesity exacerbates the age-related decline in physical function and causes frailty in older adults; however, the appropriate treatment for obese older adults is controversial.

Methods.—In this 1-year, randomized, controlled trial, we evaluated the independent and combined effects of weight loss and exercise in 107 adults who were 65 years of age or older and obese. Participants were randomly assigned to a control group, a weight-management (diet) group, an exercise group, or a weight-management-plus-exercise (diet—exercise) group. The primary outcome was the change in score on the modified Physical Performance Test. Secondary outcomes included other measures of frailty, body composition, bone mineral density, specific physical functions, and quality of life.

Results.—A total of 93 participants (87%) completed the study. In the intention-to-treat analysis, the score on the Physical Performance Test, in which higher scores indicate better physical status, increased more in the diet—exercise group than in the diet group or the exercise group (increases from baseline of 21% vs. 12% and 15%, respectively); the scores in all three of those groups increased more than the scores in the control group (in which the score increased by 1%) (P<0.001 for the between-group differences). Moreover, the peak oxygen consumption improved more in the diet-exercise group than in the diet group or the exercise group (increases of 17% vs. 10% and 8%, respectively; P<0.001); the score on the Functional Status Questionnaire, in which higher scores indicate better physical function, increased more in the diet—exercise group than in the diet group (increase of 10% vs. 4%, P<0.001). Body weight decreased by 10% in the diet group and by 9% in the diet—exercise group, but did not decrease in the exercise group or the control group (P<0.001). Lean body mass and bone mineral density at the hip decreased less in the diet—exercise group than in the diet group (reductions of 3% and 1%, respectively, in the diet-exercise group vs. reductions of 5% and 3%, respectively, in the diet group; P<0.05 for both comparisons). Strength, balance, and gait improved consistently in the diet—exercise group (P<0.05 for all comparisons). Adverse events included a small number of exercise-associated musculo-skeletal injuries.

Conclusions.—These findings suggest that a combination of weight loss and exercise provides greater improvement in physical function than either intervention alone. (Funded by the National Institutes of Health; ClinicalTrials.gov number, NCT00146107.)

▶ Obesity is a major health problem worldwide. The prevalence of obesity is around 30% to 35% in middle-aged and older adults (> 60 years). Obesity is known to increase cardiovascular disease, type 2 diabetes, and osteoarthritis, among other diseases. The older population has a high prevalence of these comorbidities, but it is not clear whether weight loss will decrease risk factors or morbidity and mortality.[1] There is evidence that being overweight (body mass index, 25-29.9 kg/m^2) is not associated with a higher mortality rate in older people.[2] Until now, few studies addressed the effect of weight loss and exercise on cardiovascular risk factors, exercise capacity, or quality of life.

This study by Villareal et al evaluated the effect of diet or exercise alone to diet and exercise in 107 obese adults older than 65 years to a control group. The primary outcome was the change in score on the modified Physical Performance Test; secondary outcomes included frailty, bone density, body composition, physical function, and quality of life. The Physical Performance Test score increased more in the diet-and-exercise group compared with the diet-alone and exercise-alone groups. All 3 groups had better results compared with the control group. Peak oxygen consumption increased more in the diet-and-exercise group compared with the diet-alone or exercise-alone groups (Fig 2 in the original article). Weight loss was similar in the diet-and-exercise and diet-alone groups, while subjects in the exercise-alone or control groups did not lose weight (Fig 3 in the original article). Lean body mass and bone mineral density decreased less in the diet-and-exercise and exercise-alone groups. Improvement in physical function was also higher in the diet-and-exercise group.

Sarcopenia is a known risk factor for frailty in the older population. In this study, a decrease in muscle mass was observed in the diet groups; this effect was attenuated in the diet-and-exercise group.

Diet and exercise provided the greatest increase in scores on the Physical Performance Tests and also improvement in balance and strength.

The negative effects observed in this study in the diet subgroups were the reductions in muscle mass and bone density. Although this effect was attenuated by exercise, it needs to be further evaluated and, if possible, prevented.

R. Ness-Abramof, MD

References

1. Witham MD, Avenell A. Inerventions to achieve long-term weight loss in obese older people. a systematic review and meta-analysis. *Age Ageing.* 2010;39: 176-184.
2. Janssen I, Mark AE. Elevated body mass index and mortality risk in the elderly. *Obes Rev.* 2007;8:41-59.

59 Reproductive Endocrinology

Parallel-Group Placebo-Controlled Trial of Testosterone Gel in Men With Major Depressive Disorder Displaying an Incomplete Response to Standard Antidepressant Treatment
Pope HG Jr, Amiaz R, Brennan BP, et al (McLean Hosp, Belmont, MA; Chaim Sheba Med Ctr, Tel Hashomer, Israel; et al)
J Clin Psychopharmacol 30:126-134, 2010

Exogenous testosterone therapy has psychotropic effects and has been proposed as an antidepressant augmentation strategy for depressed men. We sought to assess the antidepressant effects of testosterone augmentation of a serotonergic antidepressant in depressed, hypogonadal men. For this study, we recruited 100 medically healthy adult men with major depressive disorder showing partial response or no response to an adequate serotonergic antidepressant trial during the current episode and a screening total testosterone level of 350 ng/dL or lower. We randomized these men to receive testosterone gel or placebo gel in addition to their existing antidepressant regimen. The primary outcome measure was the Hamilton Depression Rating Scale (HDRS) score. Secondary measures included the Montgomery-Asberg Depression Rating Scale, the Clinical Global Impression Scale, and the Quality of Life Scale. Our primary analysis, using a mixed effects linear regression model to compare rate of change of scores between groups on the outcome measures, failed to show a significant difference between groups (mean [95% confidence interval] 6-week change in HDRS for testosterone vs placebo, -0.4 [-2.6 to 1.8]). However, in one exploratory analysis of treatment responders, we found a possible trend in favor of testosterone on the HDRS. Our findings, combined with the conflicting data from earlier smaller studies, suggest that testosterone is not generally effective for depressed men. The possibility remains that testosterone might benefit a particular subgroup of depressed men, but if so, the characteristics of this subgroup would still need to be established (Fig 2).

▶ Testosterone deficiency in men has been associated with depressed mood, depression, low energy, depressed libido, and a reduced sense of well-being. Correction of testosterone deficiency using androgen replacement therapy

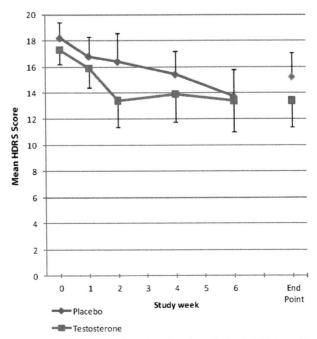

FIGURE 2.—Mean HDRS scores at each study week and at endpoint (LOCF) in participants receiving testosterone and placebo. (Reprinted from Pope HG Jr, Amiaz R, Brennan BP, et al. Parallel-group placebo-controlled trial of testosterone gel in men with major depressive disorder displaying an incomplete response to standard antidepressant treatment. *J Clin Psychopharmacol.* 2010;30:126-134.)

with various preparations of testosterone has been associated with improvement of many of these symptoms. In this study, men with major depressive disorders showing partial or no response to standard antidepressant therapy were treated with testosterone or placebo to determine whether the therapy would affect depression. The study suggests that men with depression without hypogonadism should not be treated routinely with testosterone therapy. Even in men with documented testosterone deficiency, testosterone replacement therapy does not correct all symptoms attributed to hypogonadism. In men with depression without hypogonadism, further study might identify a subpopulation of men who benefited with testosterone therapy, with resistance to standard antidepressive therapy. Any use of testosterone obviously requires a benefit-risk assessment, and until such time when benefits of relieving depression in a subgroup of men are established, testosterone is not recommended.

A. W. Meikle, MD

Determinants of Impaired Fasting Glucose Versus Glucose Intolerance in Polycystic Ovary Syndrome

Karakas SE, Kim K, Duleba AJ (Univ of California, Davis)
Diabetes Care 33:887-893, 2010

Objective.—To determine insulin resistance and response in patients with polycystic ovary syndrome (PCOS) and normal glucose tolerance (NGT), impaired fasting glucose (IFG), impaired glucose tolerance, and combined glucose intolerance (CGI).

Research Design and Methods.—In this cross-sectional study, 143 patients with PCOS (diagnosed on the basis of National Institutes of Health criteria) underwent oral glucose tolerance testing (OGTT), and 68 patients also had frequently sampled intravenous glucose tolerance tests. Changes in plasma glucose, insulin, cardiovascular risk factors, and androgens were measured.

Results.—Compared with patients with NGT, those with both IFG and CGI were significantly insulin resistant (homeostasis model assessment 3.3 ± 0.2 vs. 6.1 ± 0.9 and 6.4 ± 0.5, $P < 0.0001$) and hyperinsulinemic (insulin area under the curve for 120 min 973 ± 69 vs. $1,470 \pm 197$ and $1,461 \pm 172$ pmol/l, $P < 0.0001$). Insulin response was delayed in patients with CGI but not in those with IFG (2-h OGTT, insulin $1,001 \pm 40$ vs. 583 ± 45 pmol/l, $P < 0.0001$). Compared with the NGT group, the CGI group had a lower disposition index ($1,615 \pm 236$ vs. 987 ± 296, $P < 0.0234$) and adiponectin level (11.1 ± 1.1 vs. 6.2 ± 0.8 ng/ml, $P < 0.0096$). Compared with the insulin-resistant tertile of the NGT group, those with IFG had a reduced insulinogenic index (421 ± 130 vs. 268 ± 68, $P < 0.05$). Compared with the insulin-sensitive tertile of the NGT group, the resistant tertile had higher triglyceride and high-sensitivity C-reactive protein (hs-CRP) and lower HDL cholesterol and sex hormone—binding globulin (SHBG). In the entire population, insulin resistance correlated directly with triglyceride, hs-CRP, and the free androgen index and inversely with SHBG.

Conclusions.—Patients with PCOS develop IFG and CGI despite having significant hyperinsulinemia. Patients with IFG and CGI exhibit similar insulin resistance but very different insulin response patterns. Increases in cardiac risk factors and free androgen level precede overt glucose intolerance.

▶ Women with polycystic ovary syndrome (PCOS) often exhibit glucose intolerance, type 2 diabetes, and gestational diabetes. Compared with weight-matched controls, women with PCOS have high insulin concentrations, which can be improved with the administration of insulin sensitizers. Ovarian function, insulin sensitivity, and hyperandrogenism improve. Impaired fasting glucose (IFG, 100-125 mg/dL) is the result of hepatic insulin resistance, and impaired glucose tolerance (IGT, > 140 mg/dL) at 2 hours postglucose tolerance test results from peripheral insulin resistance. If they have both defects, it is called combined glucose intolerance. Those with IFG had an increased response to the oral glucose tolerance test compared with those with IGT, who exhibited a delayed insulin response. After 60 minutes, the insulin response changed so that those with IGT had higher insulin values than those with IFG. Patients with combined glucose intolerance have both hepatic and peripheral insulin resistance. The authors propose that IFG might precede IGT and combined glucose intolerance. In either case, improving insulin sensitivity will benefit patients with PCOS.

A. W. Meikle, MD

Low serum testosterone levels are associated with increased risk of mortality in a population-based cohort of men aged 20–79
Haring R, Völzke H, Steveling A, et al (Ernst Moritz Arndt Univ Greifswald, Germany; et al)
Eur Heart J 31:1494-1501, 2010

Aims.—Although the association of low serum testosterone levels with mortality has gained strength in recent research, there are few population-based studies on this issue. This study examined whether low serum testosterone levels are a risk factor for all-cause or cause-specific mortality in a population-based sample of men aged 20–79.

Methods and Results.—We used data from 1954 men recruited for the prospective population-based Study of Health in Pomerania, with measured serum testosterone levels at baseline and 195 deaths during an average 7.2-year follow-up. A total serum testosterone level of less than 8.7 nmol/L (250 ng/dL) was classified as low. The relationships of low serum testosterone levels with all-cause and cause-specific mortality were analysed by Cox proportional hazards regression models. Men with low serum testosterone levels had a significantly higher mortality from all causes than men with higher serum testosterone levels (HR 2.24; 95% CI 1.41–3.57). After adjusting for waist circumference, smoking habits, high-risk alcohol use, physical activity, renal insufficiency, and levels of dehydroepiandrosterone sulfate, low serum testosterone levels continued to be associated with increased mortality (HR 2.32; 95% CI 1.38–3.89). In cause-specific analyses, low serum testosterone levels predicted increased risk of death from cardiovascular disease (CVD) (HR 2.56; 95% CI 1.15–6.52) and cancer (HR 3.46; 95% CI 1.68–6.68), but not from respiratory diseases or other causes.

Conclusion.—Low serum testosterone levels were associated with an increased risk of all-cause mortality independent of numerous risk factors. As serum testosterone levels are inversely related to mortality due to CVD and cancer, it may be used as a predictive marker (Table 3).

▶ It is well documented that serum testosterone concentrations decline in men at 1% to 2% per year with aging, and many health issues have been attributed to the decline, including hypertension, abdominal obesity, insulin resistance, decreased bone mineral density, decreased libido and energy, and chronic

TABLE 3.—Hazard Ratios for Low Serum Testosterone Levels Associated with All-Cause Mortality Adjusted for Potential Mediators

	Testosterone Level <8.7 nmol/L (250 ng/dL) HR (95% CI)
Model 3[†]	2.32 (1.38; 3.89)[**]
+ Hypertension	2.36 (1.50; 3.71)[***]
+ Diabetes mellitus	2.23 (1.38; 3.59)[**]
+ Metabolic syndrome	2.36 (1.49; 4.06)[***]
+ Myocardial infarction	2.37 (1.45; 3.87)[**]
+ Renal insufficiency	2.06 (1.19; 3.53)[**]
+ Hyperlipidaemia	2.40 (1.49; 3.85)[***]
+ Cohabitation	2.41 (1.53; 3.79)[***]
+ Educational level	2.31 (1.48; 3.61)[***]
+ Stroke	2.41 (1.50; 3.89)[***]
+ DHEAS	2.77 (1.68; 4.58)[***]
+ Blood sampling time	2.13 (1.37; 3.90)[**]

Covariables were added one at a time to model 3. HR, hazard ratio; CI, 95% confidence interval; DHEAS, dehydroepian-drosterone sulfate; WC, waist circumference.
[*]*P < 0.05.
[†]Model 3: adjusted for age, WC, smoking (three categories), high-risk alcohol use, and physical activity.
[**]*P < 0.01.
[***]*P < 0.001.

fatigue. The risk of mortality has more recently been associated with low serum testosterone as reported by Haring et al. They observed that low serum testosterone was associated with all-cause mortality even after control for independent risk factors. The low testosterone was not related to a single etiology and was strongly associated with cardiovascular disease and cancer deaths. Their study does not clarify the cause-and-effect relationship of low serum testosterone and mortality. Many associated factors, such as hypertension, abdominal obesity, and insulin resistance, might be implicated as risks for cardiovascular disease mortality, but would not account for cancer mortality. Currently, it might be considered a marker of mortality and not a specific cause.

A. W. Meikle, MD

Modulatory Effect of Raloxifene and Estrogen on the Metabolic Action of Growth Hormone in Hypopituitary Women

Birzniece V, Meinhardt U, Gibney J, et al (St Vincent's Hosp, Sydney, New South Wales, Australia; et al)
J Clin Endocrinol Metab 95:2099-2106, 2010

Context.—The metabolic action of GH is attenuated by estrogens administered via the oral route. Selective estrogen receptor modulators lower IGF-I to a lesser degree than 17β-estradiol in GH-deficient women, and their effect on fat and protein metabolism is unknown.

Objective.—The aim of the study was to compare the modulatory effects of 17β-estradiol and raloxifene, a selective estrogen receptor modulator, on the metabolic action of GH.

Design.—We conducted an open-label, two-group, randomized, two-period crossover study.

Patients and Intervention.—Ten hypopituitary women received GH therapy alone (0.5 mg/d) and GH plus17β-estradiol (E₂; 2 mg/d). Eleven hypopituitary women received GH therapy alone and GH plus raloxifene (R; 60 mg/d). The treatment duration was 1 month, with a 4-wk washout period.

Main Outcome Measures.—IGF-I, IGFBP-3, resting energy expenditure, and fat oxidation were quantified by indirect calorimetry. We measured

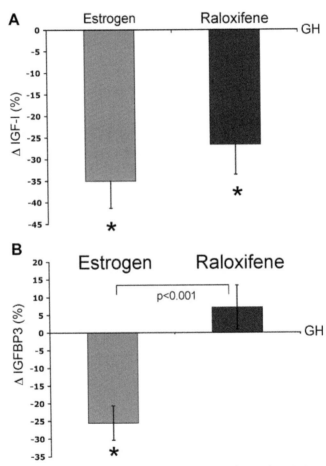

FIGURE 2.—Changes in serum IGF-I levels (A) and IGFBP-3 levels (B) in hypopituitary women after 4 wk of GH (0.5 mg/d) cotreatment with 17β-estradiol (2 mg/d) and raloxifene (60 mg/d). Data are presented as percentage change from GH treatment alone and expressed as means ± SEM. *, $P < 0.01$ compared with GH treatment alone using paired comparison. Between-group differences were analyzed using unpaired comparison. (Reprinted from Birzniece V, Meinhardt U, Gibney J, et al. Modulatory effect of raloxifene and estrogen on the metabolic action of growth hormone in hypopituitary women. *J Clin Endocrinol Metab.* 2010;95:2099-2106. Copyright © [2010], The Endocrine Society.

whole body leucine turnover from which leucine rate of appearance and leucine incorporation into protein were estimated.

Results.—GH significantly stimulated all outcome measures. During GH treatment, addition of R significantly reduced mean IGF-I but not IGFBP-3, whereas E_2 reduced both IGF-I and IGFBP-3 levels. Cotreatment with R but not E_2 significantly attenuated the stimulatory effects of GH on fat oxidation. There was a strong trend ($P = 0.08$) toward a greater reduction in leucine incorporation into protein after R compared to E_2 cotreatment.

Conclusions.—The modulatory effects of E_2 and R at therapeutic doses on GH action are different. R during GH therapy exerts a greater inhibitory effect on lipid oxidation and protein anabolism compared to E_2 (Fig 2).

▶ Growth hormone (GH) deficiency in postpubertal persons results in a reduction in muscle and bone mass and an increase in body fat by reducing fat oxidation. These adverse metabolic effects are reversed by GH replacement therapy. Orally administered estrogen suppresses serum insulin-like growth factor 1 (IGF-1) concentrations by reducing the liver's production in response to GH and reduces body fat oxidation and protein synthesis. The study by Birzniece et al compared the effects of oral estradiol-17β with raloxifene, a selective estrogen receptor modulator, in women with hypopituitarism on IGF-1, IGF binding protein-3 (IGFBP3), resting energy expenditure, and fat oxidation on the actions of GH therapy. Estradiol-17β reduced the IGF-1 and IGFBP-3 responses to GH therapy, and raloxifene only reduced IGF-1 but not IGFBP-3. Raloxifene but not estradiol-17β suppressed the fat oxidation stimulation of GH. Thus, raloxifene would not appear to have an advantage over estradiol-17β for estrogen therapy in GH-deficient women receiving GH therapy. In addition, fat accumulation over longer periods of time would be expected to be greater in women receiving raloxifene versus estradiol-17β.

A. W. Meikle, MD

Odanacatib in the Treatment of Postmenopausal Women With Low Bone Mineral Density: Three-Year Continued Therapy and Resolution of Effect
Eisman JA, Bone HG, Hosking DJ, et al (Univ of New South Wales, Sydney, Australia; Michigan Bone and Mineral Clinic, Detroit; Nottingham City Hosp, UK; et al)
J Bone Miner Res 26:242-251, 2011

The selective cathepsin K inhibitor odanacatib (ODN) progressively increased bone mineral density (BMD) and decreased bone-resorption markers during 2 years of treatment in postmenopausal women with low BMD. A 1-year extension study further assessed ODN efficacy and safety and the effects of discontinuing therapy. In the base study, postmenopausal women with BMD T-scores between −2.0 and −3.5 at the lumbar spine or femur received placebo or ODN 3, 10, 25, or 50 mg weekly. After

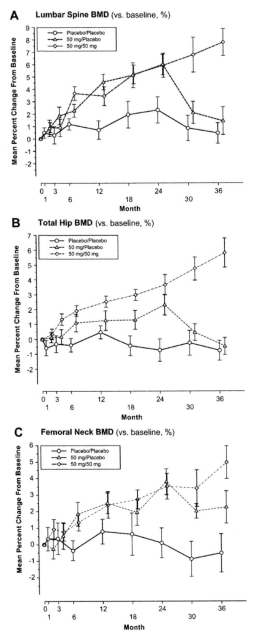

FIGURE 2.—BMD endpoints. Graphic presentation of the mean percentage change from baseline over 3 years in BMD at the specified site for the 50-mg/50-mg (ODN/ODN), 50-mg/placebo (ODN/Pbo), and placebo/placebo (Pbo/Pbo) treatment groups in the per-protocol extension population: (A) lumbar spine, (B) total hip, (C) femoral neck. (Reproduced from Eisman JA, Bone HG, Hosking DJ, et al. Odanacatib in the treatment of postmenopausal women with low bone mineral density: three-year continued therapy and resolution of effect. *J Bone Miner Res.* 2011;26:242-251, with permission from American Society for Bone and Mineral Research.)

2 years, patients ($n = 189$) were rerandomized to ODN 50 mg weekly or placebo for an additional year. Endpoints included BMD at the lumbar spine (primary), total hip, and hip subregions; levels of bone turnover markers; and safety assessments. Continued treatment with 50 mg of ODN for 3 years produced significant increases from baseline and from year 2 in BMD at the spine (7.9% and 2.3%) and total hip (5.8% and 2.4%). Urine cross-linked N-telopeptide of type I collagen (NTx) remained suppressed at year 3 (-50.5%), but bone-specific alkaline phosphatase (BSAP) was relatively unchanged from baseline. Treatment discontinuation resulted in bone loss at all sites, but BMD remained at or above baseline. After ODN discontinuation at month 24, bone turnover markers increased transiently above baseline, but this increase largely resolved by month 36. There were similar overall adverse-event rates in both treatment groups. It is concluded that 3 years of ODN treatment resulted in progressive increases in BMD and was generally well tolerated. Bone-resorption markers remained suppressed, whereas bone-formation markers returned to near baseline. ODN effects were reversible: bone resorption increased transiently and BMD decreased following treatment discontinuation (Fig 2).

▶ Osteoporosis is clinically significant in approximately 30% of postmenopausal women in the United States and Europe, and it uses considerable health care resources. Currently, therapy includes bisphosphonates, estrogens, selective estrogen receptor modulator, calcitonin, and teriparatide. These agents, except for teriparatide, reduce bone resorption and suppress markers of bone resorption but do not improve bone formation markers, such as P1NP. Teriparatide increases bone mineral density and both bone formation and bone resorption markers. Odanacatib (ODN) is an orally active selective inhibitor of cathepsin K (catK). ODN decreases bone resorption by inhibiting proteolysis of matrix protein by catK and only transiently suppresses bone formation markers. The overall effect of ODN was to increase bone mineral density (BMD) of the lumbar spine and proximal femur in postmenopausal women treated for 3 years. The benefits on BMD were largely reversed within a year of discontinuation of ODN. It was generally well tolerated, and observations on reducing fracture risk await further investigation.

A. W. Meikle, MD

Article Index

Chapter 1: Rheumatoid Arthritis

Chapter 2: Osteoarthritis

Chapter 3: Gout and Other Crystal Diseases

Chapter 4: Systemic Lupus Erythematosus

Chapter 5: Vasculitis

Chapter 6: Sjögren's Syndrome

Chapter 7: Other Topics in Rheumatology

Chapter 8: Bacterial Infections

Chapter 9: Nosocomial Infections

Chapter 10: Health Care Associated Infections

Chapter 11: Clinical Diagnostics

Chapter 12: Fungal Infections

Chapter 13: New Antibiotics

Chapter 14: Viral Infections

Chapter 15: Human Immunodeficiency Virus

Chapter 16: Vaccines

Chapter 17: Tuberculosis

Chapter 18: Breast Cancer

Chapter 23: Head and Neck Cancer

Chapter 24: Neuro-Oncology

Chapter 25: Supportive Care

Chapter 26: Thoracic Cancer

Chapter 27: Metabolic Factors and Renal Disease Progression

Chapter 28: Glomerular Diseases and Renal Injury

Chapter 29: Diabetes

Chapter 30: Clinical Nephrology

Chapter 31: Chronic Kidney Disease and Clinical Nephrology

Chapter 32: Asthma and Cystic Fibrosis

Chapter 33: Chronic Obstructive Pulmonary Disease

Chapter 34: Lung Cancer

Chapter 35: Pleural, Interstitial Lung, and Pulmonary Vascular Disease

Chapter 36: Community-Acquired Pneumonia

Chapter 37: Lung Transplantation

Chapter 38: Sleep Disorders

Chapter 39: Critical Care Medicine

Chapter 40: Cardiac Arrhythmias, Conduction Disturbances, and Electrophysiology

Chapter 41: Cardiac Surgery

Chapter 42: Coronary Heart Disease

Chapter 43: Hypertension

Chapter 44: Non-Coronary Heart Disease in Adults

Chapter 45: Esophagus

Chapter 46: Gastrointestinal Cancers and Benign Polyps

Chapter 47: Gastrointestinal Motility Disorders/Neurogastroenterology

Chapter 48: Inflammatory Bowel Disease

Chapter 49: Liver Disease

Chapter 55: Lipoproteins and Atherosclerosis

Chapter 56: Diabetes

Chapter 57: Adrenal Cortex

Chapter 58: Obesity

Chapter 59: Reproductive Endocrinology

Author Index

A

Abebe N, 63
Abnet CC, 143
Abraham B, 449
Abraham NS, 416
Abrahamsen B, 486
Accurso FJ, 263
Acuna-Villaorduna C, 111
Adachi JD, 490
Akhtar N, 11
Aksentijevich I, 28
Alali F, 290
Allen JG, 302
Allred R, 65
Almeida FM, 260
Amdur RL, 206
Amiaz R, 555
Amler LC, 156
Amodeo S, 206
Andriole GL, 146
Ang DS, 189
Ang KK, 167
Angulo P, 462
Antiga L, 222
Arbique D, 542
Aronsohn RS, 306
Arora S, 467
Arynchyn A, 266
Asike MI, 463
Astor BC, 205
Attanasio AF, 497
Austin PC, 395
Avenell A, 481
Avni T, 69
Azria D, 142

B

Bach PB, 277
Badalian SS, 447
Baer L, 235
Baigent C, 190
Bajaj JS, 465
Balinandi S, 85
Ballman KV, 122
Bangalore S, 383
Banning AP, 343
Baraf HS, 15
Baron JA, 481
Barsegyan A, 543
Barzilay JI, 217
Bash LD, 205
Bauer MP, 60

Baxter C, 75
Bayuga S, 431
Beckers AM, 499
Begh R, 278
Belanger K, 258
Bell CM, 202
Ben-Aharon I, 125
Bencsik G, 421
Berg RA, 341
Bernard JR Jr, 147
Bernstein DI, 99
Beuving J, 67
Bevilacqua J, 104
Bhala N, 462
Bhattacharjee R, 308
Bhojani N, 149
Biagi JJ, 138
Bibbins-Domingo K, 370
Biedenbender R, 104
Biesiekierski JR, 437
Bilezikian JP, 488
Birzniece V, 559
Bispo PJM, 53
Björnsdottir S, 544
Black DM, 493
Blackstone EH, 344
Blair SN, 535
Bloomfield HE, 267
Bobrow BJ, 341
Boger-Megiddo I, 381
Böhm M, 337
Bolland MJ, 481
Bolognese MA, 488
Bone HG, 561
Bongers-Schokking JJ, 507, 513
Bonilla L, 125
Borghese F, 289
Borgia F, 347
Bostom AG, 193
Boyanton BL Jr, 70
Bozja J, 105
Bradley SF, 52
Brandimarte G, 458
Brandt L, 544
Brantner TL, 471
Brassard P, 112
Brennan BP, 555
Brinjikji W, 471
Browne L, 169
Bruggeman CA, 67
Bucci J, 169
Bueno H, 351
Buijsse B, 32
Burtin M, 186

Buskirk SJ, 147
Butler LM, 85
Buys SS, 162
Buyse M, 124

C

Camargo CA Jr, 255
Camilleri M, 451
Campbell P, 214
Cannon CP, 355
Cantrell LA, 165
Cantwell MM, 143
Capitanio U, 149
Cardwell CR, 143
Carleton D, 33
Carlino A, 29
Caroli A, 222
Carpenter MA, 193
Carrizo SJ, 305
Casanueva FF, 500
Catano G, 94
Cavanaugh KL, 226
Chan PS, 339
Chandra A, 298
Chawla LS, 206
Chen W, 320
Chen Y, 438
Chertow GM, 245, 370
Chode S, 552
Chuang Y-C, 50
Church TS, 535
Chykarenko ZA, 94
Clancy JP, 263
Clark WF, 244
Clavel MA, 407
Cnattingius S, 544
Cochrane L, 505
Cockfield SM, 214
Cocreham S, 535
Coelho J, 456
Colangelo LA, 266
Cole MA, 314
Collaco JM, 261
Collins IJ, 96
Concannon TW, 349
Connolly SJ, 331
Conus S, 427
Cooper BA, 241
Cooper LA, 229
Cooper-DeHoff RM, 389
Cortes J, 117
Cosman F, 483
Costa L, 171

583

Printed and bound by CPI Group (UK) Ltd, Croydon, CR0 4YY

08/05/2025

01864677-0019